FIFTH EDITION

CASE FILES®
Family Medicine

T0200404

Eugene C. Toy, MD
Assistant Dean for Educational Programs
Director of Doctoring Courses
Professor and Vice Chair of Medical Education
Department of Obstetrics and Gynecology
McGovern Medical School at The University
of Texas
Health Science Center at Houston (UTHealth)
Houston, Texas

Donald Briscoe, MD, FAAFP
Clinical Associate Professor
Director, Longitudinal Primary Care Course
University of Houston College of Medicine
Houston, Texas

Bruce Britton, MD
Professor of Family Medicine and Community
Medicine
Vice Chair for Medical Education
Department of Family and Community
Medicine
Eastern Virginia Medical School
Norfolk, Virginia

Joel J. Heidelbaugh, MD, FAAFP, FACG
Clinical Professor
Director of Medical Student Education and
Clerkship Director
Department of Family Medicine
University of Michigan Medical School
Ann Arbor, Michigan

Mc
Graw
Hill

New York   Chicago   San Francisco   Athens   London   Madrid   Mexico City
Milan   New Delhi   Singapore   Sydney   Toronto

Notice

Medicine is an ever-changing science. As new research and clinical experience broaden our knowledge, changes in treatment and drug therapy are required. The authors and the publisher of this work have checked with sources believed to be reliable in their efforts to provide information that is complete and generally in accord with the standard accepted at the time of publication. However, in view of the possibility of human error or changes in medical sciences, neither the editors nor the publisher nor any other party who has been involved in the preparation or publication of this work warrants that the information contained herein is in every respect accurate or complete, and they disclaim all responsibility for any errors or omissions or for the results obtained from use of the information contained in this work. Readers are encouraged to confirm the information contained herein with other sources. For example and in particular, readers are advised to check the product information sheet included in the package of each drug they plan to administer to be certain that the information contained in this work is accurate and that changes have not been made in the recommended dose or in the contraindications for administration. This recommendation is of particular importance in connection with new or infrequently used drugs.

This book was set in Adobe Jenson Pro by Cenveo® Publisher Services.
The editors were Bob Boehringer and Madison Tucky.
The production supervisor was Catherine H. Saggese.
Project management was provided by Revathi Viswanathan, Cenveo Publisher Services.

Library of Congress Cataloging-in-Publication Data

Names: Toy, Eugene C., author. | Briscoe, Donald A., author. | Britton, Bruce, 1962- author. | Heidelbaugh, Joel J., author.
Title: Case files. Family medicine / Eugene C. Toy, Donald Briscoe, Bruce Britton, Joel J. Heidelbaugh.
Other titles: Family medicine
Description: Fifth edition. | New York : McGraw-Hill Education, [2021] | Includes bibliographical references and index. | Summary: "You need exposure to high-yield cases to excel in the family medicine clerkship and on the shelf exam. Case Files Family Medicine presents 60 real-life cases that illustrate essential concepts in family medicine. Each case includes a complete discussion, clinical pearls, references, definitions of key terms, and USMLE-style review questions. With this system, you'll learn in the context of real patients, rather than merely memorize facts : 60 cases with USMLE-style questions help you master core competencies to excel in the clerkship and ace the shelf exams, clinical pearls highlight key points, primer teaches you how to approach clinical problems, proven learning system maximizes your exam scores"—Provided by publisher.
Identifiers: LCCN 2020013636 | ISBN 9781260468595 (paperback ; alk. paper) | ISBN 9781260468601 (ebook)
Subjects: MESH: Family Practice—methods | Diagnostic Techniques and Procedures | Diagnosis | Therapeutics | Case Reports | Problems and Exercises
Classification: LCC R733 | NLM WB 18.2 | DDC 610—dc23
LC record available at https://lccn.loc.gov/2020013636

*To the many students throughout the world who have embraced
the Case Files approach, you are my daily inspiration.
And to the courageous doctors, nurses, and other health care providers
who valiantly walk into this COVID-19 darkness each day,
carrying the beacon of hope for the sick and helpless.
You are the real heroes.*

–ECT

*To my friends and colleagues in the new College of Medicine
of the University of Houston. Go Coogs!*

–DB

*To May and Sean: for their infinite patience and love.
And to the students, residents, faculty, and
patients of the Eastern Virginia Medical School:
the best teachers I could ever have.*

–BB

*To my students and residents at the University of Michigan
who teach me as much as I strive to teach them—Go Blue!*

*To my dedicated colleagues in academic family medicine
who inspire me to become a greater teacher, researcher, and clinician.*

To Jacqui, Gwyneth, and Lilya for loving and supporting me.

– JJH

CONTENTS

CONTRIBUTORS

Raina Advani, MS4
Medical Student
University of Michigan Medical School
Ann Arbor, Michigan
Lower Extremity Edema
Jaundice
Irritable Bowel Syndrome
Adolescent Health Maintenance

Heba Ahmad, MS3
Medical Student
McGovern Medical School at UTHealth in Houston
Houston, Texas
Manuscript Reviewer, Clinical Case Correlation

Jennifer Cavin, MD
Sentara Family Medicine Physicians
Virginia Beach, Virginia
Dementia
Abdominal Pain and Vomiting in a Child
Wheezing and Asthma

Joy Davis, MS4
Medical Student
McGovern Medical School at UTHealth in Houston
Houston, Texas
Manuscript Reviewer, Review Questions

Ayana G.R. DeGaia, MD, MPH
Medical Student
University of Michigan Medical School
Ann Arbor, Michigan
Obstructive Sleep Apnea
Fever and Rash
Palpitations

Sara M. Ehdaie, DO
Faculty Physician
Houston Methodist Family Medicine Residency Program
Houston, Texas
Musculoskeletal Injuries

Katherine M. Heckman, MS, MS4
Medical Student
University of Michigan Medical School
Ann Arbor, Michigan
Benign Breast Diseases

Kathryn T. Holt, MS4
Medical Student
University of Michigan Medical School
Ann Arbor, Michigan
Adult Female Health Maintenance
Dyspepsia and Peptic Ulcer Disease
Wheezing and Asthma

Marsha Cline Holleman, MD, MPH
Associate Professor
Houston Methodist Family Medicine Residency Program
Houston, Texas
Clinician Well-Being

Warren L. Holleman, PhD
Professor
University of Texas M D Anderson Cancer Center
Houston, Texas
Clinician Well-Being

Motaz B. Ibrahim, MD
Resident Physician
Houston Methodist Family Medicine Residency Program
Houston, Texas
Upper Respiratory and Ear Infections
Chest Pain

Linwood T. Joyner, II, MD
Riverside Eastern Shore Family Medicine
Nassawadox, Virginia
Chronic Kidney Disease
Heart Failure
Obesity
Hyperlipidemia

Omar Tareq Mahfouz, MD
Resident Physician
Houston Methodist Family Medicine Residency Program
Houston, Texas
Hematuria
Electrolyte Disorders
Geriatric Health Maintenance and End-of-Life Issues

Kyle K. McLain, MS4
Medical Student
University of Michigan Medical School
Ann Arbor, Michigan
HIV, AIDS, and Other Sexually Transmitted Infections
Adolescent Health Maintenance
Sting and Bite Injuries

Roberto Medina, MD
Resident Physician
Houston Methodist Family Medicine Residency Program
Houston, Texas
Thyroid Disorders
Dyspnea (Chronic Obstructive Pulmonary Disease)

Karo Gary Ohanian, MD
Assistant Professor
Eastern Virginia Medical School Portsmouth Family Medicine Residency Program
Portsmouth, Virginia
Pneumonia
Migraine and Other Headache Syndromes
Hypertension
Family Violence

Jessica Quirk, MD
Sentara Family Medicine Physicians
Suffolk, Virginia
Major Depression and Other Mood Disorders
Family Planning—Contraceptives
Postpartum Care
Vaginitis and Other Vaginal Infections

Nicole Thurmond, MD, MPH
Resident Physician
Houston Methodist Family Medicine Residency Program
Houston, Texas
Non-Traumatic Joint Pain and Swelling
Well-Child Care

Irene R. Sung, MD, MPH
Resident Physician
Houston Methodist Family Medicine Residency Program
Houston, Texas
Menstrual Cycle Irregularity
Autism Spectrum Disorder
Movement Disorders

Narine Topaldjikian, MD, MBA
Resident Physician
Houston Methodist Family Medicine Residency Program
Houston, Texas
Prenatal Care
Allergic Disorders, Anaphylaxis, and Conjunctivitis
Tobacco Use and Cessation

Daniel A. Nadelman, MS4
Medical Student
University of Michigan Medical School
Ann Arbor, Michigan
Adult Male Health Maintenance
Diabetes Mellitus
Acute Low Back Pain

Nathan J. Vengalil, MS4
Medical Student
University of Michigan Medical School
Ann Arbor, Michigan
Adult Male Health Maintenance
Male Genitourinary Conditions

Kevin M. Wheelock, MS4
Medical Student
University of Michigan Medical School
Ann Arbor, Michigan
Cerebrovascular Accident/Transient Ischemic Attack
Male Genitourinary Conditions

We appreciate all the kind remarks and suggestions from the many medical students over the past 3 years. Your positive reception has been an incredible encouragement, especially in light of the short life of the *Case Files*® series. In this fifth edition of *Case Files*®: *Family Medicine*, the basic format of the book has been retained. Improvements were made in updating many of the chapters. New cases include Substance Use Disorder, Asthma, Obstructive Sleep Apnea, Osteoporosis, and Opioid Use Disorder and Chronic Pain Management. We reviewed the clinical scenarios with the intent of improving them; however, their "real-life" presentations patterned after actual clinical experience were accurate and instructive. We had utilized focus groups of students to create a more user-friendly format for the digital platform such as bullet points for the case summary for faster reading and more plentiful use of subheadings throughout the text. We have used entrustable professional activities (EPA) corresponding to the learning objectives. The summary to the case scenarios are in bullet style to allow for easier reading. The multiple-choice questions (MCQs) have been carefully reviewed and rewritten to ensure that they comply with the National Board and the US Medical Licensing Examination format. Through this fifth edition, we hope that the reader will continue to enjoy learning diagnosis and management through the simulated clinical cases. It certainly is a privilege to be teachers for so many students, and it is with humility that we present this edition.

Eugene C. Toy

ACKNOWLEDGMENTS

The curriculum that evolved into the ideas for this series was inspired by two talented and forthright students, Philbert Yau and Chuck Rosipal, who have since graduated from medical school. It has been a pleasure to work with Dr. Don Briscoe, a brilliant, compassionate, and dedicated teacher and leader; Dr. Bruce Britton, who is an excellent teacher and communicator; and most recently Dr. Joel Heidelbaugh, who has an amazing breadth of knowledge and brings a fresh perspective. I am greatly indebted to my editors, Bob Boehringer, whose experience and vision helped to continue this series. I appreciate McGraw Hill's believing in the concept of teaching through clinical cases; I am also grateful to Catherine Saggese for her excellent production expertise and Madison Tucky, who has grown into a diligent and trustworthy editor, for her wonderful editing. I am thankful to Revathi Viswanathan for the outstanding and precise project management. At the University of Texas Medical School at Houston, I appreciate Dr. Patricia Butler for her encouragement, Dr. Sean Blackwell for his example, role model, and inspiration. As always, I appreciate Allison's amazing skill, knowledge, and expertise; she somehow knows how to put the electrical impulses in the authors' brains into words, phrases, and ideas without our having to saying anything—she is a medical editing wizard extraordinaire! Most of all, I appreciate my ever-loving wife, Terri, and four wonderful children, Andy and his wife, Anna; Michael and his wife, Nadine; Allison; and Christina and her husband, Andy, for their patience, encouragement, and understanding.

Eugene C. Toy

Mastering the cognitive knowledge within a field such as family medicine is a formidable task. It is even more difficult to draw on that knowledge, procure, and filter through the clinical and laboratory data, develop a differential diagnosis, and, finally, form a rational treatment plan. To gain these skills, the student often learns best at the bedside, guided and instructed by experienced teachers, and inspired toward self-directed, diligent reading. Clearly, there is no replacement for education at the bedside. Unfortunately, clinical situations usually do not encompass the breadth of the specialty. Perhaps the best alternative is a carefully crafted patient case designed to stimulate the clinical approach and decision-making. In an attempt to achieve that goal, we have constructed a collection of clinical vignettes to teach diagnostic or therapeutic approaches that are relevant to family medicine. Most importantly, the explanations for the cases emphasize the mechanisms and underlying principles, rather than merely rote questions and answers.

This book is organized for versatility to allow the student "in a rush" to go quickly through the scenarios and check the corresponding answers, as well as enable the student who wants thought-provoking explanations to take a slower path. The explanations are arranged from simple to more complex: a summary of the pertinent points, the bare answers, an analysis of the case, an approach to the topic, a comprehension test at the end for reinforcement and emphasis, and a list of resources for further reading. The clinical vignettes are purposely placed in random order to simulate the way that real patients present to the practitioner. Section II includes a listing of cases to aid the student who desires to test his or her knowledge of a certain area or to review a topic, including basic definitions. Finally, we intentionally did not primarily use MCQ format because clues (or distractions) are not available in the real world. Nevertheless, several MCQs are included at the end of each scenario to reinforce concepts or introduce related topics.

HOW TO GET THE MOST OUT OF THIS BOOK

Each case is designed to simulate a patient encounter with open-ended questions. At times, the patient's complaint is different from the most concerning issue, and sometimes extraneous information is given. The answers are organized with four different parts.

PART I

1. **Summary.** The salient aspects of the case are identified, filtering out the extraneous information. Students should formulate their summary from the case before looking at the answers. This is in bullet form now. A comparison to the summation in the answer will help to improve their ability to focus on the important data, while appropriately discarding the irrelevant information—a fundamental skill in clinical problem solving.
2. **A Straightforward Answer** is given to each open-ended question.

Table 1 • SYNOPSIS OF ENTRUSTABLE PROFESSIONAL ACTIVITIES	
EPA 1	Gather a history and perform a physical examination
EPA 2	Prioritize a differential diagnosis following a clinical encounter
EPA 3	Recommend and interpret common diagnostic and screening tests
EPA 4	Enter and discuss orders and prescriptions
EPA 5	Document a clinical encounter in the patient record
EPA 6	Provide an oral presentation of a clinical encounter
EPA 7	Form clinical questions and retrieve evidence to advance patient care
EPA 8	Give or receive a patient handover to transition care responsibly
EPA 9	Collaborate as a member of a interprofessional team
EPA 10	Recognize a patient requiring urgent or emergent care and initiate evaluation and management
EPA 11	Obtain informed consent for tests and/or procedures
EPA 12	Perform general procedures as a physician
EPA 13	Identify system failures and contribute to a culture of safety and improvement

3. The **Analysis of the Case**, which comprises two parts:
   a. **Objectives of the Case:** A listing of the two or three main principles that are crucial for a practitioner to manage the patient. Again, the students are challenged to make educated "guesses" about the objectives of the case upon initial review of the case scenario, which helps to sharpen their clinical and analytical skills. We have included the EPA(s) corresponding to the objective for instructors and curriculum overseers (see Table 1).
   b. **Considerations:** A discussion of the relevant points and a brief approach to the specific patient.

PART II

The Approach to the Disease Process, which has two distinct parts:
   a. **Definitions or Pathophysiology:** Terminology or basic science correlates that are pertinent to the disease process.
   b. **Clinical Approach:** A discussion of the approach to the clinical problem in general, including tables, figures, and algorithms.

PART III

The **Comprehension Questions** for each case is composed of several multiple-choice questions that either reinforce the material or introduce new and related concepts. Questions about material not found in the text have explanations in the answers.

PART IV

Clinical Pearls list several clinically important points that summarize the text and allow for easy review of the material, such as before an examination.

LISTING BY CASE NUMBER

LISTING BY DISORDER (ALPHABETICAL)

How to Approach Clinical Problems

Part 1. Approach to the Patient

Applying "book learning" to a specific clinical situation is one the most challenging tasks in medicine. To do so, the clinician must not only retain information, organize facts, and recall large amounts of data but also apply all of this to the patient. The purpose of this text is to facilitate this process.

The first step involves gathering information, also known as establishing the database. This includes taking the history, performing the physical examination, and obtaining selective laboratory examinations, special studies, and/or imaging tests. Sensitivity and respect should always be exercised during the interview of patients. A good clinician also knows how to ask the same question in several different ways, using different terminology. For example, patients may deny having "congestive heart failure" but will answer affirmatively to being treated for "fluid on the lungs." Starting with open-ended questions for each section of the history often can help gather large amounts of information on the patient efficiently and allow the clinician's follow-up questions to be targeted and more meaningful.

CLINICAL PEARL

▶ The history is usually the single most important tool in obtaining a diagnosis. The art of seeking this information in a nonjudgmental, sensitive, and thorough manner cannot be overemphasized.

HISTORY

1. **Basic information:**
   a. **Age:** Some conditions are more common at certain ages; for instance, chest pain in an elderly patient is more worrisome for coronary artery disease than the same complaint in a teenager.
   b. **Gender:** Some disorders are more common in men, such as abdominal aortic aneurysms. In contrast, women more commonly have autoimmune problems, such as chronic idiopathic thrombocytopenic purpura or systemic lupus erythematosus. Also, the possibility of pregnancy must be considered in any woman of childbearing age.
   c. **Ethnicity:** Some disease processes are more common in certain ethnic groups (eg, type 2 diabetes mellitus in the Hispanic population).

CLINICAL PEARL

▶ Family medicine illustrates the importance of longitudinal care, that is, seeing the patient in various phases and stages of life.

2. **Chief complaint:** What is it that brought the patient into the provider's office or hospital? Has there been a change in a chronic or recurring condition, or is this a completely new problem? The duration and character of the complaint, associated symptoms, and exacerbating/relieving factors should be recorded. The chief complaint engenders a differential diagnosis, and the possible etiologies should be explored by further inquiry.

CLINICAL PEARL

▶ The first line of any presentation should include *age, gender, marital status, and chief complaint and if applicable ethnicity.* Example: A 32-year-old, married, man complains of lower abdominal pain of 8 hours' duration.

3. **Past medical history:**
   a. Chronic conditions such as hypertension, diabetes, reactive airway disease, congestive heart failure, angina, or stroke should be detailed.
      i. Age of onset, severity, end-organ involvement.
      ii. Medications taken for the particular illness, including any recent changes to medications and reason for the change(s).
      iii. Last evaluation of the condition (eg, When was the last stress test or cardiac catheterization performed in the patient with angina?)
      iv. Which provider or clinic is following the patient for the disorder?
   b. Minor illnesses such as recent upper respiratory infections.
   c. Hospitalizations, no matter how trivial, should be queried.

4. **Past surgical history:** Date and type of procedure performed, indication, and outcome. Laparoscopy versus laparotomy should be distinguished. Surgeon and hospital name/location should be listed. This information should be correlated with the surgical scars on the patient's body. Any complications should be delineated, including anesthetic complications, difficult intubations, and so on.

5. **Allergies:** Reactions to medications should be recorded, including severity and temporal relationship to medication. Immediate hypersensitivity should be distinguished from an adverse reaction.

6. **Medications:** A list of medications, dosage, route of administration and frequency, and duration of use should be developed. Prescription, over-the-counter, supplements, and herbal remedies are all relevant. If the patient is currently taking antibiotics, it is important to note what type of infection is being treated.

7. **Immunization history:** Vaccination and prevention of disease are principal goals of the family care provider hence, recording the immunizations received, including dates, age, route, and adverse reactions, if any, is critical.

8. **Screening history:** Cost-effective surveillance for common diseases or malignancy is another cornerstone responsibility of the family care provider. Organized record-keeping is important to an efficient approach to this area.

9. **Social history:** Occupation, marital status, family support, and tendencies toward depression or anxiety are important. Use or abuse of illicit drugs, tobacco, or alcohol should also be recorded. Social history, including marital stressors, sexual dysfunction, and sexual preference, are of importance. Patients, especially older patients or those with chronic illnesses, should be asked about medical power of attorney and advance directives.

10. **Family history:** Many major medical problems are genetically transmitted (eg, hemophilia, sickle cell disease). In addition, a family history of conditions such as breast cancer and ischemic heart disease can be a risk factor for the development of these diseases.

11. **Review of systems:** A systematic review should be performed but focused on the life-threatening and the more common diseases. For example, in a young man with a testicular mass, trauma to the area, weight loss, and infectious symptoms are important to note. In an elderly woman with generalized weakness, symptoms suggestive of cardiac disease should be elicited, such as chest pain, shortness of breath, fatigue, or palpitations.

PHYSICAL EXAMINATION

1. **General appearance:** Mental status, alert versus obtunded, anxious, in pain, in distress, interaction with other family members, and with examiner.

2. **Vital signs:** Record the temperature, blood pressure, heart rate, and respiratory rate. An oxygen saturation is useful in patients with respiratory symptoms. Height and weight should be placed here with a body mass index calculated (weight in kilogram/height in meters-squared = kg/m^2).

3. **Head and neck examination:** Evidence of trauma, tumors, facial edema, goiter and thyroid nodules, and carotid bruits should be sought. In patients with altered mental status or a head injury, pupillary size, symmetry, and reactivity are important. Mucous membranes should be inspected for pallor, jaundice, and evidence of dehydration. Cervical and supraclavicular nodes should be palpated.

4. **Breast examination:** Inspection for symmetry and skin or nipple retraction, as well as palpation for masses. The nipple should be assessed for discharge, and the axillary and supraclavicular regions should be examined.

5. **Cardiac examination:** The point of maximal impulse should be ascertained and the heart auscultated at the apex and base. It is important to note whether the auscultated rhythm is regular or irregular. Heart sounds (including S_3 and S_4), murmurs, clicks, and rubs should be characterized. Systolic flow murmurs are fairly common as a result of the increased cardiac output, but significant diastolic murmurs are unusual.

6. **Pulmonary examination:** The lung fields should be examined systematically and thoroughly. Stridor, wheezes, rales, and rhonchi should be recorded. The clinician should also search for evidence of consolidation (bronchial breath

sounds, egophony) and increased work of breathing (retractions, abdominal breathing, accessory muscle use).

7. **Abdominal examination:** The abdomen should be inspected for scars, distension, masses, and discoloration. For instance, the Grey-Turner sign of bruising at the flank areas may indicate intra-abdominal or retroperitoneal hemorrhage. Auscultation should identify normal versus high-pitched and hyperactive versus hypoactive bowel sounds. The abdomen should be percussed for the presence of shifting dullness (indicating ascites). Then, careful palpation should begin away from the area of pain and progress to include the whole abdomen to assess for tenderness, masses, organomegaly (ie, spleen or liver), and peritoneal signs. Guarding and whether it is voluntary or involuntary should be noted.

8. **Back and spine examination:** The back should be assessed for symmetry, tenderness, and masses. The flank regions particularly are important to assess for pain on percussion that may indicate renal disease.

9. **Genital examination:**
   a. **Female:** The external genitalia should be inspected, then the speculum used to visualize the cervix and vagina. A bimanual examination should attempt to elicit cervical motion tenderness, uterine size, and ovarian masses or tenderness.
   b. **Male:** The penis should be examined for hypospadias, lesions, and discharge. The scrotum should be palpated for tenderness and masses. If a mass is present, it can be transilluminated to distinguish between solid and cystic masses. The groin region should be carefully palpated for bulging (hernias) upon rest and provocation (coughing, standing).
   c. **Rectal examination:** A rectal examination will reveal masses in the posterior pelvis and may identify gross or occult blood in the stool. In females, nodularity and tenderness in the uterosacral ligament may be signs of endometriosis. The posterior uterus and palpable masses in the cul-de-sac may be identified by rectal examination. In the male, the prostate gland should be palpated for tenderness, nodularity, and enlargement.

10. **Extremities and skin:** The presence of joint effusions, tenderness, rashes, edema, and cyanosis should be recorded. It is also important to note capillary refill and peripheral pulses.

11. **Neurologic examination:** Patients who present with neurologic complaints require a thorough assessment, including mental status, cranial nerves, strength, sensation, reflexes, and cerebellar function.

CLINICAL PEARL

▶ A thorough understanding of functional anatomy is important to optimally interpret the physical examination findings.

12. **Laboratory assessment depends on the circumstances:**

    a. A complete blood count (CBC) can assess for anemia, leukocytosis (infection), and thrombocytopenia.

    b. Basic metabolic panel: electrolytes, glucose, BUN (blood urea nitrogen), and creatinine (renal function).

    c. Urinalysis and/or urine culture to assess for hematuria, pyuria, or bacteriuria. A pregnancy test is important in women of childbearing age.

    d. Aspartate aminotransferase (AST), alanine aminotransferase (ALT), bilirubin, and alkaline phosphatase for liver function; amylase and lipase to evaluate the pancreas.

    e. Cardiac markers (creatine kinase myocardial band [CK-MB], troponin, myoglobin) if coronary artery disease or other cardiac dysfunction is suspected.

    f. Drug levels such as acetaminophen level in possible overdoses.

    g. Arterial blood gas measurements give information about oxygenation, carbon dioxide, and pH readings.

13. **Diagnostic adjuncts:**

    a. Electrocardiogram if cardiac ischemia, dysrhythmia, or other cardiac dysfunction is suspected.

    b. Ultrasound examination is useful in evaluating pelvic processes in female patients (eg, pelvic inflammatory disease, tubo-ovarian abscess) and in diagnosing gallstones and other gallbladder disease. With the addition of color-flow Doppler, deep venous thrombosis and ovarian or testicular torsion can be detected.

    c. Computed tomography (CT) is useful in assessing the brain for masses, bleeding, strokes, and skull fractures. CTs of the chest can evaluate for masses, fluid collections, aortic dissections, and pulmonary emboli. Abdominal CTs can detect infection (abscess, appendicitis, diverticulitis), masses, aortic aneurysms, and ureteral stones.

    d. Magnetic resonance imaging (MRI) helps to identify soft tissue planes very well. While this is not often the first test ordered, the family health care provider frequently obtains an MRI to help with the diagnosis of musculoskeletal or central nervous system conditions.

    e. Screening tests: A lipid panel can demonstrate the cholesterol level, including the low-density lipoprotein (LDL) levels, which have prognostic significance in coronary heart disease; fasting glucose and thyroid tests may be important; in many centers, dual-energy x-ray absorptiometry (DEXA) is the test of choice to monitor bone mineral density; the mammogram is the examination of choice to screen for subclinical breast cancer; fecal immunochemistry testing, flexible sigmoidoscopy, and colonoscopy are used to screen for colon cancer.

Part 2. Approach to Clinical Problem-Solving

CLASSIC CLINICAL PROBLEM-SOLVING

There are typically four distinct steps that the family health care provider undertakes to systematically solve most clinical problems:

1. Making the diagnosis

2. Assessing the severity of the disease

3. Treating based on the stage of the disease

4. Following the patient's response to the treatment

MAKING THE DIAGNOSIS

This is achieved by carefully evaluating the patient, analyzing the information, assessing risk factors, and developing a list of possible diagnoses (the differential). Usually, a long list of possible diagnoses can be pared down to a few of the most likely or most serious ones, based on the clinician's knowledge, experience, assessment of the likelihood of having a condition (pretest probability), and selective testing. For example, a patient who complains of upper abdominal pain and has a history of nonsteroidal anti-inflammatory drug (NSAID) use may have peptic ulcer disease; another patient who has abdominal pain, fatty food intolerance, and abdominal bloating may have cholelithiasis. Yet another individual with a 1-day history of periumbilical pain that now localizes to the right lower quadrant may have acute appendicitis.

> ### CLINICAL PEARL
> ▶ The first step in clinical problem-solving is making the diagnosis.

ASSESSING THE SEVERITY OF THE DISEASE

After establishing the diagnosis, the next step is to characterize the severity of the disease process, in other words, to describe "how bad" the disease is. This may be as simple as determining whether a patient is "sick" or "not sick." Is the patient with a urinary tract infection septic or stable for outpatient therapy? In other cases, a more formal staging may be used. For example, cancer staging is used for the strict assessment of extent of malignancy.

> ### CLINICAL PEARL
> ▶ The second step in clinical problem-solving is to establish the severity or stage of disease. This usually impacts the treatment and/or prognosis.

TREATING BASED ON STAGE

Many illnesses are characterized by stage or severity because this affects prognosis and treatment. As an example, a formerly healthy young man with pneumonia and no respiratory distress may be treated with oral antibiotics at home. An older person with emphysema and pneumonia would probably be admitted to the hospital for intravenous antibiotics. A patient with pneumonia and respiratory failure would likely be intubated and admitted to the intensive care unit for further treatment.

> ## CLINICAL PEARL
>
> ▶ The third step in clinical problem-solving is tailoring the treatment to fit the severity or "stage" of the disease.

FOLLOWING THE RESPONSE TO TREATMENT

The final step in the approach to disease is to follow the patient's response to the therapy. Some responses are clinical, such as improvement (or lack of improvement) in a patient's pain. Other responses may be followed by testing (eg, monitoring the anion gap in a patient with diabetic ketoacidosis). The clinician must be prepared to know what to do if the patient does not respond as expected. Is the next step to treat again, to reassess the diagnosis, or to follow up with another more specific test?

> ## CLINICAL PEARL
>
> ▶ The fourth step in clinical problem-solving is to monitor treatment response or efficacy. This may be measured in different ways—symptomatically or based on physical examination or other testing.

Part 3. Approach to Reading

The clinical problem-oriented approach to reading is different from the classic "systematic" research of a disease. Patients rarely present with a clear diagnosis; hence, the student must become skilled in applying textbook information to the clinical scenario. Because reading with a purpose improves the retention of information, the student should read with the goal of answering specific questions. There are several fundamental questions that facilitate clinical thinking. These are the following:

1. What is the most likely diagnosis?

2. How would you confirm the diagnosis?

3. What should be your next step?

4. What is the best screening strategy in this situation?

5. What are the risk factors for this condition?

6. What are the complications associated with the disease process?

7. What is the best therapy?

WHAT IS THE MOST LIKELY DIAGNOSIS?

The method of establishing the diagnosis was discussed in the previous section. One way of determining the most likely diagnosis is to develop standard "approaches" to common clinical problems. It is helpful to understand the most common causes of various presentations, such as "the worst headache of the patient's life is worrisome for a subarachnoid hemorrhage" (see the Clinical Pearls at end of each case).

The clinical scenario would be something such as this:

A 38-year-old woman is noted to have a 2-day history of unilateral, throbbing headache with photophobia. What is the most likely diagnosis?

With no other information to go on, the student would note that this woman has a unilateral headache with photophobia. Using the "most common cause" information, the student would make an educated guess that the patient has a migraine headache. If instead the patient is noted to have "the worst headache of her life," the student would use the Clinical Pearl.

The worst headache of the patient's life is worrisome for a subarachnoid hemorrhage.

HOW WOULD YOU CONFIRM THE DIAGNOSIS?

In the previous scenario, the woman with "the worst headache" is suspected of having a subarachnoid hemorrhage. This diagnosis could be confirmed by a CT scan of the head and/or lumbar puncture (LP). The student should learn the limitations of various diagnostic tests, especially when used early in a disease process.

The LP **showing xanthochromia (red blood cells) is the "gold standard" test for diagnosing subarachnoid hemorrhage, but it may be negative early in the disease course.**

WHAT SHOULD BE YOUR NEXT STEP?

This question is difficult because the next step has many possibilities; the answer may be to obtain more diagnostic information, stage the illness, or introduce therapy. It is often a more challenging question than "What is the most likely diagnosis?" because there may be insufficient information to make a diagnosis, and the next step may be to pursue more diagnostic information. Another possibility is that there is enough information for a probable diagnosis, and the next step is to stage the disease. Finally, the most appropriate answer may be to treat. Hence, from clinical data, a judgment needs to be rendered regarding how far along one is on the road of

1. Make the diagnosis → 2. Stage the disease →
3. Treat based on stage → 4. Follow response

Frequently, the student is taught "to regurgitate" the same information that someone has written about a particular disease but is not skilled at identifying the next step. This talent is learned optimally at the bedside, in a supportive environment, with freedom to make educated guesses, and with constructive feedback. A sample scenario might describe a student's thought process as follows:

1. **Make the diagnosis:** "Based on the information I have, I believe that the patient has a small bowel obstruction from adhesive disease *because* he presents with nausea and vomiting, abdominal distension, high-pitched hyperactive bowel sounds, and dilated loops of small bowel on x-ray."

2. **Stage the disease:** "I don't believe that this is severe disease as he does not have fever, evidence of sepsis, intractable pain, peritoneal signs, or leukocytosis."

3. **Treat based on stage:** "Therefore, my next step is to treat with nothing per mouth, nasogastric tube drainage, intravenous fluids, and observation."

4. **Follow response:** "I want to follow the treatment by assessing his pain (I will ask him to rate the pain on a scale of 0-10 every day), his bowel function (I will ask whether he has had nausea, vomiting, or passed flatus), his temperature, abdominal examination, serum bicarbonate (for metabolic acidemia), and white blood cell count and then reassess him in 48 hours."

In a similar patient, when the clinical presentation is unclear, perhaps the best "next step" may be diagnostic, such as an oral contrast radiologic study to assess for bowel obstruction.

CLINICAL PEARL

▶ Usually, the vague query, "What is your next step?" is the most difficult question because the answer may be diagnostic, staging, or therapeutic.

WHAT IS THE BEST SCREENING STRATEGY IN THIS SITUATION?

A major role of the family health care provider is screening for common and/or dangerous conditions where there may be interventions to alleviate disease. Cost-effectiveness, ease of the screening modality, wide availability, and presence of intervention are some of the important issues. The age, gender, and risk factors for the disease process in question play roles. In general, age is one of the most important risk factors for cancer. For instance, with breast cancer, an annual or biannual mammogram is recommended in women older than 50 years. This imaging technique is widely available, inexpensive, and safe and has been shown to decrease mortality. In the United States, screening examinations with strong evidence for effectiveness are fully covered by insurance.

WHAT ARE THE RISK FACTORS FOR THIS PROCESS?

Understanding the risk factors helps the practitioner to establish a diagnosis and to determine how to interpret tests. For example, understanding risk factor analysis may help in the management of a 55-year-old woman with anemia. If the patient has risk factors for endometrial cancer (eg, diabetes, hypertension, anovulation) and complains of postmenopausal bleeding, she likely has endometrial carcinoma and should have an endometrial biopsy. Otherwise, occult colonic bleeding is a common etiology. If she takes NSAIDs or aspirin, then peptic ulcer disease is the most likely cause.

CLINICAL PEARL

▶ Being able to assess risk factors helps to guide testing and develop the differential diagnosis.

WHAT ARE THE COMPLICATIONS OF THIS PROCESS?

Clinicians must be cognizant of the complications of a disease so that they will understand how to follow and monitor the patient. Sometimes, the student has to make the diagnosis from clinical clues and then apply his or her knowledge of the consequences of the pathologic process. For example, "A 26-year-old man complains of right lower extremity swelling and pain after a transatlantic flight," and his Doppler ultrasound reveals a deep vein thrombosis. Complications of this process include pulmonary embolism (PE). Understanding the types of consequences also helps the clinician to be aware of the dangers to a patient. If the patient has any symptoms consistent with a PE, a ventilation-perfusion scan or CT scan with angiographic imaging of the chest may be necessary.

WHAT IS THE BEST THERAPY?

To answer the question of what is the best therapy, the clinician not only needs to reach the correct diagnosis and assess the severity of the condition, but also must weigh the situation to determine the appropriate intervention. For the student, knowing exact dosages is not as important as understanding the best medication, route of delivery, mechanism of action, and possible complications. It is important for the student to be able to verbalize the diagnosis and the rationale for the therapy. It is also important that the therapy choice takes into consideration patient beliefs and desires. Evidence-based medicine combines the best available evidence, the clinician's experience, and the patient's beliefs and values.

CLINICAL PEARL

▶ Therapy should be logical and based on the severity of disease and the specific diagnosis. An exception to this rule is in an emergent situation, such as respiratory failure or shock, when the patient needs treatment even as the etiology is being investigated.

SUMMARY

1. There is no replacement for a meticulous history and physical examination.

2. There are four steps in the clinical approach to the family medicine patient: making the diagnosis, assessing severity, treating based on severity, and following response.

3. There are seven questions that help to bridge the gap between the textbook and the clinical arena.

REFERENCES

Paulman PM, Paulman AA, Jarzynka KJ, Falk NP, eds. *Taylor's Manual of Family Medicine*. Philadelphia, PA: Wolters Kluwer; 2015.

Rakel RE, Rakel D, eds. *Textbook of Family Medicine*. Philadelphia, PA: Elsevier; 2016.

Clinical Cases

A 58-year-old man comes to the office for an "annual checkup," admitting that he has not seen a health care provider in several years. He has no significant past medical history and takes no medications. His father died at age 74 years of a myocardial infarction. His mother is alive at age 70 years and has metabolic syndrome, components of type 2 diabetes mellitus, hypertension, and hyperlipidemia. He has no siblings. He has smoked a pack of cigarettes daily for 35 years, drinks moderate alcohol weekly, denies illicit drug use, and does not exercise regularly. On examination, his blood pressure is 137/88 mm Hg, pulse is 86 beats/min and regular, height is 72 inches, weight is 225 pounds, body mass index (BMI) is 30.5 kg/m², and abdominal waist circumference is 44 inches. His physical examination is unremarkable.

▶ What screening test(s) for cardiovascular disease should be recommended for this patient?
▶ What screening test(s) for other chronic diseases should be recommended for this patient?
▶ What screening test(s) for cancer should be recommended?
▶ What immunization(s) should be recommended?

ANSWERS TO CASE 1:
Adult Male Health Maintenance

Summary: A 58-year-old man presents with

- No known chronic medical problems
- Desire for an "annual checkup"
- No complaints on history
- An unremarkable physical examination

Recommended screening tests for cardiovascular conditions: Blood pressure measurement (screening for hypertension); height, weight, body mass index (BMI), and abdominal waist circumference measurements (screening for obesity); nonfasting lipid measurement (screening for hyperlipidemia).

Recommended screening tests for other chronic diseases: Fasting glucose or hemoglobin A_{1c} (screening for diabetes mellitus); hepatitis C screening for adults ages 18 to 79 years; depression screening; screening for illicit drug use.

Recommended screening tests for cancer: Colonoscopy, fecal immunochemical testing (FIT), fecal occult blood testing with colorectal neoplasia–associated DNA markers (Cologuard) or flexible sigmoidoscopy (with or without fecal occult blood testing) to screen for colorectal cancer; low-dose computed tomography (CT) for lung cancer screening; prostate-specific antigen (PSA)–based screening performed on an individualized basis determined by risk factors and patient preference to screen for prostate cancer.

Recommended immunizations: Tetanus toxoid, reduced diphtheria toxoid, and acellular pertussis vaccine (Tdap) if he has not had one before or if it has been 10 years or more since he has had a tetanus-diphtheria (Td) vaccine or if he requires booster protection against pertussis; influenza vaccine annually (per season); two-dose zoster vaccine administered 2 to 6 months apart; 23-valent pneumococcal polysaccharide vaccine (PPSV23) recommended since he is a smoker; hepatitis A and B vaccine series if indicated.

ANALYSIS

Objectives

1. List the elements of the evidence-based adult well male health maintenance examination. (EPA 1, 12)

2. Describe the recommended screening tests and immunizations for adult men. (EPA 3, 11)

Considerations

The patient described is a 58-year-old man who has not undergone an evidence-based health maintenance examination in several years. In men aged 20 to 44 years, unintentional injuries are the leading cause of mortality. In men aged 45 to 54 years, cancer is the leading cause of mortality. In men 55 years of age and older, heart disease and cancer are the leading causes of mortality, varying by ethnicity and socioeconomic factors. Assessment of cardiovascular and cancer risk is paramount in an age-stratified well-male examination. Since cardiovascular disease is the most common cause of morbidity and mortality in his age group, screening for cardiovascular disease and risk factors is appropriate. Shared decision-making is imperative when providing men with age-appropriate strategies for cardiovascular and chronic disease screening, cancer screening, and immunization updates.

APPROACH TO:
Health Maintenance in Men

DEFINITIONS

HEALTH MAINTENANCE: Systematic program or procedure planned to prevent illness, maintain maximum function, and promote health.

SCREENING TEST: Assessment device or test that should be cost-effective with high sensitivity and can be used on a large, average-risk population to identify persons with disease.

USPSTF RECOMMENDATION GRADES: Grades created by the United States Preventive Services Task Force (USPSTF) after reviewing current evidence regarding screening tests; these consist of recommendations in five categories (A, B, C, D, I) based on the strength of evidence and benefit of a screening test.

CLINICAL APPROACH

The purpose of the adult male health maintenance examination is to identify potential health concerns, manage their current medical conditions, identify risks for future health problems, perform rational and cost-effective health screening tests, and promote a healthy lifestyle. Preventive care is divided into primary prevention, secondary prevention, tertiary prevention, and quaternary prevention. **Primary prevention** is an intervention designed to prevent a disease before it occurs via identification and management of risk factors for a given disease. Examples include counseling for smoking cessation, alcohol minimization, weight optimization, and immunization against communicable disease. **Secondary prevention** is an intervention intended to promote early detection of a disease or condition so that prompt treatment can be initiated. Examples include blood pressure measurement, diabetes screening, and appropriate cancer screening. **Tertiary prevention** involves both therapeutic and rehabilitative measures once a disease has been diagnosed. Examples include achieving optimal blood pressure and diabetes control, appropriate pharmacotherapy in patients with coronary heart disease and congestive heart failure, and asthma action plans in patients with moderate-to-severe asthma. **Quaternary prevention** highlights efforts to avoid unnecessary tests and interventions since some interventions, such as premature cancer screening, are more likely to cause harm than benefit the patient and should not be utilized.

Effective disease screening should meet several established criteria. In general, the disease should be of **high enough prevalence** in the population to make the screening effort worthwhile. There should be a time frame during which the person is asymptomatic, but during which the disease or risk factor can be identified. There should be screening test(s) available for the disease that have **sufficient sensitivity and specificity,** are **cost-effective,** and are **acceptable** to patients. Screening tests should have high sensitivity to minimize risk of false-negative results. Finally, there must be an intervention that can be made during the asymptomatic period that will prevent the development of the disease or reduce the morbidity and mortality of the disease process.

The USPSTF is a panel of experts that reviews current evidence and makes recommendations on the effectiveness of clinical preventive services, specifically in the areas of screening, immunization, preventive medications, and counseling. USPSTF recommendations are considered "gold standards" for clinical preventive medicine across five categories that reflect evidence strength and overall benefit of an intervention (see Table 1-1).

Table 1–1 • USPSTF GRADING OF RECOMMENDATIONS		
Recommendation Grade	Definition	Suggestion for Practice
A	There is high certainty that the net benefit of the intervention is substantial.	**Offer** or provide this service.
B	There is high certainty that the net benefit of the intervention is moderate or moderate certainty that it is moderate to substantial.	**Offer** or provide this service.
C	There may be considerations that support providing the service in an individual patient. There is moderate or high certainty that there is no net benefit or harm.	Offer or provide the service **only if there are other considerations that support offering or providing for the individual.**
D	There is moderate or high certainty that there is no net benefit or that the harms outweigh the benefits.	**Discourage** use of this service.
I	There is insufficient evidence, or the available evidence is of such poor quality, that the balance of benefits and harms cannot be weighed and recommendations for or against the service cannot be made.	If service is offered, patients should understand the **uncertainty** about the balance of benefits and harms.

SCREENING TESTS

Cardiovascular Diseases

Diseases of the cardiovascular system are the leading cause of death in adult men over 50 years of age, and the management of risk factors reduces both morbidity and mortality. The USPSTF strongly recommends screening of adults (ages 18 years and older) for **hypertension** by measurement of blood pressure (Grade A), as the management of hypertension is effective at reducing the risk of cardiovascular diseases. **Lipid screening** should be performed in men 40 to 75 years of age (Grade B); there is insufficient evidence to support screening below this age regardless of risk. Lipid screening should include nonfasting serum total cholesterol, high-density lipoprotein (HDL) cholesterol, low-density lipoprotein (LDL) cholesterol, and triglycerides. Men 50 to 69 years of age are no longer recommended to take a baby aspirin daily to reduce the risk of a myocardial infarction, as the risk of gastrointestinal hemorrhage may outweigh potential benefit men in that age group with cardiovascular risk factors may benefit from low dose aspirin. One-time screening Doppler ultrasonography to assess for **abdominal aortic aneurysm** is recommended for men aged 65 to 75 years who have ever smoked cigarettes (Grade B), while men 65 to 75 years who have never smoked can be selectively screened (Grade C).

The routine use of electrocardiogram or exercise stress testing is not recommended for screening for **coronary artery disease** in adult men (Grade D). There is insufficient evidence for screening peripheral artery disease or coronary artery disease with ankle-brachial index, high sensitivity C-reactive protein level, or coronary artery calcium score (Grade I).

Cancer

Adult men older than 50 years are recommended to undergo screening for **colorectal cancer** (Grade A). Colonoscopy, flexible sigmoidoscopy, FIT, and Cologuard are options. Any positive result on FIT, Cologuard, or sigmoidoscopy requires follow-up colonoscopy.

The USPSTF recommends that **prostate cancer** screening should be individualized for men 55 to 69 years of age while discussing benefits versus harms of PSA screening, taking into account patient values and preferences as well as comorbid conditions (Grade C). Men at higher risk of prostate cancer (eg, family history, African American) should be offered screening through shared decision-making. Men over 70 years of age should not be screened for prostate cancer (Grade D).

Men aged 55 to 80 years with a 30 or more pack-year history who either continue to smoke or who quit fewer than 15 years ago should undergo annual low-dose CT of the chest to screen for **lung cancer** (Grade B). Screening for **testicular cancer** in asymptomatic adults is not recommended (Grade D). There is insufficient evidence to recommend **skin cancer** screening via a whole-body skin examination (Grade I).

Other Health Conditions

All adult men should be screened for **obesity** via BMI, and men with a BMI over 30 kg/m² should be offered or referred for intensive multicomponent behavioral intervention (Grade B). Men 40 to 70 years of age who are overweight or obese should be screened for **type 2 diabetes mellitus** (Grade B) via fasting glucose, hemoglobin A_{1c} or oral glucose tolerance test. **Depression** screening is recommended if there are systems in place for ensuring accurate diagnosis, treatment, and follow-up (Grade B). Routine spirometry is not recommended to screen asymptomatic patients for **chronic obstructive pulmonary disease** (Grade D).

IMMUNIZATIONS

The Centers for Disease Control and Prevention (CDC) recommends all adults between 19 and 65 years of age receive a **Tdap** booster if they have not had one at or after the age of 11. They should then get a Td or Tdap booster every 10 years.

The CDC recommends annual/seasonal **influenza** vaccination for all adults. **Pneumococcal conjugate (PCV13) and PPSV23** vaccinations are recommended for all adults aged 65 years or older. An adult aged 19 to 64 years who smokes cigarettes should receive the PPSV23 vaccination. The PCV13 and/or PPSV23 vaccination may also be recommended for men aged 2 to 64 years if immunocompromised or in the presence of certain chronic medical conditions such as chronic lung diseases and diabetes mellitus.

Other vaccinations may be recommended for specific populations of men. **Hepatitis B** vaccination should be recommended for those at high risk of exposure, including health care workers, those exposed to blood or blood products, dialysis patients, intravenous drug users, men with multiple sexual partners or recent sexually transmitted infections (STIs), and men who have sex with men. **Hepatitis A** vaccine is recommended for persons with chronic liver disease, who use clotting factors, who have occupational exposure to the hepatitis A virus, who use intravenous drugs, men who have sex with men, or who travel to countries where hepatitis A is endemic. **Varicella** vaccination is recommended for those with no reliable history of immunization or disease or who are seronegative on testing for varicella immunity. **Meningococcal** vaccine is recommended for persons in high-risk groups, such as college dormitory residents and military recruits, and for patients with certain complement deficiencies, with functional or anatomic asplenia, or who travel to countries where the disease is endemic. The CDC recommends **herpes zoster** vaccination for healthy adults over age 50, preferably with the two-dose recombinant zoster vaccine. **Human papillomavirus (HPV)** vaccination is indicated in adult men up to age 45.

HEALTHY LIFESTYLE

Screening and counseling to identify and promote cessation of **tobacco use** is strongly recommended (Grade A). Screening and counseling to identify and prevent the **overuse of alcohol** are also recommended (Grade B), with a recommendation of no more than two drinks on one occasion. Screening for **illicit substance use** should be offered when services for accurate diagnosis, effective treatment, and appropriate care can be offered or referred (Grade B).

All men between 15 and 65 years of age should be screened for **HIV** (Grade A), and those with high-risk sexual practices should also be screened for **syphilis** (Grade A). Routine screening for **STIs** should be offered for men at high risk, and behavioral counseling should be provided when appropriate (Grade B). Condoms should be recommended to prevent contraction of STIs. **Men who have sex with men** should be screened for genital, oropharyngeal, and anorectal STIs and HIV when considered to be at high risk. There is no current guideline for screening for anorectal HPV infection.

Exercise has been consistently shown to reduce the risk of cardiovascular disease, diabetes, obesity, and overall mortality. Current recommendations for exercise posit 30 minutes of moderate-intensity exercise 5 days per week. Counseling to promote a **healthy diet** centered on limiting carbohydrates and sugars, as well as reasonable portion sizes and caloric intake, in men with risk factors for cardiovascular disease or diabetes is recommended. Intensive counseling by primary care providers or, when appropriate, referral to dietary counselors or nutritionists, can improve health outcomes. Finally, all men should be encouraged to wear **seat belts and helmets, practice gun safety,** and avoid driving while under the influence of alcohol or drugs. **Suicide and accidental death due to opioid overdose** are the leading causes of mortality in men ages 18 to 45 years.

CASE CORRELATION

- See also Case 7 (Tobacco Use and Cessation), Case 18 (Geriatric Health Maintenance and End-of-Life Issues), and Case 30 (Hypertension).

COMPREHENSION QUESTIONS

1.1 A 24-year-old man who has sex with men presents for his yearly health maintenance examination. He wants to be "tested for everything" but is completely asymptomatic. His BMI is 22 kg/m^2, blood pressure is 125/76 mm Hg, and he has no significant medical history. According to the USPSTF, for which of the following should this man be screened?

    A. Testicular cancer

    B. Marijuana abuse

    C. Diabetes

    D. Hyperlipidemia

    E. Depression

1.2 A 49-year-old sedentary man has made an appointment because his best friend died of a myocardial infarction at age 50. He asks your advice about exercise and weight loss to prevent cardiovascular disease. In counseling him, which of the following statements regarding exercise is most accurate?

    A. To be beneficial, exercise must be performed for at least 15 minutes every day.

    B. Walking for exercise has not been shown to improve meaningful clinical outcomes.

    C. Counseling patients has not been shown to increase the number of patients who exercise.

    D. Intense exercise offers no health benefit over mild-to-moderate amounts of exercise.

1.3 A 52-year-old man comes into the outpatient clinic for an annual "checkup." He is in good health and has a relatively unremarkable family history. He has never smoked cigarettes. For which of the following disorders should a screening test be performed?

A. Prostate cancer

B. Lung cancer

C. Abdominal aortic aneurysm

D. Colorectal cancer

E. Skin cancer

1.4 A 62-year-old man with recently diagnosed chronic obstructive pulmonary disease presents to your office in November for a routine examination. He has not had any immunizations in more than 10 years. Which of the following immunizations would be most appropriate for this individual?

A. Tetanus-diphtheria only

B. Tdap, pneumococcal, and influenza

C. Pneumococcal and influenza

D. Tdap, pneumococcal, influenza, and meningococcal

ANSWERS

1.1 **E.** The USPSTF recommends screening for depression in this man. The USPSTF recommends against testicular cancer screening (answer A). There is insufficient evidence to recommend for or against screening for illicit substance use, including marijuana (answer B). Since this man is not obese or hypertensive and has no medical history, screening for diabetes (answer C) or hyperlipidemia (answer D) is not indicated.

1.2 **C.** Exercise decreases cardiovascular risk, increases insulin sensitivity, decreases the incidence of metabolic syndrome, and decreases cardiovascular mortality regardless of obesity. Sadly, the benefits of counseling patients regarding exercise are unclear, and counseling does not seem to increase the number of patients who exercise. Answer A (15 minutes of exercise per day) is not necessary since many studies have shown that exercise for at least three sessions per week have been effective. Answer B (walking has not been shown to improve outcomes) is incorrect since walking, especially in older adults, is associated with lower all-cause mortality. Answer D (intense exercise showing no benefits over mild or moderate levels) is incorrect since the degree of intensity of exercise does have a greater impact on mortality risk.

1.3 **D.** Colorectal cancer screening has a Grade A recommendation by the USPSTF and is routinely offered or provided to all adults older than 50 years. Lung cancer screening (answer B) should not be offered for a patient who has never smoked. Prostate cancer screening (answer A) should be individualized in men 55 to 69 years of age. Abdominal aortic aneurysm screening (answer C) is recommended in men aged 65 to 75 years who have smoked. Routine skin cancer screening (answer E) is not recommended.

1.4 **B.** In an adult with a chronic lung disease, vaccination with pneumococcal vaccine and annual vaccination with influenza vaccine are recommended. A Tdap booster should be recommended to all adults who have never had a Tdap vaccine as an adult. Therefore, answer choices A (Td only) and C (pneumococcal and influenza) are not correct. Answer D includes meningococcal vaccination, which is only recommended for high-risk groups (college dormitory residents, military recruits, and patients with certain complement deficiencies, with functional or anatomic asplenia, or who travel to countries where the disease is endemic).

CLINICAL PEARLS

▶ There is no such thing as "testing for everything" in a health maintenance examination. All screening tests should have adequate evidence to support their benefit over harm.

▶ Cardiovascular disease and cancer pose the greatest risk of mortality for men in the United States.

▶ High-quality, evidence-based recommendations for preventive health services are available at https://www.uspreventiveservicestaskforce.org/uspstf/.

▶ Evidence-based recommendations for vaccines and immunizations are available at https://www.cdc.gov/Vaccines.

REFERENCES

ASCVD Risk Calculator. http://www.cvriskcalculator.com. Accessed March 25, 2019.

Centers for Disease Control and Prevention. Leading causes of death (LCOD) by age group, all males—United States, 2017. https://www.cdc.gov/nchs/fastats/leading-causes-of-death.htm Accessed April 21, 2020.

Centers for Disease Control and Prevention. Vaccines and immunizations. https://www.cdc.gov/vaccines/. Accessed January 8, 2019.

Healthy Weight/Assessing Your Weight. https://www.cdc.gov/healthyweight/. Accessed March 25, 2019.

Heidelbaugh JJ. The adult well male examination. *Am Fam Physician.* 2018;98(12):729-737.

Martins C, Godycki-Cwirko M, Heleno, B, Brodersen J. Quaternary prevention: reviewing the concept: quaternary prevention aims to protect patients from medical harm. *Eur J Gen Pract.* 2018;24(1):106-111.

Mayo Clinic Shared Decision Making National Resource Center. Home page. https://shareddecisions.mayoclinic.org. Accessed March 25, 2019.

United States Food and Drug Administration. Use of aspirin for primary prevention of heart attack and stroke. https://www.fda.gov/drugs/drug-information-consumers/use-aspirin-primary-prevention-heart-attack-and-stroke. Accessed March 22, 2019.

United States Preventive Services Task Force. Recommendations for primary care practice. http://www.uspreventiveservicestaskforce.org/Page/Name/recommendations. Accessed September 5, 2019.

A 62-year-old man presents to your office for an acute visit because of coughing and shortness of breath. He is well known to you because of multiple office visits in the past few years for similar reasons. He has a chronic "smoker's cough" but reports that in the past 2 days his cough has increased, his sputum has changed from white to green in color, and he has had to increase the frequency with which he uses his albuterol inhaler. He denies having a fever, chest pain, peripheral edema, or other symptoms. His medical history is significant for hypertension, peripheral vascular disease, and two hospitalizations for pneumonia in the past 5 years. He has a 60 pack-year history of smoking and continues to smoke two packs of cigarettes a day.

On examination, he is in moderate respiratory distress. His temperature is 98.4 °F, his blood pressure is 152/95 mm Hg, his pulse is 98 beats/min, his respiratory rate is 24 breaths/min, and he has an oxygen saturation of 94% on room air. His lung examination is significant for diffuse expiratory wheezing and a prolonged expiratory phase of respiration. There are no signs of cyanosis. The remainder of his examination is normal. A chest x-ray done in your office shows an increased anteroposterior (AP) diameter and flattened diaphragm, but otherwise he has clear lung fields.

▶ What is the most likely cause of this patient's dyspnea?
▶ What acute treatment(s) are most appropriate at this time?
▶ What interventions would be most helpful to reduce the risk of future episodes similar to this one?

ANSWERS TO CASE 2:

Dyspnea (Chronic Obstructive Pulmonary Disease)

Summary: A 62-year-old man presents with

- A long history of smoking
- Dyspnea, coughing, and wheezing
- Increased sputum production and a change in sputum character

Most likely cause of dyspnea: Acute exacerbation of chronic obstructive pulmonary disease (COPD).

Appropriate acute treatments: Antibiotic, bronchodilators, systemic corticosteroids.

Interventions to reduce future exacerbations: Smoking cessation, long-acting bronchodilator, inhaled corticosteroid, influenza, and pneumococcal polysaccharide vaccination.

ANALYSIS

Objectives

1. Be able to diagnose and determine the stage of COPD in adults. (EPA 1, 3)
2. Know the management of stable COPD and COPD exacerbations. (EPA 4, 10)

Considerations

Dyspnea is a common symptom in many diseases. It is important to do an appropriate history, physical examination, and diagnostic testing in order to correctly identify and manage the cause. Two of the most common causes of dyspnea and wheezing in adults are asthma and COPD. There can be substantial overlap between the two diseases, as patients with asthma can develop chronic obstructive disease over time. As in most medical situations, the patient's history will usually provide the key information for the appropriate diagnosis. Asthma often presents earlier in life, may or may not be associated with cigarette smoking, and is characterized by episodic exacerbations with return to relatively normal baseline lung functioning. COPD, on the other hand, tends to present in midlife or later, is usually the result of a long history of smoking, and is a slowly progressive disorder in which measured pulmonary functioning never returns to normal.

   In the setting of an acute exacerbation, the differentiation between an exacerbation of asthma and an exacerbation of COPD is not necessary for determination of the immediate management. The assessment of the patient presenting with dyspnea should always start with the ABCs—Airway, Breathing, and Circulation. Intubation with mechanical ventilation should be performed when the patient is unable to protect his own airway (eg, when the patient has a reduced level of consciousness), when he or she is tiring because of the amount of work required to overcome the airway obstruction, or when adequate oxygenation cannot be maintained.

For both asthma and COPD exacerbations, the mainstays of medical therapy are **oxygen, bronchodilators, and steroids.** All dyspneic patients should have an assessment of their level of oxygenation. Clinical signs of hypoxemia, such as cyanosis of the perioral region or digits, should be noted on examination. Objective levels of oxygenation using pulse oximetry or arterial blood gas measurements should also be performed. Hypoxemia must be addressed by providing supplemental oxygen. Inhaled beta-2 agonists, most commonly albuterol, can rapidly result in bronchodilation and reduction in airway obstruction. The addition of an inhaled anticholinergic agent, such as ipratropium, may work synergistically with the beta-2 agonist. Corticosteroids, given systemically (orally, intramuscularly, or intravenously), act to reduce the airway inflammation that underlies the acute exacerbation. Clinically significant effects of steroids take hours to occur; consequently, steroids should be used with bronchodilators because bronchodilators act rapidly. Steroids used in combination with bronchodilators significantly improve short-term outcomes in the management of acute exacerbations of asthma and COPD.

APPROACH TO:
Chronic Obstructive Pulmonary Disease

DEFINITIONS

CHRONIC BRONCHITIS: Cough and sputum production on most days for at least 3 months during at least 2 consecutive years.

EMPHYSEMA: Shortness of breath caused by the enlargement of respiratory bronchioles and alveoli caused by destruction of lung tissue.

FEV_1: FEV stands for forced expiratory volume; FEV_1 is a value that can be used to evaluate pulmonary function, determined by the amount of forced expiratory volume in the first second of expiration.

FVC: Stands for forced vital capacity, which is a measure of the total amount of air that can be expired after a maximal inspiration.

CLINICAL APPROACH

Epidemiology

As the third leading cause of death in the United States, COPD affects more than 5% of the adult population. COPD is defined as airway obstruction that is not fully reversible, is usually progressive, and is associated with chronic bronchitis, emphysema, or both. The most common etiology is **cigarette smoking, which is associated with 80% to 90% of cases of COPD.** Other etiologies of COPD include passive exposure to cigarette smoke ("secondhand smoke") and occupational exposures to dusts (including mining, cotton, silica, and plastics); chemicals; and fumes (eg, welding, heavy metals). Patients with symptoms of COPD who do not smoke or work in high-risk occupations warrant further evaluation. A rare cause of COPD is a genetic deficiency in **alpha-1 antitrypsin,** which is more common in Caucasians and should be considered when emphysema develops at younger ages (< 45 years of age), especially in nonsmokers.

Pathophysiology

Chronic obstructive pulmonary disease is a disease of inflammation of the airways, lung tissue, and vasculature. Pathologic changes include mucus gland hypertrophy with hypersecretion, ciliary dysfunction, destruction of lung parenchyma, elastin fiber destruction, and airway remodeling. These changes result in a narrowing of the airways, causing a fixed airway obstruction, poor mucus clearance, cough, wheezing, dyspnea, and a predisposition to lung infection.

The **primary diagnostic test of lung function is spirometry.** In normal aging, both the FVC and FEV_1 reduce gradually and proportionally over time. In normal-functioning lungs, the ratio of the FEV_1 to FVC is greater than 0.7. **In COPD, both the FVC and FEV_1 are reduced, and the ratio of FEV_1 to FVC is less than 0.7,** indicating an airway obstruction. Reversibility is defined as an increase in FEV_1 of greater than 12% or 200 mL with use of a short-acting bronchodilator. Using a bronchodilator may result in some improvement of both FVC and FEV_1, but neither will return to normal, making the diagnosis of a fixed obstruction. The severity of COPD, which can help to determine treatment, can be assessed using measurements established by National Institute of Health and Care Excellence and Global Initiative for Chronic Obstructive Lung Disease (see Table 2–1).

Clinical Presentation

The most common initial symptom of COPD is cough, which is at first intermittent and then frequently becomes a daily occurrence. The cough is often productive with white, thick mucus. Patients will present with intermittent episodes of worsening cough, with change in mucus from clear to yellow/green, and often with wheezing. These exacerbations are usually caused by infection.

Table 2–1 • CLASSIFICATION OF COPD SEVERITY		
Classification	Postbronchodilator Spirometry Findings[a]	Management
Mild COPD	$FEV_1 \geq 80\%$ predicted	Pneumococcal and influenza vaccinations Reduce risk factors (exposure to tobacco smoke, occupational exposures, etc) Short-acting bronchodilators
Moderate COPD	FEV_1 50% to 79% predicted	As above + long-acting bronchodilators
Severe COPD	FEV_1 30% to 49% predicted	As above + inhaled steroids
Very severe COPD	FEV_1 < 30% predicted	As above + oxygen therapy and consideration of surgical interventions

[a]In all classifications, $FEV_1/FVC < 0.7$.
Data from Global Initiative for Chronic Lung Disease Inc. Global strategy for the diagnosis, management and prevention of chronic obstructive pulmonary disease (2019 report). Available at https://goldcopd.org/wp-content/uploads/2018/11/GOLD-2019-v1.7-FINAL-14Nov2018-WMS.pdf

As COPD progresses, lung function continues to deteriorate and dyspnea develops. **Dyspnea is the primary presenting symptom of COPD.** Dyspnea also tends to worsen over time—initially, the dyspnea will occur only with significant effort, then with any exertion, and finally at rest. **By the time dyspnea develops, lung function (as measured by FEV_1) has been reduced approximately by half, and the COPD has been present for years.** When evaluating the patient with dyspnea, it is important to consider other diagnoses. Keep in mind that 85% of dyspnea causes are one of the following conditions: congestive heart failure, COPD, asthma, interstitial lung disease, pneumonia, and psychogenic disturbances (including anxiety).

Examination of a patient with mild or moderate COPD who is not having an exacerbation is usually normal. As the disease progresses, patients are often noted to have "barrel chests" (increased AP chest diameter) and distant heart sounds caused by hyperinflation of the lungs. Breath sounds may also be distant, and expiratory wheezes with a prolonged expiratory phase of respiration may be noted. In late stages, they may develop muscle wasting and cachexia. During an acute exacerbation, patients often appear anxious and tachypneic; they may be using accessory muscles of respiration, usually have wheezes or rales, and may have signs of cyanosis.

Chest x-rays in patients with COPD are typically normal until the disease is advanced. In more severe cases, hyperinflation of the lungs with an increased posteroanterior diameter and flattening of diaphragms may be seen. Bullae—areas of pulmonary parenchymal destruction—can also be seen in x-rays in more severe disease.

Treatment of Stable COPD

Goals. The goals of COPD management are to relieve symptoms; prevent or slow disease progression; reduce and manage exacerbations; reduce, prevent, and treat complications; and prevent or reduce the frequency of hospitalizations. Several components of treatment are common to all stages of COPD, whereas pharmacologic treatment is guided by the stage of disease.

Smoking Cessation. All patients with COPD should be encouraged to quit smoking. The pulmonary function of smokers declines more rapidly than that of nonsmokers. **Although smoking cessation does not result in significant improvement in pulmonary function, smoking cessation does reduce the rate of further deterioration to that of a nonsmoker.** Cessation also reduces the risks of other comorbidities, including cardiovascular diseases and cancers. Case 7 more thoroughly discusses smoking cessation. All patients with COPD should be appropriately vaccinated, with both pneumococcal vaccination and annual influenza vaccination. Avoidance of secondhand smoke, aggravating occupational exposures, and indoor and outdoor pollution is recommended.

Short-acting Bronchodilators. Although pharmacological treatment cannot reverse lung changes or modify long-term decline in lung function, it does reduce the severity of symptoms, decrease the frequency of exacerbations, decrease hospitalizations, and improve exercise tolerance and overall health. **Short-acting bronchodilators used as needed are the recommended treatment in mild COPD.**

These include beta-2 agonists (albuterol) and anticholinergics (ipratropium). **Inhaled medications are preferred** due to their fewer side effects. The choice of specific agent is based on availability, individual response to therapy, and side effects.

Long-acting Bronchodilators. In moderate COPD, a long-acting bronchodilator should be added. Commonly used agents in the United States are salmeterol (an inhaled beta-2 agonist) and tiotropium (a long-acting inhaled anticholinergic). Oral methylxanthines (aminophylline, theophylline) are also options but have narrow therapeutic windows (high toxicity) and multiple drug-drug interactions, making their use less common. The use of long-acting bronchodilators is more convenient and more effective than using short-acting agents but is much more expensive and does not replace the need for short-acting agents for rescue therapy in exacerbations.

Steroids. Inhaled steroids (fluticasone, triamcinolone, mometasone, etc) do not affect the rate of decline of lung function in COPD but do reduce the frequency of exacerbations. For that reason, **inhaled steroids are recommended for stages severe and very severe COPD with frequent exacerbations.** Long-term treatment with oral steroids is not recommended because there is no evidence of benefit and because there can be multiple complications (myopathy, osteoporosis, glucose intolerance, etc). Although continuous prophylactic antibiotic use decreases the number of COPD exacerbations for a few years, there is no decrease in mortality, and the risk of antibiotic resistance makes this a controversial issue.

Oxygen. Oxygen therapy is recommended in **very severe** COPD if there is evidence of hypoxemia ($PaO_2 \leq 55$ mm Hg or SaO_2 [arterial oxygen saturation] $\leq 88\%$ at rest). Oxygen can also be used if the SaO_2 is $< 90\%$ and there is poly-cythemia pulmonary hypertension or peripheral edema suggesting heart failure. **Oxygen therapy is the only intervention that has been shown to decrease mortality and must be worn for at least 15 h/d.** Depending on the stage of the patient's COPD, pulmonary rehabilitation and possibly lung resection surgery should be considered with the appropriate specialists when pharmacologic therapy is not providing improvement.

Follow-up. Since COPD is a chronic condition that is expected to worsen over time, routine follow-up is imperative. Spirometry is the best method to monitor lung function. The COPD Assessment Test (CAT) is a questionnaire given to patients every 3 months. The CAT is an objective tool to assess changes over time and the impact that COPD is having on a patient's life (it can be found at https://www.catestonline.org/).

Treatment of COPD Exacerbations

Definition. An acute COPD exacerbation is defined as a change in respiratory function causing worsening of symptoms, which leads to a change in medication. Acute exacerbations of COPD are common and typically present with change in sputum color or amount, cough, tachypnea, wheezing, and increased dyspnea. Although respiratory tract infections (viral and bacterial) are the most common precipitants, air pollutants are another common cause of acute COPD exacerbations. Diagnoses that can cause similar symptoms (eg, pulmonary embolism, congestive heart failure, myocardial infarction, pneumonia, pneumothorax, pleural effusion) must be excluded so that appropriate therapy can occur.

Evaluation. The severity of the exacerbation should be evaluated by history, examination, assessment of oxygenation using pulse oximetry, and focused testing. The following questions from the medical history may help to assist in assessing the exacerbation: number of previous episodes and hospitalizations, other chronic conditions, current treatment regimen, history of intubation/mechanical ventilation, and duration of new symptoms. Signs of severity on physical examination include respiratory rate, use of respiratory muscles, worsening or new cyanosis, unstable blood pressure and heart rate, altered mental status, and peripheral edema. Oxygen should be given with a target saturation of 88% to 92% or PaO_2 levels above 60 mm Hg.

Hospitalization. Patients with more severe symptoms, comorbidities, altered mental status, an inability to care for themselves at home, or whose symptoms fail to respond promptly to office or emergency department treatments should be hospitalized. If hospitalized, a baseline arterial blood gas should be considered to evaluate for hypercapnia, hypoxemia, and respiratory acidosis. Ventilatory support with either noninvasive (nasal or face mask) or invasive (intubation) ventilation should be considered in deteriorating or critical patients.

Bronchodilators and Steroids. All acute exacerbations should be treated with short-acting bronchodilators. Combinations of short-acting agents with different mechanisms of action (ie, beta-2 agonist and anticholinergic) can be used until symptoms improve. **Systemic steroids shorten the course of the exacerbation and may reduce the risk of relapse.** A steroid dose of 40 mg prednisolone (or equivalent) for 10 to 14 days is recommended.

Antibiotics. Exacerbations associated with increased amounts of sputum or with purulent sputum should be treated with antibiotics. A sputum culture should be performed. *Pneumococcus, Haemophilus influenzae,* and *Moraxella catarrhalis* are the most common bacteria implicated. In milder exacerbations, treatment with oral agents directed against these pathogens is appropriate. In severe exacerbations, gram-negative bacteria (*Klebsiella, Pseudomonas,* or other gram-negatives) can also play a role, so antibiotic coverage needs to be broader.

Prevention. Measures taken to prevent COPD exacerbation should be discussed and reviewed at each patient encounter. The number of annual exacerbations can be reduced by receiving appropriate vaccinations (influenza and pneumococcal), smoking cessation counseling, and education about current medications and their proper use. Patients should be encouraged to discuss social concerns, psychiatric problems (eg, anxiety), and proper nutrition and exercise with their provider.

CASE CORRELATION

- See also Case 7 (Tobacco Use and Cessation), Case 19 (Upper Respiratory and Ear Infections), and Case 56 (Wheezing and Asthma).

COMPREHENSION QUESTIONS

2.1 A 38-year-old woman presents with progressively worsening dyspnea and cough. She has never smoked cigarettes, has no known passive smoke exposure, and does not have any occupational exposure to chemicals. She has a family history of cirrhosis. Pulmonary function testing shows obstructive lung disease that does not respond to bronchodilators, and a complete metabolic panel demonstrates elevation of alanine aminotransferase (ALT) and aspartate aminotransferase (AST). Which of the following is the most likely etiology?

A. Radon exposure at home

B. Neoplasm

C. Alpha-1 antitrypsin deficiency

D. Pulmonary hypertension

2.2 A 60-year-old man is diagnosed with moderately severe COPD. He admits to a long history of cigarette smoking and is still currently smoking one pack per day. In counseling him about the benefits of smoking cessation, which of the following statements is most accurate?

A. By quitting, his pulmonary function will significantly improve.

B. By quitting, his current pulmonary function will be unchanged, but the rate of pulmonary function decline will slow.

C. By quitting, his current pulmonary function and the rate of decline are unchanged, but there are cardiovascular benefits.

D. By quitting, his age-related decline in pulmonary function will slow but will not approach that of a nonsmoker of the same age.

2.3 A 68-year-old patient with known COPD has been having frequent exacerbations of his COPD. Pulmonary function testing shows a FEV_1 of 40% predicted (normal = 80% to 120%). His SaO_2 by pulse oximetry is 91%. Which of the following medication regimens is the most appropriate at this time?

A. Inhaled salmeterol twice daily and albuterol as needed

B. Oral albuterol daily and inhaled fluticasone twice daily

C. Inhaled fluticasone twice daily, inhaled tiotropium twice daily, and inhaled albuterol as needed

D. Inhaled fluticasone twice daily, inhaled tiotropium twice daily, inhaled albuterol as needed, and home oxygen therapy

2.4 A 59-year-old man with a known history of COPD presents with worsening dyspnea. On examination, he is afebrile. His breath sounds are decreased bilaterally. He is noted to have jugular venous distension (JVD) and 2+ pitting edema of the lower extremities. Which of the following is the most likely cause of his increasing dyspnea?

A. COPD exacerbation

B. Pneumonia

C. Cor pulmonale

D. Pneumothorax

ANSWERS

2.1 **C.** This patient has a fixed airway obstruction consistent with COPD. The most common cause of COPD by far is cigarette smoke (90%). Other etiologies include other environmental exposures, such as air pollutants. Alpha-1 antitrypsin deficiency should be considered in a patient who develops COPD at a young age; this condition is also associated with liver dysfunction and can cause cirrhosis. Answer A (radon exposure at home) is a very rare cause of COPD and not as common as alpha-1 antitrypsin deficiency. Answer B (neoplasm) is associated with cough, especially with bloody sputum, weight loss, and cigarette smoking. Pulmonary hypertension (answer D) would not be associated with an obstructive lung disease but presents with progressive dyspnea.

2.2 **B.** By stopping smoking, an individual's ongoing deterioration of pulmonary function will slow (the rate of decline); unfortunately, the lung damage that has occurred is not affected. Smoking cessation will not result in reversal of the lung damage that has already occurred (answer A). Answer C (cardiovascular benefits but no change in rate of pulmonary decline) is not correct since there the rate of decline does indeed slow. In fact, smoking cessation can result in the rate of decline returning to that of a nonsmoker (answer D).

2.3 **C.** This patient has severe COPD with frequent exacerbations based on his FEV_1 and history. His FEV_1 is only 40% and SpO_2 is 91%. He is best treated by a long-acting bronchodilator (eg, tiotropium) and an inhaled steroid (eg, fluticasone) used regularly, along with an inhaled, short-acting bronchodilator on an as-needed basis. He does not need long-term oxygen at this point since his SpO_2 is not below 88% (answer D). Answer A (inhaled salmeterol and albuterol as needed) would be sufficient for a patient with moderate disease (FEV_1 between 50% and 80%). Similarly, answer B (oral albuterol, which is a short-acting bronchodilator, and fluticasone, a long-acting inhaled corticosteroid) is insufficient for severe COPD.

2.4 **C.** JVD and lower extremity edema are suggestive of cor pulmonale, which is right heart failure due to chronically elevated pressures in the pulmonary circulation. Right heart failure causes increased right atrial pressures and right ventricular end-diastolic pressures, which then lead to liver congestion, jugular venous distension, and lower extremity edema. Answer A (COPD exacerbation) usually presents with dyspnea and cough without heart failure. Answer B (pneumonia) is associated with fever, cough, and dyspnea without right heart failure. Answer D (pneumothorax) may be associated with JVD due to increased intrathoracic pressure, but not pedal edema; also, the patient usually has chest pain.

CLINICAL PEARLS

▶ All smokers should be counseled on the benefits of smoking cessation before they develop symptomatic COPD; by the time symptoms develop, the patient's FEV$_1$ will have been reduced by approximately 50%.

▶ COPD is one of the leading causes of morbidity and mortality.

▶ Always remember to evaluate the ABCs—**A**irway, **B**reathing, **C**irculation—when evaluating a dyspneic patient.

▶ All acute exacerbations should be treated with short-acting bronchodilators.

▶ The primary diagnostic test for COPD is spirometry; a fixed FEV$_1$/FVC ratio < 0.7 is diagnostic.

▶ Oxygen therapy is recommended in **very severe** COPD if there is evidence of hypoxemia.

REFERENCES

Armstrong C. ACP updated guidelines on diagnosis and management of stable COPD. *Am Fam Physician*. 2012;85(2):204-205.

Gentry S, Gentry B. Chronic obstructive pulmonary disease: diagnosis and management. *Am Fam Physician*. 2017;95(7):433-441.

Global Initiative for Chronic Lung Disease Inc. Global strategy for the diagnosis, management and prevention of chronic obstructive pulmonary disease (2019 report). https://goldcopd.org/wp-content/uploads/2018/11/GOLD-2019-v1.7-FINAL-14Nov2018-WMS.pdf

Silverman EK, Crapo JD, Make BJ. Chronic obstructive pulmonary disease. In: Jameson J, Fauci AS, Kasper DL, Hauser SL, Longo DL, Loscalzo J, eds. *Harrison's Principles of Internal Medicine*. 20th ed. New York, NY: McGraw Hill. http://accessmedicine.mhmedical.com/content.aspx?bookid=2129&sectionid=192031379. Accessed May 08, 2019.

A 45-year-old man presents to your office complaining of left knee pain that started last night. The pain started suddenly after dinner and was severe within a span of 3 hours. He denies any trauma, fever, systemic symptoms, or prior similar episodes. He takes hydrochlorothiazide (HCTZ) for his hypertension. He states that he drank "a lot" of wine last night with dinner.

On examination, his temperature is 98 °F, his pulse is 90 beats/min, his respirations are 22 breaths/min, and his blood pressure is 129/88 mm Hg. Heart and lung examinations are unremarkable. The patient is reluctant to flex the left knee and winces in pain when his knee is touched. The knee is edematous, is hot to touch, and has erythema of the overlying skin. No deformity is apparent. No other joints are involved. Inguinal lymph nodes are not enlarged. Complete blood count (CBC) reveals a white blood cell count of 10,900 cells/mm^3 and is otherwise normal.

▶ What is the next diagnostic step?
▶ What is the most likely diagnosis?
▶ What is the next step in therapy?

ANSWERS TO CASE 3:

Joint Pain

Summary: A 45-year-old man presents with

- The sudden onset of monoarticular, nontraumatic joint pain
- Denial of any trauma, systemic signs of illness, or any prior episodes
- History of taking HCTZ and drinking "a lot" of alcohol the night his symptoms started
- Stable vital signs and no appearance of being systemically ill
- Pain to movement and touch of the left knee, with evident edema, erythema, and warmth of the joint
- No other joints involved
- White blood cell count that is not indicative of an acute infectious process

Next diagnostic step: Joint aspiration for examination of joint fluid to identify crystals and exclude infection.

Most likely diagnosis: Acute gout of the left knee.

Next step in therapy: Nonsteroidal anti-inflammatory drug (NSAID), analgesia, and possibly colchicine.

ANALYSIS

Objectives

1. Have a differential diagnosis for nontraumatic joint pain based on clinical presentation. (EPA 1, 2)

2. Be familiar with the most common diagnostic tests for the acute joint pain and inflammation. (EPA 3)

3. Know the most common treatment options in the acute onset of gout and infectious arthritis, as well as the chronic management of rheumatoid arthritis (RA) and osteoarthritis (OA). (EPA 4)

Considerations

This 45-year-old man presents with the sudden onset of monoarticular joint pain. **The first diagnosis that needs to be excluded is an infected joint.** A joint becomes septic by blood inoculation, by contiguous infection (eg, from bone or soft tissue), or from direct inoculation from trauma or surgery. Exclusion of an infectious etiology is paramount, as cartilage can be destroyed within the first 24 hours of infection. In this case, the patient's history and clinical scenario do not favor an infectious cause, although it cannot be excluded by history and physical examination alone.

APPROACH TO:
Nontraumatic Joint Pain/Swelling

DEFINITIONS

GOUTY ARTHRITIS: Condition of excess uric acid leading to deposition of monosodium urate (MSU) crystals in joints.

POLYARTICULAR ARTHRITIS: Arthritis involving more than three joints.

PSEUDOGOUT: Condition of joint pain and inflammation due to **calcium pyrophosphate dihydrate (CPPD) crystals in the joints,** which can be diagnosed by noting rod-shaped, rhomboid, weakly positive birefringence on crystal analysis.

CLINICAL APPROACH

Depending on the etiology, pain may be present in one, two, or more joints. Considering the patient's age, medical history and medication profile is important. The patient's lifestyle and social history should also be considered, as certain activities may predispose a patient to specific infections. Among **the major diagnoses that have to be considered in a nontraumatic swollen joint are gout (or any crystal-induced arthritis), infectious arthritis, OA, and RA.** For acute monoarticular arthritis in adults, the most common causes include trauma, crystals, and infection.

Gout

Epidemiology. Most gout attacks occur between the ages of 30 and 50 years in men and in postmenopausal women (50–70 years of age). Premenopausal women are less likely to suffer from gout due to the increased level of female sex hormones, which aid in the urinary excretion of uric acid. Genetic mutations associated with the overproduction or underexcretion of uric acid can be a contributing factor for gout attacks. African Americans have a higher risk of having a gout attack. Other factors that may also increase the risk of a gout attack include trauma, surgery, or a large meal (eg, with food high in purines such as red meat, liver, nuts, or seafood) that induces hyperuricemia. As in the scenario at the beginning of the case, a recent increase in alcohol consumption can be considered an exacerbating factor. The patient's history of taking a **thiazide diuretic** is also important, as these drugs **may induce hyperuricemia** by increasing urinary urate reabsorption. Other medications that increase the risk of a gout attack include loop diuretics and chemotherapeutic agents. Weight loss has been proven to lower the risk of gout.

Pathophysiology. Gout can be divided into four stages: (1) asymptomatic tissue deposition of crystals, (2) acute gout flares, (3) intercritical segments (occurring after an acute flare, but before the next flare), and (4) chronic gout (symptoms of chronic arthritis and/or tophi). The examination of a joint aspirate is essential for the diagnosis. The **gross appearance of fluid is not very specific,** as both a septic aspirate and a heavily condensed crystal-induced arthritis may have a thick, yellowish/chalky appearance. To diagnose crystal-induced arthritis, polarizing microscopy must reveal MSU crystals, which will look like needles and have a strong negative birefringence. Other crystals that may be seen are **CPPD, calcium hydroxyapatite, and calcium oxalate.**

- **Calcium pyrophosphate dihydrate:** Rod shaped, rhomboid, weakly positive birefringence

- **Calcium hydroxyapatite:** Seen by electron microscopy, cytoplasmic inclusions are nonbirefringent

- **Calcium oxalate:** Bipyramidal appearance, strongly positive birefringence; seen mostly in end-stage renal disease patients

In crystal-induced arthritis, the white blood cell count of the joint aspirate is on average 2000 to 60,000 cells per microliter, with less than 90% neutrophils, while a septic joint will have an average of 100,000 white blood cells per microliter (25,000–250,000 cells), with more than 90% neutrophils. Aspirate that has been determined to be crystal induced must also be cultured to rule out a coexisting infection.

Clinical Presentation. Gout's first episode can often be confused with cellulitis. It presents with swelling and pain, usually of one joint, accompanied by erythema and warmth. **Classically, a gout attack involves the metatarsophalangeal joint of the first toe,** called **podagra,** but it may involve any joint in the body. Some cases left untreated resolve spontaneously within 3 to 10 days with no residual signs or symptoms. **During an acute attack, the serum uric acid level may be normal or even low,** likely as a result of the existing deposition of the urate crystals. Uric acid levels are, however, useful in monitoring hypouricemic therapy between attacks. Radiographs may show cystic changes in the joint surface, with punched-out lesions and soft-tissue calcifications. These findings are nonspecific and are also seen in OA and RA. In patients suspected to have gout, it is important to ask about recent trauma or injury. Following a traumatic event, an increase in the concentration of urate can be seen within the synovial fluid. Although imaging studies are not often necessary for the diagnosis of gout, a history of trauma may warrant such testing to rule out a fracture.

Treatment. In the case of an acute gout attack, colchicine, NSAIDs, and glucocorticoids are the drugs mainly used. Rapid and complete resolution of symptoms from acute gout treatment should begin within 24 hours of symptom onset. NSAIDs should be used with caution or avoided entirely in elderly patients (due to the possibility of gastrointestinal complications), heart failure patients, those with peptic ulcer disease, and individuals with liver or renal disease. To reduce these risks, intra-articular steroids, ice packs, and low-dose colchicine are more often used.

In patients with recurrent gout attacks, chronic medication therapy can be used to keep serum uric acid at levels low enough to reduce acute flares. Treatment should continue for at least 3 months in patients without tophi and for at least 6 months in patients with tophi. The maintenance therapy is usually with either probenecid, which increases the urinary excretion of uric acid, or, more commonly, with allopurinol, which reduces the production of uric acid. **While treating an acute gout attack, maintenance allopurinol should be continued in those already taking it,** and it may be started during an acute attack if other acute therapies (eg, NSAIDs or colchicine) are also used. Consider short-term corticosteroids once septic arthritis is ruled out. Use immunosuppressive therapy with caution, especially in patients with diabetes mellitus.

Infectious Arthritis

Epidemiology. Risk factors for infectious arthritis include alcoholism; malignancy; diabetes; hemodialysis; immunodeficiency (eg, HIV); immunosuppressive drugs (eg, corticosteroids), chronic medical conditions (eg, endocrine, pulmonary, or hepatic disease); hemophilia; and the use of intravenous drugs. Bacterial infections of a joint occur most commonly in persons with RA. The chronic inflammation of joints coupled with the use of steroids predispose this group to *Staphylococcus aureus* infections. HIV-positive patients may develop pneumococcal, *Salmonella*, or even *Haemophilus influenzae* joint infections. Intravenous drug users are most likely to get a streptococcal, staphylococcal, gram-negative, or *Pseudomonas* infection.

Pathophysiology. An infection usually involves only one joint if it is of bacterial origin (> 90% of cases). Most cases of infectious arthritis occur in large joints, including the knee, hip, and shoulder. A chronic monoarticular arthritis or involvement of two to three joints may be caused by fungi or mycobacteria. In the case of acute polyarticular arthritis, the etiology may be from endocarditis or a disseminated gonococcal infection. The three ways that microorganisms can infect joints are (1) direct penetration (surgery, bite, and trauma); (2) hematogenous spread from a distant infectious; and (3) extension from a nearby infected joint. Along with arthrocentesis with examination of synovial fluid, a blood culture, Gram stain and culture, CBC, and erythrocyte sedimentation rate (ESR) should be obtained.

Clinical Presentation. Range of motion (ROM) of the joint is an important maneuver of the physical examination. **A septic joint will have a very limited ROM due to pain** coupled with a joint effusion and fever. However, a nearby cellulitis, bursitis, or osteomyelitis will usually maintain the ROM of a joint. The aspirate of a septic joint will have a positive culture in more than 90% of cases.

Treatment. **The preferred treatment for septic arthritis includes intravenous antimicrobials and surgery for drainage of the infected joint.** Methicillin-resistant *S. aureus* (MRSA) will usually require vancomycin, but coverage with antibiotics is dependent on the specific organisms isolated.

Osteoarthritis

Pathophysiology. Osteoarthritis is most commonly found in people older than 65 years of age and is associated with trauma, history of repetitive joint use, and obesity (specifically for knee OA). It primarily affects the cartilage but ends up damaging the bone surface, synovium, meniscus, and ligaments. The clinical presentation is usually that of a dull, deep ache. The onset is usually gradual, with activity exacerbating the pain and rest decreasing it. In the latter stages, pain is constant. On physical examination, a bony crepitus may be felt on passive ROM. There may be a small joint effusion and periarticular muscle atrophy. In the advanced stage, joint deformity with decreased ROM will be seen. **X-rays are usually normal at first,** with the gradual development of bone sclerosis, subchondral cysts, and osteophytes.

Treatment. Degenerative joint disease treatment involves mobility exercises, maintenance of adequate ROM, and weight loss, if appropriate. Intra-articular corticosteroid injections may provide relief for varying amounts of time but should only be done every 4 to 6 months to avoid cartilage destruction. Surgery, such as joint replacement, is usually reserved for people with severe disease that affects their daily functions.

Rheumatoid Arthritis

Pathophysiology. Rheumatoid arthritis (RA) is another common disorder that may affect people from any age group, but it will usually present initially in those 30 to 55 years old. It affects more women than men (3:1), and the treatment will usually depend on the stage at which the disease is diagnosed. It is thought that the increase in pro-inflammatory cytokines (eg, tumor necrosis factor [TNF] and interleukin 6) within the synovial cells of joints is responsible for the destruction of cartilage and bony erosions seen in RA.

Clinical Presentation. The presentation of RA can be varied, ranging from a monoarticular arthritis that is intermittent to a polyarthritis that progresses gradually in intensity, leading to disability. Possible abnormal laboratory tests for RA are positive rheumatoid factor (RF) and anti–cyclic citrullinated peptide (anti-CCP) antibody, elevated ESR, elevated C-reactive protein (CRP), anemia, thrombocytosis, and low albumin. The level of hypoalbuminemia usually correlates with the severity of the disease. The anti-CCP autoantibody is more specific than RF; additionally, a positive anti-CCP may precede the clinical manifestation of disease by many years.

Diagnosis. In 2010, the American College of Rheumatology/European League Against Rheumatism (ACR/EULAR) developed a new approach to diagnose RA that focuses on features found in the earlier stages of disease. According to this new classification, RA is diagnosed if a person presents with synovitis (swelling) in at least one joint, all other diagnoses for the synovitis are excluded, and there is a calculated individual score of 6 points or more (maximum of 10 points). This individual score is based upon both clinical and laboratory factors, including the number and site of involved joints, serologic abnormalities (RF and anti-CCP), elevated acute-phase response markers (CRP and ESR), and symptom duration (Table 3–1).

Treatment. Therapy for RA involves multiple modalities. Education and counseling of the patient regarding disease progression, treatment options, and implications for lifestyle are essential. Exercises that maintain joint mobility and muscle strength are very important, as the natural course of RA is to develop joint stiffness that becomes disabling. Physical therapy and occupational therapy are important to address specific areas in which the patient may need additional devices to perform activities of daily living.

Many different categories of medications are used in RA. **Disease-modifying antirheumatic drugs (DMARDs)** are the first line agent for the treatment of RA. Among the DMARDs, methotrexate is the generally recommended initial therapy. NSAIDs, glucocorticoids, anticytokines, and topical analgesics can be used with DMARDs as adjuvant medication during the first month of treatment. Infliximab and etanercept are examples of anticytokine agents. Treatment regimens

Table 3–1 • ACR/EULAR CRITERIA FOR DIAGNOSIS OF RHEUMATOID ARTHRITIS
1. Synovitis (swelling) is present in at least 1 joint.
2. All other diagnoses for clinical synovitis are excluded.
3. Individual score > 6 points is reached based on the following criteria:
a. Joint involvement: 1 large[a] joint (no points), 2-10 large joints (1 point), 1-3 small[b] joints with or without large joint (2 points), 4-10 small joints with or without large joints (3 points), > 10 joints (5 points)
b. Serology: Negative RF **and** anti-CCP (no points), low positive RF **or** anti-CCP (2 points), high positive RF **or** anti-CCP (3 points)
c. Acute-phase reactants: normal CRP **and** normal ESR (no points), abnormal CRP **or** abnormal ESR (1 point)
d. Duration of symptoms: < 6 weeks (no points), > 6 weeks (1 point)

Abbreviations: MCP, metacarpophalangeal; MTP, metatarsophalangeal; PIP, proximal interphalangeal.
[a]*Large joints include shoulders, elbows, hips, knees, and ankles.*
[b]*Small joints include wrists, MCP, PIP, 2nd to 5th MTPs, and thumb interphalangeal joints.*
Data from Aletaha D, Neogi T, Silman AJ, et al. Rheumatoid arthritis classification criteria. Arthritis Rheum. 2010;62(9):2569-2581.

are individualized and will often include a combination of two or three of these agents. Although these agents are effective, monitoring for hepatotoxicity must be performed.

COMPREHENSION QUESTIONS

3.1 A 26-year-old man presents with a fever, dysuria, and left knee pain of 3 days' duration. He reports being sexually active with a new partner as recently as 2 weeks ago. On physical examination, his temperature is 102 °F. His left knee is erythematous, warm, swollen, and tender. He denies a previous history of arthritis. Which of the following is the next best step?

A. Complete blood count with differential

B. X-ray of the knee

C. Aspiration of synovial fluid

D. Serum uric acid level

3.2 A 44-year-old woman has a 5-month history of malaise and stiff hands in the morning that improve as the day goes by. She notes that both hands are involved at the wrists. Initial laboratory tests show an elevated ESR and high positive anti-CCP. Which of the following treatments is most likely to lead to the best long-term disease outcome for this patient?

A. Allopurinol

B. Ibuprofen

C. Naproxen

D. Methotrexate

E. Intravenous ceftriaxone

3.3 A 52-year-old man complains of bilateral knee pain for about 1 year. He is noted to have a body mass index of 40 kg/m². Which of the following is the best therapy?

A. Allopurinol

B. Ibuprofen

C. Methotrexate

D. Intravenous ceftriaxone

E. Oral glucocorticoids

3.4 A 35-year-old man with hypertension presents with the sudden onset of right big toe pain. He denies trauma of the foot. On examination, he is noted to have a swollen, red, and tender base of the right great toe. Which of the following is the best treatment for the probable condition?

A. Ibuprofen

B. Methotrexate

C. Colchicine

D. Intravenous antibiotics

ANSWERS

3.1 **C.** Infectious arthritis would need to be high on the differential diagnosis because of the danger of gonococcal arthritis. The history supports this diagnosis. This patient needs a joint aspiration to look for gram-negative diplococci and crystals and to obtain a sample for culture. He will likely require surgical drainage of the swollen joint and intravenous antibiotic therapy. Even if the Gram stain shows no organisms, if there is sufficient suspicion (eg, high white cell count of joint fluid), the patient should be treated for a possibly septic joint; this is because if an infected joint is not promptly and adequately treated, there is a high risk of joint destruction. If the joint fluid cultures show no growth in 48 hours, then antibiotics may be discontinued. Answer A (CBC with differential) and answer B (x-ray of the knee) are both studies that would be performed, but they are not as important to assess for a septic joint as aspiration. Answer D (uric acid level) is to assess for possible gout, but this is not as likely since the patient has no history of joint pain.

3.2 **D.** Morning stiffness, involvement of the hands, and symmetric arthritis are common features of RA. According to the ACR/EULAR, this patient meets the criteria for the diagnosis of newly presenting RA in that she has joint involvement, positive serology, elevated acute-phase reactants, and duration of symptoms more than 6 weeks. DMARD therapy, such as the use of methotrexate, would be indicated. Methotrexate as a disease-modifying agent would alter the natural history of the disease rather than just treat the symptoms. Answer A (allopurinol) would be indicated for gout. Answer B (ibuprofen) and answer C (naproxen) are NSAIDs that could help alleviate pain in acute attacks but carry risks for gastrointestinal problems with chronic use. Answer E (intravenous ceftriaxone) could be appropriate for septic arthritis, depending on the infectious agent.

3.3 **B.** Obesity is a risk factor for OA, which is common in the knees and typically presents with a gradual onset and worsening of symptoms. Along with exercise and efforts to lose weight, an NSAID medication, such as ibuprofen, may provide symptomatic relief. Allopurinol (answer A) would be appropriate for maintenance of gout, and oral glucocorticoids (answer E) can be helpful in acute gout attacks. Methotrexate (answer C) is helpful in cases of RA. Intravenous ceftriaxone (answer D) could be appropriate for septic arthritis, depending on the infectious agent.

3.4 **C.** Gouty arthritis often initially presents in the big toe ("podagra"), and the use of HCTZ, a common treatment for hypertension, also can increase the risk. Colchicine can provide effective acute treatment. Answer A (ibuprofen) can help to alleviate the pain somewhat due to its anti-inflammatory effect, but its contribution is less than colchicine in an acute gouty attack. Answer B (methotrexate) is useful for RA of systemic lupus erythematosus, which would be unlikely in a patient without a history of arthritis; also, arthritis only affecting the great toe would be unusual for these disorders. Answer D (intravenous antibiotics) would be a treatment for a septic joint. There is no history such as trauma that would be a risk for that etiology.

CLINICAL PEARLS

▶ A red, swollen joint **must** be aspirated to rule out a joint infection.

▶ A septic joint must be promptly treated since delay beyond 24 hours is associated with joint destruction.

▶ Trauma, infection, and crystals are the most common causes of acute monoarthritis in adults.

▶ Classically, a gout attack involves the metatarsophalangeal joint of the first toe, called podagra, but it may involve any joint in the body.

▶ The preferred treatment for septic arthritis includes intravenous antimicrobials and surgery for drainage of the infected joint.

▶ In the case of an acute gout attack, colchicine, NSAIDs, and glucocorticoids are the drugs mainly used.

▶ The NSAIDs should be used with caution or avoided entirely in elderly patients (due to the possibility of gastrointestinal complications), heart failure patients, those with peptic ulcer disease, and individuals with liver or renal disease.

▶ Disease-modifying antirheumatic drugs are the first-line agents for the treatment of RA.

REFERENCES

Aletaha D, Neogi T, Silman AJ, et al. Rheumatoid arthritis classification criteria. *Arthritis Rheum.* 2010;62(9);2569-2581.

Bieber JD, Terkeltaub RA. Gout. On the brink of novel therapeutic options for an ancient disease. *Arthritis Rheum.* 2004;50:2400-2414.

Cush JJ. Approach to articular and musculoskeletal disorders. In: Jameson J, Fauci AS, Kasper DL, Hauser SL, Longo DL, Loscalzo J, eds. *Harrison's Principles of Internal Medicine.* 20th ed. New York, NY: McGraw Hill. http://accessmedicine.mhmedical.com/content.aspx?bookid=2129&sectionid=192285968. Accessed May 27, 2019.

Hainer BL, Matheson E, Wilkes RT. Diagnosis, treatment and prevention of gout. *Am Fam Physician.* 2014;90(12):831-836.

Mochan E, Ebell MH. Predicting rheumatoid arthritis risk in adults with undifferentiated arthritis. *Am Fam Physician.* 2008;77:1451-1453.

Schmitt S. Acute infectious arthritis. In: *Merck Manual Professional Version.* Last update January 2019. https://www.merckmanuals.com/professional/musculoskeletal-and-connective-tissue-disorders/infections-of-joints-and-bones/acute-infectious-arthritis?query=infectious%20arthritis. Accessed May 27, 2019.

Shah A, St Clair E. Rheumatoid arthritis. In: Jameson J, Fauci AS, Kasper DL, Hauser SL, Longo DL, Loscalzo J, eds. *Harrison's Principles of Internal Medicine.* 20th ed. New York, NY: McGraw Hill. http://accessmedicine.mhmedical.com/content.aspx?bookid=2129&sectionid=192284979. Accessed May 27, 2019.

Wasserman AM. Rheumatoid arthritis: common questions about diagnosis and management. *Am Fam Physician.* 2018;97(7):455-462.

A 22-year-old woman who has never been pregnant presents to the office after having a positive home pregnancy test. She has no significant medical history. Upon further questioning, she states that she is unsure of the date of her last menstrual period (LMP). She denies any symptoms and is worried as she has not felt the baby move thus far. She is also concerned because she recently had dental x-rays taken prior to discovering that she was pregnant. She denies the use of any drugs, alcohol, or tobacco. She inquires about when she can get an ultrasound and a genetic test to rule out Down syndrome.

▶ When is an ultrasound indicated in prenatal care?
▶ What laboratory studies are routinely indicated at an initial prenatal visit?
▶ What is the risk to the pregnancy based on the radiation exposure that the patient has encountered?
▶ When is the optimal time for a trisomy screen test?

ANSWERS TO CASE 4:
Prenatal Care

Summary: A 22-year-old woman presents with

- Primigravida status and desire for initial prenatal care visit with unknown LMP
- No significant past medical history
- Numerous questions regarding her care
- Recent history of dental x-rays

Indications for an ultrasound in pregnancy: According to the American College of Obstetricians and Gynecologists (ACOG), an ultrasound is not mandatory in routine, low-risk prenatal care. An ultrasound is indicated for the evaluation of uncertain gestational age, size/date discrepancies, vaginal bleeding, multiple gestations, or other high-risk situations.

Laboratory studies recommended at the initial prenatal visit: Confirm pregnancy with urine pregnancy test. If positive, then complete blood count (CBC), hepatitis B surface antigen (HBsAg), HIV testing, syphilis screening with a rapid plasma reagin (RPR), urinalysis and urine culture, rubella antibody, blood type and Rh status with antibody screen, Papanicolaou (Pap) smear, and cervical swab for gonorrhea and *Chlamydia*. A urine drug screen is also considered and often performed at the first prenatal visit.

Risk to the pregnancy based on the radiation exposure from dental x-rays: Risk for the baby is increased once the radiation exposure is greater than 5 rad or 50 mGy; the radiation exposure from routine dental x-rays is 0.0005 rad. ACOG states that dental x-rays are safe in pregnancy when the thyroid and the abdomen are adequately shielded.

Optimal time for the trisomy screen: Considerations for trisomy screening include

- First trimester testing for nuchal translucency (NT) via ultrasound or a combined test of NT and serum markers human chorionic gonadotropin (hCG) and pregnancy-associated plasma protein A (PAPP-A) testing between 10 and 13 weeks.

- Second-trimester triple (alpha-fetoprotein [AFP], hCG, estriol) or quadruple (triple screen and inhibin-A) screen between 16- and 18-weeks' gestation; however, it may be performed between 15- and 20-weeks' gestation, if necessary.

- Emerging evidence shows that combining results of first- and second-trimester screening tests improves the trisomy detection rate; consequently, the optimal time for screening should be discussed at the initial prenatal visit.

- Concerning results from the tests mentioned may warrant more invasive testing to confirm chromosomal abnormalities. These tests include chorionic villous sampling at 11 to 13 weeks or amniocentesis at or after 15 weeks.

ANALYSIS

Objectives

1. Learn the components of the preconception counseling and the initial prenatal visit. (EPA 12)

2. Know the recommended screening tests and visit intervals in routine prenatal care. (EPA 3, 11, 12)

3. Learn the relevant psychosocial aspects of providing prenatal care, including important counseling issues. (EPA 12)

Considerations

Prenatal, or antenatal, care affords the opportunity to both perform appropriate medical testing and provide counseling and anticipatory guidance. Pregnancy can be a time of anxiety, and patients frequently have many questions. One of the goals of prenatal care is to provide appropriate education to reduce anxiety and help women to be active participants in their own care.

APPROACH TO:

Prenatal Care

DEFINITIONS

ADVANCED MATERNAL AGE: Pregnant woman who will be 35 years or beyond at the estimated date of delivery (EDD).

ANTENATAL TESTING: A procedure that attempts to identify whether the fetus is at risk for uteroplacental insufficiency and perinatal death. Some of these tests include nonstress test (NST) and biophysical profile (BPP).

ASYMPTOMATIC BACTERIURIA (ASB): ASB is assessed as 100,000 colony-forming units per milliliter (cfu/mL) or more of a pure pathogen of a midstream voided specimen without clinical symptoms. ASB in pregnant women increases risk of acute pyelonephritis, preterm delivery, and low birth weight; therefore, early detection is paramount, and treatment is mandated.

GENETIC COUNSELING: An educational process provided by a health care professional for individuals and families who have a genetic disease or who are at risk for such a disease. It is designed to provide information about their condition or potential condition and help them make informed decisions.

ISOIMMUNIZATION: The development of specific antibodies as a result of antigenic stimulation by material from the red blood cells of another individual. For example, Rh isoimmunization occurs when an Rh-negative woman develops anti-D (Rh factor) antibodies in response to exposure to Rh (D) antigen.

VERTICAL TRANSMISSION: Infectious passage of infection from mother to fetus, whether in utero, during labor and delivery, or postpartum.

CLINICAL APPROACH

Preconception Care

In the United States, the first visit for prenatal care frequently is at 8 weeks of gestation or later, and yet it is the time preceding this that poses the greatest risk to fetal development. **A preconception visit is an ideal opportunity for the patient to discuss with her provider any issue related to possible pregnancy or contraception occurring within 1 year of pregnancy.** Providers may also take this opportunity to do counseling for inheritable conditions. The preconception visit can be included during visits for many reasons, including fertility problems, contraception, periodic health assessment, recent amenorrhea, or specifically for preconception counseling. Roughly one-half of patients with a negative pregnancy test may have some risk that could adversely affect a future pregnancy. Because approximately 50% of pregnancies are unplanned or unintended, clinicians should consider the potential of pregnancy when writing each prescription. The primary care provider should ask women of reproductive age about their intention to become pregnant. Contraceptive counseling should be given based on the patient's intentions. Women who intend to become pregnant should be advised to avoid, whenever possible, potentially harmful agents such as radiation, drugs, alcohol, tobacco, over-the-counter (OTC) medications, herbs, and other environmental agents.

Radiation. **Radiation exposure greater than 5 rad is associated with fetal harm. Most commonly performed x-ray procedures, including dental, chest, and extremity x-rays, expose a fetus to only very small fractions of this amount of radiation.** Fetuses are particularly sensitive to radiation during the early stages of development, between 2 and 15 weeks after conception. Whenever possible, the abdomen and pelvis should be shielded and x-rays performed only when the benefit outweighs the potential risk. Imaging procedures not associated with ionizing radiation, including ultrasound or magnetic resonance imaging, should be considered as alternatives to x-ray during pregnancy when appropriate.

OTC Preparations. Women should refrain from OTC medicines, herbs, vitamins, minerals, and nutritional products until cleared by their obstetric provider. The US Public Health Service and Centers for Disease Control and Prevention (CDC) recommend that all women of childbearing age take folic acid daily, and women considering conception should start a folic acid supplement at least 1 month prior to attempting to conceive. **For low-risk women, a dose of 400 to 800 micrograms of folic acid daily is recommended to reduce the risk of neural tube defects.** Higher doses are recommended in the presence of certain risk factors. For women with diabetes mellitus or epilepsy, 1 mg of folic acid a day is recommended. **A woman who has had a child with a neural tube defect should take 4 mg of folic acid daily.**

Genetic Screening. Women from certain ethnic backgrounds may be offered specific genetic screening. African and African American women may be offered sickle cell trait screening. A French Canadian or Ashkenazi Jewish background is an indication to consider screening for a Tay-Sachs carrier state. Southeast Asian and

Middle Eastern women may be offered screening for thalassemia. Ashkenazi Jews and Caucasian women may be offered screening for cystic fibrosis.

Age-Related Risk. **Women who will be 35 years old or older at the anticipated time of delivery should be educated about age-related risk,** particularly the increased risk of Down syndrome. They should be counseled about the available screening and diagnostic testing available, along with the appropriate time frame in which each test may be performed. Although invasive in nature, chorionic villous sampling or amniocentesis are recommended to be offered to women who are 35 years of age or greater during the time of pregnancy. In practice, however, screening laboratory tests usually precede invasive testing for general risk identification.

Comorbidities. Women with medical conditions such as diabetes, asthma, thyroid disease, hypertension, lupus, thromboembolism, and seizures should be referred to providers with experience in managing high-risk pregnancies. Women with psychiatric disorders should be comanaged with a psychiatrist and counselor/therapist so that the patient can benefit from pharmacologic and behavioral therapy. These patients may require more frequent visits.

Lifestyle Counseling. Pregnant women and those looking to become pregnant should be screened for tobacco use. Patients who have drug, tobacco, or alcohol dependence should be educated about the risks and referred to rehab/treatment centers to quit the drug prior to conception. Women should also be educated about proper nutrition and exercise during pregnancy. Preconception counseling may also address issues such as financial readiness, social support during pregnancy and the postpartum period, and issues of domestic violence.

Initial Prenatal Visit

The initial visit should address all the concepts in the preconception visit if no preconception counseling was done. Ideally, the initial visit should be in the first trimester. A detailed history and physical examination, initial obstetric laboratory tests, and counseling regarding the logistics for prenatal care should be done at this visit.

Last Menstrual Period. The history should begin with an assessment of the LMP and its reliability. **One of the most crucial pieces of information is the accuracy of the dating.** The first day of the LMP is used to obtain the EDD using Naegele's rule (from the first day of the LMP subtract 3 months and add 7 days). The LMP is considered reliable if the following criteria are met: the date is certain, the LMP was normal, there has been no contraceptive use in the past 1 year, the patient has had no bleeding since the LMP, and her menses are regular. If these criteria are not met, an ultrasound should be performed. The ACOG has established further criteria that can be used to ensure that a fetus is mature at the time of delivery, which include criteria such as early sonography and the timing of the positive pregnancy test.

History Components. History should also be obtained with particular attention to medical history, prior pregnancies, delivery outcomes, pregnancy complications, neonatal complications, and birth weights. Gynecologic history should focus on the menstrual history, contraceptive use, and history of sexually transmitted infections. Allergies, current medications—both prescription and OTC—and substance use should also be investigated. Social history should consider whether the pregnancy was planned, unplanned, or unintentional. A discussion of social supports for the patient during the prenatal and postpartum period is also warranted. Genetic history should be obtained for the patient and partner's family, if known.

Physical Examination. The initial examination should be thorough and should include height, weight, body mass index, blood pressure, thyroid, breast, and general physical and pelvic examinations. Pregnancy-specific examinations, including an estimation of gestational age by uterine size or fundal height measurement and an attempt to hear fetal heart tones by Doppler fetoscope, should be performed. Heart tones should be obtainable by 10 weeks' gestation using a handheld Doppler fetoscope. Pelvimetry has been removed as a recommended intervention, but it may be useful to have a subjective assessment for risks of problems during delivery.

Laboratory Screening. The initial laboratory screen (Table 4–1) should include blood type and Rh status antibody screen, rubella status, HIV, HBsAg, RPR, urinalysis, urine culture, Pap smear, cervical swab for gonorrhea and *Chlamydia*, and a CBC. The inactivated influenza vaccination should be offered to all pregnant women during flu season.

Prenatal Visit Scheduling. The logistics of the prenatal visits should be addressed. A typical protocol includes follow-up visits every 4 weeks until 28 weeks' gestation, every 2 weeks from 28 to 36 weeks' gestation, and every week from 36 weeks' gestation until delivery. More frequent visits should be performed if any problems arise or if not all issues are addressed in the scheduled visits.

Ultrasound. **The ACOG does not stipulate routine ultrasonography in patients without complications.** Ultrasound is considered accurate for establishing gestational age, fetal number, viability, and placental location. Therefore, ultrasonography should be performed in patients without reliable dating criteria, with a discrepancy between the measured and expected uterine growth, and, in the case of a postdated pregnancy, suspicion for twin gestation, placental issues, chromosomal abnormalities, or other problems. For gestational age estimations, ultrasonography is accurate to within 1 week if performed in the first trimester, 2 weeks in the second trimester, and 3 weeks in the third trimester. If the ultrasound dates and LMP are off by more than the aforementioned intervals, the due date should be recalculated based on the ultrasound findings.

Other Concerns. The visit should end with an adequate explanation of all patient/partner concerns. Women should be counseled that sexual activity is not associated with any harm during an uncomplicated pregnancy, although there may be conditions that arise during the course of a pregnancy that would make sexual activity inadvisable. A follow-up visit should be scheduled prior to her leaving the office. She should also be educated about preterm labor precautions, signs of ectopic pregnancy, and situations in which to call the provider or go to the obstetrics triage unit for evaluation.

Subsequent Prenatal Visits

Assessing for Complications. At follow-up prenatal visits, concerns or questions brought up by the patient should be addressed. The examiner should ask questions

Table 4–1 • SUMMARY OF PRENATAL LABORATORIES, RAMIFICATIONS, AND EVALUATION

Lab Test	Finding	Ramifications	Next Step	Comments
Hemoglobin	Below 10.5 g/dL	Preterm delivery Low fetal iron stores Identify thalassemia	Mild: therapeutic trial of iron Moderate: ferritin and Hb electrophoresis	
Rubella	Negative	Nonimmune to rubella	Stay away from sick individuals, vaccinate postpartum	Live attenuated vaccine in the postpartum period
Blood type	Any type	May help pediatricians identify ABO incompatibility		
Rh factor	Negative	May be susceptible to Rh disease	If antibody screen negative, give RhoGAM at 28 weeks, after any trauma, miscarriage, obstetrical complication, or invasive procedure, and if baby is Rh+, then also after delivery	RhoGAM (D immunoglobulin) 300 mcg IM × 1 dose at 28-wk gestation or within 72 h of trauma, complication, procedure, miscarriage, or delivery
Antibody screen	Positive	May indicate isoimmunization	Need to identify the antibody, and then titer	Lewis lives, Kell kills, Duffy dies (mnemonic for antibodies)
HIV ELISA	Positive	May indicate infection with HIV	Western blot or PCR, if positive then place patient on anti-HIV meds, offer elective cesarean, or intravenous ZDV (zidovudine) in labor	Intervention reduces vertical transmission from 25% to 2% Antiretroviral therapy is started in 2nd trimester
RPR or VDRL	Positive	May indicate syphilis	Specific antibody such as MHA-TP, and if positive then stage disease	Less than 1 y, penicillin IM × 1; > 1 y or unknown, penicillin IM each week × 3
Gonorrhea	Positive	May cause preterm labor, blindness	Ceftriaxone 250 mg IM × 1 dose	
Chlamydia	Positive	May cause neonatal blindness, pneumonia	Azithromycin 1 g PO × 1 or amoxicillin 500 mg PO three times daily × 7 days	
Hepatitis B surface antigen	Positive	Patient is infectious	Check LFTs and hepatitis serology to determine if chronic carrier vs active hepatitis	Baby needs HBIG and hepatitis B vaccine within 12 h of birth

(Continued)

Table 4–1 • SUMMARY OF PRENATAL LABORATORIES, RAMIFICATIONS, AND EVALUATION (continued)

Lab Test	Finding	Ramifications	Next Step	Comments
Urine culture	Positive	Asymptomatic bacteriuria may lead to pyelonephritis 25%	Treat with antibiotic and recheck urine culture	If GBS is organism, then give penicillin in labor
Pap smear	Positive	Only invasive cancer would alter management	ASC-US → repeat Pap postpartum; LGSIL, HSIL → colposcopy	Reflexive HPV not recommended with ASC-US
Nuchal translucency (NT) (10-13 wk) or combined test (NT, hCG, and PAPP-A)	Positive	May indicate trisomy	Offer karyotype, follow-up ultrasounds, chorionic villa sampling (CVS) or second-trimester screening	Increased NT means increased risk, not definitive diagnosis
Trisomy screen (15-20 wk)	Positive	At risk for trisomy or NTD	Basic ultrasound for dates; if dates confirmed offer genetic amniocentesis	Most common reason for abnormal serum screening: wrong dates
1-h diabetic screen (24-28 wk)	Positive (elevated > 135)	May indicate gestational diabetes	Go to 3-h GTT	About 15% of those screened will be positive
3-h glucose tolerance test	Two abnormal values	Gestational diabetes	Try ADA diet, monitor blood sugars; if elevated may need meds or insulin	About 15% of abnormal 1-h GCT will have gestational diabetes, lifetime risk of DM is 50%
GBS culture (35-37 wk)	Positive	GBS colonizing genital tract	Penicillin during labor	Helps to prevent early GBS sepsis, pneumonia, or meningitis of newborn

Abbreviations: ADA, American Diabetes Association; ASC-US, atypical squamous cell of uncertain significance; DM, diabetes mellitus; ELISA, enzyme-linked immunosorbent assay; GBS, group B Streptococcus; GCT, glucose challenge test; HBIG, hepatitis B immune globulin; HPV, human papilloma virus; HSIL, high-grade squamous intraepithelial lesion; IM, intramuscular; LFT, liver function tests; LGSIL, low-grade squamous intraepithelial lesion; MHA-TP, microhemagglutination assay for Treponema pallidum; NTD, neural tube defect; PCR, polymerase chain reaction; PO, by mouth (per os).
Reproduce, with permission, from Toy EC, Baker B, Ross P, Jennings J. Case Files: Obstetrics and Gynecology. 3rd ed. 2009.

specifically targeted at symptoms suggestive of complications, including gestational hypertension, preeclampsia, infections (urinary tract, vaginal, etc), fetal compromise, placenta previa/abruption, and preterm labor or premature rupture of membranes. At each visit, the patient should be asked about vaginal bleeding, loss of fluid, headaches, visual changes, abdominal pain, dysuria, facial or upper extremity edema, vaginal discharge, and subjective sensation of fetal movements.

The examination on each subsequent visit should include weight, blood pressure, fundal height measurement, and fetal heart tones by handheld Doppler. In addition, a urinalysis should be performed at every visit to assess for protein, glucose, or nitrates/leukoesterase.

Prenatal Screening and Laboratory Studies

Triple and Quad Screens. At 15 to 20 weeks' gestation (preferably between 16 and 18 weeks' gestation), a multiple-marker test, which screens for trisomy 21, trisomy 18, and neural tube defects, should be offered to patients. The two most common modalities of screening the fetus for these anomalies are the triple screen and the quad screen. The triple screen tests for serum hCG, unconjugated estriol, and AFP; the quad screen tests for those three plus inhibin-A. **The triple screen has a sensitivity of approximately 65% to 69% and specificity of 95% for detecting aneuploidy.** The quad screen increases sensitivity to approximately 80% without reducing specificity. The most common cause for a false-positive serum screen is incorrect gestational age dating. During the first trimester, fetal NT can be measured by ultrasonography combined with maternal serum analyte levels (ie, free hCG and PAPP-A). This testing can be performed at 10 to 14 weeks' gestation. Sensitivity and specificity of these tests are determined by the risk cutoff used (eg, for trisomy 21, sensitivity is 85.2% when specificity is 90.6%; at 95% specificity, the sensitivity is 78.7%). Women should be counseled about the limited sensitivity and specificity of the tests, the psychological implications of a positive test, the potential impact of delivering a child with Down syndrome, the risks associated with prenatal diagnosis and second-trimester abortion, and the delays inherent in the process. More advanced testing is also available to look for fetal DNA fragments that are present in maternal blood. These tests are high tech and not invasive, but they are expensive and insurance coverage varies.

Amniocentesis and Chorionic Villus Sampling. Women at increased risk of aneuploidy should be offered prenatal diagnosis by amniocentesis or chorionic villus sampling (CVS). Persons at increased risk include women with singleton pregnancies who will be older than 35 years at delivery, or those with twin pregnancies who will be older than 32 years at delivery; women carrying a fetus with a major structural anomaly identified by ultrasonography; women with ultrasound markers of aneuploidy (including increased nuchal thickness); women with a previously affected pregnancy; couples with a known translocation, chromosome inversion, or aneuploidy; and women with a positive maternal serum screen. Amniocentesis may be performed after 15 weeks' gestation and is associated with a 0.5% risk of spontaneous abortion. CVS is performed at 10- to 12-weeks' gestation and has a 1% to 1.5% risk of spontaneous abortion. CVS may be associated with transverse limb defects (0.3 to 1 per 1000 fetuses). Women undergoing CVS also should be offered maternal serum AFP testing for neural tube defects. Women older than age 35 years at time of delivery may opt for serum screening and ultrasonography before deciding whether to proceed with amniocentesis. **Although the risk for trisomy 21 increases with maternal age, an estimated 75% of affected fetuses are born to mothers younger than age 35 years at time of delivery.**

Gestational Diabetes. The United States Preventive Services Task Force recommends screening for gestational diabetes in asymptomatic pregnant women after

24 weeks of gestation (Grade B). At 24 to 28 weeks' gestation, patients should be screened for gestational diabetes with a 1-hour, 50-g glucose challenge test. When the screening test is positive, a 3-hour glucose tolerance test (GTT) should be performed (after an overnight fast) by giving the patient a 100-g glucose load and obtaining fasting, 1-hour, 2-hour, and 3-hour postload serum glucose samples; two out of four positive values generally establish the diagnosis of gestational diabetes. A diagnosis of gestational diabetes not only impacts the pregnancy, but it also increases the risk of type 2 diabetes in the patient throughout her life. Women diagnosed with gestational diabetes should be screened for type 2 diabetes at 12 weeks' postpartum.

Laboratory Tests at 28 Weeks. At 28 weeks' gestation, repeat RPR, HIV, and hemoglobin/hematocrit tests should be obtained in those at risk. In addition, a patient who is Rh negative should receive Rho(D) immune globulin (RhoGAM) at this time. An Rh-negative patient should also receive RhoGAM at delivery and in any instance of trauma. Nonsensitized, Rh-negative women also should be offered a dose of RhoGAM after spontaneous or induced abortion, ectopic pregnancy termination, CVS, amniocentesis, cordocentesis, external cephalic version, abdominal trauma, and second- or third-trimester bleeding. Administration of RhoGAM can be considered before 12 weeks' gestation in women with a threatened abortion and live embryo, but Rh alloimmunization is rare.

Group B Streptococcus *Screening.* The CDC and ACOG recommend that **all women be offered group B *Streptococcus* (GBS) screening by vaginorectal culture at 35 to 37 weeks' gestation,** and that colonized women be treated with intravenous antibiotics at the time of labor or rupture of membranes in order to reduce the risk of neonatal GBS infection. The **proper method of collection is to swab the lower vagina, perineal area, and rectum.** Of tested women, 10% to 30% will test positive for GBS colonization. Because GBS bacteriuria indicates heavy maternal colonization, women with GBS bacteriuria at any time during their pregnancy should be offered intrapartum antibiotics and do not require a vaginorectal culture. Similarly, women with a previous infant who was diagnosed with a GBS infection should be offered intrapartum antibiotics.

Preterm and Late Term Pregnancies

Birth before 37 weeks' gestation is considered preterm. To decrease the risk of neonatal morbidity and mortality, it is important to distinguish women with a history of preterm delivery and premature rupture of membranes. Women with either of these known risk factors should be given progesterone injections weekly from 16 to 37 weeks' gestation. Women diagnosed with a short cervix have an increased risk of preterm labor. Placing a cervical cerclage may reduce this risk, but current evidence is not definitive.

Late-term pregnancy is from 41 weeks, 0 days to 41 weeks, 6 days. Postterm pregnancy is defined as a pregnancy that has extended beyond 42 weeks or 294 days. Several studies found that induction of labor at 41 weeks reduced the need for cesarean delivery and reduced neonatal mortality and morbidity. Women who deliver postterm are at greater risk for maternal complications such as postpartum hemorrhage, dystocia, and maternal infection.

Vaccinations During Pregnancy

All pregnant women should receive the influenza vaccination at their initial prenatal visit. The influenza vaccine is safe in any stage of pregnancy provided there is no allergy to any of its components. Tetanus toxoid, diphtheria, and acellular pertussis vaccination (Tdap) should be administered between 27 and 36 weeks' gestation of each pregnancy, regardless of prior vaccination status. Varicella, rubella, and the live attenuated intranasal influenza vaccinations are not advised during pregnancy. For pregnant mothers with a rubella nonimmune status, a rubella vaccination should be given after delivery of the infant. During the first prenatal visit, the mother's history of varicella should be documented. Women with a negative varicella history should undergo serologic testing to confirm immunoglobulin G. Those not immunized to varicella should be advised to avoid exposure during pregnancy and should be offered the vaccine postpartum.

> ## CASE CORRELATION
>
> - See also Case 11 (Adult Female Health Maintenance), Case 28 (Family Planning—Contraceptives), and Case 29 (Adolescent Health Maintenance).

COMPREHENSION QUESTIONS

4.1 A 24-year-old woman presents for an initial prenatal visit. She is at 9 weeks' gestation based on her LMP, but on further questioning, she is not certain of the first day of her LMP. Which of the following would be the most accurate estimate of her gestational age?

A. Using her LMP if her uterine size is consistent

B. A first-trimester ultrasound

C. A second-trimester ultrasound

D. A quantitative serum hCG level

4.2 A 38-year-old pregnant woman presents for initial visit at 12 weeks' gestation. She requests a "genetic screen" because she is concerned about her advanced maternal age. She does not want any invasive testing that may cause a potential miscarriage but does want the test that would have the highest detection rate. Which of the following is most appropriate to offer this patient?

A. If no prior personal or family history of genetic defects, no screen is needed.

B. Draw and send blood for the triple or quad screen as patient has advanced maternal age.

C. Nuchal translucency screening and hCG and PAPP-A testing.

D. Offer the patient CVS.

E. Discuss cell-free DNA testing.

4.3 A 28-year-old woman with a history of epilepsy presents to the office for a pre-conception consultation visit. Her seizures are well controlled on medication. Which of the following is the most important advice to give to this patient?

A. Diabetes screening prior to pregnancy.

B. Electroencephalogram (EEG) reading that is normal prior to conception.

C. Preconception folate supplementation.

D. Stop epilepsy medication prior to pregnancy and through the first trimester.

4.4 A 28-year-old gravida 1, para 0 woman at 16 weeks' gestation is noted to be Rh negative. She denies any previous blood transfusion or pregnancy. Which of the following is the most appropriate next step for this patient?

A. Administer RhoGAM at this time.

B. Check the patient's antibody screen (indirect Coombs).

C. Schedule the patient for amniocentesis to assess for isoimmunization.

D. Counsel the patient to terminate the pregnancy.

ANSWERS

4.1 **B.** A first-trimester ultrasound is accurate to within ± 1 week for gestational dating and would be the most accurate assessment of gestational age of the options listed. The further into the pregnancy the ultrasound is performed, the less accurate the gestational dating is; therefore, a second-trimester ultrasound (answer C) would not be as accurate as a first-trimester ultrasound. When LMP is in question (answer A), an ultrasound is a more reliable method of gestational dating. Answer D (quantitative hCG level) does not correlate to the gestational age as accurately, and there is significant overlap among various gestational ages.

4.2 **E.** Cell-free DNA testing (looking for fetal cells within the maternal serum) has the highest sensitivity in detecting a chromosomal abnormality (aneuploidy). For example, the sensitivity in detecting Down syndrome is in the 99% range, trisomy 18 in the 96% range, and trisomy 13 in the 90% range. This modality can be performed from 10 weeks' gestation onward. Answer C (biochemical screening and NT) is performed between 10 and 13 weeks' gestational age; first-trimester trisomy screening may be performed by NT, serum hCG, and PAPP-A; the sensitivity for detecting Down syndrome is about 85% to 90%. CVS (answer D) is more invasive and is not the initial screening of choice. Not performing the screening due to a lack of personal or family history of genetic defects (answer A) would not be appropriate, especially since the patient is requesting screening.

4.3 **C.** Women with a history of epilepsy should receive 1 mg of folic acid sup-plementation daily to help prevent neural tube defects. In general, epilepsy medications should be continued (not stopped, as in answer D), although the type of medication may be changed. For instance, valproic acid has a relatively high rate of neural tube defects associated with its use, and if possible, another medication should be used. Answer A (diabetes screening before pregnancy) is indicated if a patient has significant risk factors or symptoms that are suggestive. Answer B (EEG reading) is not relevant to pregnancy considerations as long as her seizures are under control.

4.4 **B.** For women who are Rh negative, the next step is to assess the antibody screen or indirect Coombs test. Even though this patient is unaware of prior transfusion or miscarriage, there is some risk of the development of alloantibodies (against red blood cell antigens)—for example, an early miscarriage when she did not suspect she was pregnant. If the antibody screen is negative, there is no isoimmunization, and RhoGAM is given at 28 weeks' gestation and again at delivery if the baby is confirmed as Rh positive. The RhoGAM is given to prevent isoimmunization. This patient is at 16 weeks' gestation, so RhoGAM would not be given at this time (answer A). If the antibody screen is positive and the identity of the antibody is confirmed as Rh (anti-D), then assessment of its titer will assist in knowing the probability of fetal effect. A low titer can be observed, whereas a high titer should initiate further testing such as ultrasound and possibly amniocentesis (answer C). Answer D (counseling the patient to terminate the pregnancy) is not appropriate.

CLINICAL PEARLS

▶ The initial prenatal visit often is scheduled after fetal organogenesis has occurred. For this reason, a preconception visit can be very beneficial.

▶ When prescribing medications, clinicians must consider the possibility that any woman of reproductive age may become pregnant.

▶ Genetic counseling should be offered to any woman who *will be* 35 years old or older at her estimated date of confinement (EDD).

▶ Folic acid supplementation is important for every woman, and the recommended daily dose is based on individual risk factors such as anticonvulsant therapy or a previous pregnancy with a neural tube defect.

▶ If all criteria are met, Naegele's rule can be used to determine the EDD (subtract 3 months, add 7 days). If there is any uncertainty, the dating should be confirmed by ultrasound, preferably in the first trimester.

REFERENCES

American College of Obstetricians and Gynecologists Committee on Healthcare for Underserved Women. Oral health care during pregnancy and through the lifespan. Committee opinion no. 569. American College of Obstetricians and Gynecologists. *Obstet Gynecol.* 2013;122:417-422.

Centers for Disease Control and Prevention. Immunization schedules. https://www.cdc.gov/vaccines/schedules. Accessed January 27, 2019.

Committee on Obstetric Practice, the American Institute of Ultrasound in Medicine, and the Society for Maternal-Fetal Medicine. Committee opinion no. 700: methods for estimating the due date. *Obstet Gynecol.* 2017;129(5):e150-e154.

Institute for Clinical Systems Improvement (ICSI). *Health Care Guideline: Routine Prenatal Care.* Bloomington, MN: Institute for Clinical Systems Improvement (ICSI); July 2010.

Kirkham C, Harris S, Grzybowski S. Evidence-based prenatal care: part I. General prenatal care and counseling issues. *Am Fam Physician.* 2005;71(7):1307-1316.

Kirkham C, Harris S, Grzybowski S. Evidence-based prenatal care: part II. Third-trimester care and prevention of infectious diseases. *Am Fam Physician.* 2005;71(8):1555-1560.

National Collaborating Centre for Women's and Children's Health. *Antenatal Care: Routine Care for the Healthy Pregnant Woman.* London, UK: RCOG Press; June 2008.

United States Preventive Services Task Force. Gestational diabetes mellitus, screening. https://www.uspreventiveservicestaskforce.org/uspstf/recommendation/gestational-diabetes-mellitus-screening Accessed January 27, 2019.

Veterans Health Administration, Department of Defense. *DoD/VA Clinical Practice Guidelines for the Management of Uncomplicated Pregnancy, version 2.0.* Washington, DC: Department of Veteran Affairs; 2009.

Wang M. Common questions about late-term postterm pregnancy. *Am Fam Physician.* 2014; 90(3):160-165.

Wapner R, Thom E, Simpson JL, et al. First-trimester screening for trisomies 21 and 18. *N Engl J Med.* 2003;349:1405-1413.

Zolotor A, Carlough MC. Update on prenatal care. *Am Fam Physician.* 2014;89(3):199-208.

CASE 5

A 6-month-old boy is brought to your office by his mother for a routine well-child visit. His mother is concerned that he is not yet saying "mama" because her best friend's baby said "mama" by age 6 months. She also asks when she can place her son in a front-facing car seat. Your patient was born via an uncomplicated pregnancy to a 23-year-old gravida 1, para 1 mother. He was delivered by a spontaneous vaginal delivery at full term, and there were no complications in the neonatal period. You have been following him since his birth. He has had appropriate growth and development up to this age and is up to date on his routine immunizations. He had one upper respiratory infection at age 5 months that was treated symptomatically. There is no family history of any developmental, hearing, or speech disorders. He has been fed since birth with an iron-fortified infant formula. Cereals and other baby foods were added starting at age 4 months. He lives with both parents, neither of whom smokes cigarettes.

On examination, he is a vigorous infant who is at the 50th percentile for length and weight and 75th percentile for head circumference. His physical examination is normal. On developmental examination, he is seen to sit for a short period of time without support, reach out with one hand for your examining light, pick up a Cheerio with a raking grasp and put it in his mouth, and babble frequently.

▶ What immunizations would be recommended at this visit?
▶ By what age should an infant say "mama" and "dada"?
▶ What is your recommendation regarding front-facing versus rear-facing car seats?

ANSWERS TO CASE 5:

Well-Child Care

Summary: A 6-month-old healthy child presents with

- Appropriate growth and development up to this age and up-to-date status on routine immunizations
- History of an upper respiratory infection at age 5 months that was treated symptomatically
- Normal physical examination
- Concerned mother with questions about when child will say "mama" and when he can be in a front-facing car seat

Recommended immunizations: Third dose of diphtheria, tetanus, and acellular pertussis (DTaP); hepatitis B; *Haemophilus influenzae* type b (Hib); pneumococcal conjugate vaccine (PCV13); and rotavirus dose no. 3. The third dose of inactivated polio vaccine (IPV) can be given between ages 6 months and 18 months. If the encounter is during "flu season," annual influenza vaccination is recommended beginning at 6 months of age.

Age by which a child should say "mama" and "dada": Most children will start to say "dada" or "mama" nonspecifically between ages 6 and 9 months. It usually becomes specific between ages 8 and 15 months.

Recommendations for front-facing versus rear-facing car seats: A child should stay in a rear-facing car seat until the child reaches the maximum height and weight limit for the car seat.

ANALYSIS

Objectives

1. List the basic components of a well-child examination. (EPA 1, 12)
2. Know the routine immunization schedule for children. (EPA 12)
3. Know common developmental milestones for young children. (EPA 7, 12)

Considerations

The pediatric well-child examination serves many valuable purposes. It provides an opportunity for parents, especially first-time parents, to ask questions, and for the provider to address specific concerns regarding the child. It allows the clinician to assess the child's growth and development in a systematic fashion and to perform an appropriate physical examination. It also allows for a review of both acute and chronic medical conditions. When performed at recommended time intervals, it gives the opportunity to provide age-appropriate immunizations, screening tests, and anticipatory guidance. Finally, it supports the development of a good provider-patient-family relationship, which can promote health and serve as an effective tool in the management of illnesses.

APPROACH TO:
Well-Child Care

DEFINITIONS

AMBLYOPIA: Monocular childhood vision reduction caused by abnormal vision development. Strabismus is the most common cause of amblyopia.

STRABISMUS: Ocular misalignment.

CLINICAL APPROACH

Pediatric History

For the purposes of routine well-child visits, a comprehensive history should be obtained at the initial visit, with more focused, interval histories obtained at subsequent encounters. The initial history should include an opportunity for the parent to raise any questions or concerns that the parent may have. New parents, especially first-time parents and young parents, often have many questions or anxieties about their child. The ability to discuss them with the provider will help to engender a positive provider-patient-family relationship and improve the parent's satisfaction with their child's care.

Past Medical History. A complete past medical history should be obtained. This should start with a detailed prenatal and pregnancy history, including the duration of the pregnancy, any complications of pregnancy, the type of delivery performed, the child's birth weight, and any neonatal problems. Any significant chronic or acute illnesses should be recorded. The use of any medications, both prescription and over the counter, should be reviewed. Old medical records should be obtained if available. Growth charts, immunization records, results of screening tests, and other valuable information that can assist with the child's assessment can often be found and reduce the unnecessary duplication of previously performed interventions.

Family History. A detailed family history, including information (when available) on both maternal and paternal relatives, should be obtained. A thorough social history is critical in pediatric care; information such as the parents' education levels, relationships, religious beliefs, use of substances (tobacco, alcohol, drugs), and socioeconomic factors can provide significant insight into the health and development of the child.

Growth

At each well-child visit, the child's height and weight should be recorded and plotted on a standard growth chart. Head circumference is measured and plotted in children 3 years of age and younger. Children older than age 3 years should have their blood pressure recorded using an appropriate-size pediatric cuff. Significant variances from accepted, age-adjusted, population norms or predicted growth curves may warrant further evaluation. The Centers for Disease Control and Prevention (CDC) and the American Academy of Pediatrics (AAP) recommend

Table 5–1 • BMI CLASSIFICATIONS IN CHILDREN	
Definition	BMI
Obese	> 95th percentile
Overweight	85th-95th percentile
Healthy body weight	5th-85th percentile
Underweight	< 5th percentile

measuring body mass index (BMI) to screen for overweight and obese states in children age 2 years and older. The measurement of BMI in children is calculated the same way it is for adults, and it is compared to typical values for other children of the same age. Weight classifications based on BMI in children are listed in Table 5–1.

Failure to thrive is defined by some as weight below the third or fifth percentile for age and by others as decelerations of growth that have crossed two major growth percentiles in a short period of time. Either significant loss or gain of weight may prompt an in-depth discussion of nutrition and caloric intake.

Development

An assessment of the child's development in the areas of **gross motor, fine motor/ adaptive, language, and social/personal** skills is an important aspect of each well-child visit. Numerous screening tools, such as the Denver II developmental screening test, the Parents' Evaluations of Developmental Status (PEDS), and others, are available to assist with these assessments. These assessments typically involve both responses from the parents regarding the child's behavior at home and observations of the child in the office setting. Persistent delays in development, either globally or in individual skill areas, should prompt a more in-depth developmental assessment, as early intervention may effectively aid in the management of some developmental abnormalities.

Bilingual Children. Children who are raised in a bilingual environment may have some language "mixing" at first (eg, saying some words in English and some in Spanish in the same sentence). This tends to improve over time, and proficiency in both languages is often reached by age 5. The threshold for referral to a specialist should be the same for bilingual children as monolingual children. Table 5–2 summarizes many of the important motor, language, and social developmental milestones of early childhood.

Screening Tests

A variety of screening tests are used to prevent disease and promote proper developmental and physical growth. These include tests for congenital diseases, lead screening, evaluating children for anemia, and hearing and vision screens.

Newborn Screening. Each state requires screening of all newborns for specified congenital diseases; however, the specific diseases for which screening is done vary from state to state. **All states require testing for phenylketonuria (PKU) and congenital hypothyroidism,** as early treatment can prevent the development of profound

Table 5–2 • DEVELOPMENTAL MILESTONES

Age	Motor	Language	Social	Mnemonics
1 mo	Reacts to pain	Responds to noise	Regards human face Establishes eye contact	
2 mo	Eyes follow object to midline Head up prone	Vocalizes	Social smile Recognizes parent	
4 mo	Eyes follow object past midline Rolls over	Laughs and squeals	Regards hand	
6 mo	Sits well unsupported Transfers objects hand to hand (switches hands) Rolls prone to supine	Babbles	Recognizes strangers	Six strangers switch sitting at 6 mo
9 mo	Crawls Cruises (walks holding furniture) Pincer grasp (10 mo)	Says "mama," "dada," and "bye-bye"	Starts to explore	Can crawl and therefore explore It takes 9 mo to be a "mama"
12 mo	Walks Throws object	1-3 words Follows 1-step commands	Stranger and separation anxiety	Knows 1 word at 1 y
2 y	Walks up and down stairs Copies a line Runs Kicks ball	2- to 3-word phrases Half of speech is understood by strangers Refers to self by name Pronouns	Parallel play	Puts 2 words together at 2 At age 2, 2/4 (1/2) of speech understood by strangers
3 y	Copies a circle Pedals a tricycle Can build a bridge of 3 cubes Repeats 3 numbers	Speaks in sentences Three-fourths of speech is understood by strangers Recognizes 3 colors	Group play Plays simple games Knows gender Knows first and last name	Tricycle, 3 cubes, 3 numbers, 3 colors, 3 kids make a group At age 3, 3/4 of speech understood by strangers
4 y	Identifies body parts Copies a cross Copies a square (4½ y) Hops on one foot Throws overhand	Speech is completely understood by strangers Uses past tense to speak of things that happened before Tells a story	Plays with kids, social interaction	Song "head, shoulder, knees, and toes," 4 parts reminds you that at age 4 can identify body parts At age 4, 4/4 of speech is understood by strangers

(Continued)

Age	Motor	Language	Social	Mnemonics
				A 4-year-old can copy 2 lines to draw a cross and a square, which has 4 sides
5 y	Copies a triangle Catches a ball Partially dresses self	Writes name Counts 10 objects		
6 y	Draws a person with 6 parts Ties shoes Skips with alternating feet	Identifies left and right		Skips, shoes, person with parts

Table 5–2 • DEVELOPMENTAL MILESTONES (continued)

Modified with permission, from Hay WW, Hayword AR, Levin MJ, Sondheimer JM. Current Pediatric Diagnosis and Treatment. 17th ed. 2005. Copyright © McGraw Hill LLC. All rights reserved.

intellectual disability. Diseases for which testing commonly occurs include hemoglobinopathies (including sickle cell disease), galactosemia, and other inborn errors of metabolism. This screening is done by collecting blood from newborns prior to discharge from the hospital. In some states, newborn screening is repeated at the first routine well visit, usually at about 2 weeks of age.

Lead Poisoning Screening. Nationwide, the prevalence of childhood lead poisoning has declined, primarily because of the use of unleaded gasoline and lead-free paints. However, in some communities, the risk of lead exposure is higher. The AAP's Bright Futures program recommends screening all children between the ages of 6 months and 6 years for their risk of elevated blood lead levels. Those children identified as having a high risk based upon answers to a questionnaire should have blood testing (Table 5–3). Consideration should be given to test all children, regardless of risk, with blood testing at age 12 and 24 months. All children born outside of the United States should have a blood level measured on arrival to the United States.

Anemia Screening. Iron deficiency is the most common cause of anemia in children. Iron-containing formula and cereals have helped to reduce the occurrence of iron deficiency. Children at higher risk include those who drink more than 24 oz of cow's milk, have iron-restricted diets, were low birth weight or preterm, or whose mother was iron deficient. In 2010, the AAP recommended universal screening for anemia in all children at 1 year of age. Additional laboratory screening for iron deficiency is recommended at later ages in those children at high risk for iron-deficiency anemia. The American Academy of Family Physicians (AAFP) and the US Preventive Services Task Force (USPSTF) found insufficient evidence to recommend for or against screening asymptomatic children for anemia. An anemic child can empirically be given a trial of an iron supplement and dietary modification.

Table 5–3 • ELEMENTS OF A LEAD RISK QUESTIONNAIRE
Recommended questions
• Does your child live in or regularly visit a house built before 1950? This could include a day care center, preschool, the home of a babysitter or relative, and so on.
• Does your child live in or regularly visit a house built before 1978 with recent, ongoing, or planned renovation or remodeling?
• Does your child have a sister or brother, housemate, or playmate who is being followed for lead poisoning?
Questions that may be considered by region or locality
• Does your child live with an adult whose job (eg, at a brass/copper foundry, firing range, automotive or boat repair shop, or furniture-refinishing shop) or hobby (eg, electronics, fishing, stained-glass making, pottery making) involves exposure to lead?
• Does your child live near a work or industrial site (eg, smelter, battery recycling plant) that involves the use of lead?
• Does your child use pottery or ingest medications that are suspected of having a high lead content?
• Does your child have exposure to burning lead-painted wood?

Failure to respond to iron therapy should warrant further evaluation of other causes of anemia.

Hearing Screening. Most states now mandate newborn hearing screening by auditory brainstem response or evoked otoacoustic emission. All high-risk infants, regardless of requirement, should be screened. High-risk infants include those with a family history of childhood hearing loss, craniofacial abnormalities, syndromes associated with hearing loss (eg, neurofibromatosis), or infections associated with hearing loss (eg, bacterial meningitis). Older infants and toddlers can be assessed for hearing problems by questioning the parents or performing office testing by snapping fingers or by using rattles or other noisemakers. Office-based audiometry should be performed in children aged 4 years and older. Any hearing loss should be promptly evaluated and referred for early intervention, if necessary.

Vision Screening. Vision screening can also start in the newborn nursery. Evaluation of the neonate for red reflexes on ophthalmoscopy should be a standard part of the newborn examination. The presence of red reflexes helps to rule out the possibility of congenital cataracts and retinoblastoma. The evaluation of an older infant should include a subjective evaluation of the child's vision by the parent. Infants should be able to focus on a face by age 1 month and should move their eyes consistently and symmetrically by age 6 months. An examining light should reflect symmetrically off of both corneas; asymmetric light reflex may be a sign of strabismus. The cover-uncover test also is a screening examination for strabismus. The child focuses on an object with both eyes and the examiner covers one eye. Strabismus is suggested when the uncovered eye deviates to focus on the object. **Strabismus should be referred to a pediatric ophthalmologist as soon as it is detected,** as early intervention results in a lower incidence of amblyopia. After the age of

Table 5–4 • FIRST-TIME LIPID-SCREENING RECOMMENDATIONS
Perform first-time lipid screening in children ages 2-10 years if
• Family history of dyslipidemia
• Family history of premature (men < 55 y or women < 65 y) cardiovascular disease or dyslipidemia
• Parent with total cholesterol ≥ 240 mg/dL
• Patient with other cardiovascular risk factors:
• Overweight (BMI > 85th percentile and < 95th percentile)
• Obese (BMI > 95th percentile)
• Hypertension (blood pressure > 95th percentile)
• Cigarette smoking
• Diabetes mellitus

Data from Expert Panel on Integrated Guidelines for Cardiovascular Health and Risk Reduction in Children and Adolescents. National Heart, Lung, and Blood Institute, 2011. Available at: https://www.nhlbi.nih.gov/files/docs/peds_guidelines_sum.pdf.

3 years, most children can be tested for visual acuity using a Snellen chart, modified with a "tumbling E" or pictures instead of letters.

Other Screening Tests. Other screening tests may be recommended for high-risk children. Tuberculosis (TB) screening is recommended for children who were born or live in a region of high TB prevalence or who have close contact with someone known to have TB. The Mantoux test (an intradermal injection of PPD [purified protein derivative] tuberculin) is the screening test of choice. In accordance with the National Heart, Lung, and Blood Institute (NHLBI), the American Heart Association (AHA) and AAP recommend universal screening of high cholesterol for all children at least one time between the ages of 9 and 11 years and again between 17 and 21 years. Screening for hyperlipidemia should begin at age 2 in children with a family history of hyperlipidemia, premature cardiovascular disease, or other risk factors (see Table 5–4).

Dental Care. Early childhood caries are one of the most prevalent chronic conditions during childhood; therefore, it is important to discuss good oral hygiene and the establishment of a dental home during well-child visits. At the 4-month visit, sources of systemic fluoride should be assessed. One of the most effective tools to prevent teeth decay is systemic fluoride. If there are concerns with the amount of fluoride in drinking water supplies, especially well water, appropriate testing should be performed. At 6 months of age, infants should begin to receive appropriate topical (fluoride toothpaste) and systemic fluoride. By the 12-month visit, each appointment should include a complete dental screening during the physical examination and reassurance that the child has a regular source of dental care. The American Academy of Pediatric Dentistry recommends that all children see a dentist by the age of 12 months.

Anticipatory Guidance

A primary feature of the well-child visit should be education of the patient and family on issues that promote health and prevent illness, injury, or death. This anticipatory guidance should be focused and age appropriate. The use of pre-printed handouts can reinforce topics discussed in the office, address issues that could not be discussed because of time limitations, and allow for the parent to review the information as needed at home. Subjects that should routinely be addressed include injury prevention, nutrition, development, discipline, exercise, mental health issues, and the need for ongoing care (eg, immunization schedules, future well-child visits, dental care). During the well-child examination, it is important to evaluate how much time is spent watching television, using the computer, and playing video games. Screen time should be limited to 1 to 2 hours or fewer daily. The number of hours and quality of sleep should be asked at each visit. Abnormalities in sleep should be further investigated and managed appropriately.

Car Seat Recommendations. **Accidents and injuries are the leading cause of death in children older than age 1 year.** Accidents involving motor vehicles, both traffic and pedestrian accidents, are the leading cause of these accidental deaths. All states now require the use of car safety seats for children, although the regulations vary from state to state. The general recommendation is that a child should be in the back seat of the vehicle whenever possible. If there is no back seat, the child should only ride in the front seat if there is no air bag or if the air bag can be disabled.

A child should sit in a rear-facing car seat as long as possible, until the child has reached the maximum height or weight limit of the rear-facing seat. The child should then be transitioned to a forward-facing car seat. When the child reaches the weight limit for the forward-facing car seat, they should ride in a booster-type seat along with the lap and shoulder seatbelts. The child can stop using the booster when the child can sit with his or her back squarely against the back of the seat with the legs bent at the knees over the front of the seat. The child usually will need to be at least 4 feet, 9 inches. tall and 8 to 12 years of age to meet these requirements. No child should ride in the front seat unless they are 13 years of age or older and meet height and weight requirements.

Sudden Infant Death Syndrome Prevention. According to the CDC, the top three causes of death in infants younger than 1 year old are congenital abnormalities, short gestation, and **sudden infant death syndrome** (SIDS). The "Back to Sleep" campaign advises parents to place their infant on the infant's back—not abdomen or side—when the infant is put down to sleep, as this reduces the risk of dying of SIDS. In addition, the infant should be placed on a firm mattress with nothing else in the crib—this includes pillows, positioning devices, and toys. Heavy coverings and soft mattresses have been associated with an increased risk of SIDS.

Safety in the Home. As children get older, anticipatory guidance on other safety issues become important. As children learn to crawl and walk, stairwells should be blocked to reduce the risk of injuries from falling. Cleaning supplies, medications, and other potential poisons need to be stored safely out of reach of children, preferably in locked cabinets. Similarly, firearms should be stored safely, preferably unloaded and in locked cabinets or safes. Parents should be counseled on keeping matches and lighters in a safe place out of the reach of children. All families should be advised to have smoke detectors throughout the home, especially in rooms where people sleep, and to keep the hot water heater set at or below 120 °F to reduce the risk of scald injuries. The AAFP recommends that all caregivers be trained in cardiopulmonary resuscitation. When a pool or hot tub

Table 1 Recommended Child and Adolescent Immunization Schedule for ages 18 years or younger United States, 2019

These recommendations must be read with the Notes that follow. For those who fall behind or start late, provide catch-up vaccination at the earliest opportunity as indicated by the dark gray bars in Table 1. To determine minimum intervals between doses, see the catch-up schedule (Table 2). School entry and adolescent vaccine age groups are marked with a star.

Vaccine	Birth	1 mo	2 mos	4 mos	6 mos	9 mos	12 mos	15 mos	18 mos	19-23 mos	2-3 yrs	4-6 yrs	7-10 yrs	11-12 yrs	13-15 yrs	16 yrs	17-18 yrs
Hepatitis B (HepB)	1st dose	2nd dose			←——— 3rd dose ———→												
Rotavirus (RV) RV1 (2-dose series); RV5 (3-dose series)			1st dose	2nd dose	See Notes												
Diphtheria, tetanus, & acellular pertussis (DTaP: <7 yrs)			1st dose	2nd dose	3rd dose		←——— 4th dose ———→					5th dose					
Haemophilus influenzae type b (Hib)			1st dose	2nd dose	See Notes		3rd or 4th dose, See Notes										
Pneumococcal conjugate (PCV13)			1st dose	2nd dose	3rd dose		←——— 4th dose ———→										
Inactivated poliovirus (IPV: <18 yrs)			1st dose	2nd dose	←——————— 3rd dose ———————→							4th dose					
Influenza (IIV)							Annual vaccination 1 or 2 doses							Annual vaccination 1 dose only			
Influenza (LAIV)											Annual vaccination 1 or 2 doses			Annual vaccination 1 dose only			
Measles, mumps, rubella (MMR)					See Notes		←——— 1st dose ———→					2nd dose					
Varicella (VAR)							←——— 1st dose ———→					2nd dose					
Hepatitis A (HepA)					See Notes		2-dose series, See Notes										
Meningococcal (MenACWY-D ≥9 mos; MenACWY-CRM ≥2 mos)							See Notes							1st dose		2nd dose	
Tetanus, diphtheria, & acellular pertussis (Tdap: ≥7 yrs)														Tdap			
Human papillomavirus (HPV)														See Notes			
Meningococcal B															See Notes		
Pneumococcal polysaccharide (PPSV23)														See Notes			

Range of recommended ages for all children
Range of recommended ages for catch-up immunization
Range of recommended ages for certain high-risk groups
Range of recommended ages for non-risk groups that may receive vaccine, subject to individual clinical decision-making
No recommendation

02/22/19

Centers for Disease Control and Prevention | Recommended Child and Adolescent Immunization Schedule, United States, 2019 | Page 2

Figure 5–1. Recommended immunization schedule for persons aged 0 through 18 years—United States, 2019. (Reproduced with permission, from Recommended Child and Adolescent Immunization Schedule for Ages 18 Years or Younger, United States, 2020. Copyright © Centers for Disease Control and Prevention (CDC). 2020. Available at http://www.cdc.gov/vaccines/schedules/downloads/child/0-18yrs-child-combined-schedule.pdf.)

Table 2 Catch-up immunization schedule for persons aged 4 months—18 years who start late or who are more than 1 month behind, United States, 2019

The figure below provides catch-up schedules and minimum intervals between doses for children whose vaccinations have been delayed. A vaccine series does not need to be restarted, regardless of the time that has elapsed between doses. Use the section appropriate for the child's age. Always use this table in conjunction with Table 1 and the notes that follow.

Children age 4 months through 6 years

Vaccine	Minimum Age for Dose 1	Dose 1 to Dose 2	Dose 2 to Dose 3	Dose 3 to Dose 4	Dose 4 to Dose 5
Hepatitis B	Birth	4 weeks	8 weeks and at least 16 weeks after first dose. Minimum age for the final dose is 24 weeks.		
Rotavirus	6 weeks Maximum age for first dose is 14 weeks, 6 days.	4 weeks	4 weeks Maximum age for final dose is 8 months, 0 days.		
Diphtheria, tetanus, and acellular pertussis	6 weeks	4 weeks	4 weeks	6 months	6 months
Haemophilus influenzae type b	6 weeks	No further doses needed if first dose was administered at age 15 months or older. **4 weeks** if first dose was administered before the 1st birthday. **8 weeks (as final dose)** if first dose was administered at age 12 through 14 months.	No further doses needed if previous dose was administered at age 15 months or older. **4 weeks** if current age is younger than 12 months and first dose was administered at younger than age 7 months, and at least 1 previous dose was PRP-T (ActHib, Pentacel, Hiberix) or unknown. **8 weeks and age 12 through 59 months (as final dose)** if current age is younger than 12 months and first dose was administered at age 7 through 11 months; OR if current age is 12 through 59 months and first dose was administered before the 1st birthday, and second dose administered at younger than age 15 months; OR if both doses were PRP-OMP (PedvaxHIB, Comvax) and were administered before the 1st birthday.	**8 weeks (as final dose)** This dose only necessary for children age 12 through 59 months who received 3 doses before the 1st birthday.	
Pneumococcal conjugate	6 weeks	No further doses needed for healthy children if first dose was administered at age 24 months or older. **4 weeks** if first dose administered before the 1st birthday. **8 weeks (as final dose for healthy children)** if first dose was administered at the 1st birthday or after.	No further doses needed for healthy children if previous dose administered at age 24 months or older. **4 weeks** if current age is younger than 12 months and previous dose given at <7 months old; **8 weeks (as final dose for healthy children)** if previous dose given between 7-11 months (wait until at least 12 months old); OR if current age is 12 months or older and at least 1 dose was given before age 12 months.	**8 weeks (as final dose)** This dose only necessary for children age 12 through 59 months who received 3 doses before age 12 months or for children at high risk who received 3 doses at any age.	
Inactivated poliovirus	6 weeks	4 weeks	4 weeks if current age is < 4 years. 6 months (as final dose) if current age is 4 years or older.	6 months (minimum age 4 years for final dose).	
Measles, mumps, rubella	12 months	4 weeks			
Varicella	12 months	3 months			
Hepatitis A	12 months	6 months			
Meningococcal	2 months MenACWY-CRM 9 months MenACWY-D	8 weeks	See Notes	See Notes	

Children and adolescents age 7 through 18 years

Vaccine	Minimum Age for Dose 1	Dose 1 to Dose 2	Dose 2 to Dose 3	Dose 3 to Dose 4	Dose 4 to Dose 5
Meningococcal	Not Applicable (N/A)	8 weeks			
Tetanus, diphtheria, tetanus, diphtheria, and acellular pertussis	7 years	4 weeks	**4 weeks** if first dose of DTaP/DT was administered before the 1st birthday. **6 months (as final dose)** if first dose of DTaP/DT or Tdap/Td was administered at or after the 1st birthday.	**6 months** if first dose of DTaP/DT was administered before the 1st birthday. DT was administered before the 1st birthday.	
Human papillomavirus	9 years	Routine dosing intervals are recommended.			
Hepatitis A	N/A	6 months			
Hepatitis B	N/A	4 weeks	8 weeks and at least 16 weeks after first dose.		
Inactivated poliovirus	N/A	4 weeks	6 months A fourth dose is not necessary if the third dose was administered at age 4 years or older and at least 6 months after the previous dose.	A fourth dose of IPV is indicated if all previous doses were administered at <4 years or if the third dose was administered <6 months after the second dose.	
Measles, mumps, rubella	N/A	4 weeks			
Varicella	N/A	3 months if younger than age 13 years. 4 weeks if age 13 years or older.			

02/22/19

Figure 5–1. (Continued)

is accessible to children, a nearby telephone with emergency contacts should be at the poolside. All children under the age of 4 should have supervision within arm's length at all times.

Older children should be advised regarding the importance of wearing a helmet while riding a bicycle, skateboard, scooter, or other similar vehicle. The National Highway Traffic Safety Administration recommends that, in addition to helmets, bicyclists should wear clothing that is bright and reflective, ride with the flow of traffic, and obey all traffic laws.

Nutrition. Nutrition is another important area of anticipatory guidance. Infants younger than 1 year old should be breastfed or receive an iron-containing formula. Cereals, other baby foods, and water can be introduced between 4 and 6 months of age. Whole cow's milk is introduced at 12 months and continued until at least the age of 2 years, before considering changing to reduced fat milk.

Immunizations

Ensuring that each child has received age-appropriate immunizations is a key component of each well-child visit. The child's immunization status also should be reviewed at acute care visits. Minor illnesses, even those causing low-grade fevers, are not contraindications to vaccinating children, allowing an acute care visit to be an excellent opportunity to provide this service. **True contraindications to providing a vaccination include a history of an anaphylactic reaction to a specific vaccine or vaccine component or a severe illness,** with or without a fever. The recommended childhood vaccination schedule (Figure 5–1) and catch-up schedules for children who are either completely unimmunized or who have missed doses of the recommended vaccines are published by the CDC.

CASE CORRELATION

- See also Case 4 (Prenatal Care) and Case 26 (Postpartum Care).

COMPREHENSION QUESTIONS

5.1 A 7-month-old baby boy is brought into the office for a possible ear infection. When assessing the infant's posture, you note that he is not able to sit very well without support. You observe other fine motor skills and speech. Which of the following is the most accurate statement?

A. By 3 months of age, a child should be able to sit up without support.

B. By 6 months of age, a child should be able to transfer objects from one hand to another.

C. By 9 months of age, a child should be able to walk.

D. By 12 months of age, a child should be able to put two words together.

5.2 A 4-month-old infant is brought into the primary care provider's office for routine checkup and immunizations. Which of the following vaccines is routinely recommended at this time?

    A. Diphtheria, tetanus, acellular pertussis (DTaP)

    B. Oral polio vaccine (OPV)

    C. Measles, mumps, rubella (MMR)

    D. Varicella

5.3 A 5-year-old child is brought into the pediatrician's office for immunization and physical examination. The mother is concerned that her child is a little "under the weather." Which of the following is a contraindication to vaccinating the child?

    A. Acute otitis media with a temperature of 100 °F requiring antibiotic therapy

    B. Previous vaccination reaction that consisted of fever and fussiness that lasted for 2 days

    C. History of an allergic reaction to penicillin

    D. Previous vaccination reaction that consisted of wheezing and hypotension

ANSWERS

5.1 **B.** It is critical to understand the normal milestones for gross motor, fine motor, speech, and social categories. Delay in one or more areas can indicate problems that, if addressed, can alleviate long-term issues. Most 6-month-old children would be expected to sit without support (not 3-month-olds, as in answer A). Six-month-old children would also be expected to transfer objects from one hand to the other, roll from a prone to supine position, babble, and recognize strangers. Children should begin to walk (answer C) at 12 months and put two words together (answer D) at 2 years of age.

5.2 **A.** DTaP is routinely recommended at ages 2, 4, 6, and 12 to 18 months and at 4 to 6 years of age. Oral polio vaccination (answer B) is no longer routinely recommended in children; the inactivated, injectable polio vaccine is recommended in its place and is recommended at ages 2, 4, 6 to 18 months and 4 to 6 years. The MMR (answer C) and varicella (answer D) vaccinations are recommended at ages 12 to 15 months and 4 to 6 years.

5.3 **D.** A previous anaphylactic reaction is a true contraindication to vaccination. Minor illnesses (answer A) or vaccination reactions (answer B), even with fever, are not contraindications. Penicillin is not a component of vaccines and history of allergy to this medication is not a contraindication (answer C).

CLINICAL PEARLS

▶ True contraindications to providing vaccinations are rare; acute care visits are an excellent opportunity to provide childhood vaccinations.

▶ SIDS is the leading cause of death in infants younger than age 1 year. Parents should place their children on their "Back to Sleep."

▶ A variety of screening tests are used in childhood, including tests for congenital diseases, lead screening, evaluating children for anemia, and hearing and vision screens.

▶ At each well-child visit, the child's height and weight should be recorded and plotted on a standard growth chart. Head circumference is measured and plotted in children 3 years of age and younger.

▶ A comprehensive history for a pediatric patient includes prenatal and pregnancy history, past medical history of the patient, and a detailed family history.

REFERENCES

Bright Futures/American Academy of Pediatrics. Recommendations for preventive pediatric health care, 2017. https://www.aap.org/en-us/professional-resources/practice-support/Periodicity/Periodicity%20Schedule_FINAL.pdf. Accessed November 10, 2018.

Centers for Disease Control and Prevention. Vaccines and immunizations. http://www.cdc.gov/vaccines/. Accessed May 27, 2019.

Douglass JM, Douglass AB, Silk HJ. A practical guide to infant oral health. *Am Fam Physician*. 2004;70(11):2113-2120.

Durbin DR for the AAP Council on Injury, Violence and Poison Prevention. American Academy of Pediatrics policy statement: child passenger safety. *Pediatrics*. 2018;142(5):e20182461. doi:10.1542/PEDS.2018-2461

Turner K. Well-child visits for infants and young children. *Am Fam Physician*. 2018;98(6):347-353.

Warniment C, Tsang K, Galazka SS. Lead poisoning in children. *Am Fam Physician*. 2010;81(6):751-757.

A 35-year-old woman with a history of asthma presents to your office with symptoms of nasal itching, sneezing, and rhinorrhea. She states she feels this way most days, but her symptoms are worse in the spring and fall. She has had difficulty sleeping because she is always congested. She states she has taken diphenhydramine (Benadryl) with no relief. She does not smoke cigarettes and does not have exposure to passive smoke, but she does have two cats at home. On examination, she appears tired but is in no respiratory distress. Her vital signs are as follows: temperature 98.8 °F, blood pressure 128/84 mm Hg, pulse 88 beats/min, and respiratory rate 18 breaths/min. The mucosa of her nasal turbinates appears swollen (boggy) and has a pale, bluish-gray color. Thin and watery secretions are seen. No abnormalities are seen on ear examination. There is no cervical lymphadenopathy noted, and her lungs are clear.

▶ What is the most likely diagnosis?
▶ What is your next step?
▶ What are important considerations and potential complications of management?

ANSWERS TO CASE 6:

Allergic Disorders, Anaphylaxis, and Conjunctivitis

Summary: A 35-year-old woman presents with

- A history of asthma
- Complaint of chronic nasal congestion that is worse in the spring and the fall
- No exposure to cigarette smoke but does have two cats
- Normal vital signs
- Mucosa of nasal turbinates that is swollen (boggy) and has a pale, bluish-gray color
- Thin, watery secretions

Most likely diagnosis: Allergic rhinitis.

Next step: Treatment with antihistamines, decongestants, or intranasal steroids. These treatments can also be used in combination with each other. First-line treatment is intranasal corticosteroids for mild-to-moderate disease. With moderate-to-severe allergic rhinitis, antihistamines and decongestants should be added.

Considerations and possible complications of management: Recognition and reduction of potential allergen exposure will yield more success in management than pharmacotherapy alone. Excessive use of topical decongestants can cause rebound congestion.

ANALYSIS

Objectives

1. Understand the inflammatory nature of allergic rhinitis. (EPA 1, 2)
2. Recognize physical examination findings consistent with allergic rhinitis. (EPA 1)
3. Develop an approach to the management of allergic rhinitis, including the roles of pharmacotherapy and reduction of allergen exposure. (EPA 4)
4. Recognition and management of asthma. (EPA 4, 10)
5. Identification of essential features and treatment of anaphylaxis. (EPA 1, 4, 10)

Considerations

This patient presents with a classic history of allergic rhinitis. Her history of itchy eyes, nasal congestion and discharge, and seasonal nature (worse in spring and fall) are all consistent with allergic rhinitis. Her examination is also consistent with the diagnosis. The best therapy for this condition is avoidance of allergens, but due to the probable allergy to pollen, this can be very difficult. Nasal corticosteroids offer the most consistent symptomatic relief.

APPROACH TO:

Allergic Disorders, Anaphylaxis, and Conjunctivitis

DEFINITIONS

ALLERGIC RHINITIS: Inflammation of the nasal passages caused by immuno-globulin (Ig) E–mediated response to airborne substances.

ANAPHYLAXIS: Rapidly progressing, life-threatening allergic reaction, mediated by an IgE immediate hypersensitivity reaction.

CLINICAL APPROACH TO ALLERGIC DISORDERS

Epidemiology

Rhinitis is inflammation of the nasal membranes and is characterized by any combination of the following: sneezing, nasal congestion, nasal itching, obstruction, pruritus, and rhinorrhea. The eyes, ears, sinuses, and throat can also be involved. Allergic rhinitis is the most common cause of rhinitis, occurring in up to 30% of adults and 40% of children.

Pathophysiology

Allergic rhinitis involves inflammation of the mucous membranes of the nose, eyes, eustachian tubes, middle ear, sinuses, and pharynx. Inflammation of the mucous membranes is characterized by a complex interaction of inflammatory mediators but, ultimately, is triggered by an IgE-mediated response to an extrinsic protein.

IgE Production. In susceptible individuals, exposure to certain foreign proteins leads to allergic sensitization, which is characterized by the production of specific IgE directed against these proteins. This specific IgE coats the surface of mast cells, which are present in the nasal mucosa. When the specific allergen is inhaled into the nose, it can bind to the IgE in the mast cells, leading to the delayed release of a number of mediators.

Mediators. Mediators that are immediately released include histamine, tryptase, chymase, and kinase. Mast cells quickly synthesize other mediators, including leukotrienes and prostaglandin D_2. Symptoms can occur quickly after exposure. Mucus glands are also stimulated, leading to increased secretions. In response to increased inflammatory response, vasodilation occurs, causing congestion. Stimulation of sensory nerves leads to sneezing and itching. Other symptoms include the redness and tearing of eyes, postnasal drip, and ear pressure.

Over the next 4 to 8 hours, these mediators, through a complex interplay of events, recruit neutrophils, eosinophils, lymphocytes, and macrophages to the mucosa. These inflammatory cells cause more congestion and mucus production that may persist for hours or days. Systemic effects, including fatigue, sleepiness, and malaise, can result from the inflammatory response as well.

History. Obtaining a detailed history is important in the evaluation of allergic rhinitis, as specific triggers may be identified. Evaluation should include the nature, duration, and time course of symptoms. The recent use of medications is another important consideration, as are a family history of allergic diseases, environmental exposures, and comorbid conditions.

Part of the history should include the time pattern of symptoms and whether symptoms occur at a consistent level throughout the year (**perennial rhinitis**), only occur in specific seasons (**seasonal rhinitis**), a combination of the two, or in relation to a workplace (**occupational rhinitis**). Trigger factors such as exposure to pollens, mold spores, specific animals, or cleaning of the house can sometimes be identified. Irritant triggers such as smoke, pollution, and strong smells can aggravate symptoms of allergic rhinitis. Response to treatment with antihistamines supports the diagnosis of allergic rhinitis.

Causes of Allergic Rhinitis

The causes of allergic rhinitis can differ depending on whether the symptoms are seasonal, perennial, or sporadic/episodic. Some patients are sensitive to multiple allergens and can have perennial allergic rhinitis with seasonal exacerbations. Although food allergy can cause rhinitis, particularly in children, it is rarely a cause of allergic rhinitis in the absence of gastrointestinal or skin symptoms. Seasonal allergic rhinitis is commonly caused by allergy to seasonal pollens and outdoor molds.

Pollens (Tree, Grass, and Weed). Tree pollens, which vary by geographic location, are typically present in high counts during the spring, although some species produce their pollens in the fall. Grass pollens also vary by geographic location. Most of the common grass species are associated with allergic rhinitis. A number of these grasses are cross-reactive, meaning that they have similar antigenic structures (ie, proteins recognized by specific IgE in allergic sensitization). Consequently, a person who is allergic to one species is also likely to be sensitive to a number of other species. The grass pollens are most prominent from the late spring through the fall, but they can be present year-round in warmer climates.

Weed pollens also vary geographically. Many weeds (eg, short ragweed, a common cause of allergic rhinitis in much of the United States) are most prominent in the late summer and fall. Other weed pollens are present year-round, particularly in warmer climates.

Perennial allergic rhinitis is typically caused by allergens within the home, but it can also be caused by outdoor allergens that are present year-round. In warmer climates, grass pollens can be present throughout the year. In some climates, individuals may be symptomatic because of trees and grasses in the warmer months and molds and weeds in the winter.

House Dust Mites. In the United States, two major house dust mite species are associated with allergic rhinitis. These mites feed on organic material in households, particularly the skin that is shed from humans and pets. They can be found in carpets, upholstered furniture, pillows, mattresses, comforters, and stuffed toys. Exposure can be reduced by methods such as carpet removal; however, current studies have not found any benefit to using mite-proof mattresses or pillow covers.

Animals. Allergy to indoor pets is a common cause of perennial allergic rhinitis. Cat and dog allergies are encountered most commonly in clinical practice. However, allergies have been reported to occur with most of the furry animals and birds that are kept as indoor pets. Although cockroach allergy is most frequently considered to be a cause of asthma, particularly in the inner city, it can also cause perennial allergic rhinitis in infested households. Rodent infestation may also be associated with allergic sensitization.

Clinical Presentation

Symptoms that can be associated with **allergic rhinitis include sneezing, itching (of nose, eyes, or ears), rhinorrhea, postnasal drip, congestion, anosmia, headache, earache, tearing, red eyes, and drowsiness.** Common findings on examination include "allergic shiners," which are dark circles around the eyes related to vasodilation or nasal congestion. The "nasal crease" can be seen in some cases. It is a horizontal crease across the lower half of the bridge of the nose caused by repeated upward rubbing of the tip of the nose by the palm of the hand ("allergic salute").

Nose Examination. Examination of the nose may reveal **mucosa of the nasal turbinates to be swollen (boggy) and of a pale, bluish-gray color.** Assessment of the character and quantity of nasal mucus may be helpful in ascertaining a diagnosis. Thin and watery secretions are frequently associated with allergic rhinitis, whereas thick and purulent secretions are usually associated with sinusitis. The characteristic of the mucus is not always diagnostic, as thick, purulent, colored mucus can also occur with allergic rhinitis.

The nasal cavity should be inspected for growths such as polyps or tumors. Polyps are firm, gray masses that are often attached by a stalk, which may not be visible. After spraying a topical decongestant, polyps do not shrink, whereas the surrounding nasal mucosa does shrink. Examine the nasal septum to look for any deviation or septal perforation that may be present as a consequence of chronic rhinitis, granulomatous disease, cocaine abuse, prior surgery, topical decongestant abuse, or rarely, topical steroid overuse.

Otoscopy. Otoscopy should be performed to look for tympanic membrane retraction, air-fluid levels, or bubbles. Performing pneumatic otoscopy can be considered to look for abnormal tympanic membrane mobility. These findings can be associated with allergic rhinitis, particularly if eustachian tube dysfunction or secondary otitis media is present. Ocular examination may reveal findings of injection and swelling of the palpebral conjunctivae, with excess tear production. Dennie-Morgan lines (prominent creases below the inferior eyelid) are associated with allergic rhinitis.

Throat and Respiratory Examination. "Cobblestoning" of the posterior pharynx is often observed. This is caused by the presence of streaks of lymphoid tissue on the posterior pharynx. Tonsillar hypertrophy can also be seen. The neck should be examined for the presence of lymphadenopathy. The respiratory system must be examined for findings consistent with asthma. These include wheezing, tachypnea, and a prolonged expiratory phase of respiration.

Treatment

The management of allergic rhinitis consists of four major categories of treatment: patient education, allergen avoidance, pharmacologic management, and immunotherapy. All aspects of treatment are more successful when exposure to allergens is decreased. Recommendations for treatment are primarily based on symptoms and patient age. Pharmacotherapy can involve the use of **antihistamines, decongestants, intranasal corticosteroids, and, in severe cases, systemic corticosteroids.**

Antihistamines. Antihistamines competitively antagonize the receptors for histamine, which is released from mast cells. This reduces the production of symptoms mediated by the release of histamine. First-generation antihistamines, including diphenhydramine, chlorpheniramine, and hydroxyzine, are inexpensive and available over the counter. Side effects include sedation and the anticholinergic effects of dry mouth, dry eyes, blurred vision, and urinary retention; therefore, their use should be monitored in sensitive populations, such as the elderly. **Second-generation antihistamines, including loratadine, desloratadine, fexofenadine, azelastine, and cetirizine,** have a lower incidence of sedation and anticholinergic side effects; they are therefore preferred over first-generation antihistamines. Caution should be used with cetirizine because sedative side effects can occur at recommended doses. Oral antihistamines begin to take effect within 15 to 30 minutes after ingestion and are best used in persons with mild and intermittent symptoms.

Corticosteroids. **Corticosteroid nasal sprays** are the most effective treatment and first-line therapy for the long-term management of mild-to-moderate persistent symptoms of allergic rhinitis. They reduce the production of inflammatory mediators and the recruitment of inflammatory cells. Systemic absorption of the steroid is relatively low, reducing the risk of complications associated with the chronic use of systemic corticosteroids. Side effects include nosebleeds, nasal irritation, and rarely nasal septum perforation. Maximal effectiveness is achieved after 2 to 4 weeks of use.

Oral corticosteroids are potent inhibitors of cell-mediated immunity. The use of systemic steroids is limited by adverse effects, including suppression of the hypothalamic-pituitary-adrenal axis and hyperglycemia. Long-term use can lead to peptic ulcer formation, increased susceptibility to infection, poor wound healing, and the reduction of bone density. Because of these significant risks, systemic steroids are used only for severe allergies unresponsive to other pharmacological modalities or a diagnosis of nasal polyposis. Oral steroids should be used in the lowest effective dose for the shortest possible time.

Decongestants. Decongestants, given either orally or intranasally, can be used to provide symptomatic relief of nasal congestion. These alpha-adrenergic agonist agents constrict blood vessels in the nasal mucosa and reduce the overall volume of the mucosa. Common decongestants include pseudoephedrine and phenylephrine. Oral decongestants can cause tachycardia, tremors, and insomnia. Rebound hyperemia and worsening of symptoms can occur with chronic use or upon discontinuation of nasal decongestants. For this reason, it is generally not recommended to use intranasal decongestants for more than 3 days. Caution should be used in the elderly or young children, during the first trimester of pregnancy, and in individuals with cardiac arrhythmias, glaucoma, or hyperthyroidism.

Leukotriene Inhibitors. Leukotriene inhibitors (zafirlukast, montelukast, zileuton) are indicated both for allergic rhinitis and for maintenance therapy for persistent asthma. They are particularly useful in patients with both asthma and allergies or in those whose asthma may be triggered by allergens. These medications can be taken alone or in combination with antihistamines.

Desensitization Therapy. Desensitization therapy is frequently attempted in patients who remain symptomatic despite maximal medical therapy. Skin allergy testing is used to detect reactivity against specific antigens. The next step is to inject the patient with highly diluted concentrations of this antigen. The concentration of the antigen(s) in the injection is gradually increased in an effort to reduce the patient's inflammatory response to the antigen(s). Injections are typically given weekly or biweekly. This process is expensive and time consuming and requires numerous injections. Patients and physicians must be prepared to address severe, even anaphylactic, reactions that may occur during the process.

Complications

Urticaria and Angioedema. Urticaria is characterized by large, irregularly shaped, pruritic, erythematous wheals. **Angioedema** is painless, deep, subcutaneous swelling that often involves the periorbital, circumoral, and facial regions. Anaphylaxis is another dangerous complication and is discussed in depth next.

CLINICAL APPROACH TO ANAPHYLAXIS

Pathophysiology

Anaphylaxis is a systemic reaction with cutaneous symptoms that is associated with dyspnea, visceral edema, and hypotension. Insect bites or stings, foods, and medications are the most common culprits of anaphylactic reactions. The manifestations of anaphylaxis include hypotension or shock from widespread vasodilation, respiratory distress from bronchospasm or laryngeal edema, gastrointestinal and uterine muscle contraction, and urticaria and angioedema.

Treatment

Epinephrine. **At the first suspicion of anaphylaxis, aqueous epinephrine 1:1000, in a dose of 0.2 to 0.5 mg, is injected intramuscularly.** Repeated injections can be given every 5 to 15 minutes when necessary. Epinephrine administration increases peripheral resistance by causing immediate vasoconstriction.

Airway and Circulation. Airway obstruction and vascular collapse improve due to the inotropic properties of epinephrine on the heart and bronchodilator effects on the lungs. Rapid intravenous infusion of large volumes of fluids (saline, lactated Ringer solution, plasma or plasma expanders) is essential to replace loss of intravascular plasma into tissues. Airway obstruction may be caused by edema of the larynx or by bronchospasm. In addition to securing the airway, oxygen therapy should be provided. Endotracheal intubation may be required.

Antihistamines. Antihistamines may be useful as adjuvant therapy for alleviating cutaneous manifestations of urticaria or angioedema and pruritus. Caution is recommended with antihistamine use given the sedative effects, which could be problematic in compromised patients. Systemic corticosteroids can be beneficial, but they should not be used as first line due to their delayed onset of action. All patients with anaphylaxis should be monitored for a period of time, for example, 24 hours.

CLINICAL APPROACH TO CONJUNCTIVITIS

Conjunctivitis is an infection of the palpebral and/or bulbar conjunctiva. It is the most common eye disease seen in community medicine. Most cases are caused by bacterial or viral infection. Other causes include allergy and chemical irritants. The mode of transmission of infectious conjunctivitis is usually direct contact to the opposite eye or to other persons via fingers, towels, or handkerchiefs.

Bacterial conjunctivitis. The organisms isolated most commonly in bacterial conjunctivitis are *Staphylococcus*, *Streptococcus*, *Haemophilus*, *Moraxella*, and *Pseudomonas*. There is no blurring of vision and only mild discomfort. In severe cases, including those with immunocompromised patients, contact lens wearers, and failure to respond to initial treatment, cultures and examination of stained conjunctival scrapings are recommended. The disease is usually self-limited, lasting about 10 to 14 days if untreated. A sulfonamide instilled locally three times daily will usually clear the infection in 2 to 3 days.

Epidemic keratoconjunctivitis. Epidemic keratoconjunctivitis (pink eye) is highly contagious and spread by person-to-person contact or fomites. The most common cause is adenovirus. It is usually associated with pharyngitis, fever, malaise, and preauricular lymphadenopathy. Locally, the palpebral conjunctiva is red with a copious watery discharge and scanty exudates. Symptomatic treatment includes ocular decongestants, artificial tears, and cool or warm compresses to reduce the discomfort of the associated lid edema. Weak topical steroids may be necessary to treat the corneal infiltrates. The disease usually lasts at least 2 weeks.

Noninfectious conjunctivitis. Noninfectious causes of conjunctivitis include allergic and chemical irritants. Symptoms of allergic conjunctivitis include itching, tearing, redness, stringy discharge, and sometimes photophobia. In addition to avoiding the irritant, treatment can include the use of oral antihistamines or topical antihistamine or anti-inflammatory eye drops.

CASE CORRELATION

- See also Case 7 (Tobacco Use and Cessation), Case 19 (Upper Respiratory and Ear Infections), and Case 56 (Wheezing and Asthma).

COMPREHENSION QUESTIONS

6.1 A 30-year-old man has both mild persistent asthma and chronic environmental allergies. Which of the following medications is indicated for the management of this patient's conditions?

    A. Inhaled albuterol (short-acting beta-adrenergic agonist)

    B. Intranasal fluticasone (corticosteroid)

    C. Oral montelukast (leukotriene modifier)

    D. Oral cetirizine (second-generation antihistamine)

6.2 A 12-year-old adolescent male presents with eye itching and redness. He has clear drainage from his eyes but no crusting. Examination today is normal except for mildly injected conjunctiva bilaterally. Which of the following is the most appropriate treatment?

A. Antibiotic eye drops

B. Ophthalmology consultation

C. Anti-inflammatory eye drops

D. Oral leukotriene inhibitor

6.3 A 56-year-old man presents to his provider with symptoms consistent with allergic rhinitis. His past medical history is positive for benign prostatic hyperplasia. He continues to work in a warehouse as a forklift operator. Which of the following medications should be used to treat this patient?

A. Diphenhydramine

B. Hydroxyzine

C. Chlorpheniramine

D. Fexofenadine

ANSWERS

6.1 **C.** Montelukast is indicated for both the management of both persistent asthma and chronic allergies. Although it is effective, it does have a fair number of side effects, such as flu-like symptoms, skin rash, mood changes, headache, nausea, insomnia, abdominal pain, and fatigue. Nasal steroids (answer B) and oral antihistamines (answer D) are indicated only for allergies. Inhaled albuterol (answer A) is indicated for acute asthma exacerbations or episodes of shortness of breath.

6.2 **C.** This patient has allergic conjunctivitis. Topical anti-inflammatory drops are appropriate therapy. Other options would include topical or oral antihistamines. The other therapies listed (answer A, antibiotic eye drops; answer B, ophthalmology consultation; and answer D, oral leukotriene inhibitor) are not appropriate for this condition.

6.3 **D.** The second-generation antihistamines, such as fexofenadine, are less sedating and have fewer anticholinergic side effects than the first-generation antihistamines. They would be a better choice for someone who operates heavy machinery and has benign prostatic hyperplasia. However, they are no more effective at symptom relief than the first-generation antihistamines listed (answer A, diphenhydramine; answer B, hydroxyzine; and answer C, chlorpheniramine).

CLINICAL PEARLS

▶ The management of allergic rhinitis consists of four major categories of treatment: patient education, allergen avoidance, pharmacologic management, and immunotherapy.

▶ At the first suspicion of anaphylaxis, aqueous epinephrine 1:1000 in a dose of 0.2 to 0.5 mL (0.2–0.5 mg) is injected subcutaneously or intramuscularly. The airway should always be assessed and the patient intubated if necessary to secure breathing.

▶ Pharmacotherapy for allergic rhinitis can involve the use of antihistamines, decongestants, intranasal corticosteroids, and, in severe cases, systemic corticosteroids.

▶ The most common causes of conjunctivitis are bacterial or viral infection; other causes include allergies and chemical irritants.

REFERENCES

American Academy of Allergy Asthma and Immunology. Allergy testing: tips to remember. https://www.aaaai.org/conditions-and-treatments/library/allergy-library/allergy-testing. Accessed January 20, 2019.

Arnold JJ, Williams PM. Anaphylaxis: recognition and management. *Am Fam Physician.* 2011;84(10):1111-1118.

Barnes PJ. Asthma. In: Jameson J, Fauci AS, Kasper DL, Hauser SL, Longo DL, Loscalzo J, eds. *Harrison's Principles of Internal Medicine.* 20th ed. New York, NY: McGraw Hill; 2018: chap. 281. http://accessmedicine.mhmedical.com/content.aspx?bookid=2129&sectionid=186950288. Accessed May 07, 2019.

Cahill KN, Boyce JA. Urticaria, angioedema, and allergic rhinitis. In: Jameson J, Fauci AS, Kasper DL, Hauser SL, Longo DL, Loscalzo J, eds. *Harrison's Principles of Internal Medicine.* 20th ed. New York, NY: McGraw Hill; 2018: chap. 345. http://accessmedicine.mhmedical.com/content.aspx?bookid=2129&sectionid=181951047. Accessed May 07, 2019

Cronau H, Kankanala RR, Mauger T. Diagnosis and management of red eye in primary care. *Am Fam Physician.* 2010;81(2):1137-1441.

Lambert M. Practice parameters for allergic rhinitis. *Am Fam Physician.* 2009;80(1):79-85

Quillen DM, Feller DB. Diagnosing rhinitis: allergic vs. non-allergic. *Am Fam Physician.* 2006; 73(9):1583-1590.

Scow DT, Luttermoser GK, Dickerson KS. Leukotriene inhibitor in the treatment of allergy and asthma. *Am Fam Physician.* 2007;75(1):65-70.

Sur DK, Plesla M. Treatment of allergic rhinitis. *Am Fam Physician.* 2015;92(11):985-992.

Sur DK, Scandale S. Treatment of allergic rhinitis. *Am Fam Physician.* 2010;81(12):1440-1446.

A 55-year-old man comes into your office for follow-up of a chronic cough. He also complains of shortness of breath with activity. He reports that this has been getting worse over time. As you are interviewing the patient, you note that he smells of cigarette smoke. Upon further questioning, he reports smoking one pack of cigarettes per day for the past 35 years and denies ever being advised to quit. On examination, he is in no respiratory distress at rest, his vital signs are normal, and he has no obvious signs of cyanosis. His pulmonary examination is notable for reduced air movement and faint expiratory wheezing on auscultation.

▶ What would you recommend to this patient?
▶ What interventions are available to aid with smoking cessation?

ANSWERS TO CASE 7:
Tobacco Use and Cessation

Summary: A 55-year-old man presents with

- A 35 pack-year history of smoking
- A chronic cough and progressively worsening dyspnea
- Shortness of breath with activity
- Reduced air movement and faint expiratory wheezing on pulmonary examination

Recommendations to this patient: This patient should be advised to quit smoking; one strategy, using the 5 A's, is discussed further in the text.

Interventions available to help with smoking cessation: Counseling to quit smoking along with pharmacologic assistance with bupropion, varenicline, or nicotine replacement.

ANALYSIS

Objectives

1. Know the many medical conditions and complications related to tobacco use. (EPA 1, 2)

2. Develop a framework for the discussion of tobacco use and promotion of smoking cessation. (EPA 4, 5)

3. Know the currently available pharmacologic agents that are used to aid in smoking cessation. (EPA 5)

Considerations

This is a 55-year-old man with a long history of smoking who presents with a chronic cough and worsening dyspnea. The most important first steps are to address the airway and breathing and ensure that there is no respiratory emergency. Assessment of the patient's air movement, oxygenation, and degree of respiratory distress are important. After evaluating his condition and ascertaining whether it is chronic lung disease or an exacerbation such as bronchitis superimposed on chronic obstructive pulmonary disease (COPD), therapy may be enacted. Bronchodilator therapy, antibiotic therapy depending on the character of the sputum, and chest radiographic findings are typically used. One critical component of therapy includes smoking cessation. Clinician intervention is paramount, and the use of adjuvant therapies helps to increase success.

APPROACH TO:
Tobacco Use and Cessation

DEFINITIONS

PREGNANCY CATEGORY B: The Food and Drug Administration (FDA) category for use of a medication in pregnancy in which animal studies have shown no harm to a fetus but human studies are not available *or* animal studies have shown harm to a fetus but studies in pregnant women have not shown harm.

PREGNANCY CATEGORY C: Animal studies have shown adverse fetal effects, and there are no adequate studies in humans *or* no animal studies have been conducted and there are no adequate studies in humans.

PREGNANCY CATEGORY D: Human studies have shown potential adverse fetal effects; however, the benefits of therapy may outweigh the potential risks.

CLINICAL APPROACH

Epidemiology

Tobacco use is the single greatest cause of preventable death. It is responsible for increased death rates from cancer, cardiac, cerebrovascular, and chronic pulmonary diseases. Approximately 14% of the adult population reported smoking in 2017, and over 480,000 deaths per year are a result of tobacco use. Smoking also affects the health of those in close contact with people who smoke.

Secondhand Smoke. Each year, 41,000 deaths from cancer and heart disease in nonsmokers are attributable to secondhand smoke. Secondhand smoke increases a nonsmoker's risk of lung cancer up to 30%. Data pooled in 2010 by the Centers for Disease Control and Prevention showed nearly 11% of pregnant women reported tobacco use in the third trimester. Smoking in pregnancy is associated with prematurity, intrauterine growth restriction, stillbirth, spontaneous abortion, and infant death. Smoking cessation reduces all of these risks. However, despite this evidence, it is difficult for smokers to quit. Health care providers are important in the effort to reduce tobacco use and its related disease burden.

Smoking Cessation Counseling

Research indicates that physician intervention, even in brief encounters, increases the tobacco cessation rate. Furthermore, cessation rates increase with increased physician time and frequency of encounters to address tobacco use, but the optimal duration and frequency have not been defined. **The process of discussing tobacco use and cessation involves several steps; one useful framework is the "five A's"** (Table 7–1). Individuals who fail to quit smoking or those who relapse should be reassessed using the five A's framework. Once a new plan of cessation is in place, patients should determine a new quit date.

Motivation and the 5 R's. Multiple factors may be part of a patient's unwillingness to quit. **A strategy to enhance motivation (5 R's strategy)** includes discussing the specific **relevance** to the patient of smoking cessation, **risks** of ongoing tobacco use;

Table 7–1 • FIVE A'S OF TOBACCO CESSATION COUNSELING	
Ask about tobacco use	Ask the patient at each visit about current tobacco use and document the discussion.
Advise to quit through clear personalized messages	Let the patient know of his/her specific risks of tobacco use; in the sample case, talk to the patient about how the persistent cough and dyspnea can be related to the tobacco use and how cessation might be helpful.
Assess willingness to quit	Find out the patient's thoughts about quitting and if the patient is ready to proceed. Try to identify barriers and previous attempts to quit smoking while assessing for the general smoking history.
Assist to quit	Include individual, group, or telephone counseling and pharmacologic treatment. For the patient who does not desire to quit, provide interventions that increase future attempts to quit (motivational interviewing). Keep in mind and explain complications, especially withdrawal signs, and offer specialized support for those times.
Arrange follow-up and support	Schedule office visits, phone calls, or electronic communication focused specifically on tobacco cessation.

rewards of quitting (financial, health, social); **roadblocks** to quitting (withdrawal, discouragement because of failed past attempts, enjoyment of smoking); and **repetition** (readdressing the problem at each visit and reminding patients most people attempt to quit several times before being successful).

Smoking Cessation in Pregnancy. In pregnancy, it has been found to be helpful to discuss specific risks to the mother and fetus of continued tobacco use. While cessation prior to pregnancy is ideal, cessation at any time during pregnancy is associated with health benefits for the patient and fetus, so ongoing discussions are encouraged. The pregnant patient will also need ongoing support after delivery to reduce the risk of remission after delivery.

Withdrawal Symptoms. Discussing the symptoms of nicotine withdrawal prior to cessation may decrease failure rates in nicotine-dependent patients. It is not uncommon for patients to avoid smoking cessation secondary to a previous experience or fear of withdrawal symptoms. Common nicotine withdrawal symptoms include mood changes (irritability, anxiety, frustrated); difficulty concentrating; increased hunger; and restlessness.

Nonnicotine Pharmacologic Therapy

In addition to counseling and reviewing the risks and benefits of quitting, the use of pharmacologic aids can increase the likelihood of successful smoking cessation when a patient has decided to quit. There are two broad modalities approved by the FDA to assist with smoking cessation: nicotine replacement and nonnicotine medications. The approved nonnicotine medications are bupropion sustained release (brand name Zyban) and varenicline (brand name Chantix).

Bupropion. Bupropion was the first nonnicotine treatment for smoking cessation approved by the FDA. It is thought to work by blocking uptake of norepinephrine and/or dopamine. It is **contraindicated in patients with eating disorders,** monoamine oxidase inhibitor use in the last 2 weeks, or a history of seizure disorder. The usual course of treatment is 7 to 12 weeks, but it can be used for up to 6 months as maintenance therapy. This treatment can be used alone or in combination with nicotine-based treatments. According to a Cochrane Review, individuals taking bupropion for smoking cessation were two times more likely to quit compared with individuals taking a placebo. Common side effects include insomnia and dry mouth. Caution should be used in patients with established coronary heart disease; doses above the recommended amount can be cardiotoxic and lead to widened QRS complexes and subsequently fatal arrhythmias.

Varenicline. **Varenicline is a partial nicotinic receptor agonist.** The use of varenicline increases the rate of smoking cessation by three-fold when compared with a placebo. Varenicline reduces cravings for nicotine, reduces nicotine withdrawal symptoms, and blocks some of the binding of nicotine from cigarettes. Doses are reduced in patients on hemodialysis or with creatinine clearance < 30 mL/min. Varenicline has been associated with neuropsychiatric symptoms, including changes in behavior, agitation, depression, and suicidal behaviors, so it should be used with caution in anyone with a history of psychiatric disorders. Given recent studies showing a possible increased risk of cardiac events while taking varenicline, caution should be used in people with coronary artery disease. Common side effects include nausea, trouble sleeping, and abnormal, vivid, or strange dreams.

Nicotine Pharmacologic Therapy

Nicotine replacement therapies as a group increase smoking cessation rates over placebo by diminishing cravings and reducing nicotine withdrawal. They can be used in combination therapy, which may increase cessation rates over monotherapy. Specifically, the combination of a daily nicotine patch and an as-needed nicotine replacement therapy (nicotine gum, inhaler, nasal spray, or lozenge) has been shown to be more effective than the patch alone.

Nicotine Gum. Nicotine gum is available in 2 mg and 4 mg of nicotine per piece. The patient chews a piece of the gum until the patient feels a peppery taste in the mouth, "parks" the gum in a cheek until the sensation goes away, and then chews the gum again until the peppery sensation returns. The 4-mg dose is recommended for those who smoke more than 25 cigarettes per day and the 2-mg dose for those who smoke fewer than 25 cigarettes per day. Common pitfalls include not "parking" the gum (ie, chewing constantly) and not using enough pieces per day initially. Consider advising the patient initially to use the gum on a scheduled basis and then slowly taper the number of pieces per day. Common side effects, such as mouth soreness, hiccups, dyspepsia, and jaw ache, often are related to improper chewing techniques.

Nicotine Cartridge Inhaler. The nicotine cartridge inhaler is available by prescription and has also been found to be effective in increasing smoking cessation rates. Each cartridge contains 4 mg of nicotine in 80 inhalations. The recommended dose is 6 to 16 cartridges per day. The inhaler can be used over several months, with a gradual tapering of the dose. For the gum, lozenge, and inhaler, acidic beverages (coffee, soda, or juices) can reduce absorption of the nicotine from the buccal mucosa, so the patient should avoid ingestion within 15 minutes of use of these products. Common side effects, such as local irritation of the mouth and throat, coughing, and rhinitis, usually decline with continued use.

Nicotine Nasal Spray. Another therapeutic option is the nicotine nasal spray. The spray provides 0.5 mg of nicotine per inhalation and can be used at a starting rate of 1 to 2 doses per hour, for a maximum of 40 doses per day (5 doses per hour). The inhaler can also be used over months, with gradual tapering of the dose. Nasal irritation is the most common side effect. Of all the nicotine replacement products, the inhaler has the highest peak nicotine level and therefore also has the highest dependency potential.

Nicotine Lozenge. The nicotine lozenge is available over the counter in 2-mg and 4-mg nicotine doses. The 4-mg nicotine lozenge is recommended for those who smoke their first cigarette within 30 minutes of waking, and the 2-mg nicotine lozenge is for those who smoke their first cigarette more than 30 minutes after waking. The patient should allow the lozenge to dissolve in the mouth without swallowing or chewing. The recommended dose is 1 lozenge every 1 to 2 hours, not to exceed 20 lozenges a day, for the first 6 weeks and then a gradual 6-week taper for a total of 12 weeks of treatment. Common side effects include nausea, hiccups, and heartburn.

Nicotine Patch. Compared to the other methods outlined, the nicotine patch is a passive nicotine replacement system. The patches are available over the counter and in varying strengths. The patch is replaced daily, and consideration should be given to starting with higher dose patches in heavy smokers. Treatment with the patch for fewer than 8 weeks is as effective as longer treatment periods. The most common side effect is irritation of the skin at the site of the patch. When used overnight, the patch has been shown to decrease morning cravings of nicotine.

Electronic Nicotine Delivery System. Electronic nicotine delivery systems (ENDS) have become popular over the past decade or so. Specifically, the use of electronic cigarettes (also called e-cigarettes) for smoking cessation has gained popularity since introduced to the United States in 2007. These battery-operated devices convert liquid nicotine into a vapor that is inhaled. Depending on the version of e-cigarettes used, flavors, additives, herbal extracts, or vitamins may be added, and nicotine may or may not be present. There is insufficient evidence for electronic cigarettes being safer than cigarettes. Previously, they were considered a safe option, as they were free from tar or known carcinogens. Recent studies, however, have shown that the exhaled smoke is not just water vapor. It contains products that are carcinogenic to not only the smoker but also those in the smoker's immediate vicinity. It is still unclear if e-cigarettes are more effective for treating smoking cessation than traditional nicotine replacement modalities. In an effort to halt the increased use of e-cigarettes among children and adolescents, in 2014 the FDA prohibited the sale of smokeless tobacco to individuals younger than 18 years old. Caution should be used when suggesting smokeless tobacco as a means for quitting. Until further research is conducted, more familiar methods should be recommended.

Other Considerations

Pharmacologic Interventions in Pregnancy. The nicotine inhaler, nasal spray, patch, and gum are pregnancy category D drugs. Pregnant smokers should be encouraged to quit without the use of any pharmacologic agents. However, these products can be considered for use in the pregnant smoker if counseling is insufficient to promote cessation and if, in discussion with the patient, it is determined that the risks of continued smoking outweigh the risks of the medication. Bupropion and varenicline are pregnancy category C. They have not been studied in pregnancy and should only be used if the benefit justifies the potential risk to the fetus.

Screening. The United States Preventive Services Task Force strongly recommends screening all adults and pregnant patients for tobacco use and offering cessation intervention for those who use tobacco products (Grade A recommendation). For adolescent smokers, counseling has been shown to be effective, and counseling interventions should be provided to aid in quitting (Grade B recommendation). The strongest risk factor for smoking initiation among children and adolescents is parental smoking.

CASE CORRELATION

- See also Case 1 (Adult Male Health Maintenance) and Case 56 (Wheezing and Asthma).

COMPREHENSION QUESTIONS

7.1 A pregnant woman who smokes one pack of cigarettes a day asks for your advice regarding smoking cessation while she is pregnant. Which of the following statements is most appropriate?

    A. Bupropion is pregnancy category C and relatively safe in pregnancy.

    B. Varenicline is pregnancy category B and relatively safe in pregnancy.

    C. Nicotine gum delivers a lower and safer dose of nicotine than the nasal spray.

    D. The use of smoking cessation products during pregnancy frequently leads to adverse outcomes.

7.2 Which of the following statements regarding available treatments for smoking cessation is accurate?

    A. Bupropion can be used in combination with nicotine supplements.

    B. Nicotine gum is most effective if chewed continuously, to promote a constant release of the nicotine.

    C. Nicotine supplements are most effective when used as needed for withdrawal symptoms.

    D. All of the available agents are more effective when used in combinations with each other.

7.3 Which of the following counseling strategies is most likely to enhance your patients' smoking cessation rates?

 A. Discuss smoking cessation techniques only with patients who ask for your advice, as others will resent your suggestions.

 B. Emphasize primarily the health risks of smoking.

 C. Note in each patient's chart that you have discussed cessation, so that you do not repeat the message to the same patient at subsequent visits.

 D. Ask about smoking cessation at each encounter.

ANSWERS

7.1 **A.** Bupropion and varenicline are both pregnancy category C (not category B, as in answer B). Pregnant smokers should be encouraged to quit without the use of any pharmacologic agents. However, pharmacologic aids to increase the rate of smoking cessation during pregnancy can be used (answer D) after discussion with the patient of the risks and benefits of the medications and of continued smoking. Cessation of smoking at any time during the pregnancy is likely to provide health benefits for the mother and fetus. Nicotine gum (answer C) delivers higher doses of nicotine than its nasal spray counterpart.

7.2 **A.** Bupropion can be used in combination with any of the nicotine supplementation products. The nicotine products can also be used in combination with each other. While some studies have looked at the use of varenicline with nicotine replacement, the prescribing information for varenicline still states that it has not been studied for use with other smoking cessation agents and cautions against the combination (answer D). Two common pitfalls in using nicotine supplementation are using supplementation only when having withdrawal symptoms (answer C) and failing to use nicotine gum correctly. The gum should be chewed briefly and then parked in the cheek. It is less effective if chewed continuously (answer B).

7.3 **D.** Asking patients about tobacco use is a key to promoting cessation. It is important to ask all patients (not only patients who ask for advice, as in answer A) at each visit (not solely at one visit, as in answer C) and to be prepared to provide advice and assistance at any time. Motivational counseling is most effective, which means describing both the positive effects of smoking cessation and the risks (answer B).

CLINICAL PEARLS

▶ Most smokers require multiple attempts before successfully quitting for good. Remind your patients of this if they become discouraged in their efforts.

▶ Use the five A's—ask, advise, assess, assist, and arrange follow-up—to help your patients quit smoking.

▶ Common nicotine withdrawal symptoms include mood changes (irritability, anxiety, frustration), difficulty concentrating, increased hunger, and restlessness.

▶ The approved nonnicotine medications are bupropion sustained release (brand name Zyban) and varenicline (brand name Chantix).

▶ The combination of a daily nicotine patch and an as-needed nicotine replacement therapy (nicotine gum, inhaler, nasal spray, or lozenge) has been shown to be more effective than the patch alone.

REFERENCES

Centers for Disease Control and Prevention. Fast facts and fact sheets. https://www.cdc.gov/tobacco/data_statistics/fact_sheets/index.htm?s_cid=osh-stu-home-spotlight-001. Accessed May 7, 2019.

Crawford P, Cieslak D. Varenicline for smoking cessation. *Am Fam Physician.* 2017;96(5). https://www.aafp.org/afp/2017/0901/od1.html. Accessed May 7, 2019.

Drew AM, Peters GL. Electronic cigarettes: cautions and concerns. *Am Fam Physician.* 2014;90(5):282-284.

Fiore MC, Bailey WC, Cohen SJ, et al. *Treating Tobacco Use and Dependence. Clinical Practice Guideline.* Rockville, MD: US Department of Health and Human Services, Public Health Service; May 2008.

Hughes JR, Stead LF, Hartmann-Boyce J, Cahill K, Lancaster T. Antidepressants for smoking cessation. *Cochrane Database Syst Rev.* 2014;(1):CD000031. doi: 10.1002/14651858.CD000031.pub4

Larzelere MM, Williams DE. Promoting smoking cessation. *Am Fam Physician.* 2012;85(6):591-598.

Okuyemi KS, Nolen NL, Ahluwalia JS. Interventions to facilitate smoking cessation. *Am Fam Physician.* 2006;74(2):262-271.

United States Food and Drug Administration. Compliance with regulations restricting the sale and distribution of cigarettes and smokeless tobacco to protect children and adolescents. Available at: https://www.fda.gov/regulatory-information/search-fda-guidance-documents/compliance-regulations-restricting-sale-and-distribution-cigarettes-and-smokeless-tobacco-protect. Accessed April 23, 2020.

United States Food and Drug Administration. Vaporizers, e-cigarettes, and other electronic nicotine delivery systems (ENDS). Available at: https://www.fda.gov/tobacco-products/products-ingredients-components/vaporizers-e-cigarettes-and-other-electronic-nicotine-delivery-systems-ends. Accessed January 27, 2019.

United States Department of Health and Human Services. *The Health Consequences of Smoking—50 Years of Progress: A Report of the Surgeon General.* Atlanta, CA: US Department of Health and Human Services, Centers for Disease Control and Prevention, National Center for Chronic Disease Prevention and Health Promotion, Office on Smoking and Health; 2014. Available at: https://www.hhs.gov/sites/default/files/consequences-smoking-exec-summary.pdf. Accessed January 27, 2019.

United States Preventive Services Task Force (USPSTF). Tobacco smoking cessation in adults, including pregnant women: Behavioral and pharmacotherapy interventions. https://www.uspreventiveservicestaskforce.org/uspstf/recommendation/tobacco-use-in-adults-and-pregnant-women-counseling-and-interventions. Accessed April 23, 2020.

A 24-year-old medical student is about to begin her first clinical rotation and has been eagerly awaiting the chance to apply her medical knowledge to real patients. She also hopes to identify physician role models.

On her first rotation, she is disappointed to find that her attending is miserable. Scurrying between patient rooms, the attending barely has time to speak to her patients and perform a minimal examination. Instead, she mostly types and clicks on the electronic health record (EHR), rarely even looking at her patients while she talks. The attending often has to pause the visit to locate missing laboratory or imaging reports. Meanwhile, the clinic staff seems to be in perpetual crisis mode, interrupting the attending with requests for help with patient calls, emergency visit slots, refills, and patient complaints. Additionally, after the attending goes home at night, she still spends several hours charting in the EHR.

At the end of a particularly difficult day, the attending, slumped in her chair in a daze, tells the student that she regrets becoming a physician. "I used to see patients; now I stare at the computer screen. I used to be in charge of my day, but now an administrator tells us how many patients to see and how much time to spend with each one. I used to care about each and every one of my patients; now, I just want to get through the day and go home. I work so hard, but I wonder if I'm really making a difference," she says.

▶ What syndrome is the attending physician suffering from?
▶ What are some of the underlying causes of this syndrome?
▶ What are some characteristics of this syndrome?
▶ What should the medical student do to preserve her own well-being?

ANSWERS TO CASE 8:

Clinician Well-Being

Summary: A new medical student

- Is working with a physician in a dysfunctional clinic setting
- Observes the dysfunction affects not only the physician's work satisfaction but also the quality of her patient care and teaching
- Hears the attending say she regrets becoming a physician and does not know if she is making a difference

What syndrome: Job burnout.

Causes of burnout: Work overload, clinical inefficiencies, excessive time documenting on the EHR, loss of job autonomy, and not being able to focus on patient care.

Symptoms of burnout: Feeling exhausted at the end of the workday, frustration with clinical inefficiencies, loss of empathy for patients and coworkers, loss of a sense of personal accomplishment, and loss of a sense of meaning in work.

Medical student response: The student should recognize that her attending physician is stressed and demoralized because she is working in a toxic job environment. The student has an opportunity to use this unfortunate situation to learn about physician burnout, including ways that high-functioning medical organizations are creating healthier job environments. In the future, when choosing electives, her specialty, her residency, and eventually her job, she should consider the job environment.

ANALYSIS

Objectives

1. Describe health care provider burnout, including symptoms, causes, and impact. (EPA 1, 12)

2. Discuss the solutions currently proposed for burnout. (EPA 12, 13)

3. Discuss coping strategies for clinicians at risk of burnout. (EPA 12)

Considerations

The physician in the case is suffering from job burnout, a syndrome that affects her energy, mood, attitude about her patients and coworkers, and effectiveness as a physician. The source is the dysfunctional clinic organization, beginning with a mismatch between the period of time the physician needs to care well for her patients and the actual time allotted. Additional aspects of this clinic's dysfunction include the time the physician spends doing clerical work rather than patient care and the time spent after hours with the EHR. Rather than improving workflow and respecting the doctor-patient relationship, the staff hinders by interrupting the physician during visits.

In addition to having a negative impact on the physician's morale, the clinic dysfunction is likely to have a negative impact on the quality of patient care. Instead of a rich physician-patient relationship marked by trust, open communication, and attention to detail, patients will likely feel that their physician is inattentive and uncaring, and the distracted provider is likely to miss subtle communication hints and important clinical details. As for the staff, instead of being part of an efficient, productive, happy team, they may feel ignored, underutilized, and bored. Trainees observe the chaos and wonder if they chose the right profession.

Because the problem is rooted in a toxic work environment, the solutions will require a systemic approach and culture change within the health care organization. The attending physician will need to enlist help from clinical colleagues and support of organizational leadership to identify the drivers of burnout and to implement strategies for correcting them.

Although health care providers are not to blame for their high rates of job burnout, they are still the symptom bearers and thus are at risk of serious health and relationship problems. The attending physician in this case needs to pay close attention to her own self-care: sleep, exercise, diet, and relationships. Ultimately, she may need to change jobs or transition to part-time.

APPROACH TO:
Clinician Well-Being

DEFINITIONS

DEPERSONALIZATION: Treatment of patients, patients' families, and/or coworkers as objects rather than persons. It often involves a reduced capacity for empathy, clinical insight, and creative problem-solving.

PROVIDER BURNOUT: A syndrome of disengagement from work by a variety of factors such as consequence of a poorly structured clinic environment. These providers feel exhausted physically and emotionally. Instead of their work being satisfying and rejuvenating, it drains their energy and enthusiasm. Many also experience symptoms of depersonalization and a low sense of accomplishment.

CLINICAL APPROACH

Sources of Burnout

Being a health care provider has always been a demanding profession. Clinicians care for those who are most sick and vulnerable in our society. They bear a heavy burden of responsibility for the lives of others, they see disability and death on a near-daily basis, and they suffer the collateral damages of physical exhaustion and family stress due to working long hours. Job stress and workaholism have always been features of the profession.

From the physicians' perspective, there was one saving grace: Physicians were in control of their jobs, their clinics, and their hospitals. The work was hard, but it was "their" work: They controlled the appointment templates, the operating room schedule, hiring of staff, and which medical record to use. They also enjoyed consultations and camaraderie with their colleagues via phone calls, hallway conversations, lunch meetings, and breaks in the lounge. They experienced the joy and privilege of doing meaningful work: solving problems, helping people, and being part of a team of dedicated professionals. There was more physician autonomy in the past.

In the past two decades, however, the structure of health care has changed. As a consequence, physicians as a whole have less control of their jobs, clinics, and hospitals. In many settings, it appears that administrators focus on efficiency, and financial goals have shortened clinic visit times, increased numbers of patients seen per clinic session, and reduced the number of ancillary staff. Insurance companies have required clinicians to justify needed procedures or medications, a frustrating task. In an effort to increase patient safety and legibility and portability of medical records, government policies require the use of the EHR. Sadly, from the clinician's viewpoint, the typing, clicking, and peering at the computer screen in the examination room can interfere with the provider-patient relationship. In summary, today's providers not only face the burden of numerous nonclinical tasks, but they also feel that they have a reduced ability to fix problems.

Effects of Health Care Provider Burnout

Provider burnout has a negative impact on health care delivery and the health and happiness of the individual provider. Burned-out clinicians tend to deliver inferior care, make more mistakes, and are at increased risk of malpractice suits. Sensing their provider's disinterest and demoralization, patients are dissatisfied with their care and are less likely to follow their provider's advice. Burned-out providers are not as productive as healthy ones. They often work fewer hours, see fewer patients, and are more likely to leave jobs in search of something better. Burned-out providers also pay a high price in terms of their own health and well-being. They experience higher rates of depression, alcohol and substance abuse, suicide, work-home conflicts, job dissatisfaction, and career abandonment.

Solutions to Burnout

Research has shown that physician burnout can be prevented and reduced by the organizational interventions and approaches discussed next.

Addressing Local Issues at the Local Level. With the endorsement of institutional leaders, clinic- or department-based focus groups identify key drivers of burnout and are empowered to fix them for their particular unit. Typical issues and solutions include previsit planning, individualizing appointment templates, delegating clerical tasks, utilizing EHR scribes, sharing clinical care among the entire team, and improving communication and care of complex patients via team meetings.

Appointing, Training, and Empowering Physician Leaders. Physician leaders are an important component of health care organizations because they understand and embrace the values of health care rather than the values of corporate America. Empowering physicians who possess leadership skills to address problems within their domain helps reduce physician burnout.

Letting Providers Follow Their Passion. Providers who are able to identify a professional activity that gives them high levels of meaning and satisfaction and are allowed to spend at least 1 day per week focusing on that activity are less likely to experience job burnout. Such activities might include caring for a particular type of patient, teaching health care students, chairing a task force, or writing a textbook.

Building Teamwork, Community, and Camaraderie. Providers who meet together with colleagues to discuss difficult cases, to process the emotional impact of their work, and to reflect on the meaning of their work are less likely to experience job burnout.

Avoiding Productivity-Based Compensation. Studies showed that providers are motivated to provide a high quality of care, not a high quantity of care. Providers whose pay is based on productivity experience higher rates of burnout.

Promoting Work Flexibility and Work-Life Integration. Many young clinicians, particularly women, experience high rates of burnout due to the difficulty of juggling work, home, and personal needs. Those who work in organizations sensitive to these needs are less likely to experience job burnout.

Promoting Individual Wellness. While stress management training, meditation, exercise, and nutrition are not the cornerstones of burnout prevention, they do help individuals cope with the stressors of their jobs, families, and lives. Other practices that might enhance individual wellness include self-compassion in the face of bad patient outcomes, journaling about meaningful patient interactions, taking time for breaks and vacations, and reducing personal financial pressure by living a less affluent lifestyle.

Other Solutions. Other burnout solutions might include measures to reduce conflict and improve workplace civility, train and reward good mentors, and improve communication and trust within the organization.

Learning From the Problem of Burnout

While the drivers of burnout are largely beyond the control of health care students or residents, what trainees can do is understand the symptoms, causes, and solutions so that they can identify the problem in themselves and others and make wiser choices in terms of future training and practice. Since students have little control over their hours, assignments, patients, and rotations, it becomes more important to emphasize areas in which they do have some control, such as supportive relationships, regular exercise, a healthful diet, and adequate sleep. Choosing good mentors and staying active in nonmedical social groups are also helpful.

It is also important to be aware of other mental health problems with similar symptoms as job burnout. These include clinical depression, imposter syndrome, and life imbalance. **Clinical depression** can be distinguished from job burnout in that it is often driven by factors other than work or it continues after the work stressors are removed. However, burnout can be a contributing factor to clinical depression. Clinical depression is particularly troubling because of its high association with suicide. It is often associated with substance abuse as well. **Imposter syndrome** is common among students, trainees, and young professionals. Its hallmark is anxiety regarding one's ability to perform job tasks or one's overall fitness for a particular career. Imposter syndrome can be distinguished from job burnout in that it affects anxiety rather than mood and energy levels, and it is a response primarily to transitional training and work experiences. **Life imbalance** occurs when one feels compelled to focus on training or job tasks to the detriment of meeting personal and family needs and responsibilities. It can lead to feelings of depression and anxiety as well as feelings of inadequacy and guilt. Life imbalance can be distinguished from job burnout in that it involves feeling trapped in a job situation that does not allow for adequate time for self and family, whereas burnout's primary symptom is emotional exhaustion.

A study published in 2018 in the *Journal of Internal Medicine* highlights the importance for more investigation (especially longitudinal studies) in this area to better understand the problem and focus on a multiprong solution of both structural/organizational and individual physician interventions to correct this current crisis.

COMPREHENSION QUESTIONS

8.1 A 26-year-old third-year medical student awakens each day with dread as she contemplates her day on the clinical rotation. What she dreads the most are attending rounds, where she is expected to answer difficult clinical questions in front of everybody. She wonders why she ever thought she was smart enough for medical school. Which of the following is most accurate?

　A. She is suffering from imposter syndrome, a common syndrome among learners.

　B. She is definitely not suited for medical school and should drop out.

　C. While clinical environments can be difficult, this is how students learn. She should soldier on and tough out the rotation.

　D. Awakening with dread is a normal part of medical school.

8.2 A 27-year-old medical student is nearing the end of his required clinical clerkship on internal medicine. Although he began medical school with enthusiasm and eagerness to learn, now he only feels tired and wishes he could hurry up and finish the day so he can go home and rest. His current rotation includes numerous late-day admissions. He notices that at the end of a long day, he rushes and only lets his patient respond in yes–no answers to his questions, cutting off their rambling responses or added detail. He goes home exhausted and feeling guilty about interacting with his patients in this way. Which of the following statements is most accurate?

　A. This is a normal response to a busy day and hectic medical school schedule.

　B. This is a manifestation of depersonalization and may be a sign of burnout.

　C. Students should expect that a loss of enthusiasm and idealism will occur naturally through the process of medical school.

　D. Patients do not mind being interrupted. They realize that student doctors have time constraints.

8.3 Dr. Jackson is a 55-year-old man who has been in medical practice for 25 years. He used to enjoy his work greatly and feel a sense of satisfaction when he left each day, knowing that he had contributed to the well-being of his patients and staff. Recently, however, his practice was bought by a local hospital, and productivity requirements have increased. He must rush through each visit, and he finds that his work is no longer satisfying. He cannot give each patient the proper time and attention. Which of the following individual interventions would most likely be effective in this situation?

A. Spend the necessary time with patients and save charting for later.

B. Threaten to quit unless productivity targets are more reasonable.

C. Stress management and resiliency training.

D. Recommend a more efficient electronic health system.

ANSWERS

8.1 **A.** Although imposter syndrome is a normal response of a student to initial clinical rotations, as a student gains experience the sense of dread is short-lived and is replaced by a growing sense of mastery. Feeling dread does not mean she is not suited for medical school (answer B). Sustained dread of clinical work, however, is emotionally exhausting and unhealthy. Rather than soldiering through (answer C), a student is advised to seek help via formal or informal student support groups or the student dean's office. Awakening each day with dread (answer D) is not normal and should be investigated.

8.2 **B.** This medical student is clearly burned out and experiencing depersonalization, leading to cynical attitudes toward patients and a lack of empathy. He exhibits an age-old conflict: balancing good medical care with healthy self-care. As productivity pressures have increased, this conflict has escalated. When clinicians are expected to see more patients in shorter times, the conflict becomes less a situation of balancing self-care and more an institutional issue of quality care. The solutions are best done at an institutional level. Enthusiasm and idealism may be tempered and matured but are not lost during training (answer C), and patients should never have to accept poor care (answer D) on the grounds of a busy provider schedule.

8.3 **C.** Sadly, this situation of having a dramatic increase in productivity targets is a very common scenario for today's providers. There are organizational interventions that may be helpful, such as answer D (more efficient electronic health system). Threatening to quit (answer B) is not very positive. Answer A (spending more time charting later) will likely impinge on personal time and even cause more depression and burnout. The individual interventions that have been shown to effectively reduce burnout include stress management and resiliency training, positive coping strategies, and mindfulness.

CLINICAL PEARLS

▶ The prevailing symptom of provider burnout is emotional exhaustion. It sometimes also includes treating patients as objects rather than persons and having a lowered sense of personal accomplishment.

▶ Multiple studies have documented the prevalence of physical burnout symptoms at about 50% in both physicians in training and practicing physicians.

▶ Clinician burnout is a public health crisis and affects clinicians, patients, and the health care organization.

▶ It is important to address burnout so that we can more fully experience the joy, meaning, and rewards inherent in this healing profession.

▶ Every day brings new opportunities to partner with patients for healing, to be invited into their lives when help is most needed, to develop durable relationships over many years, and to be rewarded with our patients' expressions of gratitude for our role in their lives.

▶ Physician suicide rates have steadily increased over the past 15 years.

▶ The solution to clinician burnout is both a structural/organizational and an individual intervention and change.

REFERENCES

Dyrbye LN, Shanafelt TD, Sinsky CA, et al. Burnout among health care professionals: a call to explore and address this underrecognized threat to safe, high-quality care. *NAM Perspectives*. Discussion paper, National Academy of Medicine, Washington, DC. July 5, 2017. Retrieved from NAM.edu/Perspectives. https://doi.org/10.31478/201707b

Linzer M, Paplau S, Grossman E, et al. A cluster randomized trial of interventions to improve work conditions and clinical burnout in primary care: results from the Health Work Place (HWP) Study. *J Gen Intern Med.* 2015:30(8):1105-1111.

Maslach C, Leiter MP. *The Truth about Burnout: How Organizations Cause Personal Stress and What to Do About It.* San Francisco, CA: Jossey-Bass; 1997.

Nedrow A, Steckler NA, Jardman J. Physician resilience and burnout: Can you make the switch? *Fam Pract Manag.* 2013;20(1):25-30.

Shanafelt TD, Noseworthy JH. Executive leadership and physician well-being: nine organizational strategies to promote engagement and reduce burnout. *Mayo Clin Proc.* 2017:92(1):129-146. http://dx.doi.org/10.1016/j.mayocp.2016.10.004

Sinksy CA, Willard-Grace E, Schutzbank AM, et al. In search of joy in practice: a report of 23 high-functioning primary care practices. *Ann Fam Med.* 2013;11(3):272-278.

West CP, Dyrbye LN, Rabatin JT, et al. Intervention to promote physician well-being, job satisfaction, and professionalism: a randomized clinical trial. *JAMA Intern Med.* 2014;174(4):527-533.

West CP, Dyrbye LN, Shanafelt TD. Physician burnout: contributors, consequences and solutions. *J Intern Med.* 2018;283(6):516-529.

A 65-year-old woman presents to the emergency department complaining of worsening shortness of breath and palpitations for about 1 week. She reports "feeling dizzy" on and off for the past year; the dizziness is associated with weakness that has been worsening for the past month. She has been feeling "too tired" to even walk to her backyard and water her flower bed, which she used to do "all the time." She has been so dyspneic walking up the stairs at her home that she moved downstairs to the guest room about a week ago. Review of systems is significant for knee pain, for which she frequently takes aspirin or ibuprofen; otherwise, the review of systems is negative. She has no significant medical history and has not been to a doctor in several years. She had a normal well-woman examination and screening colonoscopy about 5 years ago. She occasionally has an alcoholic drink and denies tobacco or drug use. She is married and is a retired shopkeeper. On examination, her blood pressure is 150/85 mm Hg, pulse is 98 beats/min, respiratory rate is 20 breaths/min, temperature is 98.7 °F (37.1 °C), and oxygen saturation is 99% on room air. Significant findings on examination include conjunctival pallor, mild tenderness with deep palpation in the epigastric and left upper quadrant (LUQ) region of the abdomen, normal bowel sounds, and no organomegaly but a positive stool guaiac test. The remainder of the examination, including respiratory, cardiovascular, and nervous systems, is normal.

▶ What is the most likely diagnosis?
▶ What is your next diagnostic step?
▶ What is the next step in therapy?

ANSWERS TO CASE 9:
Anemia in the Geriatric Patient

Summary: A 65-year-old woman presents with

- Worsening dyspnea on exertion, fatigue, dizziness, and palpitations
- Dyspnea that has caused her to alter her lifestyle (moving downstairs, not watering plants)
- Conjunctival pallor
- Guaiac-positive stool
- Mild tenderness with deep palpation in the epigastric and LUQ region

Most likely diagnosis: Anemia secondary to gastrointestinal (GI) bleeding; other considerations should include new-onset angina, congestive heart failure, and atrial fibrillation.

Next diagnostic step: A complete blood count (CBC) to evaluate for the anemia, an electrocardiogram (ECG) and cardiac enzymes, and a prothrombin time (PT) and partial thromboplastin time (PTT) to look for coagulation abnormalities.

Next step in therapy: Further workup, including blood transfusion (if needed), completion of two more sets of cardiac enzymes, and ECGs. A gastroenterology consult for esophagogastroduodenoscopy (EGD) and colonoscopy is appropriate because of the positive guaiac findings.

ANALYSIS

Objectives

1. Know a diagnostic approach to anemia in geriatrics. (EPA 2, 3)
2. Be familiar with a rational workup for anemia of different origins. (EPA 1, 2)
3. Describe the treatment of anemia in older patients. (EPA 4)

Considerations

A 65-year-old woman who has developed worsening dyspnea and palpitations over a 1-week period of time needs to be evaluated for cardiac and respiratory problems despite the gradual onset of symptoms. Specifically, in a postmenopausal woman, signs and symptoms of angina or acute myocardial infarction may not always have a typical presentation. That the patient has been feeling weak and has conjunctival pallor warrants testing for anemia. Since evaluation with serial cardiac enzymes and ECGs is part of the workup, admission into the hospital is appropriate.

Assuming that the initial workup for cardiac and pulmonary causes is negative and that the hemoglobin and hematocrit levels are low, a thorough evaluation for the cause of the anemia is necessary. A CBC with peripheral smear, reticulocyte count, iron studies, and vitamin B_{12} and folic acid levels would provide clues to the type of anemia that this patient has. A gastroenterology consult for possible EGD and colonoscopy to further investigate the source of GI bleeding should be considered. The presence of epigastric and LUQ pain, along with long-term use of nonsteroidal anti-inflammatory drugs, should also raise a flag for testing to rule out a bleeding ulcer.

The presence of other findings may direct your workup toward other diagnoses. If this patient were from a developing country, the possibility of intestinal parasites would need to be considered. If the PT and PTT were abnormal, GI bleeding from a coagulopathy or liver disease would be possibilities. Weight loss, lymphadenopathy, and coagulopathy may warrant evaluation for nongastrointestinal malignancies, such as leukemias or lymphomas. In younger patients, sickle cell disease, thalassemias, glucose-6-phosphate dehydrogenase deficiency, and other inherited causes of anemia would be on the differential diagnosis list. These are unlikely to manifest as an initial diagnosis at the age of 65 years.

APPROACH TO:
Anemia in the Geriatric Population

DEFINITION

ANEMIA: According to the World Health Organization, a hemoglobin level of less than 12 g/dL in women and less than 13 g/dL in men. In older populations, anemia may be defined as a hemoglobin less than 12 g/dL for both men and women.

CLINICAL APPROACH

Epidemiology

The prevalence of anemia in Americans older than age 65 years is estimated at 9% to 45%. There is **a wide variation in the rates of anemia in different ethnic and racial groups,** with the National Health and Nutrition Examination Surveys data showing the highest rates in non-Hispanic blacks and lowest rates in non-Hispanic whites. These differences are reportedly a result of biologic, not socioeconomic, differences. Most studies show the rate of anemia to be higher in men than women, and there is increasing evidence for anemia as an independent risk factor for increased morbidity and mortality and decreased quality of life.

Pathophysiology

Microcytic Anemia. The most common cause of anemia with a low mean corpuscular volume (MCV), microcytic anemia, is iron deficiency. Iron deficiency could be confirmed by subsequent testing that shows a low serum iron, low ferritin, and high total iron-binding capacity (TIBC). Other causes of microcytic anemia include thalassemias and anemia of chronic inflammation. In the elderly, iron deficiency is frequently caused by chronic GI blood loss, poor nutritional intake, or a bleeding disorder. A thorough evaluation of the GI tract for a source of blood loss, usually requiring a gastroenterology consultation for upper and lower GI endoscopy, should be undertaken, as iron-deficiency anemia may be the initial presentation of a GI malignancy.

Macrocytic Anemia. **Anemia with an elevated MCV, macrocytic anemia, is most often a manifestation of folate or vitamin B_{12} deficiency;** other causes include drug effects, liver disease, and hypothyroidism. The presence of macrocytic anemia, with or without the symptoms previously mentioned, should lead to further testing to determine B_{12} and folate levels. An elevated methylmalonic acid (MMA) level can be used to confirm a vitamin B_{12} deficiency; an elevated homocysteine level can be used to confirm folate deficiency. Folate deficiency anemia is usually seen in alcoholics, whereas B_{12}-deficiency anemia mostly occurs in people with pernicious anemia, a history of gastrectomy, and diseases associated with malabsorption (eg, bacterial infection, Crohn disease, celiac disease). The long-term use of certain medications, including proton pump inhibitors and H_2 blockers, can also result in the inhibition of B_{12} absorption. Under normal conditions, the body stores 50% of its B_{12} (2–5 mg total in adults) in the liver for 3 to 5 years. A minimal amount of B_{12} is lost daily through GI secretions. B_{12}-deficiency anemia is rare but possible in long-term vegans and vegetarians. B_{12} deficiency can be distinguished clinically from folic acid deficiency by the presence of neurological symptoms in B_{12} deficiency.

Normocytic Anemia. In the elderly, anemia of chronic inflammation (formerly known as anemia of chronic disease) is the most common cause of a normocytic anemia. Anemia of chronic inflammation is anemia that is secondary to some other underlying condition that leads to increased inflammation and bone marrow suppression. Along with causing a normocytic anemia, anemia of chronic inflammation can also present as a microcytic anemia. This type of anemia can easily be confused with iron-deficiency anemia because of its similar initial laboratory picture. **In anemia of chronic inflammation, the body's iron stores (measured by serum ferritin) are normal, but the capability of using the stored iron in the reticuloendothelial system becomes decreased.** A lack of improvement in symptoms and hemoglobin level with iron supplementation is an important clue indicating that the cause is chronic disease and not iron depletion, regardless of the laboratory picture. Another cause of normocytic anemia is renal insufficiency due to decreased erythropoietin production. Although bone marrow iron store remains the gold standard to differentiate between iron-deficiency anemia and anemia of chronic inflammation, simple serum testing is still used to diagnose and differentiate these two types of anemia (Table 9–1).

Table 9–1 • LABORATORY VALUES DIFFERENTIATING IRON-DEFICIENCY ANEMIA FROM ANEMIA OF CHRONIC INFLAMMATION		
Test	Iron Deficiency	Anemia of Chronic Inflammation
Serum iron	Low	Low or normal
Total iron-binding capacity (TIBC)	High	Low
Transferrin saturation	Low	Low or normal
Serum ferritin	Low	Normal or high

Clinical Presentation

Anemia that develops slowly may be asymptomatic and found incidentally on laboratory testing. Fatigue, weakness, and dyspnea are symptoms that are commonly reported by elderly persons with anemia. These vague and nonspecific symptoms are often ignored by both patients and clinicians as symptoms of "old age." Anemia may result in worsening of symptoms of other underlying conditions. For example, the reduced oxygen-carrying capacity of the blood as a consequence of anemia may exacerbate dyspnea associated with congestive heart failure.

Certain signs found on examination may prompt a workup for anemia. **Conjunctival pallor is recommended as a reliable sign of anemia in the elderly and commonly noted in patients with hemoglobin < 9 g/dL.** Other signs may suggest a specific cause of anemia. Glossitis, decreased vibratory and positional senses, ataxia, paresthesia, confusion, dementia, and pearly gray hair at an early age are signs suggestive of vitamin B_{12}-deficiency anemia. Folate deficiency can cause similar signs, except for the neurologic deficits. Profound iron deficiency may produce koilonychias (spoon nails), glossitis, or dysphagia. Other clinical manifestations of anemia include jaundice and splenomegaly. Jaundice can be a clue that hemolysis is a contributing factor to the anemia, while splenomegaly can indicate that a thalassemia or neoplasm may be present.

Initial workup of anemia should include a CBC with measurement of red blood cell (RBC) indices, a peripheral blood smear, and a reticulocyte count. Further laboratory studies would be indicated based on the results of the initial tests and the presence of symptoms or signs suggestive of other diseases.

Treatment

The treatment of anemia is determined based on the type and cause of the anemia. Any cause of anemia that creates a hemodynamic instability can be treated with an RBC transfusion.

Correcting Blood Loss. A hemoglobin less than 7 g/dL is a commonly used threshold for transfusion; however, transfusion may be indicated at higher levels if the patient is symptomatic or has a comorbid condition such as coronary artery disease. Iron-deficiency anemia is treated first by identification and correction of any source of blood loss.

Oral Iron Supplementation. Most iron deficiency can be corrected by oral iron replacement. Oral iron is given as ferrous sulfate 325 mg (contains 65 mg of elemental iron) three times a day. In uncomplicated anemia, it is considered first-line therapy because of its low cost and easy accessibility. Adherence to oral iron may be poor due to GI side effects (dark stools, nausea, vomiting, and constipation) and the required 6 to 8 weeks of treatment needed to correct the anemia. New evidence suggests that lower oral iron doses may be as effective as higher doses and have fewer side effects.

Intravenous Iron Supplementation. Individuals with malabsorptive conditions, malignancy, chronic kidney disease, heart failure, or significant blood loss may not benefit from oral iron replacement and therefore require parenteral iron preparations. It is recommended that patients requiring parenteral administration be given iron intravenously and not intramuscularly. Given the high risk of side effects, only trained clinicians should administer intravenous iron.

Vitamin Therapy. Vitamin B$_{12}$ deficiency traditionally has been treated by intramuscular B$_{12}$ therapy with a regimen of 1000 μg IM daily for 7 days, then weekly for 4 weeks, then monthly for the rest of the patient's life. However, most patients can be successfully treated with oral B$_{12}$ therapy using 1000 to 2000 μg in a similar regimen. Folate deficiency can be treated with oral therapy of 1 mg daily until the deficiency is corrected.

Anemia of Chronic Inflammation Treatment. Anemia of chronic inflammation is managed primarily by treatment of the underlying condition in order to decrease inflammation and bone marrow suppression. When anemia of chronic inflammation is severe (hemoglobin < 10 g/dL), the risks and benefits of two modalities of treatment, blood transfusion and erythropoiesis-stimulating agents, may be considered. Of note, the goals of treatment of anemia of chronic inflammation in patients with chronic kidney disease undergoing dialysis are to maintain a hemoglobin level between 10 and 12 g/dL; higher hemoglobin levels in this patient population are associated with increased rates of death and cardiovascular events.

> ## CASE CORRELATION
> - See also Case 14 (Hematuria) and Case 23 (Lower Gastrointestinal Bleeding).

COMPREHENSION QUESTIONS

9.1 A 58-year-old woman comes to your office complaining of fatigue. She has also noticed a burning sensation in her feet over the past 6 months. A CBC shows anemia with an increased MCV. Which of the following is the most likely cause of her anemia?

    A. Lack of intrinsic factor

    B. Inadequate dietary folate

    C. Strict vegetarian diet for the past 6 months

    D. Chronic GI blood loss

9.2 A 65-year-old man with a history of rheumatoid arthritis is found to have a microcytic anemia. He had a colonoscopy 1 year ago that was normal, and a stool guaiac is negative. Which of the following is the most likely cause of his anemia?

    A. Iron deficiency

    B. Chronic disease

    C. Pernicious anemia

    D. Folate deficiency

9.3 A 68-year-old man is found to have an incidental finding of anemia while hospitalized with pneumonia. His physical examination is normal except for crackles in the left lower lobe. Serum laboratory examinations reveal a normal MMA and a decreased serum folate level. Which of the following is the best next step?

A. Administer CAGE questionnaire

B. Esophagogastroduodenoscopy

C. Serum iron assay

D. Neurology consultation

For questions 9.4 and 9.5, match the following laboratory pictures (A–D) of patients with anemia:

A. Normal MMA; decreased serum folate level

B. Elevated MMA; decreased serum B_{12} level

C. Elevated ferritin; normal MCV; decreased serum iron level

D. Decreased ferritin; decreased MCV; decreased serum iron level

9.4 A 68-year-old man has an incidental finding of anemia while in the hospital for alcohol abuse.

9.5 A 67-year-old man presents with dizziness and a positive stool guaiac test.

ANSWERS

9.1 **A.** The clinical presentation of paresthesia and CBC findings are consistent with macrocytic anemia due to B_{12} deficiency. Pernicious anemia (lack of intrinsic factor) is the most common cause; recall that intrinsic factor is critical to binding vitamin B_{12} and absorption by the terminal ileum. Also, B_{12} deficiency can rarely be seen in patients who follow a strict vegetarian diet (answer C); however, the body's B_{12} stores can last several years before they are depleted. Answer B (inadequate folate) is another cause of macrocytic anemia, but it usually does not have neurological symptoms. Answer D (chronic GI blood loss) can lead to an iron-deficiency anemia, but it usually presents with microcytic anemia and without neurological symptoms.

9.2 **B.** Anemia of chronic inflammation can cause normocytic or microcytic anemia and may be secondary to rheumatoid arthritis in the patient. Iron-deficiency anemia (answer A) is less likely to be the etiology with a normal colonoscopy and negative stool guaiac, and serum iron studies could be used to help differentiate the two. Answer C (pernicious anemia) and answer D (folate deficiency) would lead to vitamin B_{12} deficiency and a macrocytic anemia.

9.3 **A.** Alcohol abuse, which may be assessed by the CAGE questionnaire, is a common cause of folate deficiency. CAGE is an acronym that stands for "Have you ever felt that you should Cut back?", "Do you feel Annoyed when others criticize your drinking?", "Do you feel Guilty about your drinking?", and Do you ever need to have a drink in the morning to wake up (Eye-opener)?". A normal MMA level essentially rules out a concomitant vitamin B_{12} deficiency. Upper endoscopy (answer B) to look for atrophic gastritis would be indicated for pernicious anemia. A serum iron assay (answer C) would likely be high because of increased turnover of iron in patients with megaloblastic anemia due to either B_{12} or folate deficiency. A neurology consultation (answer D) would be needed if the patient had neurologic signs or symptoms of B_{12} deficiency.

9.4 **A.** Alcohol abuse is a common cause of folate deficiency. A normal MMA level essentially rules out a concomitant vitamin B_{12} deficiency.

9.5 **D.** Low serum iron, low MCV, and low ferritin levels, along with a finding of blood in the stool, are consistent with iron-deficiency anemia. A workup for the source of the GI blood loss should ensue.

CLINICAL PEARLS

▶ Conjunctival pallor is an indication for anemia workup in elderly patients.

▶ Clinical findings of anemia require investigation for underlying causes.

▶ Gastrointestinal bleeding is an important cause of iron-deficiency anemia in both female and male geriatric patients; this type of anemia mandates a GI workup in this patient population.

▶ Investigating for vitamin B_{12} and folate deficiency is of high importance in a patient with a history of heavy alcohol intake and/or abuse.

REFERENCES

Adamson JW. Iron deficiency and other hypoproliferative anemias. In: Jameson J, Fauci AS, Kasper DL, Hauser SL, Longo DL, Loscalzo J, eds. *Harrison's Principles of Internal Medicine.* 20th ed. New York, NY: McGraw Hill; 2018: chap. 93. http://accessmedicine.mhmedical.com/content.aspx?bookid=2129&sectionid=192017034. Accessed May 10, 2019.

Auerbach M, Ballard H, Glaspy J. Clinical update: intravenous iron for anaemia. *Lancet.* 2007;369:1502.

Cappellini MD, Motta I. Anemia in clinical practice—definition and classification: does hemoglobin change with aging? *Semin Hematol.* 2015;52(4):261-269.

Lanier JB, Park JJ, Callahan RC. Anemia in older adults. *Am Fam Physician.* 2018;98(7):437-442.

A 40-year-old man presents to the clinic complaining of having 10 episodes of watery, nonbloody diarrhea that started last night. He vomited twice last night but has been able to tolerate liquids today. He has had intermittent abdominal cramps as well. He reports having muscle aches, weakness, headache, and a low-grade fever. He is here with his daughter, who started with the same symptoms this morning. On questioning, he states that he has no significant medical history and no surgeries and does not take any medications. He does not smoke cigarettes, drink alcohol, use any illicit drugs, and has never had a blood transfusion. He and his family returned to the United States yesterday after a weeklong vacation in Mexico.

On examination, he is not in acute distress. His blood pressure is 110/60 mm Hg, his pulse is 98 beats/min, his respiratory rate is 16 breaths/min, and his temperature is 99.1 °F (37.2 °C). His mucous membranes are dry. His bowel sounds are hyperactive, and his abdomen is mildly tender throughout, but there is no rebound tenderness and no guarding. A rectal examination is normal, and his stool is guaiac negative. The remainder of his examination is unremarkable.

▶ What is the most likely diagnosis?
▶ What is your next step?
▶ What are potential complications?

ANSWERS TO CASE 10:

Acute Diarrhea

Summary: A 40-year-old man presents with

- Profuse, acute, nonbloody diarrhea
- Dry mucous membranes on examination, which are consistent with developing dehydration
- History of recently returning from Mexico
- An ill family member with identical symptoms, suggesting an infectious cause of this acute illness

Most likely diagnosis: Acute gastroenteritis.

Next step: Rehydration with oral fluids if possible. If unable to tolerate oral fluids, then administer intravenously; consider empiric antibiotic treatment for traveler's diarrhea.

Potential complications: Dehydration and electrolyte abnormalities.

ANALYSIS

Objectives

1. Understand when and how to do a workup for acute diarrhea, considering the most probable etiologies of diarrhea. (EPA 1, 2)

2. Understand the role of fecal leukocytes and stool occult blood in the evaluation of acute diarrhea. (EPA 3, 10)

3. Understand that volume replacement and correction of electrolyte abnormalities are key components in the treatment and prevention of diarrhea complications. (EPA 4)

Considerations

This 40-year-old man developed severe diarrhea, nausea, and vomiting. His **most immediate problem is volume depletion,** as evidenced by his dry mucous membranes. The priority is to **replace the lost intravascular volume.** In persons who are not severely dehydrated, oral rehydration is preferred. If patients are unable to tolerate fluids or are very dehydrated, intravenous fluids should be used, usually with normal saline. Electrolytes and renal function should be evaluated and abnormalities corrected.

While correcting and/or preventing further dehydration, it is vital to determine the etiology of the diarrhea. Up to **90% of acute diarrhea is infectious** in etiology. This patient does not have any history compatible with chronic diarrhea, causes of which include Crohn disease, ulcerative colitis, gluten intolerance, irritable bowel syndrome, and parasites. He had been in Mexico recently, which predisposes him to different pathogens, including *Escherichia coli*, *Campylobacter*,

Shigella, Salmonella, and *Giardia.* Bacterial infections are more likely to be the source of acute diarrhea in individuals who have recently traveled, ingested contaminated food, or have other medical conditions. He does not have bloody stools. The **presence of blood in the stool would suggest an invasive bacterial infection,** such as hemorrhagic or enteroinvasive *E. coli* species, *Yersinia* species, *Shigella,* and *Entamoeba histolytica.*

The majority of the diarrheas are viral, self-limited, and do not need further evaluation. In this particular patient, because of his recent travel to Mexico, traveler's diarrhea should be strongly considered and treated with an appropriate antibiotic.

APPROACH TO:

Acute Diarrhea

DEFINITIONS

ACUTE DIARRHEA: Diarrhea present for a duration less than 2 weeks.

CHRONIC DIARRHEA: Diarrhea present for longer than 4 weeks.

DIARRHEA: Passage of abnormally liquid or poorly formed stool in increased frequency (three or more times a day).

SUBACUTE DIARRHEA: Diarrhea present for a 2- to 4-week duration.

CLINICAL APPROACH

Pathophysiology

Infectious Etiologies. Approximately 90% of acute diarrhea is caused by infectious etiologies, with most of the remainder caused by medications, ischemia, and toxins. Infectious etiologies often depend on the patient population. **Travelers to Mexico** will frequently contract **enterotoxigenic** *E. coli* as a causative agent. **Traveler's diarrhea** is a common entity and can be induced by a variety of bacteria, viruses, and parasites (Table 10–1). Campers are often affected by *Giardia.* Contaminated food and water supplies account for the high incidence of diarrhea in developing countries.

Table 10–1 • COMMON ETIOLOGIES OF TRAVELER'S DIARRHEA		
Bacteria	Viruses	Parasites
Escherichia coli (enterotoxigenic most common, but all types may be seen)	Rotavirus	*Giardia lamblia*
	Norovirus	*Entamoeba histolytica*
Salmonella		*Cryptosporidium parvum*
Shigella		
Vibrio noncholera		
Campylobacter		

Food Consumption. Consumption of foods is also frequently a culprit. *Salmonella* or *Shigella* can be found in **undercooked chicken,** enterohemorrhagic *E. coli* in undercooked hamburger, and *Staphylococcus aureus* or *Salmonella* in **creamy foods.** Raw seafood may harbor *Vibrio, Salmonella,* or hepatitis A. Sometimes the **timing** of the diarrhea following food ingestion is helpful. For example, **illness within 6 hours of eating mayonnaise-containing food suggests** *S. aureus,* **within 8 to 12 hours suggests** *Clostridium perfringens,* **and within 12 to 14 hours suggests** *E. coli.*

Other Etiologies. Day care settings are particularly common for *Shigella, Giardia,* and rotavirus to be transmitted. Patients who were recently treated with antibiotics may develop *Clostridium difficile* colitis. Consuming cold meats, raw milk, and soft cheeses increases the risk of listeriosis. Pregnant women are advised to avoid foods associated with listeriosis because they are at a significantly higher risk of infection. Immunocompromised patients (eg, those with AIDS) are more susceptible to parasitic gastrointestinal infections.

Clinical Presentation

Most patients with acute diarrhea have self-limited processes and do not require further testing. Further workup could be indicated for children, elderly patients, immunocompromised patients, and those with profuse diarrhea, dehydration, fever exceeding 100.4 °F (38.0 °C), bloody diarrhea, severe abdominal pain, or diarrhea for more than 7 days.

History. The history should include exposures to medications and foods, close contacts with similar symptoms, and travel history. A history of a viral illness may provide a clue to the etiology. The initial evaluation should determine if the patient can tolerate oral intake. The patient who is both vomiting and having diarrhea is more prone to dehydration and more likely to need hospital admission for intravenous hydration.

Physical Examination. The physical examination should focus on the vital signs, clinical impression of the volume status, and abdominal examination. Volume status is determined by observing whether the mucous membranes are moist or dry, the skin has good turgor, and the capillary refill is normal or delayed. Traveler's diarrhea is characterized by greater than three loose stools in a 24-hour period accompanied by abdominal cramping, nausea, vomiting, fever, or tenesmus. Most cases occur within the first 2 weeks of travel.

Laboratory Results. Laboratory testing is usually not needed. Stool cultures have limited benefit due to high cost and inefficient results. The use of stool cultures should be limited to individuals with bloody diarrhea, diarrhea lasting for more than 3 to 7 days, an immunocompromised state, or evidence of systemic disease or severe dehydration. In general, ova and parasite evaluation is unhelpful unless the history strongly points toward a parasitic source or the diarrhea is prolonged.

Examination of the stool for leukocytes is an inexpensive test that helps to differentiate between the types of infectious diarrhea. If leukocytes are present in the stool, the suspicion is higher for *Salmonella, Shigella, Yersinia,* enterohemorrhagic and enteroinvasive *E. coli, C. difficile, Campylobacter,* and *E. histolytica.*

Fecal lactoferrin immunoassay testing kits have increased in popularity due to their ease of use and faster results compared to tests for fecal leukocytes. Lactoferrin is an iron-binding protein that is found in polymorphonuclear neutrophils (PMNs) and bodily secretions such as breast milk. Gastrointestinal inflammation causes immune-activated PMNs to release lactoferrin. Lactoferrin elevations in stool can be seen with irritable bowel syndrome, intestinal bacterial infections, parasitic infections, and other conditions. Lactoferrin will be low in viral infections, making the lactoferrin immunoassay a useful test for distinguishing viral from bacterial diarrhea.

Testing for C. *difficile* toxins A and B is recommended in patients who develop diarrhea within 3 days of hospitalization, during antibiotic treatment, or within 3 months of discontinuing antibiotics. Although classically associated with clindamycin, **any antibiotic can cause pseudomembranous colitis.**

Treatment

Fluid Replacement. **Most cases of diarrhea resolve spontaneously in a few days without treatment.** Replacement of fluids and electrolytes is the first step in treating the consequences of acute diarrhea. For mildly dehydrated individuals who can tolerate oral fluids, solutions such as the World Health Organization oral rehydration solution or commercially available drinks such as Pedialyte or Gatorade often are all that is needed. It is no longer recommended that patients avoid eating solid foods for 24 hours. Increased intestinal permeability caused by gastrointestinal infections can be limited by early refeeding. Those with more serious volume deficits, elderly patients, and infants generally require hospitalization and intravenous hydration.

Antibiotics. If a parasitic infection is the cause of the diarrhea, prescription antibiotics may ease the symptoms. Antibiotics sometimes, but not always, help improve symptoms of bacterial diarrhea. However, antibiotics will not help viral diarrhea, which is the most common kind of infectious diarrhea. For traveler's diarrhea, when antibiotics are indicated, therapy with a quinolone antibiotic should be started as soon as possible after the diarrhea begins. Most commonly, **ciprofloxacin (500 mg twice daily) is given for 3 days.** Quinolones cannot be used in children or pregnant women. **Azithromycin**, given as a single 1000-mg dose in adults or 10 mg/kg daily for 3 days in children, is another effective drug for the treatment of traveler's diarrhea. Azithromycin also can be used in pregnant women with traveler's diarrhea. **Rifaximin** given as 200 mg three times a day for 3 days can be used in traveler's diarrhea caused by noninvasive strains of E. *coli.* However, rifaximin is not effective against infections associated with fever or blood in the stool. Rifaximin is safe for use in children under the age of 12 years.

Treatment of most C. *difficile* infections is with oral metronidazole. Oral vancomycin or fidaxomicin may be used in moderate-to-severe infections, recurrent C. *difficile* infections, or in the case of a treatment failure with metronidazole.

Antimotility Drugs. Over-the-counter antimotility or antisecretory medications may help to slow the frequency of the stools, but they do not shorten the course of the illness. Certain infections may be made worse by over-the-counter medications because they prevent the body from getting rid of the organism that is causing the diarrhea. Better relief of acute diarrhea with excessive gas may be possible with combined loperamide and simethicone compared to either medication alone.

Supplements. Probiotics, which are supplements that contain live organisms such as *Lactobacillus* spp. or *Saccharomyces boulardii*, may reduce the incidence of antibiotic-related diarrhea and the duration/severity of all-cause infectious diarrhea. Zinc supplementation has shown promising results for decreasing the duration and severity of the diarrheal illnesses in children.

Prevention

Viral Diarrhea. **Handwashing is a simple and effective way to prevent the spread of viral diarrhea.** Adults, children, and clinic and hospital personnel should be encouraged to wash their hands. Because viral diarrhea spreads easily, children with diarrhea should not attend school or child care until their illness has resolved.

Diarrhea Due to Food. To prevent diarrhea caused by contaminated food, use dairy products that have been pasteurized. Serve food immediately or refrigerate it after it has been cooked. Do not leave food out at room temperature because it promotes the growth of bacteria.

Traveler's Diarrhea. The **best method for preventing traveler's diarrhea is to avoid contaminated food and water.** Travelers to locations where there is poor sanitation and frequent contamination of food and water (eg, developing countries) need to be cautious to reduce their risk of developing diarrhea. They should be advised to eat hot and well-cooked foods and to drink bottled water, soda, wine, or beer served in its original container. Beverages from boiled water, such as coffee and tea, are usually safe. Recommend the use of bottled water even for toothbrushing. Also recommend avoiding raw fruits and vegetables unless they are peeled by the consumer immediately before being eaten. Patients should avoid tap water and ice cubes. In all, these recommendations may reduce but not completely eliminate one's risk of developing traveler's diarrhea.

Antibiotic prophylaxis is not indicated unless the patient is at increased risk for complications from diarrhea or dehydration, such as underlying inflammatory bowel disease, renal disease, or an immunocompromised state. Studies have shown that the antibacterial and antisecretory effects of bismuth subsalicylate decrease the incidence of traveler's diarrhea. Bismuth subsalicylate should be avoided in persons allergic to aspirin, pregnant women, or those taking methotrexate, probenecid, or doxycycline for malaria prophylaxis. The evidence is insufficient regarding the efficacy of probiotics as prophylaxis for traveler's diarrhea.

CASE CORRELATION

- See also Case 17 (Electrolyte Disorders) and Case 40 (Irritable Bowel Syndrome).

COMPREHENSION QUESTIONS

10.1 Several friends develop vomiting and diarrhea 6 hours after eating food at a private party. They describe the diarrhea as watery and nonbloody. Which of the following is the most likely etiology of the symptoms?

 A. Rotavirus

 B. *Giardia*

 C. *Escherichia coli*

 D. *Staphylococcus aureus*

 E. *Cryptosporidium*

10.2 A 40-year-old man travels to South America and develops watery diarrhea 1 day after coming back to the United States. He had been in good health previously. Which of the following is the most likely etiology of the symptoms?

 A. Rotavirus

 B. *Giardia*

 C. *Escherichia coli*

 D. *Staphylococcus aureus*

 E. *Cryptosporidium*

10.3 A 18-year-old woman eats raw seafood and 2 days later develops fever, abdominal cramping, and watery diarrhea. She is being seen in the emergency center for dizziness and lightheadedness. She describes the diarrhea as profuse and continues even if she is not eating or drinking foods. Which of the following is the most likely etiology of the symptoms?

 A. Rotavirus

 B. *Giardia* species

 C. *Escherichia coli*

 D. *Shigella* species

 E. *Vibrio* species

10.4 During the winter, a young day care worker develops watery diarrhea. Which of the following is the most likely etiology of the symptoms?

 A. Rotavirus

 B. *Giardia*

 C. *Escherichia coli*

 D. *Staphylococcus aureus*

 E. *Cryptosporidium*

10.5 A 45-year-old man presents with 3 days of watery diarrhea and abdominal cramping. He has no sick contacts and has not traveled recently. He is not currently taking any medications, but he was prescribed amoxicillin 2 weeks ago for a sinus infection. Which of the following tests is most likely to identify the cause of his diarrhea?

A. Stool guaiac

B. Evaluation of stool for fecal leukocytes

C. Evaluation of stool for ova and parasites

D. *Clostridium difficile* toxin immunoassay

10.6 In the patient described in Question 10.5, which of the following is the treatment of choice for his diarrhea?

A. Ciprofloxacin

B. Azithromycin

C. Metronidazole

D. Loperamide

ANSWERS

10.1 **D.** This group of people all became ill after eating food at a party and had both emesis and diarrhea, which is consistent with food poisoning. This is most likely due to *S. aureus* toxin, which usually causes vomiting and diarrhea within a few hours of food ingestion because the toxin is preformed in the food. Answer A (rotavirus infection) typically affects children or those exposed to children and presents with anorexia, low-grade fever, watery and nonbloody diarrhea, vomiting, and abdominal cramping. The diarrhea can be profuse and is one of the most common causes of death worldwide in children under age 2 years. Answer B (*Giardia*) is usually obtained from drinking from untreated fresh water and is associated with abdominal distension, flatulence, abdominal cramping, malodorous and greasy stool, and low-grade fever. The diarrhea can be chronic as well. Answer C (*E. coli*) is the most common cause of traveler's diarrhea, presenting with watery diarrhea (enterotoxigenic *E. coli*). A variety of *E. coli* can be invasive and lead to bloody diarrhea and fever similar to *Shigella* infections. Answer E (*Cryptosporidium*) does not commonly infect immunocompetent individuals but may infect immunocompromised hosts such as those with HIV infection. Diarrhea, abdominal cramping, nausea, vomiting, and fever may occur about 2 to 10 days after being infected. It is a waterborne parasite, and ingesting contaminated water is a common mode of transmission.

10.2 **C.** *Escherichia coli* is the most common etiology for traveler's diarrhea. This is most likely enterotoxigenic *E. coli*. The other answer choices (answer A, rotavirus; answer B, *Giardia*; answer D, *S. aureus*; and answer E, *Cryptosporidium*) are generally associated with different histories and are elaborated upon in the rationale for Question 10.1.

10.3 **E.** *Vibrio* infections are a common cause of diarrhea among people who eat raw seafood. *Vibrio* species are subdivided into cholera and noncholera, and the classic presentation is a watery diarrhea, abdominal cramping, nausea, and vomiting about 1 to 2 days after eating contaminated (raw) seafood.

10.4 **A.** Rotavirus is a common etiology for watery diarrhea, especially in the winter. It is very common in children. Given this patient's employment in a day care center where rotavirus would be very common in the winter, rotavirus is the most likely cause of this infection.

10.5 **D.** Although any antibiotic can cause *C. difficile* colitis, clindamycin, cephalosporins, and penicillins are the most commonly implicated. Stool guaiac (answer A) for occult blood may be positive in patients with *C. difficile* infection, but this would be a nonspecific finding. Fecal leukocytes (answer B) are often positive in *C. difficile* infection, but this too is a nonspecific finding for any inflammatory diarrhea. Answer C (stool ova and parasites) would be negative in *C. difficile*.

10.6 **C.** Oral metronidazole is the first-line treatment for *C. difficile*. Oral vancomycin can be used in the event of failure to respond to metronidazole therapy. Ciprofloxacin (answer A) and azithromycin (answer B) can be used for treatment of traveler's diarrhea. Loperamide (answer D) can decrease the frequency of bowel movements but is contraindicated in any patient with suspected *C. difficile* colitis.

CLINICAL PEARLS

▶ Most acute diarrheas are caused by viruses and are self-limited.

▶ The history of the duration and whether it is inflammatory or osmotic or secretory helps to determine the etiology.

▶ The most common cause of traveler's diarrhea is enterotoxigenic *E. coli*.

▶ Diarrhea that develops after antibiotic use can be due to *C. difficile*; the diagnosis is made by identifying the toxin in the stool, and treatment is via oral vancomycin or fidaxomicin if severe.

▶ Be cautious when assessing diarrhea in a child, elderly patient, or immunosuppressed host.

▶ Dehydration, bloody diarrhea, high fever, and diarrhea that do not respond to treatment after 48 hours are warning signs of possible complicated diarrhea.

▶ In general, acute, uncomplicated diarrhea can be treated with oral electrolyte and fluid replacement.

REFERENCES

Barr W, Smith A. Acute diarrhea in adults. *Am Fam Physician.* 2014;89(3):180-189.

Centers for Disease Control and Prevention. *Travelers' Health—2018 Yellow Book.* http://wwwnc.cdc.gov/travel/page/yellowbook-home. Accessed May 10, 2019.

McQuaid KR. Gastrointestinal disorders. In: Papadakis MA, McPhee SJ, Rabow MW, eds. *Current Medical Diagnosis & Treatment 2019* New York, NY: McGraw Hill; 2019: chap. 15. http://accessmedicine.mhmedical.com/content.aspx?bookid=2449&sectionid=194439115. Accessed May 10, 2019.

Shane AK, Mody RK, Crump JA, Tarr PI, et al. 2017 Infectious Diseases Society of America clinical practice guidelines for the diagnosis and management of infectious diarrhea. *Clin Infect Dis.* 65(12):1963-1973. https://doi.org/10.1093/cid/cix959

Wilkins T, Sequoia J. Probiotics for gastrointestinal conditions: a summary of the evidence. *Am Fam Physician.* 2017;96(3):170-178.

Yates J. Traveler's diarrhea. *Am Fam Physician.* 2005;71:2095-2100, 2107-2108

A 45-year-old woman presents to your office for an "annual physical examination." She reports that she is very healthy and has no specific complaints. Her past medical history is significant for seasonal allergies and well-controlled, mild, intermittent asthma. She is married and has two children via normal spontaneous vaginal delivery without complication. She takes a multivitamin daily and antihistamines (as needed) and a puff of an albuterol inhaler on occasion. Her family history is significant for hypertension and type 2 diabetes mellitus in her father, depression in her mother and sister, and breast cancer diagnosed in her maternal grandmother at age 72. The patient is married and monogamous, gets regular exercise, and does not smoke cigarettes, drink alcohol, or use illicit drugs. On examination, her blood pressure is 129/79 mm Hg, pulse is 74 beats/min and regular, height is 67 inches, weight is 152 pounds, body mass index is 23.8 kg/m^2, and abdominal waist circumference is 32 inches. Her physical examination is unremarkable.

▶ What screening test(s) for cardiovascular disease should be recommended for this patient?
▶ What screening test(s) for other chronic diseases should be recommended for this patient?
▶ What screening test(s) for cancer should be recommended?
▶ What immunization(s) should be recommended?

ANSWERS TO CASE 11:

Adult Female Health Maintenance

Summary: A 45-year-old woman presents with

- Desire for an annual health maintenance examination (HME)
- A history of seasonal allergies and mild, intermittent asthma
- Medications include multivitamin daily and antihistamines (as needed) and occasionally, an albuterol inhaler
- Normal vital signs and healthy lifestyle
- Family history significant for hypertension and type 2 diabetes mellitus in her father, depression in her mother and sister, and breast cancer diagnosed in her maternal grandmother at age 72

Recommended screening tests for cardiovascular disease: Blood pressure measurement (screening for hypertension); height, weight, body mass index, and abdominal waist circumference measurements (screening for obesity); nonfasting lipid measurement (screening for hyperlipidemia).

Recommended screening tests for other chronic diseases: Fasting glucose or hemoglobin A_{1c} (screening for diabetes mellitus); hepatitis C screening for adults ages 18–79; depression screening; intimate partner violence screening.

Recommended screening tests for cancer: Mammography per interval (screening for breast cancer); Papanicolaou (Pap) smear, with or without high-risk human papilloma virus testing, per interval (screening for cervical cancer).

Recommended immunizations: Tetanus toxoid, reduced diphtheria toxoid, and acellular pertussis vaccine (Tdap) if she has not had one after the age of 11 and then a tetanus-diphtheria (Td) or Tdap vaccine every 10 years; influenza vaccine annually (per season); 23-valent pneumococcal polysaccharide vaccination (PPSV-23) if she has not had it before because of her history of asthma; hepatitis A and B vaccine series if indicated.

ANALYSIS

Objectives

1. List the elements of the evidence-based adult well female health maintenance examination (HME). (EPA 1, 12)

2. Describe the recommended screening tests and immunizations for adult women. (EPA 3, 12)

3. Counsel patients in ways to be healthier and improve health outcomes. (EPA 10, 12)

Considerations

The patient described is a 45-year-old woman who presents for an annual HME. In women aged 20 to 34 years, unintentional injuries are the leading cause of mortality.

In women aged 35 to 54 years, cancer is the leading cause of mortality. In women 55 years of age and older, heart disease is the leading cause of mortality. Shared decision-making is imperative when providing women with age-appropriate strategies for cardiovascular and chronic disease screening, cancer screening, and immunization updates.

Recommended adult immunizations are discussed in Case 1, tobacco use is discussed in Case 7, and screening and treatment for sexually transmitted infections are discussed in Case 45. The interventions discussed in this chapter are primarily based on recommendations of the United States Preventive Services Task Force (USPSTF); recommendations of other expert panels or advocacy organizations are included where appropriate.

APPROACH TO:
Health Maintenance in Women

DEFINITIONS

BRCA: Abbreviation for genes associated with breast cancer and ovarian cancer. Mutations in the *BRCA-1* or *BRCA-2* genes can be associated with a three- to seven-fold increased risk for breast cancer, along with increased risks of ovarian, tubal, peritoneal, and possibly other types of cancer.

USPSTF RECOMMENDATION GRADES: Grades created by the USPSTF after reviewing current evidence regarding screening tests; these consist of recommendations in five categories (A, B, C, D, I) based on the strength of evidence and benefit of a screening test.

WOMEN'S HEALTH INITIATIVE: A research program sponsored by the National Institutes of Health to address the most common causes of morbidity and mortality in postmenopausal women. This initiative included clinical trials of the effect of hormone therapy on the development of heart disease, fractures, and breast cancer.

CLINICAL APPROACH

Screening for Cardiovascular Disease

Many of the cardiovascular disease risk factors in women are the same as those in men but are often underappreciated with relation to morbidity and mortality risks; these risk factors include hypertension, high low-density lipoprotein cholesterol, tobacco use, diabetes mellitus, and family history of cardiovascular disease. The **USPSTF screening recommendations for cardiovascular disease for women are similar to those for men.** All women aged 18 and older should be screened for hypertension by the measurement of blood pressure (Grade A recommendation). The USPSTF recommends screening all women aged 40-75 periodically for dyslipidemia. The American Heart Association and the American College of Obstetricians and Gynecologists recommend routine lipid screening for all women.

An area of cardiovascular disease risk unique to women is in postmenopausal hormone replacement. Hormone replacement therapy is sometimes used for relief of vasomotor symptoms ("hot flashes"). Studies such as the Women's Health Initiative have shown **increased rates of adverse cardiovascular outcomes in women taking either estrogen alone or combined estrogen and progesterone.** These risks include an increased risk of coronary heart disease, stroke, and venous thromboembolic disease. For this reason, the use of hormone replacement therapy for the prevention of chronic conditions is not advised (Grade D), and **any use of hormone replacement should be of the lowest effective dose for the shortest effective time period.**

Screening for Breast Cancer

Breast cancer is second to lung cancer in number of cancer-related deaths in women. There are over 200,000 new cases and over 40,000 deaths per year from breast cancer in the United States. Incidence increases with age; other risk factors include having the first child after the age of 30, menarche before age 12 or menopause after age 55, a family history of breast cancer (particularly if in the mother or sister), personal history of breast cancer or atypical hyperplasia found on a previous breast biopsy, or a known carrier of the BRCA-1 or BRCA-2 gene.

The process of screening for breast cancer generally includes consideration of three modalities: the breast self-examination (BSE), the clinical breast examination (CBE) performed by a health care professional, and mammography. The USPSTF has determined that there is insufficient evidence to recommend CBE (Grade I) and recommends against teaching BSE (Grade D). These recommendations suggest that BSE offers no significant mortality benefit and may lead to unnecessary anxiety, biopsies, and false-positive test results. Clinicians are recommended to encourage women to be familiar with how their breasts normally appear and feel and to report any changes to their health care provider. The evidence regarding CBE suggests that as the sole screening modality it may have good detection rates, yet its benefits in conjunction with mammography are limited.

The USPSTF advises screening with mammography beginning at the age of 50 years, with a recommended interval of every 2 years (Grade B). For women aged 40 to 49, biennial screening should be an individual decision and take into account the patient's values regarding the benefits and harms (Grade C). The American Cancer Society, American Academy of Family Physicians, and American College of Obstetricians and Gynecologists advocate offering patients annual or biennial mammography starting at age 40 years and strongly encourage annual mammography after the age of 50 years. Beyond the age of 75 years, continuation of screening should be individualized based on the overall health status and probability of death from other conditions prior to the expected benefits from detection of breast cancer.

Screening for Cervical Cancer

Mortality rates from cervical cancer have decreased dramatically in recent decades as a direct result of routine cervical cancer screening via Pap smear (cytology). Risk factors for cervical cancer include early onset of sexual intercourse, multiple sexual partners, human papilloma virus (HPV) infection with high-risk subtypes of HPV (16, 18, 45, 56), and tobacco use.

Pap Smear. For any woman with a cervix, the USPSTF recommends that cervical cancer screening with Pap smear should begin at age 21 years regardless of sexual activity and should be repeated at 3-year intervals. For women over the age of 30 years desiring a longer interval between tests, cotesting for HPV can be used in conjunction with or without cytology once every 5 years (Grade A). Since the likelihood of a positive test result is higher with HPV cotesting (better sensitivity at the cost of more false positives), women should be made aware of the possibility of frequent and ongoing testing if they persistently test positive for HPV. Abnormal results should be followed per current guidelines.

Screening Intervals. **Most cases of cervical cancer occur in women who either have not been screened in over 5 years or did not have follow-up after an abnormal Pap smear.** The optimal screening interval therefore is based on providing the maximum benefit from treatment of precancerous lesions, while preventing overtreatment of HPV-related pathology that may have otherwise resolved spontaneously. Since the development of a cancerous lesion is a prolonged process, and at times treatment of cervical abnormalities is not without harm in terms of future childbearing potential, screening prior to age 21 years (regardless of sexual activity) is not recommended (Grade D).

Discontinuing Screening. For women who have had a hysterectomy for any reason other than cervical cancer, screening should be discontinued (Grade D). Women who have had a hysterectomy with retention of cervix (supracervical hysterectomy) should follow the recommendation for age-appropriate routine screening. The USPSTF recommends cessation of cervical cancer screening at age 65 years in women who have had three consecutive negative Pap results or two consecutive negative HPV results within the last 10 years (Grade D). An individualized approach should be implemented in women who have previously been treated for precancerous lesions or those who have never been tested before.

HPV Vaccination. HPV infection is the most significant cause of all cervical cancers. A vaccine against high-risk HPV subtypes is available as a two-shot series for children/adolescents who initiate the series between ages 9 and 14 and as a three-injection series for those receiving the vaccination at age 15 or older. It is indicated for use in both males and females aged 9 through 45. To date, there is no recommendation to alter the Pap smear screening intervals for women who have been vaccinated against HPV.

Screening for Osteoporosis

Osteoporosis is a condition of decreased bone mineral density associated with an increased risk of fracture. **One-half of all postmenopausal women will have an osteoporosis-related fracture in their lifetime.** Common osteoporotic fractures include hip and vertebral fractures, which are associated with higher risks of loss of independence, institutionalization, and mortality. The risk of osteoporosis is increased with advancing age, tobacco use, low body weight, poor nutrition, Caucasian or Asian ancestry, family history of osteoporosis, low calcium intake, and sedentary lifestyle.

Bone Density Measurement. Screening for osteoporosis is performed by measurement of bone density in the greater trochanter and lumbar spine via dual-energy x-ray absorptiometry (DEXA). Measurement of bone density is compared to the bone density of young adults, and the result is reported as standard deviation from the mean bone density of the young adult (T-score). **Osteoporosis is present if the patient's T-score is at or below −2.5** (ie, measurement of the patient's bone density is more than 2.5 standard deviations below the young adult mean); **osteopenia** is present if the T-score is between −1.0 and −2.5. The USPSTF recommends screening for osteoporosis via DEXA in women over the age of 65 years and considering screening in women younger than 65 years with higher risk of osteoporosis-related fractures (Grade B). There is no current recommendation on repeating screening if the initial test is normal. See Case 58 for a discussion of medications used for the prevention and treatment of osteoporosis.

Screening for Depression and Intimate Partner Violence

Depression screening is recommended if there are systems in place for ensuring accurate diagnosis, treatment, and follow-up (Grade B). Because of the prevalence of these disorders, screening and support are important.

Estimates indicate that between 1 and 4 million women are **sexually, physically, or emotionally abused by an intimate partner** each year. Women are also much more likely to be abused by an intimate partner than are men. Multiple factors are associated with intimate partner violence and include young age, low-income status, pregnancy, mental illness, alcohol or substance use by victims or partners, separated or divorced status, and a history of childhood sexual/physical abuse. The USPSTF recommends that providers should screen women between the ages of 14 and 46 years for evidence of physical, sexual, or psychological abuse by a current or former partner and to appropriately refer those with positive screens to interventional services (Grade B). There are many different screening tools available, including HITS (Hurt, Insult, Threaten, Screen), HARK (Humiliation, Afraid, Rape, Kick), and STaT (Slapped, Things, and Threaten) screens. Most of these are three- to four-item questionnaires with very high sensitivity and specificity and are available in both English and Spanish. Documentation and treatment of injuries, counseling, and information regarding protective services should be provided when domestic violence is suspected. Reporting of domestic violence is mandatory in several states; be aware of the requirements of your state.

CASE CORRELATION

- See also Case 1 (Adult Male Health Maintenance), Case 7 (Tobacco Use and Cessation), Case 22 (Vaginitis and Other Vaginal Infections), and Case 58 (Osteoporosis).

COMPREHENSION QUESTIONS

11.1 A 21-year-old woman presents for her first Pap smear. She completed the HPV vaccine series by age 19. Assuming that her examination and Pap smear results are normal, when would you recommend that she return for a follow-up Pap smear?

A. In 6 months, as the first Pap smear should be repeated within a year to reduce a potential false-negative result

B. In 1 year, as she is higher risk of cervical cancer because of her age

C. In 3 years, as the Pap smear was normal

D. In 5 years, as she is at low risk because she received the HPV vaccine

11.2 A 32-year-old G2 P1 woman is pregnant at 12 weeks' gestation. She is being seen for her prenatal visit. As you examine her, you note some bruises on her arms and neck area. She looks down at the floor and is tearful when you ask about these bruises. She confides that her husband has been violent toward her. Which of the following factors is associated with an increased risk of intimate partner violence in this patient?

A. Pregnancy

B. Older age

C. Higher income

D. Married status

11.3 Which of the following statements regarding breast cancer screening is true?

A. Breast self-examinations have been shown to decrease mortality rates

B. Clinical breast examinations in conjunction with routine mammography have been shown to improve mortality rates.

C. Most abnormalities found on routine mammography are not breast cancer.

D. Since breast cancer rates increase in older women, there is no upper age at which breast cancer screening may be discontinued.

11.4 A 48-year-old woman presents for an annual examination. She has had a supracervical hysterectomy and Pap smears with HPV cotesting every 5 years since her 20s and all were normal. She read on the Internet that women who have had a hysterectomy no longer require Pap smears. Which of the following would be your advice?

A. "You no longer need to get Pap smears since you have had a hysterectomy."

B. "You should continue to have Pap smears every 3 years since your hysterectomy is an indication to shorten the interval for testing."

C. "You should continue to have Pap smears with HPV cotesting every 5 years since your hysterectomy does not exclude you from routine screening recommendation in your age group."

D. "You should continue with annual Pap smears until the age of 50. If they are all normal, you can stop having them at that time."

ANSWERS

11.1 **C.** Per the USPSTF, screening for cervical cancer should begin at age 21 years and be repeated at 3-year intervals. After age 30, patients can be offered 5-year testing intervals (answer D) if they elect for HPV testing with or without cytology. Six-month (answer A) and one-year (answer B) intervals are inappropriate and not part of routine screening recommendations for women with normal Pap smears. The use of HPV vaccine is not an indication to alter cervical cancer screening recommendations at this time.

11.2 **A.** Intimate partner violence can occur in any relationship, but the risk is increased in certain situations, which include young age, low-income status, pregnancy, mental illness, alcohol or substance use by victims or partners, separated or divorced status, and a history of childhood sexual/physical abuse. The other answer choices (answer B, older age; answer C, higher income; and answer D, married status) are the opposite of risk factors.

11.3 **C.** Most abnormalities seen on mammography are not cancerous. They may, however, require further imaging studies, testing, or biopsy. BSE (answer A) has not been definitively shown to reduce cancer mortality. CBE (answer B) may be of benefit but likely does not impact outcome if mammography is available. The age to consider discontinuation of mammography screening (answer D) should be individualized based on the woman's risk factors and overall health status.

11.4 **C.** Women who have had a hysterectomy with removal of the cervix for benign indications can discontinue Pap smear screening. Women who still have a cervix, with or without a uterus (answer A), should continue with screening for cervical cancer as per screening recommendation for their age group. Cervical cancer screening can be discontinued at age 65 years if the patient has had adequate screening for the last 10 years, which is defined as three consecutive normal Pap smears or two consecutive normal cotesting screens, with the most recent one being in the last 5 years. A hysterectomy is not an indication for more frequent testing (answer B). Pap smears are not indicated yearly (answer D).

CLINICAL PEARLS

▶ Cancer and cardiovascular disease pose the greatest mortality risk for women in America.

▶ Risk factors for cardiovascular diseases in women need to be managed as aggressively as they are in men.

▶ Human papilloma virus infection is the most significant cause of all cervical cancers. An HPV vaccine is available; however, vaccination status has no bearing on cervical cancer screening recommendations.

▶ Women of childbearing age should be screened for intimate partner violence.

REFERENCES

American Cancer Society. *Cancer Facts & Figures 2018*. Atlanta, GA: American Cancer Society; 2018.

American College of Obstetricians and Gynecologists. Breast cancer risk assessment and screening in average-risk women. *Obstetrics and Gynecology*; 2017;30(1):e1-e16.

Centers for Disease Control and Prevention. *HPV Vaccine*. Atlanta, GA: Centers for Disease Control and Prevention; 2014.

Centers for Disease Control and Prevention. Leading causes of death. https://www.cdc.gov/nchs/fastats/leading-causes-of-death.htm. Accessed April 30, 2020.

United States Preventive Services Task Force (USPSTF). BRCA Related Cancer: Risk Assessment, Genetic Counseling, and Genetic Testing. August 20, 2019. https://www.uspreventiveservicestaskforce.org/uspstf/recommendation/brca-related-cancer-risk-assessment-genetic-counseling-and-genetic-testing. Accessed April 30, 2020.

United States Preventive Services Task Force (USPSTF). Recommendations for primary care practice. https://www.uspreventiveservicestaskforce.org/uspstf/topic_search_results?topic_status=P&searchterm=. Accessed April 30, 2020.

Women's Health Initiative. https://www.nhlbi.nih.gov/science/womens-health-initiative-whi. Accessed April 30, 2020.

A 25-year-old man presents to your office on a Monday morning with ankle pain. He was playing in his usual Saturday afternoon basketball game when he injured his right ankle. He says that he jumped for a rebound and landed on another player's foot. His right ankle "rolled over," he fell to the floor, and his ankle immediately started to hurt. He did not hear or feel a pop. He was able to stand and walk with a limp, but he was unable to continue playing. His ankle swelled over the next day in spite of rest, icing, and elevation. He suffered no other injury from the fall. On examination, he is a healthy-appearing man with normal vital signs. The lateral aspect of the right ankle is swollen. The right ankle has normal dorsiflexion and plantar flexion, and there is no focal tenderness to palpation of the fibula, malleoli, or foot. No ligamentous laxity is noted on testing. He can bear weight with minimal pain. There is normal sensation and capillary refill in the foot. The remainder of his examination is normal.

▶ What is the most likely diagnosis of this injury?
▶ What further diagnostic testing is needed at this time?
▶ What is the most appropriate therapy?

ANSWERS TO CASE 12:

Musculoskeletal Injuries

Summary: A 25-year-old man presents with

- An inversion injury of his right ankle that occurred during a basketball game
- A swollen ankle but with the ability to bear weight
- No focal tenderness and no ligament laxity

Most likely diagnosis: Sprain of the right ankle.

Further diagnostic testing needed: None at this time.

Most appropriate therapy: "PRICE" therapy: Protection, Rest, Ice, Compression, and Elevation; a nonsteroidal anti-inflammatory drug (NSAID) or acetaminophen as needed for pain and early mobilization.

ANALYSIS

Objectives

1. Describe the diagnostic approach to musculoskeletal injuries. (EPA 1, 2)

2. Describe when to order imaging tests and which test to order to evaluate musculoskeletal complaints. (EPA 3)

3. Describe how to manage common musculoskeletal injuries and scenarios. (EPA 4)

Considerations

Ankle sprains are the most common acute, sports-related injury, and they are a common reason for visits to primary care providers, urgent care centers, and emergency departments. As in this case, **most ankle sprains are the result of landing on an inverted foot that is plantar flexed,** such as landing on another player's foot in basketball, stepping in a hole or on uneven ground when running, or missing a curb while walking. Management of ankle sprains are geared toward decreasing pain and swelling, speeding recovery, providing appropriate ankle support, and protecting against a recurrence of the sprain in the future. An easy way to remember the cornerstone of management of ankle sprains is by the mnemonic PRICE.

APPROACH TO:

Musculoskeletal Injuries

DEFINITIONS

OTTAWA ANKLE RULES: A decision model designed to aid a provider in determining which patients with ankle injuries need an x-ray.

PRICE: A mnemonic to remember how to treat musculoskeletal injuries. The letters stand for the following: Protection from further injury, relative Rest, Ice to reduce swelling and pain, Compression, and Elevation to reduce edema.

SPRAIN: A stretching or tearing injury of a **ligament.**

STRAIN: A stretching or tearing injury of a **muscle** or **tendon.**

CLINICAL APPROACH

Pathophysiology

More than 20,000 people sprain their ankles every day in the United States. The lateral ankle is injured much more commonly than the medial ankle, with around 85% of all sprains involving the lateral structures. This is because the bony anatomy of the tibiotalar joint and the very strong deltoid ligament complex protect the medial ankle from injury. The lateral ligaments responsible for resistance against inversion and internal rotation—anterior talofibular ligament (ATFL), calcaneofibular ligament (CFL), and posterior talofibular ligament (PTFL)—are relatively weaker and more commonly injured. The **ATFL is the most commonly injured ligament,** followed by the CFL. Some common risk factors include previous ankle fracture, excess body weight, and an unconditioned body.

Ankle sprains are graded as grade 1, 2, or 3 according to degree of severity. A grade 1 sprain is characterized by a stretch of a single ligament, most commonly the ATFL, but with minor swelling, no mechanical instability, and without significant loss of function. The patient can usually bear weight with, at most, mild pain. The history and examination of the patient in the case presented is consistent with a grade 1 ankle sprain. A grade 2 sprain represents a partial ligamentous tear. This injury causes more severe pain, swelling, and bruising. There is mild-to-moderate joint instability, significant pain with weight-bearing, and loss of range of motion (ROM). A grade 3 sprain is a complete ligamentous tear. This injury causes significant joint instability, swelling, loss of function, and inability to bear weight.

Clinical Presentation

As in all areas of medicine, the history of the presenting illness will guide the diagnostic workup. Examination of the musculoskeletal system should include documentation of inspection, palpation, ROM, strength, neurovascular status, and, where appropriate, testing specific for the involved joint.

History. In the history of a patient with musculoskeletal complaints, important information to gather includes whether the primary symptom is pain, limited movement, weakness, instability, or a combination of symptoms. The onset of the symptoms—whether acute, chronic, or an acute worsening of a chronic problem—can be significant. The location, severity, and pattern of radiation of pain should be delineated. Associated symptoms, such as numbness, should be identified. Efforts should be made to identify as specifically as possible the mechanism of any injury that led to the complaint. Interventions that have already been made, such as ice or heat, medications, splinting, and whether or not the interventions helped, should be noted.

Physical Exam. **Inspection** should note the presence of swelling, bruising, deformity, and the use of any supports or assistive devices (eg, splints, crutches, bandages) that the patient is already using. **Examination of the unaffected limb can provide a good comparison and allow for subtle changes to be more easily identified.** Documentation should also be made of the patient's general functioning and mobility—Does the patient walk with a limp? Can the patient easily rise from a chair? Is there difficulty getting on the examining table? Is the patient's arm moving freely or held tightly to the patient's chest? and so on.

Palpation. **Palpation** of the affected and surrounding areas can help to localize and confirm the presence of a specific injury. A focal area of bony tenderness may lead to the consideration of a fracture, whereas a tender, tight muscle may be more suggestive of a strain. The presence of joint effusions or soft-tissue swelling should be documented and may lead to consideration of specific injuries. Notation should be made of sensation, peripheral pulses, and capillary refill in the involved extremity. Absent pulses and delayed capillary refill, especially if the extremity is cool or cold, should prompt emergent evaluation and management of vascular insufficiency.

Range of Motion. **Range of motion** should be tested both passively and actively. Active ROM tests the patient's ability to move a joint. It tests the structural integrity of the joint, muscles, tendons, and neurologic impulses to the area and can be limited by problems with any of them or by the presence of pain. Passive ROM tests the movement that an examiner can elicit in a relaxed patient. The presence of a dislocated joint or significant joint effusion may lead to limitations in both passive and active ROM, where a torn tendon or muscle injury may have limited active, but preserved passive, ROM. Tables 12–1, 12–2, and 12–3 list differential diagnosis, physical examination findings, and management for common musculoskeletal complaints.

Imaging. Following the history and examination, the provider must decide when it is necessary to perform x-rays or other imaging tests. Validated decision rules include the Ottawa ankle rules for the determination of when an x-ray is necessary in an ankle injury. The Ottawa ankle rules have been validated for nonpregnant adults who have a normal mental status, no other significant concurrent injury, and are evaluated within 10 days of the injury. When properly applied, the **Ottawa ankle rules have a sensitivity approaching 100% in ruling out significant malleolar and midfoot fractures.** These rules state that x-rays of the ankle should be performed if there is bony tenderness of the posterior edge or tip of the distal 6 cm of either the medial or lateral malleolus; tenderness in the midfoot coupled with point tenderness over the bony aspects of base on fifth metatarsal or the navicular; or if the patient is unable to bear weight immediately or when examined. Negative findings on Ottawa ankle rules safely eliminate the need for an x-ray. The patient presented, who has no bony tenderness, no limitation in weight-bearing, and no contraindication to the application of the decision rules, does not need imaging of his ankle or foot. These rules, however, have a specificity of 30% to 50%, indicating that positive findings do not necessarily confirm a fracture, but confirm the need for x-ray to evaluate the possibility of a fracture. **In general, bony tenderness and severe restriction in motion after injury are signs that an x-ray would be helpful in diagnosis.**

Table 12–1 • LOWER EXTREMITY PAIN

Differential Diagnosis	Pertinent Historical Clues	Physical Examination	Diagnostic/Treatment Plan
Ligament sprain	ACL injury associated with loud pop and acute swelling of anterior knee Meniscus tear acute from twisting injury or chronic from repetitive motion; report knee "locking up" (as part of torn cartilage flips into knee joint during ambulation)	Anterior knee swelling for ACL and joint line tenderness for meniscus injury, tender on collaterals if MCL or LCL tear *Special tests* for increased ligament laxity. **Laxity of ligament when compared to contralateral joint can be a sign of a torn ligament:** Lachman's—ACL: flex knee to 20 degrees, stabilize upper leg, and pull forward on tibia Anterior drawer—ACL: flex knee to 90 degrees, pull forward on upper tibia while stabilizing upper leg McMurray—Menisci: flex knee past 90 degrees, abduct and externally rotate lower leg, feeling for palpable clunk on medial meniscus as you fully extend the leg from initial position; for lateral meniscus, start with knee adducted and internal rotated Valgus—MCL: 30-degree knee flexion, medial-directed force on knee, lateral-directed force on ankle Varus—LCL: 30-degree knee flexion, lateral-directed force on knee, medial-directed force on ankle Anterior drawer for ATFL of ankle: stabilize ankle with one hand and pull forward on heel with other hand	*Short term:* PRICE (protection, rest, ice, compression, and elevation)/NSAIDs Protect (air stirrup brace for ankle, knee immobilizer) *X-ray:* Follow Ottawa rules for ankle and knee *Long term:* Stabilization, strengthening, PT; consider MRI if not improved in 6 weeks of conservative care Ligament tears frequently require surgical repair

(Continued)

Table 12–1 • LOWER EXTREMITY PAIN (continued)

Differential Diagnosis	Pertinent Historical Clues	Physical Examination	Diagnostic/Treatment Plan
Tendon rupture or muscle strain	Acute injury	Ecchymosis, edema, erythema, tenderness Lack of movement of associated muscle: patellar tendon rupture—lack of quadriceps extension Achilles tendon rupture associated with lack of plantar flexion (Thompson test)	*Short term:* RICE (rest, ice to reduce swelling and pain, compression, and elevation) NSAIDs; consider x-ray. Tendon rupture often requires surgical repair *Long term:* Stabilization, strengthening, PT; MRI if not improved in 6 weeks of conservative care
Septic joint (emergency)	Acute timeline, fever, joint pain and swelling, and decreased mobility: recent skin infection or joint surgery	Edema, erythema, tenderness, warmth to palpation	Ultrasound Joint aspiration and fluid analysis for WBCs, Gram stain and culture, crystal analysis, intravenous antibiotics, and surgical debridement
Osteoarthritis of knee and hip	Chronic pain	Knee crepitus, restricted ROM Hip examination elicits groin pain on **F**lexion, **A**bduction, and **E**xternal **R**otation (FABER test)	Acetaminophen, NSAIDs, weight loss if overweight Joint steroid or hyaluronic acid injections PT with straight leg raises for quad strengthening Joint replacement for lifestyle-limiting chronic pain

Abbreviations: ACL, anterior cruciate ligament; LCL, lateral collateral ligament; MCL, medial collateral ligament; MRI, magnetic resonance imaging; NSAIDs, nonsteroidal anti-inflammatory drugs; PT, physical therapy; ROM, range of motion; WBC, white blood cell.

Table 12–2 • SHOULDER PAIN

Differential Diagnosis	Pertinent Historical Clues	Physical Examination	Diagnostic/ Treatment Plan
Rotator cuff tear or tendinopathy, which can cause impingement syndrome when involving supraspinatus muscle Impingement syndrome refers to narrowing of the space between the head of the humerus and the acromion, which then causes pain	Acute injury: hurts to sleep on shoulder, especially with acute rotator cuff tears	Swelling and tenderness Passive maneuvers to check for impingement: Hawkins test: pain with passive flexion of shoulder to 90 degrees and internal rotation (brings the head of the humerus closer to the acromion to exacerbate impingement syndrome) Neers test: abduct and internally rotate shoulder to elicit pain; Hawkins is more sensitive and specific than Neers Empty can test: resisted abduction of both arms with thumbs pointed down; arms are placed in 90-degree abduction and 30-degree forward flexion prior to testing muscle strength; weakness suggests supraspinatous tendinopathy	Therapy includes steroid injection into the subacromial space or glenohumeral joint to decrease the effect of the subacromial bursitis and supraspinatus tendonopathy PT may be required Consider MRI if not improved with conservative care in 6 weeks Surgery is saved for recalcitrant cases and involves decompression of the narrowed space by cutting part of the acromion
Bicipital tendonitis	Acute or chronic injury	Speeds test: pain with resisted biceps flexion—patient palm up and elbow flexed 20 degrees and arm forward flexed to 60 degrees; provider pushes down on forearm as patient forward flexes	NSAIDs, PT, *avoid* steroid injection into tendons
Osteoarthritis	Chronic swelling, pain, stiffness	Crepitus, grinding, with or without edema	Acetaminophen/ NSAIDs Joint steroid injection PT with rotator cuff strengthening
Frozen shoulder (adhesive capsulitis): fibrous adhesions form in the joint capsule due to lack of motion, further impeding motion	Chronic shoulder pain and severe restriction in motion, especially abduction and internal rotation; predisposing history may include underlying rotator cuff injury or severe osteoarthritis limiting motion	Even passive motion is met with restriction and pain—restriction in active motion, especially forward flexion and internal rotation, which cannot be corrected with passive motion	Joint steroid injections followed by PT and strengthening exercises Osteopathic manipulation also helps increase range of motion Recalcitrant cases may require surgery involving manipulation of the shoulder under anesthesia to break up the fibrous adhesions

Abbreviations: MRI, magnetic resonance imaging; NSAIDs, nonsteroidal anti-inflammatory drugs; PT, physical therapy.

Table 12–3 • LUMBAR PAIN			
Differential Diagnosis	Pertinent History	Physical Examination	Diagnostic/ Treatment Plan
Spondylolisthesis: slippage of the vertebral body posterior to the vertebral body above it	Repetitive backward bending as in gymnastics	Mild-to-moderate tenderness on palpation of spinous process	Lumbar x-ray, *avoid* bed rest and overexertion
Osteoarthritis of lumbar spine (degenerative disk disease)	Older age or early arthritis as a consequence of motor vehicle accident or other trauma to back	Stiffness in lumbar flexion and sometimes decreased ROM to less than 75 degrees of lumbar flexion	Stabilization, strengthening via home exercises or PT Consider imaging if not improved in 6 weeks
Spinal stenosis: narrowing of the spinal canal as occurs with facet arthropathy, hypertrophy, spondylosis associated with advanced arthritis	Pain improves with bending forward (lumbar flexion) as this action opens the spinal canal	Pain improves with bending forward (lumbar flexion)	Stabilization, strengthening, PT MRI if not improved in 6 weeks of conservative care Consider surgical decompression of lumbar spine if severe pain
Herniated lumbar disk with or without radiculopathy	Pain worsens with lumbar flexion (bending forward, sitting, lifting leg up from sitting or supine position)	Perform SLR: provider raises straightened leg of patient to increase lumbar flexion; positive SLR is pain shooting down leg to below the knee; SLR test has high sensitivity for herniated disk	Avoid overexertion, but avoid extended bed rest as this worsens condition; NSAIDs, stabilization, PT (McKenzie exercises) Consider imaging if not improved in 6 weeks of conservative care Consider surgical diskectomy if severe
Thoracic or lumbar strain	Acute injury: patient felt "pull on back" when lifting or pulling object	Tenderness to palpation; muscle spasms with overlying edema and warmth during acute phase Palpation reveals muscle spasms with texture of a tight rope down the back and is often cool to touch when pain becomes chronic	Avoid overexertion, but avoid extended bed rest as this worsens condition; NSAIDs, stabilization, strengthening, home exercises, or PT Imaging if not improved in 6 weeks of conservative care
Cauda equina syndrome	History of herniated disk or back injury with sudden onset of bowel or bladder incontinence, saddle anesthesia, and severe limp	Loss of rectal tone, decreased sensation in the groin and perianal area (saddle anesthesia); severe limp	Emergent MRI and emergent neurosurgical consultation to prevent paralysis from occurring

(Continued)

Table 12–3 • LUMBAR PAIN (continued)			
Differential Diagnosis	Pertinent History	Physical Examination	Diagnostic/ Treatment Plan
Malignancy: may be primary (eg, multiple myeloma) OR metastatic	Weight loss, advanced age, severe back pain, possible history of pathological fractures	Severe bony tenderness in spine (which may be present due to bony lytic lesions or pathologic fractures)	Blood work: elevated protein X-ray/MRI/bone scan Multimodal treatment for the malignancy
Infectious etiology (diskitis: spinal disk infection or osteomyelitis)	Fever and severe pain Direct or hematogenous spread from infectious source (wound, ulcer, etc)	Fever, bony tenderness at site of infection	Blood work: elevated WBCs and ESR X-ray and/or MRI of involved area with or without biopsy and culture Intravenous antibiotics; consider diskectomy or surgical debridement

Abbreviations: ESR, erythrocyte sedimentation rate; MRI, magnetic resonance imaging; MVA, motor vehicle accident; NSAID, non-steroidal anti-inflammatory drug; PT, physical therapy; ROM, range of motion; SLR, straight leg raise; WBC, white blood cell.

When a decision is made to perform an imaging test, whether to acutely rule out a fracture or to evaluate an injury that is failing to improve, the **initial imaging study of choice is the plain x-ray.** At minimum, an x-ray series should include at least two views at 90-degree angles to each other. In patients with normal x-rays and continued symptoms despite an adequate trial of conservative management or who have suspected disk, ligament, or tendon injuries, magnetic resonance imaging (MRI) has largely supplanted other modalities as the imaging method of choice. MRI is highly sensitive and specific for articular or soft-tissue abnormalities, including ligament, tendon, and cartilage tears.

Treatment

PRICE. The initial management of most acute sprains and strains is PRICE—protection from further injury, relative rest, ice to reduce swelling and pain, compression, and elevation to reduce edema. **Protection** by appropriate splinting or casting can help to prevent further injury. Although initial **rest** during the acute phase marked by maximal pain and swelling is common sense, evidence has shown that prolonged rest is in fact inferior to early functional mobilization. Additionally, ROM exercises started early in the recovery period allow for a quicker recovery and return to activities than otherwise. **Ice** applied as soon as possible after the injury helps to minimize swelling and relieve pain. Cryotherapy is now recommended in the first 3–7 days for short-term pain relief and improved functionality. **Compression and elevation** with an air stirrup brace with an elastic compression wrap also promote reduction of swelling. In most cases, NSAIDs or acetaminophen are adequate for pain control, with narcotics used only if intolerance or contraindication to other medications exists.

Mobilization. Numerous studies showed that early mobilization of injured ligaments actually promotes healing and recovery. ROM exercises should be started at 48 to 72 hours after injury in patients with sprains and strains. For lower extremity injuries, protected weight-bearing with orthotics is allowable, with advancement to unsupported weight-bearing as tolerated. Crutches may be necessary initially because of painful weight-bearing. Lace-up or semirigid ankle supports have been shown to be superior to tape and elastic bandages and provide stability to the injured ankle.

The **most common cause of persistently stiff, painful, or unstable joints following sprains is inadequate rehabilitation.** All patients with musculoskeletal injuries should be educated on the importance of rehabilitative exercises and avoiding bed rest. When possible, handouts with a specific exercise program should be given to the patient when the patient is evaluated. If the patient is unsuccessful in accomplishing this on his own, referral for a formal physical therapy program can be beneficial.

Surgery. Surgery is rarely needed for sprains, and its use is controversial even in the presence of chronic pain or persistent functional instability. Surgery for ankle sprains has been shown to increase stiffness in the joint, lead to longer recovery times, and result in impaired mobility when compared to conservative treatment only; however, it is the joint that may require surgery after conservative therapy if there is persistent instability, for example. In general, surgical consideration should be a last resort when all else has failed and should be discussed in a case-by-case manner.

CASE CORRELATION

- See also Case 37 (Limping in Children) and Case 58 (Osteoporosis).

COMPREHENSION QUESTIONS

12.1 A 57-year-old man with well-controlled diabetes presents to the office with more than 3 months of right shoulder pain. He notes that he stopped moving it because it hurt to do so after he hit his shoulder. He can no longer raise his arm. You are the first health care provider he has told about this. On examination, he can actively forward flex his left shoulder to 180 degrees but cannot abduct right arm past 110 degrees. With passive ROM, you cannot abduct his right shoulder past 135 degrees, as you meet strong resistance. He is also restricted in internal rotation. He has pain when you flex his shoulder to 90 degrees with internal rotation and has decreased strength with arm abduction against resistance. The rest of the examination is unremarkable. A shoulder x-ray in your office is normal. What would you recommend as initial therapy?

A. Ibuprofen taken regularly for 6 weeks

B. Glenohumeral steroid joint injection followed by 3 weeks in a sling

C. Glenohumeral steroid joint injection followed by physical therapy

D. MRI and manipulation of shoulder under anesthesia

12.2 A 38-year-old woman who works as a cashier on her feet all day has gradually developed pain in the medial aspect of her left knee. She says the knee sometimes buckles or locks up on her, and the medial side of the knee swells by the end of the day. On examination, she has a slight limp, medial joint line tenderness, and a positive McMurray sign. Her examination is otherwise unremarkable, with normal Lachman and varus/valgus testing. What is her most likely diagnosis?

    A. Medial collateral ligament (MCL) injury

    B. Anterior cruciate ligament (ACL) injury

    C. Medial meniscus tear

    D. Lateral meniscus tear

12.3 A 45-year-old pipe fitter complains of severe back pain after heavy lifting this morning. Sharp, shooting pain radiates down his right leg, especially when he is sitting. He has no loss of bowel or bladder function and no saddle anesthesia. On examination, he has a significant right-sided limp, tenderness at the L4/L5 intervertebral disk at the level of the iliac crest on the right side, and lumbar flexion limited to 45 degrees secondary to pain. Extension is normal. Muscle strength is 5/5 on the left and 4/5 on the right secondary to pain; reflexes are 2+ and equal bilaterally. Sensation is decreased on the lateral calf of the right leg. The supine straight leg raise (SLR) is positive at 30 degrees for re-creating the radiculopathy down his right leg. What is your initial management?

    A. Since the pain is severe, start an oral narcotic and order a lumbar x-ray.

    B. Start NSAIDs and physical therapy.

    C. Complete bed rest for 6 weeks until pain free.

    D. Stat MRI and referral for emergent surgical intervention.

ANSWERS

12.1 **C.** This patient has a frozen shoulder (adhesive capsulitis) with the underlying cause related to an injury that stopped him from moving his shoulder. He may have an underlying rotator cuff impingement, as evidenced by a positive Hawkins maneuver. The goal in management is to improve pain and restore motion. Glenohumeral steroid injection will help pain but is not adequate by itself. It should be followed by immediate mobilization and physical therapy. The joint should not be immobilized in a sling (answer B). MRI and surgical manipulation (answer D) may be appropriate options later if he does not improve with the initial management. Ibuprofen (answer A) is not sufficient treatment for this condition.

12.2 **C.** Medial joint line tenderness with a positive McMurray test is consistent with a diagnosis of medial meniscus tear, which can be a chronic or acute injury. It is unlikely that the patient had an ACL tear (answer B), as she did not have acute injury with immediate large swelling at her anterior knee.

MCL injury (answer A) is less likely since valgus stress testing is negative. MCL injury will also not cause the locking up of the knee, which is caused as a flap of torn cartilage from the meniscus flips inside the patellofemoral joint. Lateral meniscus tears (answer D) are less common than medial meniscus tears and would present with pain or tenderness at the lateral aspect.

12.3 **B.** This patient likely has a herniated lumbar disk secondary to a heavy lifting injury, as evidenced by aggravated pain with lumbar flexion as occurs with sitting or during supine SLR. First-line management is NSAIDs or acetaminophen and physical therapy exercises. NSAIDs are used if there are no contraindications, such as a peptic ulcer. Complete bed rest (answer C) will worsen back pain and increase risks of deep venous thrombosis. There are no red flags for emergent MRI or surgery (answer D). In the absence of red flag signs, conservative management for 6 weeks with physical therapy is warranted before obtaining imaging studies. Answer A (oral narcotic and lumbar x-ray) is not warranted and can lead to a patient becoming habituated on opioids; nonopioid anti-inflammatory agents should be tried first.

CLINICAL PEARLS

▶ A complete history and physical examination is essential in diagnosing and treating musculoskeletal injuries.

▶ Use the uninjured, contralateral extremity as a comparison for your examination of an injured extremity.

▶ Always be sure to examine the joint above and below the site of injury.

▶ Order x-rays with at least two views at 90 degrees to each other; otherwise, you may miss a fracture.

▶ The mainstay of treatment is early remobilization and therapy to improve muscle strength, flexibility, endurance, and proprioception.

▶ PRICE is a mnemonic to remember how to treat musculoskeletal injuries and stands for protection from further injury, relative rest, ice to reduce swelling and pain, compression, and elevation to reduce edema.

REFERENCES

Brigham and Women's Hospital, Department of Rehabilitation Services. Standard of care: ankle sprain. 2010. https://www.brighamandwomens.org/assets/BWH/patients-and-families/rehabilitation-services/pdfs/ankle-sprain-bwh.pdf. Accessed April 30, 2020.

Burbank KM, Stevenson JH, Czarnecki GR, Dorfman J. Chronic shoulder pain: part I. Evaluation and diagnosis. *Am Fam Physician.* 2008;77:453-460.

Burbank KM, Stevenson JH, Czarnecki GR, Dorfman J. Chronic shoulder pain: part II. Treatment. *Am Fam Physician.* 2008;77:493-497.

Childress MA, Beutler A. Management of chronic tendon injuries. *Am Fam Physician*. 2013: 87(7):486-490.

Hockenberry RT, Sammarco GJ. Evaluation and treatment of ankle sprains. *Phys Sports Med*. 2001;29(2):57-64.

Jones BQ, Covey CJ, Sineath MH, Nonsurgical management of knee pain in adults. *Am Fam Physician*. 2015:92(10):875-883.

Monica J, Vredenburgh Z, Korsh J, Gatt C. Acute shoulder injuries in adults. *Am Fam Physician*. 2016;94(2):119-127.

Ramirez J. Adhesive capsulitis: diagnosis and management. *Am Fam Physician*. 2019;99(5):297-300.

Tiemstra JD. Update on acute ankle sprains. *Am Fam Physician*. 2012;85(12):1170-1176.

Trojian TH, McKeag DB. Ankle sprains: expedient diagnosis and management. *Phys Sports Med*. 1998;26(10):29-40.

Will JS, Bury DC, Miller JA. Mechanical low back pain. *Am Fam Physician*. 2018;98(7):421-428.

A 45-year-old woman presents to your office concerned about a "mole" on her face. She says that it has been present for years, but her husband has been urging her to have it checked. She denies any pain, itching, or bleeding from the site, and the mole has not changed in size. She has no significant past medical history, takes no medications, and has no allergies. She has no history of skin cancer in her family. She is an accountant by occupation.

On examination, the patient is normotensive, afebrile, and in no distress. The physical examination reveals a nontender, symmetric, 4-mm papule that is uniformly reddish-brown in color and located in the right nasolabial fold region. The lesion is well circumscribed, and the surrounding skin is normal in appearance. There are no other lesions in the area.

► What is the most likely diagnosis?
► What features indicate a benign versus malignant condition?
► What is your next step?

ANSWERS TO CASE 13:
Skin Lesions

Summary: A 45-year-old healthy woman presents with

- No significant past medical history
- A skin lesion that is symmetric, with well-defined borders, relatively small (< 6 mm), and with uniform coloration
- No obvious growth of the skin lesion and no history of itching or bleeding at the site
- No family history of skin cancer

Most likely diagnosis: Benign nevus.

Features indicating benign versus malignant condition: Signs that are reassuring of a benign condition include:

- Size less than 6 mm
- Symmetric, uniform color
- Well-defined borders

Malignancy would be indicated by larger size, asymmetric appearance and irregular borders.

Next step: Reassurance and surveillance.

ANALYSIS

Objectives

1. Describe an approach to the evaluation of skin lesions. (EPA 1, 2)
2. Describe the features of a skin lesion in dermatologic terms. (EPA 1)
3. Describe which features of a lesion are typically benign and which are concerning for malignancy or potential malignancy. (EPA 1, 10)

Considerations

This case represents a typical scenario seen in primary care medicine: "I have this mole. Is it cancer?" Although simplified, this is what the patient is most concerned about and wants to know. The **role of the provider is to determine the likelihood of malignancy or premalignancy and to define a course of action that is appropriate.** In this particular case, there are several features that reassure a benign condition that can be monitored without the need for a biopsy. There was neither a family medical history of skin cancer nor a history of skin cancer in the patient. She has an occupation that does not expose her to harmful chemicals or the sun on a regular basis. On examination, the lesion has typically benign features (size < 6 mm, symmetric, uniform color, well-defined borders).

In this case, it would be appropriate to make a note (or possibly even a photograph) in the patient's chart describing the characteristic features of the lesion and monitor for changes in the lesion at periodic health evaluations. The patient should also be educated in self-examination of the skin, with an emphasis on what to look for and when to come to the clinician's office for an evaluation of a new or changing skin lesion. Finally, it should be understood that many otherwise benign-appearing moles might have an atypical characteristic that warrants further investigation.

The **criteria that are used to predict the likelihood of a benign versus malignant lesion are only guidelines;** to be sure, not all malignant skin lesions present in the same manner, and a malignant melanoma is not always visibly pigmented. The bottom line is that all tools available should be used—the history of present illness, medical history of the patient, the family medical history, social and occupational history, and a pertinent review of systems—to arrive at a conclusion that is consistent with the physical examination.

APPROACH TO:
Skin Lesions

DEFINITIONS

ABSCESS: A closed pocket containing pus.

BULLA: A blister greater than 0.5 cm in diameter (plural: bullae).

CYST: A closed, saclike, membranous capsule containing a liquid or semisolid material.

MACULE: A discoloration on the skin that is neither raised nor depressed.

NODULE: An elevated mass of rounded or irregular shape that is greater than 1 cm in diameter.

PAPULE: A small, circumscribed elevated lesion of the skin that is less than 1 cm in diameter.

PLAQUE: A plateau-like, raised, solid area on the skin that covers a large surface area in relation to its height above the skin.

ULCER: A lesion through the skin or mucous membrane resulting from loss of tissue.

VESICLE: A small blister less than 0.5 cm in diameter.

CLINICAL APPROACH

Epidemiology

There has been an increase in the morbidity and mortality of skin cancer in the past few decades in the United States. The American Academy of Dermatology estimated that almost 192,000 new cases of melanoma would be diagnosed in 2019, and the incidence is increasing. When considering nonmelanoma skin cancers, including basal cell carcinoma (BCC) or squamous cell carcinoma, approximately 5.5 million new cases of skin cancer are diagnosed annually.

The **single most important risk factor for the development of skin cancer is expo-sure to natural and artificial ultraviolet (UV) radiation.** It is also one of the only risk factors that can be avoided, and avoiding it can potentially prevent millions of new cases of skin cancer every year. Other risk factors include a prior history of skin cancer; a family history of skin cancer; fair skin; red or blonde hair; a propensity to burn easily; chronic exposure to toxic compounds such as creosote, arsenic, or radium; and a suppressed immune system.

Pathophysiology

Melanoma In Situ. No invasion has occurred in this type of melanoma, as the malig-nant melanocytes are localized to the epidermis. If diagnosed early, this type of lesion should be excised with 5- to 10-mm borders.

Superficial Spreading Melanoma. This is the **most common type of melanoma** in both sexes. As its name implies, this lesion spreads superficially along the top layers of skin before penetrating into the deep layers. The superficial, or radial, growth phase is slower than the vertical phase, which is when the lesion grows into the dermis and can invade other tissues or metastasize. Men are more commonly affected on the upper torso, whereas women are affected mostly on the legs. Common clinical features include raised borders, comprised of dark and light brown color, and also sometimes pinks, whites, grays, or blues.

Lentigo Maligna. Similar to the superficial spreading type, this lesion is **most often found in the elderly (commonly diagnosed in the seventh decade of life),** usually on chronic sun-damaged skin such as the face, ears, arms, and upper trunk. It is the **least common of the four types of melanoma.** Clinically, they are characterized as tan-to-brown lesions with very irregular borders.

Amelanotic Melanoma. This is an uncommon (less than 5%) melanoma that is nonpigmented and can clinically present as many other types of noncancerous con-ditions, including eczema, fungal infections, or basal or squamous cell carcinoma. Because of its lack of pigmentation, this type of melanoma usually remains undiag-nosed until a more invasive stage as compared to other melanomas.

Acral Lentiginous Melanoma. This lesion is similar to the other two superficial melanomas in that it begins in situ, but it differs in many ways. This is the **most common melanoma found in African Americans and Asians.** This melanoma is usu-ally found under the nails, on the soles of the feet, and on the palms of the hands; common clinical features include flat, irregular lesions that are dark brown to black.

Nodular Melanoma. This melanoma, unlike the others, is usually invasive at the time of diagnosis. This is the **most aggressive and second most common type of mela-noma** (Figure 13–1). It is clinically characterized as mostly black, but occasionally brown, blue, gray, red, or tan, lesions that arise from nevi or normal skin.

Clinical Presentation

In 1985, it was noted by clinicians studying melanoma that there were several char-acteristic features of skin lesions that correlated with melanoma. Specifically, color variegation, border irregularity, asymmetry, and size greater than 6 mm in diameter were consistently observed with melanoma. This led to the **ABCD acronym,** which has been used extensively to determine the likelihood of a cancerous skin lesion (Table 13–1).

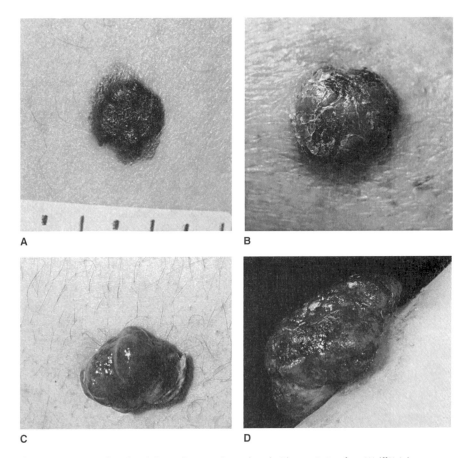

A   B

C   D

Figure 13–1. **Examples of nodular melanoma.** Reproduced with permission, from Wolff K, Johnson R, Saavedra AP, et al., eds. *Fitzpatrick's Color Atlas and Synopsis of Clinical Dermatology,* 8th ed. 2017. Copyright © McGraw Hill LLC. All rights reserved.

Table 13–1 • CLASSIC ABCDE CRITERIA FOR SUSPICIOUS SKIN LESIONS			
Acronym	**Characteristic**	**More Likely Benign**	**More Likely Malignant**
A	Asymmetry	Symmetric (right half looks like left half)	Asymmetric (in > 2 axes)
B	Borders	Well defined	Ragged or blurred
C	Color	Uniform color	Variegated (2 or more colors)
D	Diameter	< 6 mm (6 mm = size of pencil eraser)	> 6 mm
E	Elevation Evolving	Flat surface Stable in size and appearance	Raised surface Enlargement, changes in thickness, or bleeding

One other criterion that is often used is the change in the size or appearance of the skin lesion. This is sometimes cited as E in the ABCD criteria and referred to as evolving and elevation. Benign lesions may present at birth, or any time thereafter, and several benign lesions may also present near the same point in time. However, a benign lesion, once present, will usually remain stable in size and appearance, whereas a malignancy will present as increasing in size or changing in appearance. Thus, it is useful to ask whether a "mole" has recently changed in appearance or has grown in size.

The "ugly duckling sign" may guide physical examination of skin lesions, as it is easy to remember and teach. Simply, as the name suggests, this alludes to the blatantly different appearance of the melanoma as compared to the other lesions the patient may have.

Another procedure that may aid the detection of melanoma in the family care provider's office is dermoscopy. This is a magnification technique by which a skin lesion can be visualized for more detail regarding its pigment and structure. The dermascopic properties of a lesion may guide management in terms of either observing its evolution or performing a biopsy for further evaluation.

Treatment

Benign nevi need only be monitored visually. The patient can accomplish this after education on what to look for and when to come back for reevaluation.

Excision. In general, any preexisting nevus that has changed or any new pigmented lesion that exhibits any of the ABCDE signs should be excised completely with a 2- to 3-mm margin around the lesion. Larger lesions that may be cosmetically difficult to completely excise may be biopsied in several areas. If the pathology indicates a malignancy, the lesion should then be completely excised with appropriate margins by a physician trained in plastic surgical technique. Complete excision of malignant melanomas requires at least a 5 mm, and sometimes larger, margin. Once a patient has been identified as having a malignant skin lesion, the patient should be observed on an annual basis for any new or changing skin lesions. Excisional biopsies with narrow margins should be performed for suspicious lesions. If the entire lesion cannot be removed due to size or location, biopsies should be taken from the most suspicious parts of the lesion.

Prognosis. The prognosis of a patient with melanoma is based on the TNM stage of the disease. T stands for thickness in millimeters, N for the presence of metastatic lymph nodes, and M for the presence of distant metastases.

Prevention. Prevention is aimed at reducing exposure to UV radiation. When possible, avoid the sun between 10 AM and 4 PM; wear sun-protective clothing when exposed to sunlight; wear a sunscreen with a sun protection factor (SPF) of at least 15; and avoid artificial sources of UV radiation. The US Preventive Services Task Force (USPSTF) recommends behavioral counseling of young adults, adolescents, children, and parents of young children regarding minimizing exposure to UV radiation to reduce risk of skin cancer (Grade B). For adults over the age of 24, the USPSTF recommends selective counseling for those with fair skin types to reduce exposure to UV radiation (Grade C). The USPSTF, however, finds insufficient evidence to assess the balance of benefits and harms routine screening with whole-body examination in the general population for the early detection of skin cancer in adults (Grade I). It should be kept in mind that these recommendations are for the general population. Special populations, including those with family history of skin cancers, prior history of benign or malignant cancer, and other risk factors, should be examined and managed appropriately on an individual basis.

Nonmelanoma Skin Cancers

Both basal cell and squamous cell carcinomas arise from the epidermal layer of the skin. The primary risk for these types of skin cancers is exposure to UV radiation, not only sun exposure but also tanning bed use. A history of actinic keratoses and human papillomavirus infection of the skin also raises the risk of squamous cell carcinomas.

Basal cell carcinomas (BCCs) are the most common of all cancers. They typically appear as pearly papules, often with a central ulceration or with multiple telangiectasias. Patients typically present with a growing lesion and sometimes complain that it bleeds or itches. BCCs rarely metastasize but can grow large and can be locally destructive. The primary treatment is excision.

Squamous cell carcinomas have a higher rate of metastasis than BCCs, but the risk is still low. These lesions are often irregularly shaped plaques or nodules with raised borders. They are frequently scaly, ulcerated, and bleed easily. Complete excision is the treatment of choice.

CASE CORRELATION

- See also Case 1 (Adult Male Health Maintenance), Case 11 (Adult Female Health Maintenance), and Case 48 (Fever and Rash).

COMPREHENSION QUESTIONS

13.1 A 36-year-old man is noted to have a bothersome "mole" that on biopsy reveals malignant melanoma. The pathologist comments that this histology is a very rare type of melanoma and usually escapes diagnosis until a more advanced stage. Which of the following is the most likely diagnosis?

  A. Melanoma in situ

  B. Superficial spreading melanoma

  C. Amelanotic melanoma

  D. Nodular melanoma

13.2 A 73-year-old woman presents to the office due to concern about several tan-colored moles on her arms, face, and ears that have progressively grown over the past 6 months. Upon further examination, the moles are determined to be between 6 and 8 mm with very irregular borders. The clinician decides to obtain an excisional biopsy. Which of the following skin lesions should the provider be most suspicious of based on the history and physical examination?

A. Benign nevus

B. Superficial spreading melanoma

C. Lentigo maligna melanoma

D. Acral lentiginous melanoma

13.3 A 45-year-old African American woman presents for a routine examination. You notice a 9-mm diameter lesion on the palm of her right hand that is dark black and slightly raised and has a notched border. When asked about it, she says that it has been present for about a year and is growing. A friend told her not to be concerned because, "Black people don't get skin cancer." Which of the following is your advice?

A. Her friend is correct, and this is nothing to worry about.

B. While anyone can get skin cancer, this lesion has primarily benign features and can be safely observed.

C. This lesion is suspicious for cancer, but this is most likely a metastasis from breast cancer.

D. This lesion is suspicious for a primary melanoma and needs further evaluation immediately.

13.4 A 70-year-old woman presents for evaluation of a lesion on her left cheek. It has been present for several months. It is slowly enlarging and bleeds if she scratches it. On examination, you find a 7-mm diameter, pearly appearing papule with visible telangiectasias on the surface. Which of the following is the appropriate management of this lesion?

A. Close observation and reexamination in 3 months

B. Reassurance of the benign nature of the lesion

C. Excision

D. Local destruction by freezing with liquid nitrogen

ANSWERS

13.1 **C.** Amelanotic melanoma is an uncommon type of melanoma and because of the lack of pigmentation, it often goes undiagnosed until it is more invasive and has progressed to an advanced stage. Answer A (melanoma in situ) is an intraepithelial lesion (stage 0) and consists of pigmented neoplastic cells that have not yet spread and therefore would not be advanced. Answer B (superficial spreading melanoma) is the most common type of melanoma (accounting for about 70% of cases) and spreads horizontally before penetrating deeper; therefore, it is less likely to metastasize. Answer D (nodular melanoma) is a dangerous and rapidly growing type of melanoma that is responsible for about half of melanoma deaths; although it is one that is advanced at the time of diagnosis, this is more due to its rapid growth than "escaping detection." Nodular melanomas are not rare and account for 15% of melanomas.

13.2 **C.** Lentigo maligna is most often found in the elderly, usually on chronic sun-damaged skin such as the face, ears, arms, and upper trunk. Think of this type as tan-colored lesions on sun-damaged skin that have very irregular borders. A benign nevus (answer A) would typically have regular, well-defined borders. Answer B (superficial spreading melanoma) is usually a slow-growing lesion and would not be as consistent with the history of a more rapidly progressive lesion. Answer D (acral lentiginous melanomas) usually presents on the extremities, soles, and hands and under the nails.

13.3 **D.** The lesion described is suspicious for an acral lentiginous melanoma, which commonly occurs on the extremities, such as the palms and soles, and needs immediate evaluation. While skin cancers are more common in persons with lighter skin, they can occur in persons with any skin color or tone; acral lentiginous melanomas especially have a higher risk in more darkly pigmented individuals. Therefore, answer A (her friend believes there is nothing to worry about) is incorrect since the lesion may lead to metastases. Answer B (lesion has benign features) is incorrect since the lesion has features that are concerning, such as notched borders and being raised. Answer C (metastatic from breast cancer) would be an unusual presentation as a pigmented lesion. Also, the most common areas for metastases from breast cancer are the chest wall, local lymph nodes, lungs, and liver.

13.4 **C.** The lesion is most likely a BCC, which is the most common type of skin cancer, and should be treated with excision. BCCs appear as red patches, open sores, or shiny bumps with rolled edges or central indentation. They often occur on sun-exposed parts of the body. The description of a smooth, pearly tumor with telangiectasia is also a classic description. While the likelihood of metastatic spread is low, these lesions can grow and be locally destructive. The lesion does not appear to be benign (answer B) and should not merely be observed (answer A). Local destructive techniques (answer D) are best for the extremity or trunk because hypertrophic scars or hypopigmentation may occur; thus, local destructive techniques are usually not used on the face.

CLINICAL PEARLS

▶ The preventable risk factor common to all skin cancers is sun exposure. Recommend that your patients limit exposure to sunlight in the middle of the day, wear appropriate protective clothing, and use sunscreen.

▶ The use of tanning beds is a risk factor for skin cancer.

▶ There is no such thing as a "healthy tan."

▶ Clinicians should be aware that fair-skinned men and women older than 65 years, patients with atypical moles, and those with more than 50 moles constitute known groups at substantially increased risk for melanoma.

▶ Excisional biopsy should be done for any lesion suspicious for melanoma. If the entire lesion cannot be removed due to size or location, full-thickness biopsies should be taken from the most suspicious parts of the lesion.

REFERENCES

Abbasi NR, Shaw HM, Rigel DS, et al. Early diagnosis of cutaneous melanoma: revisiting the ABCD criteria. *JAMA*. 2004;292:2771-2776.

Ebell M. Clinical diagnosis of melanoma. *Am Fam Physician*. 2008;78(10):1205-1208.

Melanoma precursors and primary cutaneous melanoma. In: Wolff K, Johnson R, Saavedra AP, Roh EK, eds. *Fitzpatrick's Color Atlas and Synopsis of Clinical Dermatology*. 8th ed. New York, NY: McGraw Hill. http://accessmedicine.mhmedical.com/content.aspx?bookid=2043&sectionid=154898647. Accessed May 10, 2019.

Rager EI, Bridgeford EP, Ollila DW. Cutaneous melanoma: update on prevention, screening, diagnosis and treatment. *Am Fam Physician*. 2005;72(2):269-276.

Shenenberger DW. Cutaneous malignant melanoma: a primary care perspective. *Am Fam Physician*. 2012;85(2):161-168.

Skin Cancer Foundation. Skin cancer facts & statistics. https://www.skincancer.org/skin-cancer-information/skin-cancer-facts. Accessed May 10, 2019.

Stern RS. Prevalence of a history of skin cancer in 2007: results of an incidence-based model. *Arch Dermatol*. 2010;146(3):279-282.

US Preventive Services Task Force. Skin cancer prevention: behavioral counseling. 2018. https://www.uspreventiveservicestaskforce.org/uspstf/recommendation/skin-cancer-counseling. Accessed May 4, 2020.

US Preventive Services Task Force. Skin cancer screening: 2016. https://www.uspreventiveservicestaskforce.org/uspstf/recommendation/skin-cancer-screening. Accessed May 4, 2020.

A 40-year-old man with no past medical history presents to the clinic to establish care. He reports that he had a urinalysis (UA) 1 week ago that revealed blood as an incidental finding. The UA was done as a standard screening test by his former employer. He denies ever seeing any blood in his urine and denies any voiding difficulties, dysuria, sexual dysfunction, or any history or risk factors for sexually transmitted infections. His review of systems is otherwise negative. He has smoked a half-pack of cigarettes per day for the past 10 years and exercises by jogging 15 minutes and performing lightweight training daily. On examination, his vital signs are normal, and the entire physical examination is unremarkable. A complete blood count (CBC) and a chemistry panel (electrolytes, blood urea nitrogen, and creatinine) are normal. The results of a UA done in your office are as follows: specific gravity, 1.015; pH 5.5; leukocyte esterase, negative; nitrites, negative; white blood cell count (WBC), 0; red blood cell count (RBC), 4 to 5 per high-power field (hpf).

▶ What is the most likely diagnosis?
▶ How would you approach this patient?
▶ What is the optimal workup and plan for this patient?
▶ What are the concerns, and how would you counsel the patient?

ANSWERS TO CASE 14:

Hematuria

Summary: A 40-year-old man presents with

- An incidental finding of RBCs in his urine sample on a UA 1 week ago
- History of smoking a half pack of cigarettes per day for 10 years
- Specific gravity of 1.015; pH 5.5; leukocyte esterase, negative; nitrites, negative; WBC, 0; RBC, 4 to 5 per hpf
- Denial of ever seeing blood in his urine, voiding difficulties, dysuria, sexual dysfunction, or history/risk factors for sexually transmitted infections (STIs)
- Normal vital signs and physical examination

Most likely diagnosis: Asymptomatic microscopic hematuria.

Approach to this patient: Repeat the UA, assess for risk factors and possible reversible causes (eg, urinary tract infection [UTI], vigorous exercise, or recent urologic procedure); perform renal function testing; and then depending on low or high risk of malignancy, perform additional imaging of lower and/or upper urinary tract.

Optimal workup and plan: Rule out infection by performing a urine culture; obtain further history, including exercise routine or recent urologic procedures; perform renal function testing to rule out renal disease. If all of this is negative, evaluate for malignancy by imaging of the upper urinary tract via computed tomographic (CT) urography and the lower urinary tract via cystoscopy.

Concerns and counseling: The primary concern is to rule out malignancy, including renal cell carcinoma and transitional cell carcinoma. Counsel the patient on the importance of an appropriate workup, but reassure the patient about the low prevalence of the condition.

ANALYSIS

Objectives

1. Describe the significance of microscopic hematuria. (EPA 3, 10)
2. Describe an evidence-based approach to work up asymptomatic microscopic hematuria. (EPA 3, 7)
3. Describe the differential diagnosis of microscopic hematuria. (EPA 1, 2, 3)
4. Describe the recommendations for follow-up on patients with hematuria after a negative workup. (EPA 3, 4, 12)

Considerations

This patient has asymptomatic microscopic hematuria, as opposed to gross hematuria. The American Urological Association (AUA) defines significant microscopic hematuria as > 3 RBCs/hpf on UA with microscopy. Although he is asymptomatic, this patient deserves a thorough workup in order to determine an etiology, if possible, and to rule out malignancy. The management guidelines differ in the workup of microscopic hematuria with less than 3 RBCs/hpf versus more than 3 RBCs/hpf.

The patient's history should be reviewed with specific questions to determine any risks for STIs, occupational exposures to chemicals, strenuous exercise, drugs, medications, and herbal/nutritional supplements. For a result of < 3 RBCs/hpf, a UA should be repeated three times at 6-week intervals. If these are negative (consistently < 3 RBCs/hpf), the workup is complete, and the patient should be reassured. For a primary result of > 3 RBCs/hpf, a urine culture should be sent to evaluate for UTI. If a source is found, a repeat UA with microscopy should be done 6 weeks after the etiology has been resolved (for UTI or STI) or the offending agent has been removed (exposure, strenuous exercise, medications, etc).

At this point, if the condition persists, renal function testing should be done to evaluate for possible renal disease. This may include a basic metabolic panel to check the blood urea nitrogen (BUN) and creatinine levels, as well as the glomerular filtration rate. If there are abnormalities in renal function testing, a nephrology referral should be generated immediately. If, however, no renal abnormalities are found or the patient has risk factors for malignancy, imaging with CT urography and cystoscopy should be done. The patient should be informed that a complete workup is necessary to evaluate for conditions such as infections or tumors since as many as 30% to 40% of people with gross hematuria and about 5% of those with microscopic hematuria are found to have a malignancy.

APPROACH TO:
Hematuria

DEFINITIONS

GROSS HEMATURIA: The presence of enough blood in a urine sample to be visible to the naked eye.

LOWER URINARY TRACT: The urinary bladder and urethra.

MICROSCOPIC HEMATURIA: The presence of three or more red blood cells per hpf on two or more properly collected UAs.

UPPER URINARY TRACT: The kidneys and ureters.

CLINICAL APPROACH

Epidemiology

Asymptomatic Microscopic Hematuria. The prevalence of asymptomatic microscopic hematuria is roughly 2% to 31% in the adult population in the United States. There are many possible causes; risk factors should guide the specific workup for the individual patient. Although some elements of the workup are standard for everyone, other more detailed and expensive tests can be deferred for those at low risk. The presence of significant proteinuria, red cell casts, renal insufficiency, or a predominance of dysmorphic RBCs in the urine should prompt an evaluation for renal parenchymal disease or referral to a nephrologist. In general, glomerular bleeding is associated with more than 80% dysmorphic RBCs, whereas lower urinary tract bleeding is associated with more than 80% normal RBCs.

Bladder Cancer. Because of the possibility of bladder cancer, the AUA recommends that a single positive result for hematuria on UA with microscopy warrants further workup. There are certain risk factors that are associated with a higher probability of bladder cancer that should be explored and should serve as an impetus for timely and efficient workup and referrals. Risk factors include smoking, occupational exposure to chemicals or dyes (benzenes or aromatic amines), history of gross hematuria, age over 40 years, history of urologic disorder or disease, history of irritative voiding symptoms, history of UTI, analgesic abuse, or history of pelvic irradiation.

Pathophysiology

Hematuria is divided into glomerular, renal (nonglomerular), and urologic etiologies. Glomerular hematuria typically is associated with significant proteinuria, erythrocyte casts, and dysmorphic RBCs. Renal (nonglomerular) hematuria is secondary to tubulointerstitial, renovascular, and metabolic disorders. Like glomerular hematuria, it often is associated with significant proteinuria; however, there are no associated dysmorphic RBCs or erythrocyte casts. Urologic causes of hematuria include tumors, calculi, infections, trauma, and benign prostatic hyperplasia (BPH). Urologic hematuria is distinguished from other etiologies by the absence of proteinuria, dysmorphic RBCs, and erythrocyte casts.

Gross Versus Microscopic Hematuria. Hematuria in adults should first be defined as gross hematuria or microscopic hematuria. Gross hematuria denotes that the patient is able to visualize blood in his voided specimen. Patients most often describe their urine as having a reddish or brownish color. Patients are commonly concerned about malignancy or kidney stones. In contrast, microscopic hematuria is usually asymptomatic and often discovered incidentally. **Although malignancy may be found in 5% of adults with asymptomatic microscopic hematuria, the United States Preventive Services Task Force (USPSTF) advises that there is insufficient evidence to recommend for or against routine screening for bladder cancer (Grade I).** Hematuria can be measured quantitatively by any of the following methods:

- Determination of the number of RBCs per milliliter of urine excreted (chamber count)
- Direct examination of the centrifuged urinary sediment (sediment count)
- Indirect examination of the urine by dipstick (the simplest way to detect microscopic hematuria)

Given the limited specificity of the dipstick method (65% to 99% for 2-5 RBCs per high-power microscopic field), the initial **finding of hematuria by the dipstick method should be confirmed by microscopic evaluation of urinary sediment.** The limited specificity is due to the fact that the urine dipstick lacks the ability to distinguish RBCs from myoglobin or hemoglobin.

Clinically significant microscopic hematuria is defined as three or more RBCs per hpf on microscopic evaluation of urinary sediment from a properly collected specimen. The initial determination of microscopic hematuria should be based on microscopic examination of urinary sediment from a freshly voided, early morning, clean-catch, midstream urine specimen. Urine must be refrigerated if it cannot be examined promptly because delays of more than 2 hours between collection and examination often cause unreliable results.

Urinary Sediment Evaluation. Evaluation of the **urinary sediment** can allow for the diagnosis of patients with renal parenchymal disease. This analysis **will often also allow for distinction between glomerular disease and interstitial nephritis.** The presence of red blood cell casts and dysmorphic RBCs is suggestive of renal glomerular disease. Interstitial nephritis, often caused by analgesics or other drugs, is suggested by the presence of eosinophils in the urine.

Transient Hematuria. A complete evaluation for microscopic hematuria starts with a detailed history and physical examination, appropriate laboratory testing, and imaging of the upper and lower urinary tract. If the UA with microscopy shows significant microscopic hematuria, further history should be obtained to rule out benign causes such as menstruation, strenuous exercise, recent urologic procedures, medications, and the like. If a probable cause is determined, UA with microscopy should be repeated 6 weeks after discontinuation of the cause.

If the repeat UA is negative and the patient remains asymptomatic, no further workup is required for low-risk patients. Transient microscopic hematuria can be caused by sexual intercourse, heavy exercise, a recent digital prostate examination, other urologic procedures, or contamination by menses. The repeat UA should be done after avoidance of any of these potential confounders. Exercise-induced hematuria usually resolves spontaneously in 72 hours in the absence of other coexisting conditions. In addition, careful attention should be taken in women to ensure the blood is not from the vaginal or rectal areas. In men, one should also exclude local trauma to the foreskin. If in doubt, a catheterized specimen should be obtained, taking care not to induce trauma during the procedure.

Laboratory Studies. The laboratory studies should start with UA with microscopy and evaluation of centrifuged urinary sediment. The urine should be examined for number of RBCs per hpf, dysmorphic RBCs, and presence of casts and eosinophils. UTI should be ruled out by urine culture. A serum creatinine level should also be obtained to assess renal function, with comparison to old records if available. If the laboratory evaluation reveals elevated creatinine or red blood cell casts, the workup should focus on renal parenchymal disease and possible etiologies, such as hypertension, diabetes, or autoimmune diseases. Referral to a nephrologist should be considered. Renal biopsy may be appropriate for certain individuals. Patients with risk factors should also undergo cytologic evaluation of the urine to assess for transitional cell carcinoma. Although voided urine cytology may not pick up low-grade carcinoma, it is fairly reliable for high-grade lesions, especially if repeated.

Imaging. Numerous options exist for imaging of the upper urinary tract. Despite many studies comparing the radiographic methods, there are no evidence-based guidelines on which modality is most efficient. Choice of imaging modality should take into account any contraindications the patient may have, including renal insufficiency, contrast allergy, or pregnancy. CT urography (with and without intravenous contrast) has high sensitivity and specificity for imaging the upper urinary tract and is generally the initial modality of choice unless a contraindication exists. Urine cytology and urine markers should only be used in patients with risk factors for bladder cancer.

The lower urinary tract should be examined by cystoscopy for transitional cell carcinoma in all patients who are older than 35 years or who present with risk factors for lower urinary tract malignancies. In the absence of risk factors in selected patients younger than 35 years or with a negative history, examination, laboratory workup, and upper tract imaging, cystoscopy may be deferred or individualized at the discretion of the treating provider.

Treatment

If an infection is present, it should be appropriately treated and the UA repeated in 6 weeks. If the **hematuria resolves with treatment of the UTI, no further workup is needed.**

In patients with a thorough but negative workup, UA with microscopy should be repeated annually for two consecutive years. For those with persistent asymptomatic microscopic hematuria, the AUA recommends repeat evaluation within 3–5 years of the initial evaluation. For those with two consecutively negative results on annual UA with microscopy, workup can be stopped. However, if the patient develops gross hematuria, voiding difficulties, pain, or any abnormal cytology, immediate urologic reevaluation and urologic consultation is warranted. Patients who develop hypertension, proteinuria, glomerular casts, or abnormal renal function should be referred to a nephrologist for consultation.

CASE CORRELATION

- See also Case 16 (Male Genitourinary Conditions) and Case 45 (HIV, AIDS, and Other Sexually Transmitted Infections).

COMPREHENSION QUESTIONS

14.1 A 60-year-old man with past medical history of BPH presents to you with painless gross hematuria for 1 day. He states this has never happened before and denies strenuous exercise. Upon further questioning, he reveals that 2 days ago he had a bladder catheterization to evaluate his postvoid residual. He denies smoking, family history of cancers, or chemical exposures. Which of the following is the most appropriate management at this time?

   A. Counsel patient on the high likelihood of gross hematuria after a urologic procedure and that this will likely subside. Let him know no test is required today.

   B. Do a urine dipstick first. If blood is present, then proceed to UA with microscopy and have patient return in a few weeks for a repeat UA with microscopy.

   C. Discuss with patient the high likelihood of malignancy with gross hematuria especially given his age and past history and recommend imaging upper and lower urinary tracts.

   D. Tell him that he likely needs urine cytology today to rule out malignancy.

14.2 A 54-year-old postmenopausal woman with past medical history of hypertension is incidentally found to have significant microscopic hematuria on a UA that was done as part of her annual hypertension labs. She denies dysuria, gross hematuria, fevers, chills, nausea, and vomiting. Her physical examination is negative for suprapubic tenderness and flank pain. What would be the next best step in the management of this patient?

   A. Repeat UA with microscopy in 3 months at her next follow-up visit for hypertension.

   B. Perform a urine culture and if positive, treat immediately. Repeat UA posttreatment.

   C. Order renal function testing to rule out medical renal disease as an etiology.

   D. Repeat UA with microscopy in 6 weeks.

14.3 A 65-year-old man with past medical history of hypertension, coronary artery disease, chronic kidney disease (CKD), and a pacemaker presents to your office with complaint of "dark urine" for many weeks now. He states he has been evaluated by several other clinicians who did "several tests" that all came back negative. He states he has never had any imaging done and would like you to "take a look at what is going on in there." When accessing his medical records, you see that he has already had several UAs with microscopy, which were all positive for microscopic hematuria; renal function testing, which was significant for elevated BUN and creatinine and decreased glomerular filtration rate; and negative urine cultures. At this time, what would be the most appropriate imaging modality and management for this patient?

A. Counsel the patient against imaging at this time, as any imaging may worsen his CKD.

B. Order magnetic resonance urography since the patient is unable to undergo CT urography given his renal insufficiency and urgently refer to urology.

C. Order a combined renal ultrasound and retrograde pyelogram for maximum visualization of the upper urinary tract, along with an urgent urology referral.

D. Order urine cytology and urine markers, as this are the least invasive tests of choice at this time.

ANSWERS

14.1 **B.** Although it is very likely that the patient's hematuria is secondary to the recent urologic procedure, it is not good practice to simply assume the cause and not do appropriate initial evaluation for hematuria (answer A). The initial step in this case would be to do a urine dipstick, which if positive in the office would warrant a UA with microscopy. If this shows 3 or more RBCs per hpf, one would immediately perform a thorough workup. However, if UA with microscopy shows less than 3 RBCs per hpf, the patient should be asked to return in 6 weeks for a repeat UA. It is appropriate to discuss with the patient that his gross hematuria, given his lack of risk factors for malignancy, is most likely caused by the recent bladder catheterization; however, as stated, this is not a reason to dismiss further evaluation. Since there is a probable cause for this patient's hematuria, one would not immediately begin workup to rule out malignancy (answers C and D). Certainly, if his gross hematuria continues after several weeks, it would be imperative to conduct further evaluation.

14.2 **D.** This patient does not have signs or symptoms of a UTI, and additional workup looking for an infection (answer B) will not change management, as asymptomatic bacteriuria need not be treated except in pregnancy. As per the current guidelines, this patient needs a repeat UA with microscopy in 6 weeks before beginning workup to rule out medical renal disease (answer C). A 3-month interval between repeat UA testing (answer A) is not an appropriate interval.

14.3 **C.** This patient has two simultaneous contraindications to imaging modalities preferred in the workup of microscopic hematuria, but not all imaging is contraindicated (answer A). Due to his renal insufficiency, he should not have CT urography, and due to his pacemaker, he should not undergo MRI/ magnetic resonance urography (answer B). For this reason, the next best imaging modality would be a renal ultrasound, which when combined with a retrograde pyelogram would provide maximum information about the upper urinary tract. This would have to be done with a concurrent urology referral. Urine cytology and urine markers (answer D), although noninvasive, are not currently recommended in the routine evaluation of microscopic hematuria.

CLINICAL PEARLS

▶ Hematuria in adults should always be evaluated. If no source is found on a thorough initial workup, patients should be followed for at least 3 years to monitor for an underlying condition.

▶ Hematuria is subdivided into gross hematuria (visible to the naked eye) versus microscopic hematuria.

▶ Microscopic hematuria is defined as more than 3 RBCs/hpf on a properly collected specimen, measured twice.

▶ Microscopic hematuria may be due to infection, inflammation, glomerular diseases, kidney stones, or tumor.

▶ One of the most concerning causes of hematuria is renal cell carcinoma, which is the most common type of primary kidney malignancy.

▶ In every case of a first-time microscopic hematuria, a repeat UA with microscopy is required at a 6-week interval before any other management is done.

REFERENCES

Cohen RA, Brown RS. Microscopic hematuria. *N Engl J Med.* 2003;348:2330-2338.

Davis R, Jones SJ, Barocas DA, et al. Diagnosis, evaluation and follow-up of asymptomatic microhematuria (AMH) in adults: AUA guideline. https://www.auanet.org/guidelines/asymptomatic-microhematuria-(amh)-guideline. Accessed May 9, 2019.

Meng MV, Walsh TJ, Chi TD. Urologic disorders. In: Papadakis MA, McPhee SJ, Rabow MW, eds. *Current Medical Diagnosis & Treatment 2019.* New York, NY: McGraw Hill; 2019: Chap. 23. http://accessmedicine.mhmedical.com/content.aspx?bookid=2449&sectionid=194575332. Accessed May 09, 2019.

O'Connor OJ, McSweeney SE, Maher MM. Imaging of hematuria. *Radiol Clin North Am.* 2008;46:113.

Sharp VJ, Barnes KT, Erickson BA. Assessment of asymptomatic microscopic hematuria in adults. *Am Fam Physician.* 2013;88(11):747-754.

A 27-year-old woman presents to your office complaining of progressing nervousness, fatigue, palpitations, and the recent development of a resting hand tremor. She also states that she is having difficulty concentrating at work and has been more irritable with her coworkers. Additionally, the patient notes that she has developed a persistent rash over her shins that has not improved with the use of topical steroid creams. All of her symptoms have come on gradually over the past few months and continue to get worse. Review of systems also reveals an unintentional weight loss of about 10 lb over 4 weeks, insomnia, and amenorrhea for the past 2 months (the patient's menstrual cycles are usually quite regular). The patient's past medical history is unremarkable, and she takes no oral medications. She does not drink alcohol, smoke, or use any illicit drugs. On examination, she is afebrile. Her pulse varies from 70 to 110 beats/min, and her blood pressure is 138/92 mm Hg. She appears restless and anxious. Her skin is warm and moist. Her eyes show evidence of exophthalmos and lid retraction bilaterally, although fundoscopic examination is normal. Neck examination reveals symmetric thyroid enlargement, without any discrete palpable masses. Cardiac examination reveals an irregular rhythm. Extremity examination reveals an erythematous, thickened rash on both shins. Neurologic examination is normal except for a fine resting tremor in her hands when she attempts to hold out her outstretched arms and brisk deep tendon reflexes. Initial laboratory tests include a negative pregnancy test and an undetectable level of thyroid-stimulating hormone (TSH).

▶ What is the most likely diagnosis?
▶ What imaging study is most appropriate at this time?
▶ What is the definitive nonsurgical treatment of this condition?

ANSWERS TO CASE 15:
Thyroid Disorders

Summary: A 27-year-old woman presents with

- Progressively worsening anxiety, palpitations, tremor, menstrual irregularities, and weight loss
- Unremarkable medical history, no oral medications, and no alcohol, smoking, or illicit drug use
- Exophthalmos and bilateral lid retraction, but normal fundoscopic examination
- Symmetric thyroid enlargement without palpable masses
- Irregular heart rhythm
- Warm, moist skin and an erythematous, thickened rash on both shins
- Normal neurologic examination, except for a fine resting tremor in her hands when she attempts to hold out her outstretched arms and brisk deep tendon reflexes
- Suppressed TSH level, confirming the presence of hyperthyroidism

Most likely diagnosis: Hyperthyroidism secondary to Graves disease.

Most appropriate imaging study: Nuclear medicine thyroid scan with uptake.

Definitive nonsurgical treatment: Thyroid ablation with radioactive iodine.

ANALYSIS

Objectives

1. List the most common conditions that cause hyper- and hypothyroidism and diagnostic strategy. (EPA 2, 3)

2. Interpret the common tests used to evaluate thyroid function. (EPA 3)

3. Describe the modalities of treatment for disorders of the thyroid. (EPA 4)

4. Counsel patients on the significance of their thyroid disease and importance of adherence to treatment. (EPA 4, 12)

Considerations

This patient has symptoms and signs consistent with hyperthyroidism, including warm, moist skin caused by excessive sweating and cutaneous vasodilation; a resting tremor; an enlarged thyroid gland; weight loss; and tachycardia. Her irregular heartbeat may be a manifestation of atrial fibrillation, which occurs in approximately 10% of hyperthyroid patients. Eye abnormalities are common in hyperthyroid states, especially Graves disease. Retraction of the upper lid, resulting in the "thyroid stare" is common. Graves disease has a unique ophthalmopathy that may cause a prominent exophthalmos, which is due to orbital tissue expansion (retro-orbital fibroblasts) (Figure 15–1).

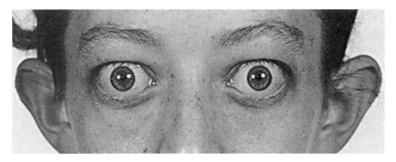

Figure 15–1. Graves ophthalmopathy, also known as "thyroid stare." Reproduced with permission, from Kasper DL, Braunwald E, Fauci A, et al. *Harrison's Principles of Internal Medicine*, 16th ed. 2005. Copyright © McGraw Hill LLC. All rights reserved.

APPROACH TO:
Thyroid Disease

DEFINITIONS

GRAVES DISEASE: An autoimmune thyroid disorder in which autoantibodies to the TSH receptors on the thyroid gland result in hyperfunctioning of the thyroid gland.

THYROID STORM: An acute hypermetabolic state associated with the sudden release of large amounts of thyroid hormone into circulation, leading to autonomic instability and central nervous system dysfunction with symptoms and signs such as arrhythmias, hypertension, high fever, altered mental status, coma, or seizures. This condition has a significant mortality risk. It can be triggered by thyroid or nonthyroid surgery, trauma, infection, iodinated contrast dye, or childbirth.

CLINICAL APPROACH TO HYPERTHYROIDISM

Pathophysiology

The most common cause of noniatrogenic hyperthyroidism is Graves disease, an autoimmune thyroid disorder. Autoantibodies to the TSH receptors on the thyroid gland cause hyperfunctioning of the gland, with the result that the thyroid gland functions outside the usual control of the hypothalamic-pituitary axis. Graves disease commonly occurs in reproductive-age women and is much more common in women than men.

The second most common cause of hyperthyroidism is a benign, autonomous thyroid nodule that secretes thyroxine (T_4). These nodules do not rely on TSH stimulation and continue to excrete large amounts of T_4 despite low or nonexistent circulating TSH levels. Hyperthyroidism can also be caused by the acute release of thyroid hormone in the early stages of thyroiditis. In such cases, symptoms are generally transient and resolve within weeks of onset. Iatrogenic hyperthyroidism can occur secondary to the overuse of T_4 supplementation.

Clinical Presentation

Signs and Symptoms. Hyperthyroidism usually presents with progressive nervousness, palpitations, weight loss, fine resting tremor, diarrhea (hyperdefecation), dyspnea on exertion, difficulty concentrating, and heat intolerance. Physical findings include a rapid pulse rate and elevated blood pressure, with the systolic pressure increased to a greater extent than the diastolic pressure, creating a widened pulse pressure. Examination findings can include atrial fibrillation, a fine resting tremor, and hyperreflexia. Approximately **50% of patients with Graves disease also have exophthalmos.**

Laboratory Values and Imaging. Hyperthyroidism can be diagnosed by a decreased TSH level with a corresponding increased free T_4 level. Once it has been identified, further testing for autoimmune antibodies and radionucleotide scanning of the thyroid can help to determine whether the problem is Graves disease, an autonomous nodule, or thyroiditis. Radionucleotide imaging provides a direct scan of the gland and an indication of its functioning. Imaging is performed using either an isotope of technetium-99m (^{99m}Tc) or iodine-123 (^{123}I). After the administration of one of these agents, imaging the thyroid allows visualization of active and inactive areas, as well as an indication regarding the level of activity in a particular area. **In patients with Graves disease, there will be diffuse hyperactivity** with large amounts of uptake. In contrast, **thyroiditis demonstrates patchy uptake** with overall reduced activity, reflecting the release of existing hormone rather than the overproduction of new T_4. The detection of serum thyroid receptor antibodies is a specific diagnostic test for Graves disease.

Treatment

The treatment of Graves disease includes antithyroid drugs and/or beta-blockers to block some of the peripheral effects of excessive T_4. However, these are only temporary measures used to give patients symptomatic relief.

Radioactive Iodine. The definitive treatment is radioactive iodine, which destroys the thyroid gland. **Radioactive iodine is the treatment of choice for Graves disease in adult patients who are not pregnant.** Radioactive iodine therapy is contraindicated in pregnant women, as the isotope can cross the placenta and cause fetal thyroid ablation. It should also not be used in children or breastfeeding mothers. **At least 40% of patients who receive radioactive iodine eventually become hypothyroid** and will need thyroid hormone replacement.

Antithyroid Drugs. Antithyroid drugs are also well tolerated and successful at blocking the production and release of thyroid hormone in patients with Graves disease. Some examples of these drugs include propylthiouracil (PTU), methimazole, and carbimazole. These drugs work by inhibiting the organification of iodine, and PTU also prevents the peripheral conversion of T_4 to triiodothyronine (T_3), its more active form.

In April 2010, the Food and Drug Administration added a "black box" warning to the labeling of PTU because of the risk of hepatotoxicity. For this reason, methimazole should be considered the first-line agent except when the patient is pregnant. Due to adverse effects on fetal development, methimazole is not used during first trimester of pregnancy. Most experts agree that PTU should be used in the first trimester, and methimazole can be safely used in second and third trimesters. Nevertheless, because of greater experience, PTU remains the preferred agent for pregnant women. Another serious potential side effect of these drugs is agranulocytosis, which occurs in 3 per 10,000 treated patients per year. **Antithyroid drugs are especially useful in treating adolescents,** in whom Graves disease may go into spontaneous remission after 6 to 18 months of therapy.

Surgical Management. Surgery is reserved for patients in whom medications and radioactive iodine ablation are unacceptable treatment modalities or in whom a large goiter is present that is either compressing nearby structures (causing dyspnea, dysphagia, hoarseness, or lightheadedness) or is disfiguring. Surgical removal of the thyroid gland is another option for pregnant patients.

Complications

Thyroid storm is an acute hypermetabolic state associated with the sudden release of large amounts of thyroid hormone into circulation. It occurs most often in patients with Graves disease but can also occur in acute thyroiditis conditions. Symptoms include fever, confusion, restlessness, and psychotic-like behavior. Examination may demonstrate tachycardia, elevated blood pressure, fever, and dysrhythmias. Patients can also have other signs of high-output heart failure, such as dyspnea on exertion and peripheral vasoconstriction, and may exhibit signs of cerebral or cardiac ischemia. **Thyroid storm is a medical emergency** that requires prompt attention and reversal of the metabolic demands of acute hyperthyroidism.

Aggressive initial therapy is essential to prevent complications of thyroid storm. Treatment should include the administration of high doses of PTU or methimazole and beta-blockers (to control tachycardia and other peripheral symptoms of thyrotoxicosis). Hydrocortisone is given to prevent possible adrenal crisis and because it has some effects blocking peripheral conversion of thyroid hormone.

CLINICAL APPROACH TO HYPOTHYROIDISM

Pathophysiology

Several different conditions can cause hypothyroidism. The **most common non-iatrogenic condition causing hypothyroidism in the United States is Hashimoto thyroiditis,** an autoimmune thyroiditis. Iatrogenic causes include post–Graves disease thyroid ablation and surgical removal of the thyroid gland. Another cause is secondary hypothyroidism related to hypothalamic or pituitary dysfunction. These conditions are primarily found in patients who have received intracranial irradiation or surgical removal of a pituitary adenoma.

Clinical Presentation

Signs and Symptoms. Patients with hypothyroidism can present with a wide range of symptoms, including lethargy, weight gain, hair loss, dry skin, slowed mentation or forgetfulness, constipation, intolerance to cold, and a depressed affect. **In older patients, hypothyroidism can be confused with Alzheimer disease** and other conditions that cause dementia. In women, it is often confused with depression. Physical findings that can present in hypothyroid patients include low blood pressure, bradycardia, nonpitting edema, hair thinning or loss, dry skin, and a diminished relaxation phase of reflexes.

Laboratory and Imaging Evaluation. **In primary hypothyroidism, the TSH level is elevated,** indicating insufficient thyroid hormone production to meet metabolic demands. Free thyroid levels are low. The pituitary has increased its TSH release in an attempt to increase the production of thyroid hormones, but the thyroid gland does not respond. In contrast, patients with secondary hypothyroidism have low or undetectable TSH levels. **Once the diagnosis of primary hypothyroidism is made, further imaging or serologic testing is unnecessary if the thyroid gland is normal on physical examination.** In cases of secondary hypothyroidism, however, further testing is needed to determine whether the cause is a hypothalamic or pituitary problem. This can be done by using a thyrotropin-releasing hormone (TRH) test. Endogenous TRH is released by the hypothalamus and stimulates the pituitary to release TSH. When TRH is injected intravenously, a normally functioning pituitary will result in an increase of TSH that can be measured in about 30 minutes. No increase in TSH after injection of TRH suggests a malfunctioning pituitary gland. In cases where pituitary dysfunction is suspected, imaging of the pituitary gland to detect microadenomas and testing of other hormones that are dependent on pituitary stimulation are indicated.

Treatment

Most healthy, nonpregnant adults with hypothyroidism require about 1.6 µg/kg of thyroid hormone replacement daily. The recommendation in patients over 50 years of age is to start with a dose between 25 and 50 µg daily and increase by 25 µg every 3 to 4 weeks until an optimal dose is reached. The same recommendation exists for those younger than 50 with ischemic heart disease. In pregnancy, thyroid hormone replacement needs may increase by approximately 30%. This can be met by having the woman take nine doses of her prepregnancy dose of levothyroxine weekly. A referral to an endocrinologist may also be indicated.

Thyroxine is usually dosed once daily, although some evidence suggests that weekly dosing may also be effective. In patients with an intact hypothalamic-pituitary axis, the adequacy of thyroid replacement can be followed with serial TSH measurements. Evaluation of TSH levels should be performed 4 to 6 weeks after an adjustment in medication has been made. If TSH is > 5 mU/L, underreplacement or nonadherence to medication should be suspected. If underreplaced, increase the levothyroxine dose by 12.5 to 25 µg per day. If TSH < 0.35 mU/L, the patient is being overreplaced, and a daily dose decrease by 25 µg is required. With increased age, thyroid binding decreases as a consequence of a drop in serum albumin level, and the medication dosage may need to be reduced by up to 20%. Annual monitoring of the TSH level in the elderly is necessary to avoid overreplacement.

Screening. Screening asymptomatic adults for thyroid disorder is controversial. The US Preventive Services Task Force reports insufficient evidence for or against routine screening. The American Academy of Family Physicians does not recommend screening in asymptomatic adults. The American Thyroid Association recommends screening all adults age 35 and above every 5 years.

CLINICAL APPROACH TO NODULAR THYROID DISEASE

Epidemiology

Thyroid nodules are more prevalent in women and increase in frequency with age. **Further workup of identified nodules is indicated, as the incidence of malignancy in solitary nodules is estimated at 5% to 6%.** The incidence of malignancy is higher in children, adults younger than 30 or older than 60 years, and patients with a history of head or neck irradiation. Other historical risk factors include a family history of thyroid cancer, the presence of cervical lymphadenopathy, and the recent development of hoarseness of the voice, progressive dysphagia, or shortness of breath.

Pathophysiology

Thyroid nodules, both solitary and multiple, are common and are often found incidentally on physical examination, ultrasonography, or computed tomography. Although their pathogenesis is not clear, nodules are known to be associated with iodine deficiency, higher gravidity, and the ingestion of goitrogens.

Laboratory Values and Imaging. Initial assessment of thyroid nodules should include evaluation of thyroid function and ultrasonography to assess for the size of the nodule. Thyroid function can be assessed by measuring the TSH level. Ultrasonography is the imaging test of choice for assessment of the size of a thyroid nodule, its characteristics (solid or cystic), the overall size of the thyroid, and the presence of other nodules that may not have been previously identified.

Functional adenomas that present with hyperthyroidism are rarely malignant. These represent less than 10% of all nodules. A patient who has a thyroid nodule and is found to be hyperthyroid should have a radioactive iodine uptake study to confirm functionality of the nodule.

Nodules measuring greater than 1 cm by ultrasonography in a person with a normal or elevated TSH require biopsy. This can be done by fine-needle aspiration (FNA), which is a highly sensitive test. Ultrasound findings suggestive of malignancy include irregular margins, intranodular vascular spots, and microcalcifications. Results of the FNA determine further management and treatment. Cytologic evaluation of FNA specimens is reported as nondiagnostic, benign, follicular lesions of undetermined significance, follicular neoplasms, suspicious for malignancy, or malignant. **Follicular cell malignancy cannot be distinguished cytologically from its benign equivalent** and thus is often read as a follicular lesion of undetermined significance. These patients should be referred to surgery to obtain a definitive evaluation. Papillary, medullary, and anaplastic thyroid carcinomas can be diagnosed accurately by FNA.

Treatment

Hyperfunctioning nodules are treated with surgery or radioactive ablation therapy, depending on the level of hyperthyroidism. Patients with thyroid malignancy are treated by thyroidectomy followed by radioactive ablation. These patients will require long-term follow-up by an endocrinologist.

Thyroid nodules discovered during pregnancy are handled similarly, except that radioisotope scanning is contraindicated. FNA is safe during pregnancy, and thyroidectomy can be performed relatively safely during the second and third trimesters. However, because thyroid cancer is relatively indolent, it may be wise to defer definitive diagnosis and treatment until the postpartum period in patients with indeterminate lesions on FNA.

CASE CORRELATION

- See also Case 25 (Major Depression and Other Mood Disorders) and Case 30 (Hypertension).

COMPREHENSION QUESTIONS

15.1 A 28-year-old woman is noted to have had a 10-lb unintended weight gain, hair loss, dry skin, and fatigue. She is diagnosed with probable hypothyroidism. Which of the following laboratory test results is most consistent with hypothyroidism?

　A. Normal TSH and elevated T_4/T_3 levels

　B. Elevated TSH levels and low T_4/T_3

　C. Elevated TSH levels and normal T_4/T_3

　D. Low TSH and elevated T_4/T_3 levels

15.2 A 35-year-old gravida 2, para 1001 at 11 weeks' gestation presents with complaint of palpitations, weight loss, nervousness, and tremor. She denies prior history of thyroid problems. Laboratory studies confirm that TSH is severely suppressed. Which of the following is the best treatment for this patient at this time?

　A. Propylthiouracil

　B. Alpha-adrenergic antagonist

　C. Levothyroxine

　D. Methimazole

15.3 A 24-year-old woman who is 8 weeks' pregnant is found to have a thyroid nodule. A biopsy is performed, and malignancy of the thyroid is diagnosed. Which of the following management options is most appropriate?

　A. Confirm the diagnosis of cancer using radioisotope scanning.

　B. Perform an immediate thyroidectomy.

　C. Follow clinically until after delivery of child.

　D. Treat with radioactive iodine ablation in the second or third trimester.

15.4 A 28-year-old man presents to his provider for a health maintenance visit. He feels well and does not report changes in his appetite, weight, energy, or bowel movements. A firm nodule is palpated in the left lobe of his thyroid. The nodule is confirmed on ultrasound and measures 0.8 cm and is cystic. Which of the following is the next step in the workup of this nodule?

A. Radioactive iodine uptake study

B. Fine-needle aspiration

C. Repeat ultrasound in 6 months

D. Referral to surgeon for open biopsy

ANSWERS

15.1 **B.** Hypothyroidism is marked by low levels of circulating thyroid hormones. In this situation, the usual thyroxine which exerts a negative feedback to TSH is absent; this leads to an increase pituitary secretion of TSH. Therefore, hypothyroidism presents with an increased TSH and low serum T_3/T_4. The other laboratory values (answer A, normal TSH and elevated T_3/T_4; answer C, elevated TSH and normal T_3/T_4; and answer D, low TSH and elevated T_3/T_4) are not seen with hypothyroidism.

15.2 **A.** Experts agree that due to adverse effects of methimazole (answer D) on fetal development, PTU should be used in the first trimester of pregnancy and methimazole in the second and third trimesters. Answer B (alpha-adrenergic antagonist) is not used for hyperthyroidism, but rather beta-blocking agents are used to control the tachycardia and tremor and anxiety. Answer C (levothyroxine) treats hypothyroidism, not hyperthyroidism.

15.3 **C.** Thyroid cancer detected during pregnancy can usually be observed until after the pregnancy is complete. If needed, thyroid surgery (answer B) can be performed safely in the second and third trimesters. The use of radioactive iodine (answers A and D) is contraindicated in pregnancy.

15.4 **C.** For thyroid nodules that are < 1 cm, benign appearing, and without the presence of positive clinical history of thyroid cancers, observation and repeat thyroid ultrasound in 6 months is appropriate. Thyroid nodules > 1 cm should undergo FNA (answer B), as this is a sensitive and specific test for thyroid nodules and can help to determine whether it is malignant. Assessment for function (answer A) or referral for surgery (answer D) is not indicated with a small nodule with benign appearances.

CLINICAL PEARLS

▶ The most common forms of both hyper- and hypothyroidism are autoimmune: Graves disease causing hyperthyroidism and Hashimoto thyroiditis causing hypothyroidism.

▶ The best initial test in assessing thyroid function is a TSH level.

▶ Once a thyroid nodule is palpated on examination, the first steps are to obtain a TSH level and a thyroid ultrasound.

▶ Thyroid disease in pregnancy needs to be evaluated and treated appropriately, as both hypothyroidism and hyperthyroidism can have serious effects on fetal development.

▶ Thyroid nodules greater than 1 cm in size should be biopsied if the TSH level is normal or high.

▶ Approximately 50% of patients with Graves disease also have exophthalmos.

▶ Radioactive iodine is the treatment of choice for Graves disease in adult patients who are not pregnant.

▶ Thyroid storm is a medical emergency; it is an acute hypermetabolic state associated with the sudden release of large amounts of thyroid hormone into circulation.

▶ Once the diagnosis of primary hypothyroidism is made, further imaging or serologic testing is unnecessary if the thyroid gland is normal on physical examination.

▶ Functional adenomas that present with hyperthyroidism are rarely malignant.

REFERENCES

Baloch ZW, LiVolsi VA, Asa SL, et al. Diagnostic terminology and morphologic criteria for cytologic diagnosis of thyroid lesions: a synopsis of the National Cancer Institute Thyroid Fine-Needle Aspiration State of the Science Conference. *Diagn Cytopathol.* 2008;36:425.

Fitzgerald PA. Endocrine disorders. In: Papadakis MA, McPhee SJ, Rabow MW, eds. *Current Medical Diagnosis & Treatment 2019.* New York, NY: McGraw Hill; 2019: Chap. 26. http://accessmedicine.mhmedical.com/content.aspx?bookid=2449&sectionid=194577758. Accessed May 08, 2019.

Gaitonde DY, Rowley KD, Sweeney LB. Hypothyroidism: an update. *Am Fam Physician.* 2012; 86(3):244-251.

Jameson J, Mandel SJ, Weetman AP. Hypothyroidism. In: Jameson J, Fauci AS, Kasper DL, Hauser SL, Longo DL, Loscalzo J, eds. *Harrison's Principles of Internal Medicine.* 20th ed. New York, NY: McGraw Hill; 2018: Chap. 376. http://accessmedicine.mhmedical.com/content.aspx?bookid=2129&sectionid=179924583. Accessed May 27, 2019.

Kravets I. Hyperthyroidism: diagnosis and treatment. *Am Fam Physician.* 2016;93(5):363-370.

A 74-year-old man comes to your office complaining of trouble sleeping. Further questioning reveals that he awakens three to four times each night to urinate. This problem has been noticeably worse over the past year. He has noticed that he has to strain to initiate voiding, especially in the morning, and that his urine stream is weak. He complains of "dribbling" at the end of urination, and at times he is uncertain if he has completely emptied his bladder. He also notes occasional feelings of urgency and has experienced urinary incontinence twice over the past month. He denies any fevers, dysuria, hematuria, pain, urethral discharge, or any changes in his bowel habits. He has a history of prediabetes, hypertension, and hyperlipidemia; these medical problems are well controlled.

On examination, his temperature is 98.3 °F, blood pressure is 126/78 mm Hg, pulse is 84 beats/min, and respirations are 14 breaths/min. Abdominal examination is without tenderness, guarding, mass, or organomegaly. There is no suprapubic fullness or tenderness. On digital rectal examination, his prostate is smooth, nonnodular, nontender, and moderately enlarged.

▶ What is the most likely diagnosis?
▶ What is the appropriate diagnostic workup?
▶ What is the next step in therapy?

ANSWERS TO CASE 16:

Male Genitourinary Conditions

Summary: This 74-year-old man presents with

- Lower urinary tract symptoms (LUTS)
- Nocturia, weak stream and difficulty initiating voiding, sensation of incomplete emptying of his bladder, and urgency
- A nontender, nonnodular yet moderately enlarged prostate

Most likely diagnosis: Benign prostatic hyperplasia (BPH).

Diagnostic workup: Measurement of postvoid residual (PVR) volume of urine, urinalysis, serum creatinine, serum prostate-specific antigen (PSA), frequency-volume chart for evaluation of nocturia.

Next step in therapy: Initial therapy consists of lifestyle modifications, followed by drug treatment with alpha-1-adrenergic antagonists or 5-alpha-reductase inhibitors. Incorporating patient preference guides how aggressive therapy for BPH will be.

ANALYSIS

Objectives

1. Recognize common male genitourinary (GU) conditions. (EPA 1)

2. Know the diagnostic workup and basic management for common male GU conditions. (EPA 3, 4)

3. Recognize complications associated with common male GU conditions. (EPA 1, 4, 12)

Considerations

Therapy for BPH is almost entirely symptom driven: A significantly enlarged prostate gland in an asymptomatic patient requires no treatment, while a less enlarged gland in a patient with severe obstructive symptoms may require surgery. First-line therapy includes alpha-1-adrenergic antagonists, which reduce sympathetic tone to the bladder outlet, reducing resistance to flow. The 5-alpha-reductase inhibitors are slower acting medications that work by reducing the size of the prostate to relieve urethral obstruction. In cases of obstruction and acute urinary retention, indwelling catheterization is recommended. Surgical therapy for BPH is second line and typically undertaken only after a failed trial of medications. Patients with symptomatic BPH symptoms and/or prostate enlargement should undergo PSA testing to evaluate for possible prostate cancer.

APPROACH TO:
Male Genitourinary Conditions

DEFINITIONS

BENIGN PROSTATIC HYPERPLASIA: A histologic diagnosis marked by proliferation of smooth muscle and epithelial cells in the transitional zone of the prostate. Clinically, it presents with LUTS with risk of bladder outlet obstruction.

EPIDIDYMITIS/ORCHITIS: Inflammation of the epididymis and/or testicle, most commonly due to infectious etiology.

ERECTILE DYSFUNCTION: Consistent or recurrent inability to acquire or sustain an erection of sufficient rigidity and duration for sexual intercourse.

PREHN SIGN: Pain relief with testicular elevation.

CLINICAL APPROACH TO BPH

Epidemiology

The prevalence of LUTS increases as men age; nearly one-half of men experience moderate-to-severe LUTS by the eighth decade of life. LUTS is also associated with diabetes, cardiovascular disease, obesity, sedentary lifestyle, and erectile dysfunction (ED). Symptoms of LUTS are measured using the American Urological Association's Symptom Index (AUA-SI), which allows response to therapy to be assessed more objectively.

Pathophysiology

BPH is a pathologic enlargement of the prostate gland that contributes to the development of LUTS in men. LUTS is a nonspecific term that encompasses all symptoms related to impaired urine storage or voiding. LUTS can be divided into obstructive symptoms (eg, hesitancy, straining, weak stream, dribbling) and irritative symptoms (eg, frequency, urgency, nocturia, urge incontinence). Although rare, untreated BPH can lead to more serious conditions, including acute urinary retention, recurrent urinary tract infections (UTIs), hydronephrosis, and renal failure. There is no current evidence to support a link between BPH and prostate cancer. Given its increased prevalence, BPH should be considered in any older male patient who presents with LUTS, and a digital rectal examination should be performed.

Clinical Presentation

BPH may be asymptomatic, and symptoms do not necessarily correlate with the degree of prostatic enlargement. Symptoms typically develop slowly and may progress over a period of years. However, not all patients experience progression of symptoms; in about one-third of patients, symptoms may improve without any treatment. LUTS are typically divided into problems with voiding (eg, hesitancy, straining, weak stream, dribbling) and storage (eg, increased frequency, urgency, nocturia, urge incontinence). Microscopic or gross hematuria may be present; gross hematuria warrants additional workup and should not be assumed to be due to BPH (see Case 14).

Documentation of symptoms is important prior to treatment. The AUA-SI is a commonly used tool for tracking clinical improvement. The AUA recommends applying the frequency-volume chart in patients who complain of nocturia, as this helps guide lifestyle modification therapy.

Differential Diagnosis. The symptoms of BPH can be similar to those caused by a number of other conditions, including urethral strictures, prostate cancer, UTI, acute prostatitis, and neurogenic bladder. A careful history and physical along with a few laboratory tests are helpful to differentiate BPH from these other diseases.

- **Urethral strictures** should be considered in any patient who has a **history of prior urethral instrumentation or urogenital trauma.**

- **UTI and acute prostatitis** typically present with dysuria, urinary frequency, and occasionally suprapubic or pelvic pain. A urinalysis with significant nitrites and leukocyte esterase as well as a positive urine culture are indicative of this diagnosis.

- **Neurogenic bladder** presents with **urinary retention and incontinence** and is associated with a history of multiple sclerosis or spinal cord injury.

- **Bladder cancer** should be considered when history includes smoking along with hematuria.

- **Anticholinergics, antiemetics, and antihistamines** may contribute to LUTS and can lead to urinary obstruction.

- **Prostate cancer** is generally asymptomatic, although it can cause ureteral obstruction similar to BPH. Digital rectal examination is useful in differentiating these conditions. BPH typically presents with a smooth, diffusely enlarged prostate, while prostate cancer may have asymmetry and nodules.

A urinalysis and testing for PSA are recommended by the AUA for the workup of BPH. Urinalysis is helpful for the detection of blood or an infection. Although a serum creatinine level is also often obtained, the AUA does not recommend this in patients for whom there is no suspicion of obstructive nephropathy.

Additional testing may be obtained depending on the patient. Renal and bladder ultrasonography can rule out obstruction in men with renal dysfunction. Obtaining the PVR urine volume may be helpful before starting an anticholinergic in men who have suspected neurogenic bladder. A PVR < 200 mL is typically not considered concerning for chronic urinary retention. Finally, urethrocystoscopy can detect urethral strictures, bladder calculi, and bladder cancer and can provide a direct visualization of intraurethral prostate enlargement.

Treatment

Treatment of BPH includes conservative management, medical management, and surgery. The goal of therapy is to improve symptoms and quality of life, as most patients do not experience any of the serious complications of BPH. In patients who have mild, uncomplicated BPH, "watchful waiting" and behavioral modifications alone may be sufficient. Helpful behavioral interventions include reducing fluid intake prior to bedtime, reducing consumption of weak diuretics such as alcohol and caffeine, and double voiding to empty the bladder more effectively.

Should conservative management fail to improve symptoms, the next step in treatment is medical management. The mainstay medication classes used in BPH treatment are alpha-1-adrenergic antagonists (alpha-blockers) and 5-alpha-reductase inhibitors. It is reasonable to start patients on monotherapy with an alpha-blocker. Common alpha-blockers include terazosin, doxazosin, tamsulosin, alfuzosin, and silodosin. These agents are similarly efficacious, although side-effect profiles vary somewhat. 5-Alpha-reductase inhibitors (eg, finasteride, dutasteride) can have additional benefit over alpha-blockers in patients with large prostates because, over time, they cause shrinkage of the prostate. These medications may take 6 to 12 months to achieve their full effect and are not ideal as a monotherapy, particularly in a patient who is having moderate-to-severe BPH symptoms at presentation. Some evidence exists to suggest a lower risk of development of prostate cancer with use of 5-alpha-reductase inhibitors, while other evidence suggests an increased risk of development of high-grade prostate cancer. Surgical management of BPH should generally be reserved for patients who have failed medical therapy or developed a BPH-related complication such as acute urinary retention.

CLINICAL APPROACH TO OTHER COMMON GENITOURINARY DISEASES

Testicular Torsion

Pathophysiology. Testicular torsion is the most serious cause of acute testicular pain and must be excluded in any patient who presents with acute scrotal pain. It is caused by twisting of the spermatic cord and its contents, causing ischemia and potential loss of the affected testicle. The age distribution of testicular torsion is bimodal, with one peak in the neonatal period and the second peak around puberty. Torsion is a surgical emergency that requires prompt recognition and treatment within 6 hours to preserve testicular function.

Clinical Presentation. Patients with testicular torsion typically present with very sudden onset unilateral scrotal pain of high severity. Nausea and vomiting often occur. Patients may also have nonspecific symptoms such as fever, urinary frequency, and dysuria. While there are no clear precipitating factors, many patients describe recent history of trauma or strenuous physical activity. Physical examination may reveal a high-riding testicle with an abnormal horizontal orientation, and the overlying skin may be indurated, erythematous, and warm. Cremasteric reflex is absent, as a light stroke to the superior/medial thigh does not elicit the ipsilateral testicle to move superiorly.

Treatment. **In patients with a history and physical examination suggestive of torsion, imaging should not be performed; immediate surgical exploration should occur.** If findings are less clear, ultrasound should be performed. Absent blood flow on color Doppler is consistent with torsion, and immediate surgical exploration should be done. There is typically a 4- to 6-hour window before significant ischemic damage occurs. During surgery, detorsion of the affected spermatic cord is performed until no twists are visible, and testicular viability is then assessed. If still viable, orchiopexy is performed, in which the testicle is permanently fixed within the scrotum.

Acute Epididymitis or Epididymo-orchitis

Pathophysiology. Acute epididymitis or acute epididymo-orchitis is the most common cause of scrotal pain in adults. It is caused by inflammation of the epididymis, which carries sperm from the seminiferous tubules to the vas deferens. Inflammation can frequently spread to the testicle, causing epididymo-orchitis. The most probable cause of inflammation differs based on the age of the patient. In patients aged 14 to 35 years old, *Neisseria gonorrhoeae* or *Chlamydia trachomatis* infection is most probable. In patients < 14 years old or ≥ 35 years old, common urinary tract pathogens, including *Escherichia coli*, are most likely.

Clinical Presentation. Diagnosis is made primarily by history and physical examination, as well as by ruling out other cases requiring urgent intervention (eg, testicular torsion). Patients commonly present with gradual increasing pain that can radiate to the lower abdomen. Patients also often have symptoms of a lower UTI (eg, urgency, frequency, dysuria). On physical examination, patients have localized pain to the posterior aspect of the testicle that can progress to swelling and tenderness. Patients have a normal cremasteric reflex and also have a positive Prehn sign (pain relief with testicular elevation). In all suspected cases of epididymitis, urinalysis, urine culture, and testing for *N. gonorrhoeae* and *C. trachomatis* should be performed. If findings are less clear, scrotal ultrasound should be performed to confirm the diagnosis, which commonly demonstrates an enlarged/thickened epididymis with increased blood flow on color Doppler.

Treatment. Treatment usually involves oral antibiotics, nonsteroidal anti-inflammatory drugs (NSAIDs), local application of ice, and scrotal elevation. Oral antibiotic choice is also stratified based on age/risk factors. In patients who are under 35 or who are at risk for sexually transmitted infections (STIs), ceftriaxone (250 mg IM for one dose) plus doxycycline (100 mg orally twice daily for 10 days) is recommended. For patients ≥ 35 years of age and with low risk of STI, recommended treatment is levofloxacin (500 mg orally once daily for 10 days).

Prostatitis

Prostatitis can be due to **inflammation or infection of the prostate and can be acute or chronic in nature.** Infection is commonly due to coliform bacteria, followed by *N. gonorrhoeae* and *C. trachomatis*. Affected patients present with dysuria, pain on ejaculation, and dull pain in less severe cases, while in acute cases patients may be febrile and have malaise. Diagnosis is often clinical and should include a digital rectal examination, which often reveals a boggy and tender prostate. Urinalysis may show leukocyte esterase and/or nitrates when infection contaminates the urine, and a urine culture should be obtained. Rarely, prostate massage for examination and culture of seminal fluid may aid in diagnosis. Treatment of acute and suspected infectious cases includes a 4-week course of trimethoprim-sulfamethoxazole, doxycycline, or ciprofloxacin and NSAIDs. Cases thought to be noninfectious generally improve with NSAIDs alone.

Erectile Dysfunction

Pathophysiology. ED is a common occurrence in men, with a prevalence that increases with age. There are numerous causes for this, including vascular, psychological, neurologic, and hormonal factors. Rapid clinical assessment of ED can be performed with the five-question International Index of Erectile Function (IIEF-5), which includes questions about confidence, ability to penetrate, maintenance of erection, ability to ejaculate, and satisfaction. Further clarification of the etiology of ED is based on history and physical examination, including genital examination and assessment of secondary sex characteristics.

History taking can help to differentiate psychogenic causes from organic medical causes. Young age, preserved nocturnal erections, and partner conflict support ED of psychogenic nature. A nocturnal penile tumescence test, an overnight test to check for sleep erection, can help clarify this. Men with ED should be evaluated for potential underlying cardiovascular disease due to the common pathophysiologic etiology of endothelial dysfunction. Laboratory evaluation of patients with ED should include fasting glucose or hemoglobin A_{1c} testing, lipid panel, and morning testosterone evaluation.

Treatment. Treatment includes optimizing the management of concomitant medical diagnoses, such as diabetes mellitus, hyperlipidemia, hypogonadism, and metabolic syndrome, while eliminating tobacco and minimizing alcohol. Medications that may contribute to ED include beta-blockers, calcium channel blockers, antidepressants, antihistamines, antipsychotics, and some diuretics. First-line therapy includes lifestyle modifications, medication changes, and oral phosphodiesterase type 5 inhibitors (PDE-5 inhibitors; eg, sildenafil). Other therapies include injectable or intraurethral alprostadil, vacuum pump erection devices, or surgically implantable penile prostheses. Testosterone replacement therapy may improve erectile function in some patients. **PDE-5 inhibitors are contraindicated in patients taking nitrates, as life-threatening hypotension can occur.**

CASE CORRELATION

- See also Case 14 (Hematuria) and Case 45 (HIV, AIDS, and Other Sexually Transmitted Infections).

COMPREHENSION QUESTIONS

16.1 A 60-year-old man reports increased urinary frequency and has been having decreased flow of his urinary stream. He has a history of hypertension controlled with hydrochlorothiazide but has been otherwise healthy. He reports that his father had a similar issue in his 70s. Rectal examination reveals a grossly enlarged prostate without any tenderness, nodules, or asymmetry. Which of the following is a reasonable initial therapy for treatment of this patient's symptoms?

A. Referral for prostatectomy

B. Terazosin 1 mg at bedtime

C. Oxybutynin 5 mg twice daily

D. Empiric antibiotic therapy for presumed infection

16.2 A 21-year-old man reports scrotal pain over the past 4 days. The pain has been radiating to his lower abdomen. He has been sexually active for a few weeks with a new female partner. On physical examination, he has a normal cremasteric reflex and has some relief of pain upon elevation of the scrotum. What is an appropriate choice for empiric antibiotics?

A. Azithromycin 1 g orally one time

B. Ceftiraxone 250 mg IM one time and doxycycline 100 mg orally twice daily for 10 days

C. Levofloxacin 500 mg orally daily for 10 days

D. Ofloxacin 300 mg orally twice daily for 10 days

16.3 A 27-year-old man reports issues obtaining erections during sexual intercourse. He has no significant past medical history. He reports obtaining erections at nighttime. His general physical examination and GU exam are normal. What is the most appropriate initial step in management?

A. Start on sildenafil 50 mg 1 hour before sexual activity as needed

B. Prescribe sublingual nitroglycerin

C. Ask about his relationship and potential stressors

D. Prescribe supplemental intramuscular testosterone 75 to 100 mg/week

ANSWERS

16.1 **B.** This patient most likely has BPH—he is an older man with increased frequency, difficulty voiding, and a symmetrically enlarged prostate without nodularity on examination. Initial therapy often involves lifestyle modification, such as fluid restriction at night, and the use of an oral alpha-blocker, such as terazosin. This agent also has the benefit of treating the hypertension. Answer A (referral for prostatectomy) is indicated for acute urinary retention, persistent or recurrent urinary infections, recurrent hematuria, and renal insufficiency due to chronic bladder outlet obstruction.

The patient does not have any of these findings. Answer C (oxybutynin) can help with some of the symptoms of frequency but does not decrease the size of the prostate or affect blood pressure. Answer D (empiric antibiotics) is not indicated since the patient has no symptoms of infection, such as dysuria, urgency, or fever.

16.2 **B.** This patient most likely has epididymitis. In his age group and with the history of a new sexual partner, gonorrhea or chlamydia is the most likely causes. The most appropriate antibiotic is a combination of ceftriaxone and doxycycline to cover both bacteria. Azithromycin (answer A) is a good alternative if the patient cannot tolerate doxycycline; however, this would not cover *N. gonorrhea.* Levofloxacin (answer C) and ofloxacin (answer D) are both reasonable options if the patient were ≥ 35 years old and not at high risk for an STI.

16.3 **C.** This patient is presenting with ED. It is important to understand what the etiology might be. He is young and healthy and has preserved nighttime erections, which are all factors that favor psychogenic ED. The next step would be to probe about relationship issues and other stressors. Sildenafil (answer A) is a first-line drug for ED that is due to an organic medical cause (ie, coronary artery disease). Nitrates (answer B) are drugs commonly prescribed for angina and are contraindicated when on PDE-5 inhibitors like sildenafil. Testosterone (answer D) would only have some efficacy if the patient had a proven low testosterone level.

CLINICAL PEARLS

▶ BPH is the most common cause of LUTS in older men. Its management is completely based on symptoms.

▶ If testicular torsion is likely, do not waste time with ultrasound; surgical exploration is imperative.

▶ Patients with epididymitis demonstrate a positive Prehn sign and have a cremasteric reflex, which are both absent in testicular torsion.

▶ Psychogenic ED usually can be distinguished from ED of organic medical causes by a patient history of preserved nocturnal erections.

REFERENCES

Dahm P, Brasure M, MacDonald R, et al. Comparative effectiveness of newer medications for lower urinary tract symptoms attributed to benign prostatic hyperplasia: a systematic review and meta-analysis. *Eur Urol.* 2017;71:570-581.

McConaghy JR, Panchal B. Epididymitis: an overview. *Am Fam Physician.* 2016;94(9):723-726.

McVary KT, Roehrborn CG, Avins AL, et al. Association guideline: management of benign prostatic hyperplasia. American Urological Association; 2010. https://www.auanet.org/documents/education/clinical-guidance/Benign-Prostatic-Hyperplasia.pdf. Accessed May 27, 2019.

Platz EA, Joshu CE, Mondul AM, et al. Incidence and progression of lower urinary tract symptoms in a large prospective cohort of United States men. *J Urol.* 2012;188:496-501.

Rew KT, Heidelbaugh JJ. Erectile dysfunction. *Am Fam Physician.* 2016;94(10):820-827.

Scher HI, Eastham JA. Benign and malignant diseases of the prostate. In: Jameson J, Fauci AS, Kasper DL, Hauser SL, Longo DL, Loscalzo J, eds. *Harrison's Principles of Internal Medicine.* 20th ed. New York, NY: McGraw Hill; 2018: Chap. 83. http://accessmedicine.mhmedical.com/content.aspx?bookid=2129&sectionid=192016319. Accessed May 27, 2019.

Serlin DC, Heidelbaugh JJ, Stoffel, JT. Urinary retention in adults: evaluation and initial management. *Am Fam Physician.* 2018;98(8):496-503.

Sharp VJ, Kieran K, Arlen AM. Testicular torsion: diagnosis, evaluation, and management. *Am Fam Physician.* 2013;88(12):835-840.

Trojian, TH, Lishnak TS, Heiman D. Epididymitis and orchitis: an overview. *Am Fam Physician.* 2009;79(7):583-587.

A 58-year-old woman presents to your office for follow-up of an emergency department visit. She was seen 1 week earlier in the emergency department for abdominal pain and was diagnosed with nephrolithiasis. Ultimately, she was sent home with pain medications and given instructions to strain her urine for stones and to follow up with her primary care provider. Today, she is asymptomatic. She takes no medications on a regular basis. Her family history is significant only for a father with high blood pressure. She had several routine laboratory tests drawn in the emergency department, copies of which she brings with her. Upon your review of the laboratory values, you note the following (normal values are in parentheses): sodium 142 mEq/L (135-145); potassium 4.0 mEq/L (3.5-5.0); chloride 104 mg/dL (95-105); bicarbonate 28 mEq/L (20-29); blood urea nitrogen (BUN) 20 mg/dL (7-20); creatinine 0.9 mg/dL (0.8-1.4); calcium 12.5 mg/dL (8.5-10.2); and albumin 4.2 g/dL (3.4-5.4). The complete blood count (CBC) was within normal limits.

The renal calculus was detected by helical computed tomographic (CT) scanning without contrast and was located in the right midureter. Your patient has brought with her the stone that she has strained from the urine. Upon questioning, you learn that she has had multiple episodes of "kidney stones" in the past 2 years. You send the stone to the laboratory for analysis and order a repeat serum calcium level. The results show that the stone is made of calcium oxalate, and the patient's serum calcium is still elevated at 11.9 mg/dL.

▶ What is the most likely diagnosis?
▶ What is the most likely cause?
▶ What is the next step?

ANSWERS TO CASE 17:

Electrolyte Disorders

Summary: This 58-year-old woman presents with

- A history of recurrent nephrolithiasis, presenting for follow-up
- Calcium oxalate stones
- An initial serum calcium level that was elevated, as was the repeat serum calcium 1 week later
- Asymptomatic presentation
- No medications and a family history only significant for hypertension

Most likely diagnosis: Hypercalcemia and recurrent nephrolithiasis.

Most likely cause: Hyperparathyroidism.

Next step: Further laboratory workup, including serum parathyroid hormone (PTH) level.

ANALYSIS

Objectives

1. Be able to list common causes of calcium, sodium, and potassium disorders. (EPA 1, 2)

2. Describe the workup and management of common electrolyte disorders. (EPA 4, 10)

Considerations

This patient illustrates one common presentation of hypercalcemia. Many times, patients with hypercalcemia are asymptomatic, and an elevated calcium level is found unexpectedly on routine laboratory studies. The diagnostic workup begins with a careful review of the patient's history, as clues to its etiology may often be elicited here. The diagnostic workup is designed to distinguish parathyroid dysfunction from other etiologies so that optimal treatment and management can be pursued.

APPROACH TO:

Electrolyte Disorders

DEFINITIONS

HYPERPARATHYROIDISM: Condition of elevated PTH usually due to excessive production by the parathyroid glands, leading to hypercalcemia.

SECONDARY HYPERPARATHYROIDISM: Condition that occurs as the parathyroid glands overproduce PTH to respond to low serum calcium levels. This may occur as a response to low dietary calcium intake or a deficiency of vitamin D.

TERTIARY HYPERPARATHYROIDISM: Elevated PTH in patients who have renal failure.

CLINICAL APPROACH TO HYPERCALCEMIA

Calcium Homeostasis

Before discussing the differential diagnosis of hypercalcemia, it is essential to review the basic mechanism by which normal calcium levels are maintained in the body. **Most of the calcium in the body is found in the skeleton** (approximately 98%). The remaining calcium is found in circulation. Of this remaining 2%, about half is bound to albumin and other proteins, and half is "free," or ionized. It is the ionized calcium that has physiologic effects. Because the serum calcium is partially bound to albumin, abnormally low serum albumin levels will affect the measurement of calcium, thus causing a misinterpretation of an abnormal calcium level. With patients found to have a concomitant hypoalbuminemia, the ionized calcium can be measured directly. However, there is a useful formula that can correct for this error. A "corrected" serum calcium is provided by the formula

Corrected serum calcium =
[0.8 × (Normal albumin) − (Patient's albumin level)] + (Serum calcium)

PTH, calcitonin, and 1,25-dihydroxyvitamin D_3 (calcitriol) are responsible for regulating calcium levels and maintaining calcium homeostasis. **Causes of hypercalcemia include an increase in calcium resorption from bone, a decrease in renal excretion of calcium, or an increase in calcium absorption from the gastrointestinal (GI) tract.** When calcium levels increase, calcitonin, produced by the thyroid parafollicular cells, attempts to lower calcium levels through renal excretion of calcium and by opposing osteoclast activation. When calcium is excreted through this pathway, phosphate is also excreted. Conversely, low levels of circulating calcium normally result in PTH secretion. This promotes osteoclast activation, which mobilizes calcium from bone and affects calcium resorption at the kidneys, thereby retaining circulating calcium. While PTH will increase the calcium in the blood, it has the opposite effect on serum phosphate levels. PTH also increases calcitriol levels, which act at the GI tract to promote both calcium and phosphate absorption.

Pathophysiology of Hypercalcemia

Any process that increases GI calcium absorption, decreases renal excretion, or activates osteoclastic activity will raise serum calcium levels. If this occurs beyond the normal bounds of maintaining calcium homeostasis, hypercalcemia will occur. **The most common cause of hypercalcemia in the ambulatory patient is hyperparathyroidism.** Cancer is the second leading cause. Hyperparathyroidism and cancer combined account for 90% of hypercalcemia cases. It is useful to categorize the etiologies of hypercalcemia into five main areas: PTH, malignancy, renal failure, high bone turnover, and those related to vitamin D (Table 17–1).

Table 17–1 • COMMON CAUSES OF HYPERCALCEMIA		
Condition	Specific Example	Pathophysiology
Increased Bone Resorption		
Primary hyperparathyroidism	Sporadic or familial; multiple endocrine neoplasia (MEN) types 1 and 2	
Malignancy	Solid tumors of lung; squamous carcinoma of head and neck; renal carcinoma	Tumor secretion of PTH-rP
	Breast cancer; multiple myeloma; prostate cancer	Direct osteolysis
Hypervitaminosis A (vitamin A intoxication)	Includes both vitamin A and its analogs (used to treat acne)	Increased bone resorption
Immobilization	Less common than above causes	Increased risk when underlying disorder of high bone turnover (eg, Paget disease)
Increased Calcium Absorption		
Hypervitaminosis D (vitamin D intoxication)		Increased calcitriol level leads to increased GI absorption of calcium and phosphate
Granulomatous disease	Tuberculosis; sarcoidosis; Hodgkin disease	Increase extrarenal conversion of 25-hydroxyvitamin D_3 to calcitriol
Milk-alkali syndrome		Excessive intake of calcium-containing antacids
Miscellaneous		
Medications	Thiazide diuretics; lithium	Reduced urinary excretion of calcium; increased PTH secretion
Rhabdomyolysis		Calcium released from injured muscle
Adrenal insufficiency		Increased bone resorption and increased protein binding of calcium
Thyrotoxicosis (usually mild hypercalcemia)		Increased bone resorption

Abbreviation: PTH-rP, parathyroid hormone-related peptide.

History. The first step in the evaluation is a careful history to try to establish a cause and to assess for manifestations. The history should include family history of calcium disorders, such as renal stones or malignancy. The patient's risk factors for malignancy, such as smoking, should be investigated. The chronicity of symptoms should be taken into account; more acute symptoms suggest malignancy over hyperparathyroidism and vice versa. A careful review of medications should also take place, including not only prescription medications but also over-the-counter supplements. Dietary intake of vitamin D and calcium should be questioned. Furthermore, history of immobilization secondary to a hospital stay or recent injury should be looked into since prolonged immobilization can cause massive bone demineralization and hypercalcemia. At this point, if the hypercalcemia is mild and

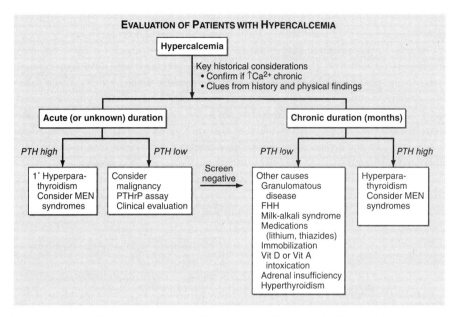

Figure 17–1. Algorithm for the evaluation of hypercalcemia. Reproduced with permission, from Jameson J, Fauci AS, Kasper DL, et al. *Harrison's Principles of Internal Medicine*, 20th ed. 2018. Copyright © McGraw Hill LLC. All rights reserved.

the patient asymptomatic, it is acceptable to stop any suspect medication(s) and repeat the serum calcium level. An algorithm for the assessment of hypercalcemia is shown in Figure 17–1.

Parathyroid Hormone Levels. If a causative medication is not found, a serum intact PTH level should be measured. This level will be suppressed, normal, or elevated. As with many endocrine disorders, **it is useful not to think of normal or abnormal values; rather, one should understand what is appropriate for a given situation.** For example, in normal subjects, an increased calcium load will normally depress the PTH hormone level; thus a low PTH level in this situation is *normal,* or appropriately suppressed. If a patient has an elevated calcium level and the PTH is "normal," it is said to be inappropriately normal because in the face of hypercalcemia it should be low, or suppressed.

Primary Hyperparathyroidism. If a patient with hypercalcemia has a normal or elevated PTH level, then the normal feedback loop is not responding. This defines hyperparathyroidism. Primary hyperparathyroidism occurs when the parathyroid gland overproduces PTH and does not respond to the negative feedback of elevated calcium levels. **The vast majority of primary hyperparathyroidism is caused by an adenoma (benign tumor) of one of the four parathyroid glands.**

Secondary and Tertiary Hyperparathyroidism. Secondary hyperparathyroidism occurs as the parathyroid glands overproduce PTH to respond to low serum calcium levels. This may occur as a response to low dietary calcium intake or a deficiency of vitamin D. Tertiary hyperparathyroidism occurs in patients who have renal failure. Patients in renal failure initially present with *hypo*calcemia, hyperphosphatemia, and low vitamin D levels. If untreated, it leads to hyperplasia of the parathyroid glands, increased PTH secretion, and subsequent hypercalcemia.

Familial Hypocalciuric Hypercalcemia. Familial hypocalciuric hypercalcemia (FHH) is a condition that can produce inappropriately high PTH levels unrelated to the parathyroid production. FHH is a genetic disorder related to a defect in a gene that codes for a calcium-sensing receptor. Consequently, simply measuring PTH alone may confound this diagnosis, which may be mistaken for primary hyperparathyroidism. To distinguish these entities, a 24-hour urinary calcium level is obtained. In hyperparathyroidism, the kidneys spill calcium into the urine at a normal or elevated level. With FHH, the urinary calcium level is low.

Cancer. A low PTH level with elevated serum calcium suggests that the parathyroid gland is responding appropriately to the high calcium environment. This is seen when tumors produce a hormone that mimics the active site of the PTH molecule. This molecule is called PTH-related peptide (PTH-rP). PTH-rP is produced by some lung cancers, squamous cell cancers of the head and neck, and renal cell cancer. PTH-rP affects osteoclastic bone resorption, increases calcitriol, and promotes calcium resorption from the kidneys, resulting in increased levels of serum calcium. The continued production of PTH-rP effectively takes the parathyroid gland out of the loop in calcium homeostasis. Because cancer is a common etiology for hypercalcemia, the **search for malignancy is paramount at this step in diagnosis before other, less common disorders are considered.**

Other Etiologies. If a malignancy is not found, other etiologies must be considered. These fall into the category of endocrine disorders other than those involving the parathyroid and include hyperthyroidism, adrenal insufficiency, and acromegaly. The workup thus includes thyroid-stimulating hormone (TSH), a cortisol level, and a pituitary imaging study, respectively.

Clinical Presentation of Hypercalcemia

Normal values of serum calcium range from 8 to 10 mg/dL. Levels of serum calcium between 10.5 and 12 mg/dL are classified as mild hypercalcemia, and patients are typically asymptomatic at these levels. As calcium levels increase, physical manifestations may become apparent. The classic mnemonic "stones, bones, psychic groans, and abdominal moans" is useful to categorize the constellation of physical symptoms associated with hypercalcemia (Table 17–2). Other clinical manifestations include the cardiac sequelae of a shortening QT interval and arrhythmias.

Treatment

Preventive Measures. The **treatment of hypercalcemia is directed at the underlying disorder.** Patients with mild hypercalcemia may be treated with preventive

Table 17–2 • PHYSICAL MANIFESTATIONS OF HYPERCALCEMIA	
Stones	Renal calculi
Bones	Bone pain, including arthritis and osteoporosis
Psychic groans	Poor concentration, weakness, fatigue, stupor, coma
Abdominal moans	Abdominal pain, constipation, nausea, vomiting, pancreatitis, anorexia

measures aimed at avoiding aggravating factors. These measures include adequate hydration (dehydration aggravates nephrolithiasis), avoiding thiazide diuretics or other offending medications, encouraging physical activity, and avoiding prolonged inactivity.

Surgery. For the treatment of primary hyperparathyroidism, surgical parathyroidectomy is the definitive treatment. Surgery is appropriate for patients with symptomatic hyperparathyroidism. Surgery may be an option for selected asymptomatic patients, including those who have developed osteoporosis or renal insufficiency, who have markedly elevated calcium levels, or who are younger than 50 years of age.

Complications

The most serious manifestations of hypercalcemia occur in the form of dysrhythmias and coma. In situations like these, it is imperative to correct the hypercalcemia while simultaneously performing a workup to understand the etiology. Management includes rehydration as the first step with intravenous 0.9% saline, 4 to 6 L/24 h. After rehydration, intravenous bisphosphonates should be used, keeping in mind that the dose and time over which these are administered must be decreased in renally impaired patients.

CLINICAL APPROACH TO SODIUM DISORDERS

Hyponatremia

Pathophysiology. Hyponatremia is defined as a plasma $Na^+ < 135$ mEq/L. It is a disorder of water balance that primarily causes neurologic symptoms due to a lowered serum osmolality that promotes water movement into brain cells. In hyponatremic states, total body sodium and total body water can be low, normal, or high, so assessment of the patient's overall volume state and osmolality is critical to the diagnosis and management.

Clinical Presentation. Although most patients with hyponatremia are asymptomatic, early symptoms may manifest as nausea, vomiting, or lethargy in acute cases. As most cases of hyponatremia present with a low serum osmolality (< 280 mOsm/kg), evaluation of the patient's volume status will help determine possible causes and guide therapy, as presented in the material that follows.

Hypovolemic Hyponatremia. This type of hyponatremia exhibits signs of volume depletion on physical examination, with urinary sodium levels < 20 mEq/L. Common causes include cerebral salt wasting, skin loss, diuretic use, GI losses, mineralocorticoid deficiency, and third spacing of fluids. The treatment is volume repletion with normal saline and addressing the underlying condition. Severe symptomatic hyponatremia, which can manifest as confusion, coma, or seizures, is usually observed with serum sodium < 125 mEq/L and warrants urgent treatment with hypertonic (3%) saline. Often, very small corrections in serum sodium will improve the symptoms. It is recommended to correct the sodium level slowly to avoid the risk of osmotic demyelination, which can result in permanent neurologic injury and death.

Hypervolemic Hyponatremia. Hypervolemic hyponatremia exhibits signs of volume expansion on examination due to decreased renal excretion of water. Common

Table 17–3 • CAUSES OF SYNDROME OF INAPPROPRIATE ADH SECRETION

Central nervous system disorders
  Head trauma
  Stroke
  Subarachnoid hemorrhage
  Hydrocephalus
  Brain tumor
  Encephalitis
  Guillain-Barré syndrome
  Meningitis
  Acute psychosis
  Acute intermittent porphyria

Pulmonary lesions
  Tuberculosis
  Bacterial pneumonia
  Aspergillosis
  Bronchiectasis
  Neoplasms
  Positive-pressure ventilation

Malignancies
  Bronchogenic carcinoma
  Pancreatic carcinoma
  Prostatic carcinoma
  Renal cell carcinoma
  Adenocarcinoma of colon
  Thymoma
  Osteosarcoma
  Lymphoma
  Leukemia

Drugs
  Increased ADH production
    Antidepressants: tricyclics, monoamine oxidase inhibitors, SSRIs
    Antineoplastics: cyclophosphamide, vincristine
    Carbamazepine
    Methylenedioxymethamphetamine (MDMA; ecstasy)
    Clofibrate
    Neuroleptics: thiothixene, thioridazine, fluphenazine, haloperidol, trifluoperazine
  Potentiated ADH action
    Carbamazepine
    Chlorpropamide, tolbutamide
    Cyclophosphamide
    NSAIDs
    Somatostatin and analogs
    Amiodarone

Others
  Postoperative
  Pain
  Stress
  AIDS
  Pregnancy (physiologic)
  Hypokalemia

Abbreviations: ADH, antidiuretic hormone; NSAIDs, nonsteroidal anti-inflammatory drugs; SSRIs, selective serotonin reuptake inhibitors.
Reproduced with permission, from Papadakis MA, McPhee SJ, Rabow MW. CURRENT Medical Diagnosis & Treatment. 2015. Copyright © McGraw Hill LLC. All rights reserved.

causes include heart failure, cirrhosis, and nephrosis. The treatment is use of diuretics and restriction of fluid and sodium intake.

Euvolemic Hyponatremia. Antidiuretic hormone (ADH) is normally secreted in response to low-volume states, resulting in retention of free water. The syndrome of inappropriate antidiuretic hormone secretion (SIADH) occurs when ADH is secreted independently of the volume status, resulting in the inappropriate retention of free water with resultant hyponatremia and hypotonicity. SIADH is a common complication of many conditions, including infections, malignancies, medications, and central nervous system disorders (see Table 17–3). The treatment of SIADH involves fluid restriction and, when possible, correction of the underlying condition. Less common causes of euvolemic hyponatremia include water intoxication, hypothyroidism, and low solute intake.

Pseudohyponatremia. Pseudohyponatremia is another cause of low plasma Na$^+$ that should be considered. In this scenario, the observed low sodium levels may be appropriate for the given clinical situation, such as in the setting of hyperglycemia, hypertriglyceridemia, hyperproteinemia, laboratory errors, or mannitol use. In this situation, patients usually have a normal volume status with normal osmolality.

Hypernatremia

Pathophysiology. Hypernatremia is defined as a plasma Na$^+$ > 145 mEq/L and reflects a state of increased serum osmolality that promotes water movement out of cells. The condition is usually due to net water loss that is often associated with an impaired thirst response or restricted access to water (eg, in the elderly, young infants, intubated patients).

Clinical Presentation. Symptoms are primarily neurologic, just like hyponatremia, and manifest as anorexia, muscle weakness, nausea, vomiting, and lethargy, which may lead to seizures and coma in severe cases. The most important first step in assessing patients with hypernatremia is to check the urine osmolality. A high urine osmolality (> 400 mOsm/kg) suggests that the body's ability to conserve water is intact and that water losses are due to hypotonic fluid loss (eg, excessive sweating, GI losses, etc). A low urine osmolality (< 300 mOsm/kg) suggests pure water loss as seen in diabetes insipidus (DI), which is further broken down into nephrogenic DI (renal resistance to action of ADH) and central DI (lack of ADH production).

Treatment. Treatment involves correcting the underlying condition and correcting the deficit in water. As with hyponatremia, hypernatremia should be cautiously corrected, as rapid correction leads to cerebral edema due to intracellular fluid shifts.

CLINICAL APPROACH TO POTASSIUM DISORDERS

Hypokalemia

Pathophysiology. Hypokalemia is defined as a plasma K$^+$ < 3.5 mEq/L. The potential causes of hypokalemia are numerous but are generally broken down into several categories: decreased net intake; intracellular shifts (eg, alkalosis, excess insulin); and renal losses or extrarenal losses (see Table 17–4).

Table 17–4 • CAUSES OF HYPOKALEMIA

I. Decreased Potassium Intake

II. Potassium Shift into the Cell
Increased postprandial secretion of insulin
Alkalosis
Trauma (via beta-adrenergic stimulation)
Periodic paralysis (hypokalemic)
Barium intoxication

III. Renal Potassium Loss
Increased aldosterone (mineralocorticoid) effects
    Primary hyperaldosteronism
    Secondary aldosteronism (dehydration, heart failure)
    Renovascular hypertension
    Malignant hypertension
    Ectopic ACTH-producing tumor
    Gitelman syndrome
    Bartter syndrome
    Cushing syndrome
    Licorice (European)
    Renin-producing tumor
    Congenital abnormality of steroid metabolism (eg, adrenogenital syndrome, 17-alpha-hydroxylase defect, apparent mineralocorticoid excess, 11-beta-hydroxylase deficiency)
Increased flow to distal nephron
    Diuretics (furosemide, thiazides)
    Salt-losing nephropathy
Hypomagnesemia
    Unreabsorbable anion
    Carbenicillin, penicillin
Renal tubular acidosis (type I or II)
    Fanconi syndrome
    Interstitial nephritis
    Metabolic alkalosis (bicarbonaturia)
Congenital defect of distal nephron
    Liddle syndrome

IV. Extrarenal Potassium Loss
Vomiting, diarrhea, laxative abuse
Villous adenoma, Zollinger-Ellison syndrome

Reproduced with permission, from Papadakis MA, McPhee SJ, Rabow MW. CURRENT Medical Diagnosis & Treatment. 2015. Copyright © McGraw Hill LLC. All rights reserved.

Clinical Presentation. Patients present with fatigue, muscle aches, ascending muscular weakness, or cramps that, in severe cases, can lead to paralysis or rhabdomyolysis. Electrocardiographic (ECG) changes may be seen in hypokalemia but are not well correlated with serum potassium concentration. Hypokalemia can lead to ST-segment depression, flattened T waves, and prominent U waves.

Treatment. The therapeutic goals are to prevent life-threatening complications (eg, arrhythmias, respiratory failure); correct the potassium deficit; and identify and treat the underlying condition. In most cases, potassium deficits are best corrected by oral potassium replacement. Intravenous potassium should be reserved for profound deficits and for persons unable to take oral medications.

Hyperkalemia

Pathophysiology. Hyperkalemia is defined as a plasma $K^+ > 5.0$ mEq/L. Causes of hyperkalemia are commonly caused by

- Medications: including angiotensin-converting enzyme inhibitors, angiotensin receptor blockers, potassium-sparing diuretics

- Shifts from intracellular to extracellular spaces: including acidosis, insulin deficiency, burns

- Reduced renal excretion of potassium: including renal insufficiency/failure, Addison disease, renal tubular acidosis type IV

It is also important to consider pseudohyperkalemia as a possible cause of elevated plasma potassium, especially in the setting of possible laboratory error, hemolysis, or traumatic venipuncture.

Clinical Presentation. Symptoms that may be present in true hyperkalemia include weakness, ascending flaccid paralysis, paresthesias, areflexia, and ileus; severe cases can lead to respiratory failure. The most serious effect of hyperkalemia is the risk of cardiac arrhythmias. ECG changes may include peaked T waves, flattening of P waves, and widening of QRS complexes.

Treatment. Acute management of hyperkalemia in the setting of ECG changes, rapid rise in plasma potassium levels, and the presence of significant acidosis include (1) stabilizing the myocardium with intravenous calcium to decrease the risk of arrhythmias; (2) shifting potassium into cells to decrease plasma concentration by the administration of glucose and insulin; and (3) eventually lowering total body K^+ with sodium polystyrene (Kayexalate), loop diuretics, or dialysis. Long-term treatment of hyperkalemia should address the underlying cause (eg, discontinuation of a suspect medication) and address patient counseling on low-potassium diets and use of diuretics to promote excretion of potassium.

CASE CORRELATION

- See also Case 10 (Acute Diarrhea), Case 21 (Chronic Kidney Disease), and Case 42 (Palpitations).

COMPREHENSION QUESTIONS

17.1 A 56-year-old woman with history of hypertension, diabetes, and newly diagnosed polycystic kidney disease presents for follow-up for hypertension. Routine laboratory work shows elevated calcium of 13 mg/dL and an elevated phosphate level. The patient denies weight loss, is taking only metoprolol for her blood pressure, and denies recent history of immobilization. Given these findings, which etiology of hypercalcemia would you be most concerned about in this patient?

A. Primary hyperparathyroidism, as this is the most common etiology of hypercalcemia

B. Iatrogenic hypercalcemia secondary to medications

C. A primary vitamin D deficiency, given her age

D. Secondary hyperparathyroidism due to renal disease

17.2 A 48-year-old man presents for follow-up of an elevated calcium level of 12.3 mg/dL found on routine screening laboratory tests at his last health maintenance visit. He takes no medications other than an occasional antihistamine for allergies. He recently started smoking a half-pack of cigarettes per day. He was prompted to attend to today's health maintenance visit by his wife, who claims that he has become forgetful, has a decreased appetite, and has had a 10-lb weight loss over the past 2 months. As part of his follow-up laboratory tests, you obtain a serum PTH, which comes back within the normal range. Which of the following is the next step in diagnosis?

A. Chest x-ray

B. Repeat calcium after hydration

C. Measurement of PTH-rP levels

D. Measurement of urinary calcium excretion

17.3 An 80-year-old woman is brought to the emergency department with altered mental status and fever. She is awake and cooperative but is not oriented to time or place. Her blood pressure is normal, her pulse is normal, and her temperature is 101 °F. She is found to have pneumonia. Laboratory testing reveals a sodium level of 130 mEq/L but otherwise normal electrolytes. Which of the following is the most appropriate treatment?

A. Intravenous antibiotic only

B. Intravenous antibiotic and aggressive rehydration with intravenous normal saline

C. Intravenous antibiotic and fluid restriction

D. Intravenous antibiotic and intravenous 3% saline

17.4 A 65-year-old dialysis patient is found to have a serum potassium level of 6.8 mEq/L, which is verified on a stat repeat level. An ECG shows peaked T waves and a widened QRS complex. What is the first intervention that should be made at this point?

A. Intravenous glucose and insulin administration

B. Arrangement for a dialysis treatment

C. Oral sodium polystyrene (Kayexalate)

D. Intravenous furosemide

E. Intravenous calcium

ANSWERS

17.1 **D.** Secondary hyperparathyroidism occurs in patients with early renal disease as a consequence of hyperphosphatemia, hypocalcemia, and impaired production of 1,25-dihydroxyvitamin D by the failing kidneys; PTH levels increase abnormally, causing in turn elevated levels of calcium. Therefore, in this disorder you would see increased PTH and increased calcium, signaling a disruption of the normal feedback cycle. The serum phosphate levels are increased due to inability of the kidneys to excrete phosphate. Answer A (primary hyperparathyroidism) is associated with elevated calcium but decreased phosphate levels. Answer B (iatrogenic hypercalcemia secondary to medications) may be due to vitamin D toxicity, for example, but the patient has no history of these medications. Answer C (primary vitamin D deficiency) would lead to hypocalcemia and not hypercalcemia.

17.2 **D.** This patient has symptomatic hypercalcemia. The high serum calcium level should have suppressed the serum PTH level; the patient has an inappropriately normal PTH level. The next step is to measure a 24-hour urinary calcium excretion to determine if this condition represents primary hyperparathyroidism (most common) or FHH (rare).

17.3 **C.** This is a common presentation of SIADH due to pneumonia. Treatment of the underlying pneumonia is key, so antibiotics must be given. This patient is euvolemic, so aggressive rehydration (answer B) is not necessary. With a sodium level of 130 mg/dL, the use of 3% saline (answer D) is not necessary. The electrolyte abnormality should correct with treatment of the pneumonia and with fluid restriction, since the mild hyponatremia is likely due to SIADH.

17.4 **E.** This patient has hyperkalemia with cardiac changes—an acute, life-threatening condition. The first intervention should be to give intravenous calcium to stabilize the cardiac membranes and reduce the risk of arrhythmia. After this, interventions can be made to lower the potassium level and are represented in the other answer choices (answer A, glucose and insulin; answer B, dialysis; answer C, oral sodium polystyrene; and answer D, furosemide).

CLINICAL PEARLS

▶ Be sure to question any patient with hypercalcemia regarding all medications—both prescription and over the counter—as both mega-dose vitamins (A and D) and excessive use of calcium carbonate antacids may play a role.

▶ Hypercalcemia with a suppressed PTH should be considered malignancy until you can prove otherwise.

▶ Assess the volume status in patients with hyponatremia to help determine the cause and guide therapy.

▶ ECG changes in the setting of hyperkalemia require urgent treatment.

REFERENCES

Bartstow C, Braun M, Psyzocha N. Diagnosis and management of sodium disorders: hyponatremia and hypernatremia. *Am Fam Physician*. 2015;91(5):299-307.

Michels TC, Kelly KM. Parathyroid disorders. *Am Fam Physician*. 2013;88(4):249-257.

Potts JT Jr, Jüppner HW. Disorders of the parathyroid gland and calcium homeostasis. In: Jameson J, Fauci AS, Kasper DL, Hauser SL, Longo DL, Loscalzo J, eds. *Harrison's Principles of Internal Medicine*. 20th ed. New York, NY: McGraw Hill; 2018: Chap. 403. http://accessmedicine.mhmedical.com/content.aspx?bookid=2129&sectionid=192530415. Accessed May 9, 2019.

Viera AJ, Wouk N. Potassium disorders: hypokalemia and hyperkalemia. *Am Fam Physician*. 2015;92(6):487-495.

Walsh J, Gittoes N, Selby P, Society for Endocrinology Clinical Committee. Society for Endocrinology endocrine emergency guidance: emergency management of acute hypercalcaemia in adult patients. *Endocr Connect*. 2016;5(5):G9-G11.

A 75-year-old man presents for a health maintenance checkup. The patient has stable hypertension but has not seen a physician in more than 2 years. He denies any particular problems. He lives alone. He takes an aspirin a day and is compliant with his blood pressure medication (hydrochlorothiazide). The patient is accompanied by his son, who fears that his father is either experiencing a stroke or getting Alzheimer disease because his father is having trouble understanding what family members are saying, especially during social events. The son reports no noticeable weakness or gait impairment. On physical examination, the patient's blood pressure is 130/80 mm Hg. Examination of the ears shows no cerumen impaction and normal tympanic membranes. His general examination is normal. Laboratory studies, including a thyroid-stimulating hormone (TSH) level, are normal.

▶ What is the most likely diagnosis?
▶ What is the next step?

ANSWERS TO CASE 18:
Geriatric Health Maintenance and End-of-Life Issues

Summary: A 75-year-old man presents with

- Loss of speech discrimination
- Complaint of difficulty understanding speech and conversation in noisy areas
- Daily medications of aspirin and hydrochlorothiazide
- No noticeable weakness or gait impairment
- No cerumen impaction, normal tympanic membranes, and normal TSH and blood pressure

Most likely diagnosis: Presbycusis.

Next step: Presbycusis is a diagnosis of exclusion. Hearing aids are underused in presbycusis but are potentially beneficial for most types of hearing loss, including sensorineural hearing loss. Consequently, referral to an audiologist for testing and consideration of amplification with a hearing aid may be an important next step.

ANALYSIS

Objectives

1. Be familiar with geriatric health maintenance. (EPA 1, 12)

2. Be aware of the importance of geriatric screening. (EPA 3, 11, 12)

Considerations

The patient described in the case is a 75-year-old man who has difficulty with speech discrimination. His son reports that the patient has difficulty understanding speech and conversation in noisy areas. He most likely has presbycusis, which is an age-related sensorineural hearing loss typically associated with both selective high-frequency loss and difficulty with speech discrimination. Physical examination of the ears in patients with presbycusis is normal. Other conditions in the differential diagnosis include cerumen impaction, otosclerosis, and central auditory processing disorder (CAPD). Cerumen impaction and otosclerosis can be diagnosed by otoscopy. CAPD is diagnosed when the patient can hear sounds without difficulty but has difficulty understanding spoken words.

> # APPROACH TO:
> ## Health Maintenance in the Elderly and End-of-Life Issues

DEFINITIONS

FUNCTIONAL ASSESSMENT: An evaluation process that gauges a patient's ability to manage tasks of self-care, household management, and mobility.

PRESBYCUSIS: An age-related sensorineural hearing loss typically associated with both selective high-frequency loss and difficulty with speech discrimination.

CLINICAL APPROACH TO GERIATRIC HEALTH MAINTENANCE

By the year 2030, the number of people aged 65 years and older is expected to double from what it was in 1999, increasing from 34 million to 69 million. Geriatric health maintenance provides screening and therapy with the goal of enhancing function and preserving health in the elderly. Screening is not indicated unless early therapy for the screened condition is more effective than late therapy or no therapy. **Preventive services for the elderly include goals of the optimization of quality of life, satisfaction with life, and maintenance of independence and productivity.** Most recommendations for patients older than age 65 years overlap recommendations for the general adult population. Certain categories are unique to older patients, including sensory perception and falling. The primary care provider can perform effective health screening using simple and relatively easily administered assessment tools (Figure 18–1).

Functional Assessment

Functional assessment gauges a patient's ability to manage tasks of self-care, household management, and mobility. Impairment in activities of daily living (ADL) results in an increased risk of falls, hip fracture, depression, and institutionalization. An estimated **25% of patients older than age 65 years have impairments in their instrumental activities of daily living (IADL) or ADL** (Table 18–1). Persons who are unable to perform IADL independently are far more likely to have dementia than their independent counterparts.

Vision Screening

Visual impairment is an independent risk factor for falls, which has a significant impact on quality of life. The majority of conditions leading to vision loss in the elderly are presbyopia, macular degeneration, glaucoma, cataracts, and diabetic retinopathy. Risk factors for cataracts and age-related macular degeneration (AMD) in older patients include vision changes, smoking, diabetes, steroid use, and family history. For these patients, visual acuity testing with the Snellen chart would be of benefit for identifying visual impairment and is a reasonable initial test to do in the primary care setting. However, the US Preventive Services Task Force (USPSTF) has found insufficient evidence regarding beneficial functional outcomes in the elderly who routinely undergo visual acuity testing. Visual acuity testing does not accurately identify ocular diseases that affect the elderly, including

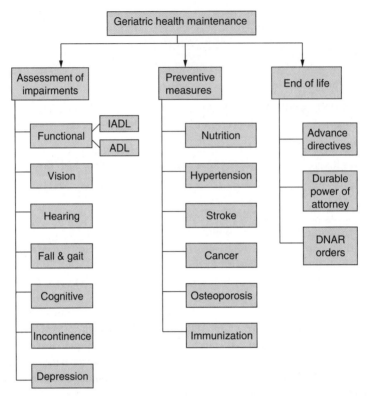

Figure 18–1. Approach to geriatric health maintenance. ADL, activities of daily living; DNAR, do not attempt resuscitation; IADL, instrumental activities of daily living.

cataracts, glaucoma, and AMD, so routine referrals for ophthalmologic examination should be considered.

Presbyopia and AMD. The incidence of presbyopia increases with age. Patients have difficulty focusing on near objects while their distant vision remains intact. **AMD is the leading cause of severe vision loss in the elderly.** AMD is characterized

Table 18–1 • INSTRUMENTAL ACTIVITIES OF DAILY LIVING (IADL) AND ACTIVITIES OF DAILY LIVING (ADL)	
IADL	**ADL**
Transportation	Bathing
Shopping	Dressing
Cooking	Eating
Using the telephone	Transferring (eg, from bed to chair)
Managing money	Continence
Taking medications	Toileting
Housecleaning	Grooming
Laundry	

by atrophy of cells in the central macular region of the retinal pigment epithelium, resulting in the loss of central vision. Treatment options for exudative AMD include laser photocoagulation and intravitreal injections of vascular endothelial growth factor.

Glaucoma. Glaucoma is characterized by a group of optic neuropathies that can occur in all ages. Although glaucoma is most often associated with elevated intraocular pressure, it is the optic neuropathy that defines the disease. For patients who are asymptomatic, the USPSTF found insufficient evidence to routinely screen for glaucoma. However, for elderly patients with risk factors, including increased intraocular pressure, family history, vision changes, or African American race, screening is beneficial.

Cataracts. A cataract is any opacification of the lens. Age-related, or senile, cataracts account for 90% of all cataracts. **Cataract disease is the most common cause of blindness worldwide.** The definitive treatment for cataracts is surgery. Diabetic retinopathy is the leading cause of blindness in working-age adults in the United States. It is important to consider diabetic retinopathy in geriatric vision screening.

Hearing Screening

More than one-third of persons older than age 65 years and half of those older than age 85 years have some hearing loss. This deficit is correlated with social isolation and depression. The whispered voice test has sensitivities and specificities ranging from 70% to 100%. The initial office screening for general hearing loss can be reliably performed with a questionnaire such as the HHIE-S (Hearing Handicap Inventory for the Elderly Screening Version). Limited office-based pure-tone audiometry is more accurate in identifying patients who would benefit from a more formal audiometry.

The majority of patients with hearing impairment will present with complaints unrelated to their sensory deficit. In a quiet examination room with face-to-face conversation, patients can overcome significant hearing loss and avoid detection from a health care provider. Family members are often more concerned about the hearing loss than the patient. **Common causes of geriatric hearing impairments are presbycusis, noise-induced hearing loss, cerumen impaction, otosclerosis, and CAPD.**

Presbycusis. Presbycusis is age-related sensorineural hearing loss usually associated with both selective high-frequency loss and difficulty with speech discrimination. Presbycusis is the most common form of hearing loss in the elderly. Because it often goes unrecognized, exact prevalence data are lacking. Presbycusis is a diagnosis of exclusion. Complete deafness is not an expected end result of presbycusis.

Noise-Induced Hearing Loss. Noise-induced hearing loss is essentially a wear-and-tear phenomenon that can occur with either industrial or recreational noise exposure. Patients will typically present with tinnitus, difficulty with speech discrimination, and problems hearing background noise.

Cerumen Impaction. Cerumen impaction in the external auditory canal is a common, frequently overlooked problem in the elderly that may produce a transient, mild conductive hearing loss. It is estimated that 25% to 35% of institutionalized or hospitalized elderly are affected by impacted cerumen.

Otosclerosis. Otosclerosis is an autosomal dominant disorder of the bones in the inner ear. It results in progressive conductive hearing loss, with onset most commonly in the late 20s to the early 40s. Speech discrimination is typically preserved. Geriatric patients with hearing loss may have otosclerosis complicating their presentation.

Central Auditory Processing Disorder. CAPD is the general term for conditions involving hearing impairment that results from central nervous system dysfunction. The patient with CAPD will have difficulty understanding spoken language but may be able to hear sounds well.

Evidence for Screening. Just as with visual acuity testing, the USPSTF did not find sufficient evidence to justify the use of routine screening tests for hearing loss in the elderly. Since the last recommendation, evidence of routine screening has become available that shows the widespread use of hearing aids after objective hearing loss was identified via in-office tests did not benefit those who did not self-report hearing loss. In other words, only those who had subjective hearing loss seemed to benefit from hearing aids. This raises the question of the benefit of routine hearing loss screening in a population in which this problem is so prevalent secondary to the natural process of aging. However, this recommendation does not apply to elderly patients with symptoms of hearing loss, cognitive impairment, or psychosocial complaints indicating other diagnoses.

Fall Assessment

Falls are the leading cause of nonfatal injuries in the elderly. The associated complications are the leading cause of death from injury in those older than age 65 years. Hip fractures are common precursors to functional impairment and nursing home placement. Approximately **30% of the noninstitutionalized elderly fall each year.** The annual incidence of falls approaches 50% in patients older than 80 years of age. Factors contributing to falls include age-related postural changes, alterations in visual ability, certain medications, and diseases affecting muscle strength and coordination. Due to the far-reaching consequences that falls have on both the patient and the health care system, the American Geriatric Society recommends clinicians ask their elderly patients about history of falls and balance problems. Additionally, the USPSTF recommends exercise interventions to prevent falls in community-dwelling elders at increased risk (Grade B).

Cognitive Screening

The prevalence of dementia doubles every 5 years after age 60, so that by age 85 approximately 30% to 50% of individuals have some degree of impairment. Patients with mild or early dementia frequently remain undiagnosed because their social graces are retained. **The combination of the "clock draw" and the "three-item recall" is a rapid and fairly reliable office-based screening for dementia.** When patients fail either of these screening tests, further testing with the Folstein Mini-Mental State questionnaire should be performed (see Case 32 for more detailed discussion).

Incontinence Screening

Incontinence in the elderly is common. Incontinence is estimated to affect 11% to 34% of elderly men and 17% to 55% of elderly women. Continence problems are frequently treatable and have major social and emotional consequences, but they are often not raised by patients as a concern.

Depression Screening

Depressive symptoms are more common in the elderly despite major depressive disorder being slightly lower in prevalence when compared with younger populations. **Unlike dementia, depression is usually treatable.** Depression significantly increases morbidity and mortality, yet it is often overlooked by health care providers. A simple two-question screen (*Have you felt down/depressed/hopeless in the last 2 weeks?* and *Have you felt little interest or pleasure in doing things?*) shows high sensitivity. Positive responses can be followed up with the Geriatric Depression Scale, a 30-question instrument that is sensitive, specific, and reliable for the diagnosis of depression in the elderly.

Nutrition Screening

Approximately 15% of older outpatients and half of the hospitalized elderly are malnourished. **A combination of serial weight measurements obtained in the office and inquiry about changing appetite are likely the most useful methods of assessing nutritional status in the elderly.** Adequate calcium intake for women is advised. Supplementation with a multivitamin formulated at about 100% daily value can decrease the prevalence of suboptimal vitamin status in older adults and improve their micronutrient status to levels associated with reduced risk for several chronic diseases. Malnutrition is common in nursing homes, and protein undernutrition has a prevalence of 17% to 56% in this setting. Protein undernutrition is associated with an increased risk of infections, anemia, orthostatic hypotension, and decubitus ulcers.

Hypertension Screening

Treatment of hypertension is of substantial benefit in the elderly. Heart disease and cerebrovascular disease are leading causes of death in the elderly. Treatment of hypertension has contributed to a reduction in mortality from both stroke and coronary artery disease. Lifestyle modifications are recommended for all hypertensive patients. Thiazides are the drugs of choice unless a comorbid condition makes another medication preferable.

Stroke Prevention

The incidence of stroke in older adults roughly doubles with each 10 years of age. The greatest risk factor is hypertension, followed by atrial fibrillation. Anticoagulation with warfarin or newer agents, including dabigatran, rivaroxaban, and apixiban, reduces the risk of strokes in people with atrial fibrillation. However, many elderly patients are not anticoagulated because of the fear of injuries from falls. In most instances, the benefits of anticoagulation are likely to outweigh the increased risk of fall-related bleeding, unless the patient has multiple falls, high-risk falls, or a very low risk of stroke.

Cancer Screening

Screening men over the age of 75 for prostate cancer is not routinely recommended (Grade D), as it has not been definitively shown to prolong life and because of the risk of incontinence or erectile dysfunction caused by the treatments. The decision to screen men between the age of 50 and 75 for prostate cancer should be individualized (Grade C). An older woman should undergo annual mammography until her life expectancy falls below 5 to 10 years; however, the USPSTF states that there is insufficient evidence for or against screening in women over the age of 75. The decision to screen for colon cancer in men and women between 65 and 75 years of age should be individualized, with those who had not been screened before likely to benefit most (Grade C). Screening for cervical cancer can be stopped in women older than 65 who have had adequate prior screening and are not at high risk for cervical cancer.

Osteoporosis Screening

The prevalence of low bone mineral density in the elderly is high, with osteopenia found in 37% of postmenopausal women. Primary prevention of osteoporosis begins with identification of risk factors, which include older age, female gender, white or Asian race, low calcium intake, smoking, excessive alcohol use, and chronic glucocorticoid use. Calcium carbonate (500 mg three times daily) and vitamin D (400-800 IU/d) reduce the risk of osteoporotic fractures in both men and women. Bone mineral density testing, using dual-energy x-ray absorptiometry (DEXA), in patients with multiple risk factors may uncover asymptomatic osteoporosis. The USPSTF recommends osteoporosis screening for women 65 years and older and those younger than 65 years of age with increased risks.

Immunizations

Everyone over the age of 6 months should receive an annual influenza vaccination. Persons older than age 65 should receive one dose of the pneumococcal conjugate vaccine (PCV 13) and one dose of the pneumococcal polysaccharide vaccine (PPSV 23). They should also get a single booster dose of tetanus, diphtheria, and pertussis vaccine. Vaccination for herpes zoster is recommended, with the preferred regimen being two doses of the recombinant zoster vaccine (Shingrix) after the age of 50. The less effective alternative is one dose of the live zoster vaccine (Zostavax) after the age of 60.

CLINICAL APPROACH TO END-OF-LIFE ISSUES

Advance Directives

Well-informed, competent adults have a right to refuse medical intervention, even if refusal is likely to result in death. To further patient autonomy, providers are obligated to inform patients about the risks, benefits, alternatives, and expected outcomes of end-of-life medical interventions such as cardiopulmonary resuscitation (CPR), intubation and mechanical ventilation, vasopressor medication, hospitalization and admission to the intensive care unit, and artificial nutrition and hydration. **Advance directives are oral or written statements made by patients when they**

are competent; the directives are intended to guide care should they become incompetent. Advance directives allow patients to project their autonomy. Although oral statements about these matters are ethically binding, they are not legally binding in all states. Written advance directives are essential to give effect to the patient's wishes in these matters.

Durable Power of Attorney for Health Care

A durable power of attorney for health care allows the patient to designate a surrogate decision-maker. The responsibility of the surrogate is to provide "substituted judgment" to decide as the patient would, not as the surrogate wants. In the absence of a designated surrogate, providers turn to family members or next of kin, under the assumption that they know the patient's wishes.

Do Not Attempt Resuscitation Orders

Clinicians should encourage patients to express their preferences for the use of CPR. Despite the favorable portrayal of CPR in the media, **only approximately 15% of all patients who undergo CPR in the hospital survive to hospital discharge.** DNAR ("do not attempt resuscitation") is the preferred term over DNR ("do not resuscitate") to emphasize the low likelihood of successful resuscitation. In addition to mortality statistics, patients deciding CPR preferences should also be informed about the possible consequences of surviving a CPR attempt. CPR may result in fractured ribs, lacerated internal organs, and neurologic disability. There is also a high likelihood of requiring other aggressive interventions if CPR is successful. For some patients at the end of life, decisions about CPR may not be about whether they will live but about how they will die.

CASE CORRELATION

- See also Case 32 (Dementia).

COMPREHENSION QUESTIONS

18.1 A third-year medical student is researching various recommendations for the care of the geriatric patient. Which of the following statements is most accurate?

    A. The USPSTF recommends routine screening for colorectal cancer for adult men starting at the age of 50 and for women starting at the age of 65.

    B. The USPSTF recommends continuing screening for cervical cancer with Papanicolaou (Pap) smear in all women until the age of 75.

    C. The USPSTF recommends that all men should be screened for prostate cancer with prostate-specific antigen (PSA) testing annually starting at the age of 50.

    D. Herpes zoster vaccination is recommended for all adults over the age of 50.

18.2 A 70-year-old man is having difficulty hearing his family members' conversations. He is diagnosed with presbycusis. Which of the following statements regarding his condition is most accurate?

A. Presbycusis does not respond to hearing aid use.

B. Presbycusis is usually caused by a conductive disorder.

C. Presbycusis usually results in loss of speech discrimination.

D. Presbycusis usually results in unilateral hearing loss.

E. Presbycusis usually results in low-frequency hearing loss.

18.3 Which one of the following recommendations is accurate regarding the current USPSTF recommendation for osteoporosis screening in the elderly?

A. All women with strong risk factors, regardless of age, should be screened for osteoporosis.

B. Only women above the age of 65 years should be screened for osteoporosis.

C. Men and women above the age of 65 years should be screened for osteoporosis.

D. African American race is an independent risk factor for osteoporosis and should warrant screening regardless of other risk factors.

ANSWERS

18.1 **D.** The recombinant zoster vaccine is recommended for all adults starting at the age of 50. There is no recommendation for universal PSA testing (answer C) for prostate cancer screening; the decision to screen men between 50 and 75 should be individualized. Pap smears (answer B) can be safely discontinued in women over the age of 65 who have had adequate prior screening. Colorectal cancer screening (answer A) is recommended to start at age 50 for both men and women.

18.2 **C.** Up to one-third of persons older than age 65 years suffer from hearing loss. Presbycusis typically presents with symmetric high-frequency hearing loss (not low frequency, as in answer E). There is loss of speech discrimination, so that patients complain of difficulty understanding rapid speech, foreign accents, and conversation in noisy areas. The mechanism is sensorineural rather than a conductive problem (answer B). Presbycusis responds to hearing aid use (answer A) and generally affects both ears (not unilateral hearing loss, as in answer D).

18.3 **A.** The USPSTF recommends screening for osteoporosis in all women above 65 years of age AND women younger than 65 years of age with risk factors (answer B). Therefore, considering age as a risk factor, essentially all women with risk factors must be screened for osteoporosis with bone mineral density test or DEXA scan. The current recommendation applies only to women (answer C), as there is insufficient evidence to support screening in men, and the race most at risk is Caucasian (not African American race, as in answer D).

CLINICAL PEARLS

▶ Protein undernutrition is associated with an increased risk of infections, anemia, orthostatic hypotension, and decubitus ulcers.

▶ Smoking is associated with osteoporosis.

▶ If "osteoporotic" fractures, such as vertebral compression fractures, occur in conjunction with osteopenia on x-ray, the diagnosis of osteoporosis is almost certain.

▶ Hearing loss and sensory impairments, in general, can be confused with cognitive impairment or an affective disorder.

▶ Presbyopia, macular degeneration, glaucoma, cataracts, and diabetic retinopathy account for the majority of conditions leading to vision loss in the elderly.

▶ A durable power of attorney for health care allows the patient to designate a surrogate decision-maker.

▶ DNAR ("do not attempt resuscitation") is the preferred term over DNR ("do not resuscitate").

REFERENCES

Centers for Disease Control. Recommended adult immunization schedule, United States—2019. https://www.cdc.gov/vaccines/schedules/downloads/adult/adult-combined-schedule.pdf. Accessed May 9, 2019.

Harper G, Johnston C, Landefeld C. Geriatric disorders. In: Papadakis MA, McPhee SJ, Rabow MW, eds. *Current Medical Diagnosis & Treatment 2019*. New York, NY: McGraw Hill; 2019: Chap. 4. http://accessmedicine.mhmedical.com/content.aspx?bookid=2449&sectionid=194431416. Accessed May 9, 2019.

Kudrimoti AM, Perman SE. Hearing & vision impairment in the elderly. In: South-Paul JE, Matheny SC, Lewis EL, et al., eds. *Current Diagnosis & Treatment: Family Medicine*. 4th ed. New York, NY: McGraw Hill; 2015: Chap. 45. http://accessmedicine.mhmedical.com/content.aspx?bookid=1415&Sectionid=77059868. Accessed May 9, 2019.

Rabow MW, Pantilat SZ, Steiger S, Naidu RK. Palliative care & pain management. In: Papadakis MA, McPhee SJ, Rabow MW, eds. *Current Medical Diagnosis & Treatment 2019*. New York, NY: McGraw Hill; 2019: Chap. 5. http://accessmedicine.mhmedical.com/content.aspx?bookid=2449&sectionid=194431700. Accessed May 9, 2019.

Rosenfeld KE, Wenger NS, Kagawa-Singer M, et al. End-of-life decision making: a qualitative study of elderly individuals. *J Gen Intern Med*. 2000;15:620.

State-specific advance directives forms. https://www.nhpco.org/patients-and-caregivers/advance-care-planning/advance-directives/downloading-your-states-advance-directive/ Accessed May 9, 2020.

Tatum PE, Talebreza S, Ross JS. Geriatric assessment: an office-based approach. *Am Fam Physician*. 2018;97(12):776-784.

Tulsky JA, Fischer GS, Rose MR, et al. Opening the black box: how do physicians communicate about advance directives? *Ann Intern Med*. 1998;129:441.

United States Preventive Services Task Force. Published guidelines. https://www.uspreventiveservices taskforce.org/uspstf/topic_search_results?topic_status=P. Accessed May 9, 2020.

A 45-year-old man presents to the clinic with a cough productive of purulent sputum of 3 weeks' duration. He says that he had just gotten over a cold a few weeks prior to this episode. He occasionally has fevers, and he coughs so much that he has chest pain. He reports having a mild sore throat and nasal congestion. He has no history of asthma or any chronic lung diseases. He denies nausea, vomiting, diarrhea, and any recent travel. He denies any smoking history. On examination, his temperature is 98.6 °F (37.0 °C), pulse is 96 beats/min, blood pressure is 124/82 mm Hg, respiratory rate is 18 breaths/min, and oxygen saturation is 99% on room air. Head, ears, eyes, nose, and throat (HEENT) examination reveals no erythema of the posterior oropharynx, tonsillar exudates, uvular deviations, or significant tonsillar swelling. Neck examination is negative. The chest examination yields occasional wheezes, but normal air movement is noted.

▶ What is the most likely diagnosis?
▶ What is your next step?
▶ What are some common noninfectious causes of cough?

ANSWERS TO CASE 19:

Upper Respiratory and Ear Infections

Summary: A 45-year-old man presents with

- No history of lung disease or smoking
- 3 weeks of productive cough following an upper respiratory infection
- History of occasional fever and coughing so much that he has chest pain
- Normal HEENT examination
- Occasional wheezes but normal air movement on chest examination

Most likely diagnosis: Acute bronchitis.

Next step: Bronchodilators, analgesics, and antitussives. Antibiotics have not been consistently shown to be beneficial. The illness is usually self-limited.

Common noninfectious causes of cough: Asthma, chronic obstructive pulmonary disease (COPD), malignancy, postnasal drip, gastroesophageal reflux disease (GERD), medication side effect (eg, angiotensin-converting enzyme inhibitors), congestive heart failure.

ANALYSIS

Objectives

1. Develop a differential diagnosis of cough persisting for 3 weeks or more. (EPA 1, 2)

2. Understand that most upper respiratory infections are self-limited illnesses. (EPA 2)

3. Develop an approach for rational prescription of antibiotics for respiratory infections. (EPA 4)

Considerations

The patient described in the case is a 45-year-old man with no prior history of lung disease, immunocompromised state, or tobacco use. These risk factors are important considerations since respiratory complaints in the setting of COPD, HIV, or a smoking history require a higher index of suspicion of lower respiratory tract infections such as pneumonia. As with any respiratory complaint, the ABCs (airway, breathing, circulation) should be considered. In the ambulatory setting, a very quick assessment of the patient's distress level, respiratory use or nonuse of accessory muscles, anxiety level, stridor, and ability to speak sentences helps to distinguish acute emergency situations from conditions that allow for a more relaxed assessment. The individual described is afebrile, has a normal respiratory rate, and appears to be comfortable. The lung examination reveals some slight wheezes but otherwise normal breath sounds and air movement. The most likely diagnosis in this setting is acute bronchitis. Chest radiography is not necessarily indicated; however, since the complaint has persisted for 3 weeks, any other abnormal finding such as dullness on percussion of the chest, history of fever, or clinical suspicion would be sufficient reason for chest x-ray. Most acute bronchitis is caused by viruses, and antibiotic therapy is not helpful. It is important to remember that acute bronchitis is a diagnosis of exclusion. By definition, a diagnosis of acute bronchitis should not be made in the presence of clinical or radiographic evidence of pneumonia and should only be made after ruling out other etiologies such as GERD, asthma, and the common cold. The patient with true acute bronchitis is best treated with bronchodilator therapy such as albuterol and antitussive agents and follow up in 2 to 3 weeks.

APPROACH TO:
Upper Respiratory and Ear Infections

DEFINITIONS

ACUTE BRONCHITIS: Inflammation of the tracheobronchial tree.

PNEUMONIA: Inflammation or infection of the lower respiratory tract involving the distal bronchioles and alveoli.

CLINICAL APPROACH TO ACUTE BRONCHITIS

Pathophysiology

Acute bronchitis refers to inflammation of the tracheobronchial tree. The inflammatory response to the trigger, whether infectious, allergic, or irritant, leads to increased mucus production and airway hyperresponsiveness. As bronchitis most commonly occurs in the setting of an upper respiratory illness, it is seen more frequently in the winter. Influenza, parainfluenza, adenovirus, rhinovirus, other viruses, *Mycoplasma pneumoniae*, and *Chlamydia pneumoniae* have been implicated as causes.

Clinical Presentation

As the primary symptoms are nonspecific, other etiologies can be mistakenly diagnosed as acute bronchitis. In one study, one-third of patients who had been determined to have recurrent bouts of acute bronchitis were eventually identified as having asthma. Occupational history may be important in determining whether irritants play a role.

There are no specific diagnostic criteria for acute bronchitis, although productive cough with purulent sputum is the most common presentation. Other symptoms are often present, including fever, malaise, rhinorrhea or nasal congestion, sore throat, wheezing, dyspnea, chest pain, myalgias, or arthralgias. The sputum produced can be of variable color and consistency; **the color of sputum is not diagnostic of the presence of a bacterial infection.**

The physical examination in bronchitis is typically nonspecific and frequently is normal. The presence of fever, tachypnea, tachycardia, and blood pressure abnormalities should be noted. In persons with underlying pulmonary or cardiac conditions or in persons with more severe symptoms, oxygen saturation by pulse oximetry may be warranted. Examination of the lungs may reveal rales, rhonchi, or wheezes, but in most cases it is unremarkable.

Bronchitis is nearly always self-limited in an otherwise healthy individual. Although most acute bronchitis lasts for less than 2 weeks, in some cases the cough can last for 2 months or more. Severe cases occasionally produce deterioration in patients with significant comorbid conditions.

Alternate Diagnoses. Occasionally, findings on examination may suggest a particular etiology or an alternate diagnosis. Prolonged fever, tachycardia, tachypnea, hypotension, and signs of consolidation on pulmonary examination may suggest a diagnosis of pneumonia. Pneumonia may present atypically in the elderly and in persons with chronic lung disease. Clinicians must have a higher index of suspicion in these populations. When pneumonia is suspected, a chest radiograph should be obtained to confirm the diagnosis. Conjunctivitis and adenopathy suggest adenoviral infection, although these findings are not specific.

Laboratory Analysis. There is no requirement for obtaining viral cultures, serologic testing, or sputum analyses in a suspected case of acute bronchitis since the organism responsible is rarely identified and, more importantly, since these tests have no effect on the subsequent management.

Treatment

The use of antibiotics has not been shown consistently to alter the natural history of acute bronchitis, except in the case of infection with *Bordetella pertussis*. While frequently prescribed for the diagnosis of bronchitis, studies have shown that antibiotics reduce symptoms by approximately 12 hours. Patients with abnormal vital signs (pulse $\geq$ 100 beats/min, respirations $\geq$ 24 breaths/min, temperature $\geq$ 100.4 °F [38.0 °C]), and examination findings consistent with pulmonary consolidation should be evaluated further for the diagnosis of pneumonia and treated appropriately, if confirmed.

As some of the symptoms of bronchitis are caused by airway hyperreactivity, bronchodilator therapy has been shown in some studies to offer benefit in reducing symptoms. Antitussives, such as dextromethorphan and codeine, may have modest benefits in reducing the cough associated with this illness. Mucokinetic agents have not been shown to be beneficial and are therefore not recommended.

CLINICAL APPROACH TO OTHER UPPER RESPIRATORY INFECTIONS

The most common cause of chronic cough in healthy nonsmokers with a normal chest x-ray is the encompassing diagnosis of upper airway cough syndrome (UACS). This diagnosis encompasses a variety of upper respiratory conditions, which are distinguished from one another by physical examination findings, signs and symptoms, and sometimes after a trial of therapy. Some conditions under this umbrella diagnosis are allergic rhinitis and bacterial sinusitis.

Rhinosinusitis

Pathophysiology. Rhinosinusitis is the inflammation/infection of the nasal mucosa and of one or more paranasal sinuses. Sinusitis occurs with obstruction of the normal drainage mechanism. It is traditionally subdivided into acute (symptoms lasting < 4 weeks), subacute (symptoms lasting 4-12 weeks), chronic (symptoms lasting > 12 weeks), recurrent acute rhinosinusitis (four or more episodes of acute rhinosinusitis per year, with interim resolution of symptoms), and acute exacerbation of chronic sinusitis.

Streptococcus pneumoniae and *Haemophilus influenzae* are the organisms most commonly responsible for acute bacterial sinusitis in adults; *S. pneumoniae*, *H. influenzae*, and *Moraxella catarrhalis* are most common in children. In chronic sinusitis, the infecting organisms are variable, with a higher incidence of anaerobic organisms seen (eg, *Bacteroides*, *Peptostreptococcus*, and *Fusobacterium* species).

Clinical Presentation. The signs and symptoms of rhinosinusitis are nonspecific and similar to other general upper respiratory tract infection symptoms. As most viral upper respiratory tract infections improve in 7 to 10 days, expert opinion suggests considering a diagnosis of bacterial rhinosinusitis after 7 days of symptoms in adults and 10 days in children. The diagnosis is suggested by the presence of purulent nasal discharge, maxillary tooth or facial pain, unilateral maxillary sinus tenderness, and worsening of symptoms after initial improvement.

Treatment. Treatment of acute sinusitis should be directed at the likely causative agents. Amoxicillin and trimethoprim-sulfamethoxazole are widely used first-line agents, typically for 10- to 14-day regimens. Second-line antibiotics are used for those who fail to improve on the initial regimen or who have recurrent or severe disease; these antibiotics include amoxicillin-clavulanic acid; second- or third-generation cephalosporins (cefuroxime, cefaclor, cefprozil, and others); fluoroquinolones; or second-generation macrolides (azithromycin, clarithromycin). Adjunctive therapy with oral or topical decongestants may provide symptomatic relief. Topical decongestants should not be used for more than 3 days to avoid the risk of rebound vasodilation with resultant worsening of symptoms. Nonsteroidal anti-inflammatory drugs and acetaminophen may provide symptomatic relief of pain and fever.

Pharyngitis

Pathophysiology. Pharyngitis is an inflammation or irritation of the pharynx and/or tonsils. In adults, the **vast majority of pharyngitis is viral**. It can also be bacterial or allergic in origin; trauma, toxins, and malignancy are rare causes. Since most cases of pharyngitis in adults are benign and self-limited, a focus of the examination of a patient with symptoms of pharyngitis should be to rule out more serious conditions, such as epiglottitis or peritonsillar abscess, and to diagnose group A beta-hemolytic *Streptococcus* (GAS) infection.

Pharyngitis occurs with much greater frequency in the pediatric population, with a peak incidence between 4 and 7 years of age. *M. pneumoniae*, *C. pneumoniae*, and *Arcanobacterium haemolyticus* are common causes of pharyngitis in teens and young adults. GAS causes 15% of all adult pharyngitis and approximately 30% of pediatric cases.

Clinical Presentation. The cause of pharyngitis cannot always be distinguished based on history or examination. Sore throat associated with cough and rhinorrhea is more likely to be viral in origin. The presence of tonsillar exudates does not distinguish bacterial from viral causes because GAS, Epstein-Barr virus (infectious mononucleosis), mycoplasma, *Chlamydia*, and adenoviruses, among others, can all cause exudates.

Infectious mononucleosis, caused by infection with Epstein-Barr virus, **is extremely difficult to distinguish clinically from GAS infection.** Exudative pharyngitis is prominent. Features suggestive of mononucleosis include retrocervical or generalized adenopathy and hepatosplenomegaly. Atypical lymphocytes can be seen on peripheral blood smear. The associated splenomegaly can be significant, as it predisposes to splenic rupture in response to trauma (even minor trauma). A patient with splenomegaly from mononucleosis should be restricted from activities, such as sports participation, in which abdominal trauma may occur.

On examination, the **patency of the airway must be addressed first.** The presence of stridor, drooling, and a toxic appearance suggest **epiglottitis.** Patients with epiglottitis are sometimes seen leaning forward on their outstretched arms, the so-called tripod position. Patients with suspected epiglottitis need to be managed in a setting where the airway can be emergently secured, via intubation or cricothyroidotomy. Epiglottitis is a rare infection and is becoming even rarer, with near-universal immunization for *H. influenzae*, type B.

Swelling of the peritonsillar region, with the associated tonsil pushed toward the midline and with contralateral deviation of the uvula, is consistent with a **peritonsillar abscess.** This can be seen either as the initial complaint of sore throat, frequently with associated trismus (pain with chewing), or as a complication of streptococcal pharyngitis. Suspicion of peritonsillar abscess should prompt immediate referral for surgical drainage of the abscess.

Findings frequently associated with GAS infections include an abrupt onset of sore throat and fever, tonsillar and/or palatal petechiae, tender cervical adenopathy, and the absence of cough. GAS can also cause an erythematous, sandpaper-like (scarlatiniform) rash. The diagnosis of GAS infection can be made by rapid antigen testing or throat culture. **Rapid antigen tests** can be conducted in a few minutes in the office or emergency department setting. They are **highly specific but have a lower sensitivity than throat culture.** A positive rapid antigen test would prompt antibiotic treatment; a negative test should be followed by a throat culture. **Throat cultures are considered the gold standard** for diagnosis of GAS infections, although the sensitivity and specificity of rapid antigen detection testing have improved significantly. Cultures can take 24 to 48 hours, but this is acceptable in most instances, as the risk of complication from GAS infections is low if treatment is instituted within 10 days of onset of symptoms.

Treatment. Several clinical guidelines have been proposed to aid in the rapid diagnosis and management of patients presenting with pharyngitis. One of the most widely used is the Modified Centor Criteria. In this guideline, a patient is given a point for each of the following criteria: absence of cough; enlarged/tender anterior cervical adenopathy; fever of 100.4 °F or higher; and tonsillar swelling/exudates. One point is also awarded if the patient is age 3 to 14, and one point is

Table 19–1 • CLINICAL DECISION RULE BASED ON CENTOR SCORE	
0-1	No further testing and no antibiotic indicated
2-3	Perform rapid strep or throat culture and treat with antibiotic if positive
4 or more	Consider empiric antibiotic treatment

deducted for the age of 45 years or higher. Based on the number of points assessed, the following decision guidelines are proposed (see Table 19-1).

Penicillin is the antibiotic of choice for GAS pharyngitis. Oral therapy requires a 10-day course of penicillin V. Intramuscular (IM) therapy with 1.2 million units of penicillin G benzathine is used for adults and children weighing more than 27 kg. Children who weigh less than 27 kg can receive 600,000 units of penicillin IM. In penicillin-allergic patients, treatment options include cephalosporins and macrolides.

Complications. **Complications from untreated GAS infections are rare** but include rheumatic fever, glomerulonephritis, toxic shock syndrome, peritonsillar abscess, meningitis, and bacteremia. Rheumatic fever, which may complicate up to 1 in 400 untreated cases of GAS pharyngitis, can cause permanent cardiac and neurologic sequelae. Glomerulonephritis results from antigen/antibody complex deposition in the glomeruli. **Poststreptococcal glomerulonephritis may occur whether or not the patient receives appropriate antibiotic treatment.**

CLINICAL APPROACH TO INFECTIONS OF THE EAR

Otitis Externa

Pathophysiology. Otitis externa (OE) is an infection of the external auditory canal. The tympanic membrane may be uninvolved. The most common pathogens include staphylococci, streptococci, and other skin flora. Some cases have been associated with the use of swimming pools or hot tubs. This infection (swimmer's ear) is usually caused by *Pseudomonas aeruginosa*.

Clinical Presentation. Patients with OE complain of ear pain and, sometimes, itching. The pain from OE can be severe. Examination shows an inflamed, swollen, external ear canal, often with exudates and discharge. Movement of the external ear is usually quite painful.

Treatment. Irrigation and administration of topical antibiotics, frequently combined with a steroid, are usually successful. **Patients with diabetes mellitus are at risk for an invasive external otitis** (malignant OE) caused by *P. aeruginosa*. Treatment for this condition involves surgical debridement of necrotic tissue and 4 to 6 weeks of intravenous antibiotics if cranial bones are involved.

Otitis Media

Pathophysiology. Otitis media (OM) is an infection of the middle ear seen primarily among preschool children, but occasionally in adults as well. Infection of the middle ear space, caused by upper respiratory tract pathogens, is promoted by edematous, congested Eustachian tubes that obstruct drainage. Viral infection with serous otitis may predispose to acute bacterial OM. *S. pneumoniae, H. influenzae,* and *M. catarrhalis* are the most common bacterial pathogens.

Clinical Presentation. Fever, ear pain, diminished hearing, vertigo, and tinnitus are common presenting symptoms. On examination, the tympanic membrane may appear red, but the presence of decreased membrane mobility or fluid behind the tympanic membrane is necessary for the diagnosis.

Treatment. **Most cases of acute OM will resolve spontaneously.** Indications for treatment with antibiotics include prolonged, recurrent, or severe symptoms. Numerous antibiotics can be used for treatment. Amoxicillin remains the recommended initial therapy. Alternative treatments include amoxicillin-clavulanic acid, trimethoprim-sulfamethoxazole, or second- and third-generation cephalosporins. Complications are uncommon but include mastoiditis, bacterial meningitis, brain abscess, and subdural empyema.

CASE CORRELATION

- See also Case 2 (Dyspnea [Chronic Obstructive Pulmonary Disease]), Case 24 (Pneumonia), and Case 56 (Wheezing and Asthma).

COMPREHENSION QUESTIONS

19.1 A 30-year-old woman with no past medical history presents with a productive cough of 2 weeks' duration. She states she also has had a runny nose, body aches, congestion, and fevers for the past week. In the office, she is normotensive, with a normal pulse and a temperature of 101.2 °F. Her physical examination is significant for sinus tenderness, boggy nasal turbinates, and crackles in the left lower lobe lung fields. Which of the following is the best initial step in management?

   A. Reassure the patient that she likely has a viral infection, and it will resolve on its own

   B. Order a rapid strep test and treat if positive

   C. Prescribe amoxicillin for a likely bacterial infection

   D. Order chest x-ray to rule out possible pneumonia

19.2 A 5-year-old boy is brought to the clinic with cough, congestion, runny nose, and low-grade fever for the past 3 days. He has been treated with acetaminophen for fever and given honey for his cough. He has been eating well and has been active at home. On examination, his temperature is 99.7 °F, and his vital signs are otherwise normal. He is active, playful, and smiles during the encounter. You note that his right tympanic membrane is red and bulging, but the left tympanic membrane is normal. His examination is otherwise normal. At this time, the best step in management is which of the following?

   A. Prescription for amoxicillin for OM

   B. Reassurance with a follow-up visit if not improving in the next 10 days

   C. Referral for a hearing test

   D. Prescription for ciprofloxacin otic drops for OE

19.3 A 13-year-old girl presents with fever and sore throat of 48 hours' duration. She has a temperature of 101 °F in the office and is tachycardic, with a pulse of 118 beats/min. Her physical examination is positive for tender, enlarged left cervical lymphadenopathy and tachycardia. Her pharynx is erythematous with tonsillar enlargement or exudate. She has had no cough. What is the best step in management?

A. Treat empirically with antibiotics

B. Order rapid strep test and, if positive, treat with antibiotics

C. Neither further testing nor antibiotics

D. Order throat culture and, if positive, treat with antibiotics

ANSWERS

19.1 **D.** Acute bronchitis is a diagnosis of exclusion in the absence of clinical or radiographic findings concerning for pneumonia. In this patient with fevers, productive cough, and rales on lung examination, it is important to rule out pneumonia and not merely assume it is a self-limited viral infection (answer A). If there is a strong clinical suspicion of community-acquired pneumonia, a chest x-ray is not necessary, and outpatient treatment with antibiotics can be initiated; however, amoxicillin is not a good choice, as there is high resistance to this agent (answer C). The diagnosis of streptococcal pharyngitis is made with a rapid strep test or throat culture (answer B), and the decision to order these in the office is guided by the Modified Centor Criteria based on the following factors: age, presence of tonsillar exudates, fever, and absence of cough.

19.2 **B.** The incidental physical finding of a red tympanic membrane is common in a child with an upper respiratory infection. This is consistent with an OM, but at this time it does not require antibiotic treatment (answers A). Most OM spontaneously resolves. In the absence of prolonged or severe symptoms, watchful waiting is the most appropriate management at this time. This presentation is not consistent with OE (answer D). Hearing loss (answer C) is not generally associated with OM.

19.3 **A.** Management of strep pharyngitis is frequently guided by the Modified Centor Criteria, which calculate a probability of strep throat based on a scoring system. This patient gets one point each for the presence of fever, tender cervical adenopathy, erythematous pharynx and tonsillar exudate, absence of cough, and age, which is a score of 5. You could reasonably consider an empiric antibiotic treatment for GAS since the likelihood of streptococcal pharyngitis would be about 50%. Thus, the other answer choices (answer B, rapid strep test and antibiotics; answer C, no further testing or antibiotics; and answer D, throat culture and antibiotics) would not be as applicable with such a high likelihood of GAS.

CLINICAL PEARLS

► The main concerns with pharyngitis include ruling out more serious conditions, such as epiglottitis or peritonsillar abscess, and diagnosing group A beta-hemolytic streptococcal infections.

► UACS is an umbrella term that encompasses a variety of upper respiratory conditions, including rhinitis and sinusitis.

► A tonsillopharyngeal exudate does not differentiate viral and bacterial causes.

► The vast majority of pharyngitis is viral.

► On examination, the patency of the airway must be addressed first. The presence of stridor, drooling, and a toxic appearance suggest epiglottitis.

► The Modified Centor Criteria are a tool that aids in the rapid diagnosis and management of pharyngitis. Points are given for absence of cough; enlarged/tender anterior cervical adenopathy; fever of 100.4 °F or higher; tonsillar swelling/exudates; and age 3 to 14. A point is deducted for age > 45 years.

► Patients with diabetes mellitus are at increased risk for invasive external otitis.

REFERENCES

Aring AM, Chan MM. Acute rhinosinusitis in adults. *Am Fam Physician*. 2011;83(9):1057-1063.

Benich JJ, Carek PJ. Evaluation of the patient with chronic cough. *Am Fam Physician*. 2011;84(8): 887-892.

Choby BA. Diagnosis and treatment of streptococcal pharyngitis. *Am Fam Physician*. 2009;79(5): 383-390.

Evans AT, Husain S, Durairaj L, Sadowski LS, Charles-Damte M, Wang Y. Azithromycin for acute bronchitis: a randomised, double-blind, controlled trial. *Lancet*. 2002;359(9318):1648-1654.

Gonzales R, Bartlett JG, Besser RE, et al. Principles of appropriate antibiotic use for treatment of uncomplicated acute bronchitis: background. *Ann Intern Med*. 2001;134(6):521-529.

Irwin RS, Baumann MH, Bolser DC, et al. Diagnosis and management of cough executive summary: ACCP evidence-based clinical practice guidelines. *Chest*. 2006;129(1 suppl):1S-23S.

Kinkade S, Long NA. Acute bronchitis. *Am Fam Physician*. 2016;94(7):560-565.

Rosenfeld RM, Andes D, Bhattacharyya N, et al. Clinical practice guideline: adult sinusitis. *Otolaryngol Head Neck Surg*. 2007;137:1S.

A 56-year-old man is brought to the emergency department complaining of chest discomfort for about 90 minutes. He has had occasional symptoms for a month, but it is worse today. Today's symptoms began while he was walking his dog and decreased slightly with rest but have not resolved. He describes the feeling as a pressure sensation in the left substernal area of his chest associated with shortness of breath and mild diaphoresis. He does not have any radiation of the discomfort today, but he has experienced radiation to the left upper extremity in the past. The patient denies any health problems, but his wife reports that he has not seen a physician in years. His wife made him come in because his younger brother had a heart attack 6 months ago. The patient is a vice president of a bank and lives with his wife and three daughters. He has smoked 1½ packs of cigarettes per day for more than 30 years and denies drinking alcohol or any drug use.

On physical examination he is an anxious, obese gentleman who appears pale and has a moist brow. His temperature is 98.8 °F (37.1 °C), his pulse is 105 beats/min, his respirations are 18 breaths/min, his blood pressure is 190/95 mm Hg, his height is 74 inches, his weight is 250 lb, and his oxygen saturation is 97%. Cardiac examination reveals a regular rhythm without murmur, but he has an S_4 gallop. His lungs are clear to auscultation, and his neck is without carotid bruits or jugular venous distension. His abdomen is normal. He does have a right femoral bruit. Extremities show trace edema but no clubbing or cyanosis. He has 2+ pulses in radial and dorsal pedalis arteries. Rectal examination reveals no masses or tenderness and a normal prostate, and he is guaiac negative.

► What is the most likely diagnosis?
► What is your next diagnostic step?
► What is the next step in therapy?

ANSWERS TO CASE 20:
Chest Pain

Summary: A 56-year-old man presents with

- Chest discomfort—a pressure sensation in the left substernal area of his chest associated with shortness of breath and diaphoresis
- Symptoms that began with minimal exertion
- No prior medical care
- Family history of coronary artery disease (CAD) and a history of heavy tobacco use
- Hypertension, tachycardia, and a cardiac gallop
- Trace edema in the lower extremities and a femoral bruit
- Obesity

Most likely diagnosis: Unstable angina pectoris; must rule out myocardial infarction (MI).

Next diagnostic step: Complete blood count (CBC), electrolytes, blood urea nitrogen (BUN), creatinine, prothrombin time (PT), partial thromboplastin time (PTT), international normalized ratio (INR), glucose, 12-lead electrocardiography (ECG), and chest x-ray (CXR); markers of myocardial damage, including creatine kinase (CK) and MB isoenzyme (CK-MB), troponin T and troponin I to be done stat and every 6 to 10 hours for three cycles; oxygen saturation must be monitored as well. Studies that can be performed later include fasting lipids, liver function tests, magnesium, homocysteine level, urine drug screen, urinalysis, and myoglobin.

Next step in therapy: MONA therapy: Morphine, Oxygen, Nitroglycerin, Aspirin.

ANALYSIS

Objectives

1. Understand a diagnostic approach to chest pain and how to reduce potential damage to myocardium by implementing rapid evaluation. (EPA 3, 10)

2. Know the acute evaluation of chest pain and how to best implement the primary and secondary treatment of chest pain. (EPA 4, 10)

3. Identify the risks and the need to educate patients to reduce their risks. (EPA 12)

4. Be familiar with the differential diagnosis of chest pain and how to best rule in and out the more life-threatening problems. (EPA 1, 2, 3)

Considerations

This 56-year-old man has unstable angina with a variety of risk factors for CAD. All patients who present to primary care providers with chest pain are immediate challenges. Most resources emphasize the life-threatening etiologies; however, the non–life-threatening etiologies are far more common in presentation. Providers must master a cost-effective approach to diagnosing the various etiologies of chest pain, determining which patients warrant further evaluation; a thorough history and physical examination are crucial. The cause of this patient's symptoms must be determined as soon as possible. If the etiology is determined to be cardiac, there are medications and interventions that can dramatically reduce both morbidity and mortality. A complete history and physical examination can give information that can help determine if and when other more expensive and invasive tests are necessary. The patient's most immediate problem is his acute symptoms. His anxiety will decrease slightly when he perceives that he is getting adequate care and information.

The first priority is to obtain the ECG and CXR, while giving medications to decrease the damage caused to his myocardium and simultaneously reducing his blood pressure. Nitroglycerin and beta-adrenergic antagonists will begin achieving these goals. He will need constant monitoring and continuous telemetry. Oxygen needs to be continued as well. Before the ECG and CXR have been completed, aspirin, oxygen, nitroglycerin, morphine, and a beta-adrenergic antagonist should be given. To limit possible morbidity and mortality to the patient, providers must assume there is a cardiac etiology until it has been effectively ruled out.

The laboratory tests previously listed need to be drawn, at which time intravenous access can be started in two places. The results of the tests will determine if the patient has other risk factors in addition to his known hypertension, family history of CAD, tobacco abuse, and obesity. If he routinely walks his dog, his lifestyle contains at least minimal physical activity.

APPROACH TO:
Chest Pain

DEFINITIONS

ANGINA PECTORIS: Severe pain around the heart caused by a relative deficiency of oxygen supply to the heart muscle.

MYOCARDIAL INFARCTION: Cardiac muscle death caused by partial or complete occlusion of one or more of the coronary arteries.

NEW YORK HEART ASSOCIATION FUNCTIONAL CLASSIFICATION OF ANGINA:

Class I—Angina only with unusually strenuous activity

Class II—Angina with slightly more prolonged or slightly more vigorous activity than usual

Class III—Angina with usual daily activity

Class IV—Angina at rest

UNSTABLE ANGINA: Angina of new onset, angina at rest or with minimal exertion, or a crescendo pattern of angina with episodes of increasing frequency, severity, or duration.

CLINICAL APPROACH

Epidemiology

Nearly 1½ million people in the United States experience an MI each year. **Every 34 seconds, one American has a coronary event.** This is fatal approximately one-third of the time. However, there has been a continuous decline in the mortality rate over the past three decades because of a better understanding of the etiology and pathophysiology of MI and because of advances in therapeutic treatments.

Chest pain or discomfort is still one the most common complaints in both the outpatient and emergency settings, and assessing the cause of such symptoms in a rapid fashion is of utmost importance. It is important to identify risk factors for CAD in patients, the presence of which would indicate an increased suspicion for an acute MI. Male gender; age older than 60 years; diaphoresis; radiation of pain to neck, arm, shoulder, or jaw; and a past history of angina or acute MI are all considered risk factors.

Pathophysiology

Atherosclerosis leading to plaque rupture and then cascading to coronary artery thrombosis is the cause of an acute MI approximately 90% of the time, but **many different conditions can be the culprit for angina.** Coronary artery spasm, including cocaine-induced injury, can cause angina. Aortic dissection extending into a coronary artery will cause extensive damage. An embolus to a coronary artery can be caused by endocarditis, prosthetic heart valves, or myxoma. Embolism can also cause cerebral vascular accidents, increasing the extent of the initial evaluation that is warranted.

If the patient is experiencing myocardial ischemia or infarction, time is myocardium. Initial evaluation should be done within 10 minutes of presentation, and the goal of this evaluation should be to determine the need for further testing, such as cardiac enzymes, stress test, or angiography.

The changes seen in an ECG that are indicative of angina include ST-segment elevation or depression and/or T-wave inversion. MIs include these changes plus elevated CK-MB and/or troponin levels. Pathologic Q waves may also indicate cardiac pathology, but they typically represent myocardial tissue necrosis from a completed infarction. When Q waves are present, the benefits of thrombolytic therapy are uncertain. **Not all MIs will have ECG changes.** A normal ECG reduces the likelihood of MI but does not rule out cardiac pathology.

Any person with symptoms of angina who has a left bundle branch block (LBBB) on ECG must have serum cardiac enzymes drawn, as there is a high degree of correlation between LBBB and organic heart disease, especially CAD. LBBB can mask signs of myocardial pathology, as it can mimic both acute and chronic ischemic changes. All of the listed ECG changes have a differential diagnosis that includes MI. The clinical picture is of utmost importance, again demonstrating the need for a complete history and physical examination.

Clinical Presentation

History. The history should focus on onset and evolution of the chest pain. The cardinal features of all chief complaints should be followed, paying attention to the patient's description of the pain/discomfort, location, radiation of pain, quality of pain, quantity of pain, duration, associating factors, and aggravating and/or alleviating factors (Table 20–1). **Many people do not describe angina as chest pain.**

Table 20–1 • DIFFERENTIAL DIAGNOSIS OF CHEST PAIN		
Disorder	Symptoms/Findings	Studies
Angina	Substernal pressure for duration < 30 min	ECG, CXR, serum values
	Radiation to arm, neck, jaw ± dyspnea, N/V, diaphoresis ↑ with exertion; ↓ with rest and NTG	
MI	Anginal symptoms but duration > 30 min	ECG, CXR, serum values
Pericarditis	Sharp pain radiates to trapezius ↑ with respiration; ↓ with sitting forward	Friction rub, ECG, ± pericardial effusion
Aortic dissection	Sudden onset of tearing pain with radiation to back	CXR, widened mediastinum CT, TEE, MRI
Heart failure	Exertional chest pain and dyspnea (uncommon cause of angina, but often patients may also have CAD)	CXR, displaced apical impulse, edema (pulmonary, lower extremities), JVD, cardiac gallop, murmurs
Pneumonia	Dyspnea, fever, and cough; pleuritic pain	CXR, egophony, dullness to percussion
Pneumothorax	Unilateral sharp pleuritic pain of sudden onset, CXR findings	Unilateral ↓ breath sounds and/or hyperresonance
Pulmonary embolism	Sudden onset of pleuritic pain, tachycardia, tachypnea, hypoxemia	D-dimer, V/Q scan, CT chest, pulmonary angiogram
Gastroesophageal reflux	Burning epigastric/substernal pain, acid taste in mouth, ↑ with meals; ↓ with PPIs or antacids	Endoscopy, esophageal pH probe
Peptic ulcer disease	Epigastric pain ↓ with antacids and PPIs	Endoscopy, *Helicobacter pylori* test
Pancreatitis	Severe epigastric and back pain	↑ amylase and lipase, abdominal CT
Costochondritis	Localized pain that is easily reproducible, tender to palpation	Tenderness to palpation
Anxiety	"Tightness" sensation of chest, SOB, tachycardia	Ask screening questions for anxiety and panic
Herpes zoster	Pain often presents prior to rash	Unilateral pain in dermatomal distribution

Abbreviations: ↓, decreasing; ↑, increasing; CAD, coronary artery disease; CT, computed tomography; CXR, chest x-ray; ECG, electrocardiogram; JVD, jugular venous distension; MI, myocardial infarction; MRI, magnetic resonance imaging; NTG, nitroglycerin; N/V, nausea and vomiting; PPI, proton pump inhibitor; SOB, shortness of breath; TEE, transesophageal echocardiogram.

It is more effective to ask the patient to describe the discomfort. Some describe it as pressure, squeezing, crushing, or smothering. Some may use a "Levine sign," a fist held firmly against the chest. The discomfort is usually central and substernal. It may radiate to the jaw, shoulder, arm, or hand, usually to the left side. Cardiogenic nausea and vomiting are associated with larger MIs.

Angina and Exertion. The relationship of the symptoms to exertion is very important. Exertion, emotional stress, or other situations that either increase myocardial oxygen demand or decrease oxygen supply can increase symptoms. **Stable angina usually responds promptly to measures that reduce myocardial oxygen demand,** such as rest. The pain typically resolves in less than 5 minutes. If angina persists for longer than 20 to 30 minutes, an MI is more likely. In this setting, hospitalization and further evaluation are warranted.

History of Myocardial Infarction. The targeted history in patients with angina needs to ascertain whether the patient has had prior episodes of myocardial ischemia (stable or unstable angina, MI, interventions such as bypass surgery or angioplasty). Evaluation of the patient's complaints should focus on chest discomfort, associated symptoms, gender and age-related differences in presentation, hypertension, diabetes mellitus, possibility of aortic dissection, risk of bleeding, and clinical cerebrovascular disease (amaurosis fugax, face/limb weakness or clumsiness, face/limb numbness or sensory loss, ataxia, or vertigo).

Physical Examination. The physical examination needs to concentrate on evidence that supports or disproves a diagnosis of cardiovascular disease. General appearance and vital signs can reveal much about the patient and the patient's stability. Hypertension, evidence of elevated lipids, changes consistent with diabetes mellitus, and signs of peripheral vascular disease all increase the risk of CAD.

Fundoscopic examination can show signs of chronic hypertension or diabetes mellitus. All blood vessels must be auscultated for bruits, a direct sign of atherosclerotic disease. Diminished peripheral pulses are also a sign of atherosclerotic disease. Signs of heart failure include pulmonary edema, rales, jugular venous distension, and hepatojugular reflux. New gallops or murmurs can signal myocardial ischemia. Shallow, painful breathing suggests chest pain with a pleural cause. Asymmetric expansion of the chest with unilateral hyperresonance to percussion and diminished breath sounds are indicative of a possible pneumothorax.

Cardiac Examination. The cardiac examination requires careful evaluation. **Unequal carotid pulses or upper extremity pulses can indicate aortic dissection, but most patients with dissection will not have pulse deficit.** The murmur of aortic stenosis can be significant, as aortic stenosis can present with angina, which can then lead to syncope and heart failure.

The patient's chest wall should be palpated. If this examination reproduces the chest pain, costochondritis becomes more likely. **Musculoskeletal causes of chest pain are the most common etiology in an outpatient setting.**

Abdominal Examination. An abdominal examination is also important, as a gastrointestinal etiology is the second most common culprit for chest pain in an outpatient setting. Careful examination of both upper quadrants and the epigastric area must be done. The abdominal aorta warrants careful examination.

Psychogenic Evaluation. Additionally, panic disorder and anxiety can cause chest pain, tightness, and shortness of breath. Clinicians should use a questionnaire to evaluate any possible psychogenic causes when this is suspected.

Primary Treatment

All patients who rule in for MI should receive aspirin and an antithrombotic treatment if there are no contraindications. Aspirin and heparin reduce the risk of subsequent MI and cardiac death in patients with unstable angina. Heparin usually should be continued for 48 hours or until angiography is performed. Patients suffering from unstable angina with ECG changes should also be given platelet glycoprotein (GP) IIb/IIIa receptor inhibitors. **GP IIb/IIIa inhibitors** reduce the end point of death or recurrent ischemia when given in addition to standard therapy for patients with high-risk unstable angina or non–ST-elevation MI treated with percutaneous coronary intervention or who are refractory to prior treatment.

Clopidogrel. Studies present different recommendations for using clopidogrel (Plavix) in addition to aspirin and heparin. It is reasonable to give clopidogrel 300 mg orally to patients with suspected acute coronary syndrome (ACS) (without ECG or cardiac marker changes) who are either allergic to or have gastrointestinal intolerance of aspirin. Current American College of Cardiology/American Heart Association recommendations advise withholding clopidogrel for 5 to 7 days before planned bypass surgery.

Other Acute Treatments. Additional acute treatment options include supplemental oxygen, nitroglycerin, intravenous morphine, beta-blockers, angiotensin-converting enzyme (ACE) inhibitors or angiotensin receptor blockers, and statins. The mnemonic MONA can be used to remember treatment for MI (see Table 20–2). Nitroglycerin is best given intravenously initially because of the ability to achieve predictable blood levels rapidly. Once stabilized after 24 hours, the asymptomatic patient should be switched to a long-acting oral or transdermal nitrate. Unless contraindicated, a beta-adrenergic antagonist should also be given to reduce myocardial damage and possibly limit infarct size. The **combination of nitroglycerin and a beta-adrenergic antagonist reduces the risk of subsequent MI.** Beta-adrenergic antagonists decreased mortality and reduced infarct size in many clinical trials.

Table 20–2 • "MONA" TREATMENT FOR ACUTE MYOCARDIAL INFARCTION	
Morphine	• Can achieve adequate analgesia that decreases levels of circulating catecholamines, thus reducing myocardial oxygen consumption • Must be initiated rapidly if nitroglycerin cannot alleviate the discomfort
Oxygen	• Administration is 2 to 4 L/min by nasal cannula • May be discontinued after 6 hours if oxygen saturation remains normal without other complications
Nitroglycerin	• Given sublingually initially every 5 minutes for a total of three doses (in the absence of hypotension or contraindications such as sildenafil [Viagra] use) • It is then advanced to intravenous or transdermal routes
Aspirin	• 325 mg should be chewed and swallowed • Clopidogrel may be used if allergy to aspirin exists

Angiotensin-Converting Enzyme Inhibitors. **ACE inhibitors reduce short-term mortality when started within 24 hours of acute MI.** Postinfarction ACE inhibitors prevent left ventricular remodeling and recurrent ischemic events. It is reasonable to recommend their indefinite use in the absence of any contraindications. All trials with oral ACE inhibitors have shown benefit from their early use, including those in which early entry criteria included clinical suspicion of acute infarctions.

Magnesium Sulfate and Calcium Channel Blockers. Magnesium sulfate should be given if levels are low, as hypomagnesemia can increase the incidence of torsade de pointes–type ventricular tachycardia. Despite the widespread use of calcium channel blockers both during and after myocardial ischemia, no evidence exists supporting any benefit when taking these medications. Rapid-release dihydropyridines (eg, short-acting nifedipine) are contraindicated because they increased mortality in multiple trials.

Stress Test and Angiography. Patients who are asymptomatic after 48 hours of drug therapy can perform a modified Bruce protocol stress test. Patients who have a markedly positive stress test should be referred for angiography. There is some debate concerning when angiography should be done. One approach shows that an early invasive approach with angiography within 24 to 48 hours is beneficial, whereas a more conservative approach recommends doing angiography only if recurrent ischemia is present or a positive stress test is done. There is no clear consensus as to which approach is superior.

Lifestyle Changes. All patients admitted for angina or MI should receive a reduced saturated fat and cholesterol diet. These patients may benefit from nutrition counselors to help them develop healthy lifestyle changes.

Reperfusion Therapy. In the event of an MI, **percutaneous cardiac intervention** (PCI; previously known as angioplasty) is considered the primary method of reperfusion. Since time to reperfusion is critical, if a patient is brought initially to a hospital that cannot perform PCI, selecting a reperfusion strategy requires considering multiple factors, including the condition of the patient, the time required for transfer, the time since symptom onset, and the risk of bleeding with fibrinolysis. Fibrinolysis should be administered to patients with an ST-segment elevation MI (STEMI) at non–PCI-capable hospitals if it is expected that the patient cannot be transferred and undergo PCI within 120 minutes. Special consideration should be given to women with STEMI because they have shown an improved response with PCI compared with fibrinolysis.

Secondary Treatment

Risk Factor Modification. Primary prevention of CAD must be encouraged for all patients. **Risk factors for CAD include diabetes mellitus, dyslipidemia, age, hypertension, tobacco abuse, family history of premature CAD, male gender, postmenopausal status, left ventricular hypertrophy, and homocystinemia** (Table 20–3). Modification of risk factors has a direct link to reduce morbidity and mortality. Patient education is particularly important.

Medications. **Aspirin, nitrates, and beta-adrenergic antagonists have proven benefits for both primary and secondary treatment.** Prolonged treatment with aspirin reduces risks for both CAD and cerebrovascular disease. Beta-adrenergic antagonist use reduces first-year mortality. If no adverse effects are experienced, patients

Table 20-3 • RISK FACTORS FOR CAUSES OF CHEST PAIN	
Risk Factor	Event
Age/gender: male > 40 y old	CAD
Hypertension	CAD and aortic dissection
Tobacco abuse	CAD, thromboembolism, aortic dissection, pneumothorax, and pneumonia
Diabetes mellitus	CAD
Cocaine use	MI

Hyperlipidemia
    Elevated TC, TG, LDL
    Low HDL
	MI

Left ventricular hypertrophy	MI
Family history of premature CAD	MI
Blunt trauma to chest	Pneumothorax, myocardial or pulmonary contusion, chest wall injury

Abbreviations: CAD, coronary artery disease; HDL, high-density lipoprotein; LDL, low-density lipoprotein; MI, myocardial infarction; TC, total cholesterol; TG, triglyceride.

should continue a beta-adrenergic antagonist 2 to 3 years or longer. Long-acting nitrates can treat angina symptoms.

Beta-hydroxy-beta-methylglutaryl-coenzyme A reductase inhibitors (statins) have documented a consistent decrease in the incidence of major adverse cardiovascular events when given within a few days after onset of ACS. It is safe and feasible to start statin therapy early (within 24 hours) in patients; once started, statin therapy should continue uninterrupted. The American College of Cardiology/American Heart Association recommendations are for all persons with known atherosclerotic cardiovascular disease to be treated with high-intensity statin therapy.

Hypertension must be treated using agents that reduce cardiac complications, as previously discussed. If further reduction is necessary, many medications treat hypertension and angina. Blood pressure and coronary pathology have a linear relationship; as blood pressure is reduced, the risk, morbidity, and mortality of cardiac disease are also reduced. Agents used often depend on a patient's comorbid conditions.

Lifestyle Changes. Physical activity is an important component of lifestyle change. Recommendation of a minimum goal of 30 minutes of exercise on most days should be given to all patients. Weight management is also encouraged but often requires numerous interventions. A minimum of a 5% reduction in weight will provide benefits to the patient. Body mass index needs to become part of the vital signs examined at every visit.

CASE CORRELATION

- See also Case 30 (Hypertension) and Case 35 (Hyperlipidemia).

COMPREHENSION QUESTIONS

20.1 A 58-year-old man presents to his provider for follow-up of his hypertension and hyperlipidemia. He also reports chest pain and feeling short of breath after climbing two flights of stairs or walking three to four blocks. The symptoms resolve after several minutes of rest. Which of the following drugs would **not** be indicated as a first-line agent in the treatment of this patient's condition?

A. Atorvastatin

B. Nitroglycerin

C. Enalapril

D. Doxazosin

E. Aspirin

20.2 Which one of the following patients presenting with chest pain is at the highest risk for an acute MI?

A. A 40-year-old woman on a proton pump inhibitor for reflux disease

B. A 75-year-old man with parasternal chest pain, lipid abnormalities, and no past history or cardiac disease

C. A 23-year-old man recently diagnosed with hypertrophic cardiomyopathy

D. A 67-year-old man with a history of a prior angioplasty, with chest pain radiating to the neck and complaint of diaphoresis

20.3 Which of the following ECG changes makes the determination of acute MI the most difficult?

A. Q wave

B. ST-segment elevation

C. Left bundle branch block

D. First-degree atrioventricular block

E. T-wave inversion

20.4 A 64-year-old woman with a history of hypertension and angina pectoris presents with chest pain for the last 3 hours. She describes the pain as "sharp"; it is worse when she inhales deeply, and it is not relieved by sublingual nitroglycerin. The pain improves if she sits up and leans forward. Her ECG shows ST elevation in most leads. Cardiac enzymes are negative. Which of the following is the most likely diagnosis in this patient?

A. Unstable angina pectoris

B. Myocardial infarction

C. Aortic dissection

D. Heart failure

E. Pericarditis

ANSWERS

20.1 **D.** This patient has a new onset of angina on top of his hypertension and hyperlipidemia. Aspirin (answer E), statins (answer A), beta-blockers (answer C), ACE inhibitors, and nitroglycerin (answer B) would all be indicated for these conditions. Doxazosin (answer D), an alpha-blocker, would not be of benefit in this situation.

20.2 **D.** Risk factors for increased likelihood of acute MI are male gender; age older than 60 years; chest pain radiating to neck, jaw, arm, or shoulder; and a prior history of angina or acute MI. Proton pump inhibitors (answer A) and hypertrophic cardiomyopathy (answer C) are not risk factors.

20.3 **C.** The changes of LBBB make the determination of an acute MI by an ECG extremely difficult. In these patients, it is particularly important to obtain serum markers of myocardial damage.

20.4 **E.** This patient likely has pericarditis. The pain is described as sharp in nature rather than dull, aching, pressure of angina (answer A and B). The pain is exacerbated by inspiration, and there is global ST-segment elevation noted on the ECG. The pain of pericarditis tends to decrease when the patient sits upright and leans forward. Aortic dissection (answer C) would present with an excruciating and severe "tearing pain" and associated with distress. Heart failure would present with dyspnea, tachypnea, pedal edema, and jugular venous distension.

CLINICAL PEARLS

▶ Angina pectoris is the most frequent symptom of intermittent ischemia.

▶ Targeted history and physical examinations of patients with angina are vital to expedite proper diagnosis and treatment of patients. The patient's description of their discomfort is key; history must be given attention because it is the most important diagnostic factor.

▶ Physical examination may be normal in many patients with angina.

▶ Aspirin, nitrates, beta-adrenergic antagonists, and statins are the backbone in treatment and prevention of myocardial pathology, having proven benefit for both primary and secondary treatment.

▶ Time is myocardium. Initial diagnosis and treatment must be done as soon as possible.

▶ Be mindful of polypharmacy, as many drugs have side effects that can exacerbate myocardial damage.

▶ The most common etiology of chest pain in the primary care setting is musculoskeletal. However, it is imperative to rule out a cardiac cause of chest pain before making a musculoskeletal-related diagnosis.

REFERENCES

McConaghy JR, Oza RS. Outpatient diagnosis of acute chest pain in adults. *Am Fam Physician.* 2013;87(3):177-182.

Mehta LS, Beckie TM, DeVon HA, et al. Acute myocardial infarction in women: a scientific statement from the American Heart Association. *Circulation.* 2016;133(9):916-947.

O'Gara PT, Kushner FG, Ascheim DD, et al. 2013 ACCF/AHA guideline for the management of ST-elevation myocardial infarction: a report of the ACCF/AMA Task Force on Practice Guidelines [published correction appears in *Circulation.* 2013;128(25):e481]. *Circulation.* 2013;127(4): e362-e425.

Smith JN, Negrelli JM, Manek MB, et al. Diagnosis and management of acute coronary syndrome: an evidence-based update. *J Am Board Fam Med.* 2015;28(2):283-293.

Switaj TL, Christensen SR, Brewer DM. Acute coronary syndrome: current treatment. *Am Fam Physician.* 2017;95(4):232-240.

A 46-year-old woman presents to the clinic for the first time, complaining of decreased urinary output with a foamy appearance for 5 months. She also complains of swelling in both legs and nonbloody, nonbilious emesis a few times a week. She was diagnosed with type 2 diabetes 10 years ago and has been taking insulin for 2 years. She does not check her sugar levels at home. When asked about her diet, she states that she eats the best she can for what she can afford but often has very little appetite and vomits sometimes. The patient last saw her health care provider 8 months ago, and insulin is her only medication.

On examination, the patient is an obese woman. Her temperature is 99 °F (37.2 °C), heart rate is 108 beats/min, blood pressure is 198/105 mm Hg, respirations are 19 breaths/min, and oxygen saturation is 94% on room air. She has periorbital edema. Her skin is hyperpigmented on both lower extremities. Her heart is tachycardic with an S_4 gallop auscultated and without murmurs or rubs. When palpating the heart's point of maximal impulse (PMI), it is lateral to the left midclavicular line. There are vesicular breath sounds throughout both lungs. Her neck reveals no jugular venous distension (JVD), and there are no carotid bruits. The lower extremities reveal pitting pretibial edema with a pit recovery time less than 40 seconds. Laboratory studies in your office include a urinalysis showing hyaline casts, 3+ proteinuria, and glucose, but negative for ketones. Her hemoglobin is 10.9 g/dL, and her hematocrit is 32% with a mean corpuscular volume (MCV) of 82.3 fL.

► What is the most likely diagnosis?
► What is your next diagnostic step?
► What is the next step in therapy?

ANSWERS TO CASE 21:
Chronic Kidney Disease

Summary: A 46-year-old woman presents with

- A history of uncontrolled diabetes and currently-uncontrolled hypertension
- Periorbital edema and long-standing lower extremity edema
- An S$_4$ heart sound and displaced PMI, indicating left ventricular hypertrophy (LVH) with diastolic dysfunction
- Central obesity
- Urinalysis showing hyaline casts, 3+ proteinuria and glucose, and negative ketones
- Hemoglobin 10.9 g/dL with an MCV of 82.3 fL

Most likely diagnosis: Acute worsening of chronic kidney disease (CKD).

Next diagnostic step: Measurement of serum electrolytes, blood urea nitrogen (BUN), and creatinine (Cr); imaging of the kidneys.

Next step in therapy: Further history to identify and remove any offending agents (eg, nonsteroidal anti-inflammatory drugs [NSAIDs]) and implement measures to control blood pressure and diabetes; she may require dialysis if she develops complications such as pulmonary edema, severe hyperkalemia, or anuria.

ANALYSIS

Objectives

1. Be able to list the common risk factors for developing CKD. (EPA 1, 12)
2. Be able to name common tests used to evaluate CKD. (EPA 3)
3. Be able to report outpatient management strategies and medications for patients with CKD. (EPA 4)
4. Be able to report common complications associated with CKD. (EPA 1, 2, 10)

Considerations

This 46-year-old patient presents with a concerning symptom of a decrease in urination with a change in the appearance of the urine. The most immediate concern is how often she is urinating and to what degree is she urinating less. A significant reduction requires immediate evaluation of renal function (serum creatinine) and volume status. **Volume status is assessed clinically by skin turgor, mucous membranes, specific gravity in the urinalysis, and orthostatic blood pressure.** A low-volume status with an elevated Cr requires that the patient be given intravenous fluids to see if there can be any recovery of kidney function. The patient's uncontrolled diabetes and hypertension predispose her to kidney damage. Another common offender in a patient with this history is the use of NSAIDs. This will increase the patient's already high risk of damage.

With CKD, patients are often able to compensate for the metabolic imbalances that occur, such as hyper- or hyponatremia, hyperkalemia, elevated uric acid levels, and metabolic acidosis. Patients may also experience secondary hyperparathyroidism. Significantly elevated potassium levels require treatment with sodium polystyrene sulfonate (Kayexalate), insulin with glucose, and retention enemas, depending on the degree of elevation. When the patient is no longer compensating, there are symptoms of pulmonary edema, which include shortness of breath, lower extremity edema, JVD, and abnormal lung sounds (rales).

This patient was compensating and mostly demonstrated the result of a hypoalbuminemic state from the loss of protein in the urine. She had lower extremity edema with a long pit time that reflected her low albumin state. Her occasional emesis reflected high levels of urea and other toxins. Persistent emesis mandates treatment. Her normocytic anemia was the result of reduced erythropoietin from the kidneys. In this setting, treatment with exogenous erythropoietin improves prognosis for cardiovascular mortality. The hyaline casts reflected the long-standing damage to the kidneys.

Increasing the patient's chance of improved kidney function requires glucose and blood pressure control, removing offenders such as NSAIDs and diuretics (if allowable), maintaining normal volume status (which is difficult with a low albumin state), and adding agents that both treat blood pressure and improve kidney and cardiovascular function, such as angiotensin-converting enzyme (ACE) inhibitors or angiotensin receptor blockers (ARBs). CKD itself is a cardiovascular risk factor. Patients are more likely to die from cardiovascular disease than to develop end-stage renal disease (ESRD) requiring dialysis. The patient's gross proteinuria of 3+ reflects her high risk for cardiovascular disease.

APPROACH TO:
Chronic Kidney Disease

DEFINITIONS

CHRONIC KIDNEY DISEASE: A spectrum of processes associated with abnormal kidney function and progressive decline in glomerular filtration rate (GFR) that are present for > 3 months.

END-STAGE RENAL DISEASE: The irreversible loss of kidney function such that the patient is permanently dependent on renal replacement therapy (dialysis or transplantation). Also defined as a GFR of less than 15 mL/min.

CLINICAL APPROACH

Epidemiology

Chronic kidney disease is becoming more common in the United States. **The most common etiologies are diabetes, hypertension, and glomerulonephritis.** Diabetic kidney disease occurs in 30% to 40% of type I diabetics, in 25% of type 2 diabetics, and in 24% of hypertensive patients. Within the diabetic patient population, 20% to 60% have hypertension. Many patients develop ESRD after years of poor control

Table 21-1 • STAGES OF CHRONIC KIDNEY DISEASE	
Stage 1	GFR more than 90 mL/min in the presence of signs of kidney disease, such as proteinuria, hematuria, or abnormal renal structure
Stage 2	GFR of 60-89 mL/min
Stage 3a **Stage 3b**	GFR of 45-59 mL/min GFR of 30-44 mL/min
Stage 4	GFR of 15-29 mL/min
Stage 5	GFR less than 15 mL/min or dialysis

of their hypertension and diabetes, which is why good control of these medical conditions has such a priority with new insurance payment mechanisms, such as Medicare's Merit Incentive Payment System (MIPS). Underlying causes may be ascertained through clinical presentation, symptomatology, and past medical and family history.

Pathophysiology

The Kidney Disease Outcomes Quality Initiative (KDOQI) from the National Kidney Foundation (NKF) recommends both a serum Cr to estimate GFR and a random urinalysis for albuminuria in those groups at risk for CKD. The stage of CKD is based on the GFR, which is normally between 90 and 120 mL/min (see Table 21–1). The GFR can be estimated with a random Cr level calculated with one of two commonly used equations:

Modification of diet in renal disease (MDRD) equation:

$$\text{GFR (mL/min/1.73 m}^2) = 175 \times (\text{SCr})^{-1.154} \times (\text{age})^{-0.203}$$
$$\times (0.742, \text{if female}) \times (1.210, \text{if black})$$

Cockcroft-Gault equation:

$$\text{CCr (mL/min)} = \{(140 - \text{age}) \times \text{weight [kg]}\}/(72 \times \text{SCr}) \times (0.85, \text{if female})$$

(SCr = serum creatinine concentration; CCr = creatinine clearance).

The Cockcroft-Gault equation is preferred for older patients and in renal dosing of medications. It is important to note that these equations do not give an accurate calculation of GFR in the setting of an acute change in renal function, such as acute kidney injury. Serial measurements of renal function are recommended for newly diagnosed cases to determine the pace of renal deterioration and whether the disease is truly chronic, as opposed to acute or subacute. A 24-hour urine collection is recommended for persons with extremes of age and weight, malnutrition, skeletal muscle disease, paraplegia or quadriplegia, or a strict vegetarian diet.

Imaging. The evaluation in all patients with CKD includes renal imaging (typically with renal ultrasound). Treatment may be more successful in patients with normal-size kidneys. **Small kidneys are a sign of irreversible disease.** Asymmetry suggests renovascular disease.

Urine Evaluation. Evidence of proteinuria or microalbuminuria should be evaluated in all patients with CKD. If the urine dipstick does not reveal gross proteinuria, a sample should be sent to evaluate for microalbumin. A test is positive if there is more than 30 mg of microalbumin per gram Cr. In the case of less than 200 mg of protein per gram Cr, it is recommended that the test be repeated yearly. Any patient with more than 200 mg of protein per gram Cr will need diagnostic evaluation and treatment. The protein-to-Cr ratio in an early morning random urine sample may be used instead of a 24-hour urine protein excretion.

Laboratory Values. Some common laboratory studies include ANA (antinuclear antibody), antiphospholipid antibodies, C3, C4, ESR (erythrocyte sedimentation rate) and/or CRP (C-reactive protein) (looking for lupus nephritis); hepatitis panel and HIV test (looking for infectious etiologies); serum and urine protein electrophoresis (looking for multiple myeloma) for those patients older than age 35; hemoglobin A_{1c}; fasting blood sugar; and analysis of urine sediment.

Biopsy. Renal biopsy, if not contraindicated by comorbidities, is indicated in patients with unknown etiology after history and laboratory evaluation, if parenchymal disease is suspected, or if treatment or prognosis will be based on the biopsy. However, biopsy is contraindicated if bilateral small kidneys are seen on imaging, as there is a low likelihood of improving outcome due to the presence of late-stage disease. Patients should be tested for common conditions associated with CKD, such as anemia and hyperphosphatemia.

Treatment

Treating Reversible Causes. Managing CKD includes treatment of reversible causes. Hypovolemia, hypotension, infection leading to sepsis, and drugs that lower the GFR all reduce renal perfusion. History and physical examination allow for this diagnosis, and a trial of fluids may improve kidney function. Drugs such as NSAIDs, ACE inhibitors, ARBs, aminoglycosides at full strength, and radiographic contrast material can affect kidney function. Urinary tract obstruction, commonly caused by prostate enlargement in elderly men, is a potentially reversible cause.

Controlling Blood Pressure. Nonproteinuric renal disease requires strict blood pressure control. The Eighth Joint National Committee (JNC 8) guidelines recommend a blood pressure goal of less than 140/90 mm Hg in all patients age 18 years or older with CKD. Multiple guidelines recommend a blood pressure goal of less than 130/80 mm Hg, especially if there is diabetes or proteinuria. Another goal is the reduction of protein excretion to less than 500 to 1000 mg/d (or at least 60% of the baseline value). JNC 8 guidelines recommend starting with an ACE inhibitor or an ARB for blood pressure control in patients with CKD, followed by a thiazide diuretic or calcium channel blocker if the blood pressure goal is not achieved. When using ACE inhibitors or ARBs, be aware that a Cr increase of less than 30% is considered acceptable, as this lowers the pressure in the glomerulus. Beta-blockers may also be considered as a second- or third-line treatment for blood pressure control. **Combining an ACE inhibitor with an ARB is not recommended.**

Phosphate Binders. When the GFR is below 25 to 30 mL/min, oral phosphate binders are usually required. Caution is used when treating hyperphosphatemia in stages 3 to 5 of CKD. It is suggested that calcium intake not exceed 2000 mg/d, as this may contribute to cardiovascular disease.

Treating Anemia. Guidelines suggest evaluation of anemia with a hemoglobin less than 12 g/dL in women and 13.5 g/dL in men. This should include evaluation for nonrenal causes of anemia. In patients with CKD whose hemoglobin is less than 10 g/dL, treatment with erythropoietin is helpful, with a goal of 12 mg/dL in low-risk patients and 13 mg/dL in those at risk for stroke and cardiovascular events. This may reduce symptoms of anemia, show cardiovascular improvement, and possibly decrease mortality.

Other Treatments. Other treatments may be beneficial in CKD. Dietary protein restrictions of 0.8 to 1.0 mg/kg/d may be beneficial. Statins are recommended for treatment of hyperlipidemia in most CKD patients not on dialysis. The volume overload associated with CKD responds well to sodium restriction and loop diuretics. Hyperkalemia may be prevented by a low-potassium diet, avoiding drugs such as NSAIDs, and adding diuretics to the regimen of patients on ACE inhibitor/ARB therapy. Metabolic acidosis may be treated with sodium bicarbonate, with a goal of maintaining a concentration of 22 mEq/L. Dietary phosphate restriction may limit the development of secondary hyperparathyroidism in these patients. There is evidence for vitamin D supplementation reducing all-cause mortality. Patients should also have influenza and pneumococcal vaccinations. Those with a high risk of progression should also receive hepatitis B vaccination.

Renal Replacement Therapy. Ultimately, the patient who is proceeding toward ESRD must be identified and adequately prepared for renal replacement therapy. It is recommended that patients with a GFR < 30 mL/min, difficult-to-control comorbidities, or significant proteinuria or sudden worsening of renal function be referred to a nephrologist for evaluation and preparation for possible dialysis. Patients with ESRD have high rates of medical complications and therefore are ideal patients for interprofessional care management.

CASE CORRELATION

- See also Case 30 (Hypertension) and Case 51 (Diabetes Mellitus).

COMPREHENSION QUESTIONS

21.1 A 56-year-old man with known CKD presents to the emergency center with a 3-day history of shortness of breath and rapid weight gain. On examination of the heart, you are able to auscultate an S_3 heart sound and hear crackles at the lung bases. You also see moderate JVD. The oxygen saturation is 90% on room air. Which of the following is your next step in evaluation?

    A. Order an echocardiogram.

    B. Order a chest x-ray.

    C. Measure a Cr to calculate GFR.

    D. Order a computed tomographic (CT) angiograph of the chest.

21.2 A 39-year-old woman with hypertension and type 2 diabetes has been noted to have progressively worsening renal insufficiency. Which of the following measures is most important in the prevention of ESRD?

  A. Tobacco cessation

  B. Triglyceride control

  C. Glycemic control

  D. Weight control

  E. Dietary sodium restriction

21.3 A 72-year-old man with a long history of hypertension presents to the emergency department complaining of not being able to urinate for the last 36 hours. He also has a 1-day history of nausea, vomiting, and abdominal pain. He states that his urinary stream has been decreasing over the past 2 years. On examination, the abdomen is firm and tender, and the prostate is enlarged. His serum Cr level is 3.4 mg/dL. Which of the following is the best next step?

  A. Give intravenous fluids and see if he begins to make urine.

  B. Perform a renal ultrasound in the emergency department.

  C. Maintain tight control of his blood pressure.

  D. Place an indwelling Foley catheter.

21.4 A 45-year-old woman with type 2 diabetes presents to the clinic for follow-up. She states that over the past year, she has decreased vision in the left eye. She also has had some occasional chest pain for the past 2 months. On examination, the blood pressure is 145/92 mm Hg. The cardiac and lung examinations are normal. Laboratory tests show the urinalysis reveals 1+ proteinuria. Serum laboratory tests reveal a baseline Cr of 1.6 mg/dL, a low-density lipoprotein (LDL) cholesterol level of 135 mg/dL. Which of the following is the best medication to start the patient on at this time?

  A. ACE inhibitor

  B. Hydralazine

  C. Oral nitrate

  D. Thiazide diuretic

ANSWERS

21.1 **B.** This patient has CKD with volume overload, as evidenced by symptoms of shortness of breath, weight gain, the presence of an S_3, crackles, and moderate JVD. Because oxygenation is the most important first priority, respiratory status should be addressed first. A quick and simple first step is to do a chest x-ray to confirm what you already suspect—pulmonary edema. After initiating furosemide (Lasix), the chest x-ray may be repeated to see to what degree the diuresis has improved the overload. Echocardiography (answer A) may be indicated but would not be the first test performed. Answer C (measure Cr to calculate GFR) is also an important point, but not as important as addressing the respiratory status. Rather than simply fluid overload, another potential problem is acute myocardial infarction, so an electrocardiogram and cardiac enzyme values are also indicated.

21.2 **C.** Optimal control of high blood pressure, acidosis, volume depletion, and cholesterol is important to prevent worsening renal function. Diabetes is a leading cause of ESRD. Tight glycemic control can prevent the microvascular complications of diabetes, such as diabetic nephropathy, though it has not been shown to decrease significantly the occurrence of macrovascular complications of diabetes, such as coronary artery disease or peripheral vascular disease. Treating secondary hyperparathyroidism prevents complications such as renal osteodystrophy. The patient's weight (answer D) does not impact renal function substantially. Smoking (answer A) has numerous health risks but does not tend to impact kidney function directly; nevertheless, its effect on the cardiovascular system may impact the kidneys. Answer B (triglyceride control) is not as important as hypertension and diabetes control; also, the LDL cholesterol more closely correlates to cardiovascular events. Answer E (dietary sodium intake) can help to avoid fluid overload, but it is control of protein in the diet that is more important in slowing the progression of kidney disease.

21.3 **D.** This patient has an enlarged prostate that has caused urinary obstruction and potentially reversible renal failure, depending on when the obstruction is resolved. Placing the Foley catheter usually allows for significant reversal of an elevated Cr. Following catheter placement, the urine output needs to be carefully monitored and evaluation of the Cr repeated later. Another clue to the diagnosis of urinary obstruction is the tense lower abdomen, which is caused by a very enlarged bladder. When evaluating for a cause, it is especially important to rely on clinical examination skills in elderly patients who have less-than-optimal communication skills as a consequence of dementia or who have a history of stroke. Importantly, when there is relief of postobstructive kidney insufficiency, profuse diuresis is common. Answer A (intravenous fluids) would be indicated in a prerenal situation, where the patient is volume depleted, but intravenous fluids would only make the distended bladder even more distended in this case. Answer B (perform renal ultrasound in the emergency department) is something that should be done at some time in the next 24 hours, but it is not as important as relieving the urinary obstruction. Answer C (maintain control of blood pressure) is important in preserving kidney function on a chronic basis.

21.4 **A.** ACE inhibitors would help in hypertension treatment and protect renal function in this patient. Both diabetes and CKD are known to be cardiovascular risk equivalents. Other factors, such as uncontrolled blood pressure and cholesterol, add to the patient's high risk, which is why it is so important for all diabetics and CKD patients to improve all modifiable risk factors. The goals become much more stringent when looking at these two groups of patients. Answer B (hydralazine) will not help with cardiac risk and will not protect the kidneys. Answer C (oral nitrate) may help with occasional chest pain but will not affect survival. The patient should have a cardiac stress test to evaluate the chest pain. Answer D (thiazide diuretic) may possibly worsen the renal insufficiency, worsen the diabetes, and not protect the kidneys.

CLINICAL PEARLS

▶ Small kidneys on imaging usually reflect irreversible disease. Small kidneys should rarely be biopsied since the result of the biopsy usually will not alter the treatment or prognosis of the condition.

▶ Calculation of the estimated GFR using the Cockcroft-Gault formula is an important process because, especially in older persons, a seemingly normal serum Cr could reflect a significant reduction in GFR and could affect dosing of medications.

▶ Volume status is assessed clinically by skin turgor, mucous membranes, specific gravity in the urinalysis, and orthostatic blood pressure.

▶ The most common etiologies of CKD are diabetes, hypertension, and glomerulonephritis.

▶ Patients with a GFR < 30 mg/dL, difficult-to-control comorbidities, significant proteinuria, or sudden worsening of renal function should be referred to a nephrologist for evaluation and preparation for possible dialysis.

REFERENCES

ADVANCE Collaborative Group; Patel A, MacMahon S, et al. Intensive blood glucose control and vascular outcomes in patients with type 2 diabetes. *N Engl J Med.* 2008;358(24):2560-2572.

Bargman JM, Skorecki KL. Chronic kidney disease. In: Jameson J, Fauci AS, Kasper DL, Hauser SL, Longo DL, Loscalzo J, eds. *Harrison's Principles of Internal Medicine.* 20th ed. New York, NY: McGraw Hill; 2018: Chap. 305. http://accessmedicine.mhmedical.com/content.aspx?bookid=2129&sectionid=186950702. Accessed May 3, 2019.

Fowler M. Microvascular and macrovascular complications of diabetes. *Clin Diabetes.* 2008;26:2. http://clinical.diabetesjournals.org/content/26/2/77.full.pdf+html. Accessed May 3, 2019.

Gaitonde DY, Cook DL, Rivera IM. Chronic kidney disease: detection and evaluation. *Am Fam Physician.* 2017;96(12):776-783.

James PA, Oparil S, Carter BL, et al. 2014 evidence-based guideline for the management of high blood pressure in adults: report from the panel members appointed to the Eighth Joint National Committee (JNC 8). *JAMA.* 2014;311(5):507-520.

Kidney Disease: Improving Global Outcomes (KDIGO) Lipid Work Group. KDIGO clinical practice guideline for lipid management in chronic kidney disease. *Kidney Int.* 2013;3(suppl):259-305.

Kliger AS, Foley RN, Goldfarb DS, et al. KDOQI US commentary on the 2012 KDIGO clinical practice guideline for anemia in CKD. *Am J Kidney Dis.* 2013;62(5):849-859.

National Kidney Foundation. KDOQI clinical practice guideline for diabetes and CKD: 2012 update. *Am J Kidney Dis.* 2012;60(5):850-886.

A 25-year-old woman presents to the office with 1 week of vaginal discharge. She describes this as green-yellow in color with a bad odor. She has never had this before. She says the symptoms started along with vaginal soreness after she had sexual intercourse. She denies any itching, abdominal pain, nausea, vomiting, fever, or chills. She is sexually active and prevents pregnancy with an intrauterine device (IUD). She has been with one male partner for the past 3 months, and he has no symptoms. She states she first had intercourse at age 15 and has had multiple sexual partners. She had a chlamydial infection 2 years ago that was treated with oral antibiotics. Her last menstrual period was 2 weeks ago and was normal. She denies any recent antibiotic treatment. On examination, she is afebrile, has normal vital signs, and is well appearing. Her general physical examination is normal. On pelvic examination, she has normal external genitalia. She has a small amount of frothy, homogenous green-gray discharge at the introitus. The cervix has a "strawberry"-red appearance with a slight amount of discharge noted coming from the os. The IUD string is in place. *Chlamydia* and gonorrhea specimens are obtained from the cervical os, and a sample of the vaginal discharge is collected for microscopic evaluation. Bimanual examination shows no cervical motion tenderness and a normal uterus and adnexa.

▶ What organism is the most likely cause of her symptoms?
▶ What would you expect to see on microscopic examination of the vaginal discharge?
▶ What is the recommended treatment for this infection?

ANSWERS TO CASE 22:

Vaginitis and Other Vaginal Infections

Summary: A 25-year-old woman presents with

- A foul-smelling vaginal discharge and vaginal soreness after sexual intercourse
- Greenish, frothy discharge and a "strawberry cervix" noted on examination
- Denial of any itching, abdominal pain, nausea, vomiting, fever or chills, or recent antibiotic use
- Sexual history includes one male partner (with no symptoms) for the past 3 months, first intercourse at age 15, and multiple sexual partners in the past
- An IUD with string in place and last menstrual cycle 2 weeks ago
- Chlamydial infection 2 years ago that was treated with oral antibiotics
- Normal bimanual examination

Organism most likely to cause this infection: *Trichomonas vaginalis.*

Expected microscopic examination findings: Motile, flagellated trichomonads and many white blood cells.

Recommended treatment: Metronidazole 2 g by mouth in a single dose for both the patient and her sexual partner. Metronidazole 500 mg twice a day for a week is an alternate regimen.

ANALYSIS

Objectives

1. Be able to create a differential for common presentations of vaginitis on the basis of clinical information and laboratory testing. (EPA 1, 2)

2. Describe the diagnostic strategy for vaginal infections. (EPA 1, 2, 3)

3. Be able to state current recommendations for treatment of the various etiologies of vaginitis. (EPA 4)

Considerations

Women with vaginitis may present with a variety of symptoms, including vaginal discharge, itching, odor, and dysuria. There are many potential causes of vaginal discharge, including sexually transmitted pathogens and overgrowth of the normal vaginal flora.

Certain historical information may lead a clinician to suspect a specific cause of vaginitis in a given patient. For example, a history of recent antibiotic use may predispose to a *Candida* vaginitis, as the antibiotic may alter the normal vaginal flora and allow the overgrowth of a fungal organism. Women with diabetes mellitus are also more predisposed to developing yeast infections. A history of multiple sexual partners may raise the likelihood of a sexually transmitted infection (STI), such as trichomonas vaginitis (trichomoniasis).

The patient's symptoms and signs may also suggest a specific organism as the cause of her vaginitis. Fungal infections tend to have thick discharge and cause significant pruritus. The discharge of bacterial vaginosis (BV) is often thinner and patients complain of a "fishy" odor. Trichomoniasis produces a discharge that is usually frothy, and the patient's cervix is frequently very erythematous.

The key test to determining the cause of vaginal discharge, which guides the specific treatment, is microscopic examination of the discharge. A sample of the discharge is examined both as a "wet mount" (ie, mixed with a small amount of normal saline) and as a "KOH prep" (ie, mixed with a small amount of 10% potassium hydroxide). On wet mount, the examiner can evaluate the normal epithelial cells and look for white blood cells, red blood cells, clue cells, and motile trichomonads. The hyphae or pseudohyphae of *Candida* are best seen on KOH prep.

APPROACH TO:
Vaginal Infections

DEFINITIONS

BACTERIAL VAGINOSIS: Condition of excessive anaerobic bacteria in the vagina, leading to a discharge that is alkaline.

CANDIDA **VULVOVAGINITIS:** Vaginal and/or vulvar infection caused by *Candida* species, usually with heterogeneous discharge and inflammation.

TRICHOMONAS **VAGINITIS:** Infection of the vagina caused by the protozoa *T. vaginalis*, usually associated with a frothy yellow/green discharge and intense inflammatory response.

CLINICAL APPROACH

Vulvovaginal Candidiasis

A vulvovaginal candidiasis infection is typically caused by *C. albicans*, although other species are occasionally identified. **More than 75% of women have at least one episode during their lifetime.** The presenting symptom is a thick, sometimes curd-like, whitish discharge that has no odor. The patient usually complains of significant pruritus of the external and internal genitalia. On physical examination, the vaginal area can be edematous with erythema present. The discharge has a pH between 4.0 and 5.0. The diagnosis is confirmed by wet mount or KOH preparation showing budding yeast or pseudohyphae. **Fungal cultures are not needed to confirm the diagnosis,** but they are useful if the infection recurs or is unresponsive to treatment. Numerous treatment options are available for patients with vulvovaginal candidiasis, including over-the-counter and prescription medications. Uncomplicated candidiasis can be treated effectively with short-term intravaginal preparations (creams or vaginal suppositories) or single-dose oral therapies (fluconazole 150 mg). Treatment of complicated or recurrent infection should begin with an intensive regimen for 10 to 14 days followed by

6 months of maintenance therapy to reduce the likelihood of recurrence. Treatment of sexual partners is not indicated unless they are symptomatic (eg, male partners with balanitis).

Trichomoniasis

Trichomoniasis infection is caused by the protozoan *T. vaginalis* and is sexually transmitted. The incubation period is 3 to 21 days after exposure. **Certain factors predispose to infection, such as multiple sexual partners, pregnancy, and menopause.** The presenting complaint is copious amounts of a thin, frothy, green-yellow or gray, malodorous vaginal discharge. Women can also have vaginal soreness or dyspareunia. Symptoms may start or be exacerbated during the time of their menses. Vaginal examination may reveal that the **cervix has a "strawberry" appearance** (red and inflamed with punctations) or that redness of the vagina and perineum is present. Microscopically, the **wet mount preparation can demonstrate motile trichomonads and many white blood cells,** although cultures or polymerase chain reaction (PCR) may be necessary because of the significant number of false-negative results. The recommended treatment for trichomoniasis is a single 2-g oral dose of metronidazole or 1-week regimen of 500 mg twice a day for the patient and her sexual partner. **It is important to screen for other STIs and to remember to treat the partner to ensure better cure rates.**

Bacterial Vaginosis

Bacterial vaginosis arises when normal vaginal bacteria are replaced with an **overgrowth of anaerobic bacteria and *Gardnerella vaginalis*.** Although not sexually transmitted, it is associated with having multiple sexual partners. **Diagnosis can be based on the presence of three of four clinical criteria:** (1) a thin, homogenous vaginal discharge; (2) a vaginal pH more than 4.5; (3) a positive KOH "whiff" test (a fishy odor present after the addition of 10% KOH to a sample of the discharge); and (4) the presence of clue cells in a wet mount preparation (Figure 22–1). Culture is generally not needed. Treatment options include both oral and topical vaginal preparations of metronidazole or clindamycin. There are no advantages to any of these regimens with regard to cure rates or recurrence, although patients do report more satisfaction with the vaginal preparations. **Treatment of BV in pregnant women may reduce the incidence of miscarriage and postpartum endometritis.** Treatment of sexual partners is not necessary and does not reduce the risk of recurrent infection.

Chlamydia trachomatis and Neisseria gonorrhea

Approximately 50% of gonococcal infections and 70% of chlamydial infections are asymptomatic in women. For this reason, the US Preventive Services Task Force recommends screening for these infections in sexually active women < 25 years old and in older women if at higher risk. **The Centers for Disease Control and Prevention (CDC) recommends nucleic acid amplification tests (NAAT) as the test of choice, which can be done with either urine or cervical specimens.** Symptomatic women may present with mucopurulent cervicitis or vaginal discharge. **As it may take a few days to get a test result, empiric treatment should be considered in symptomatic women**

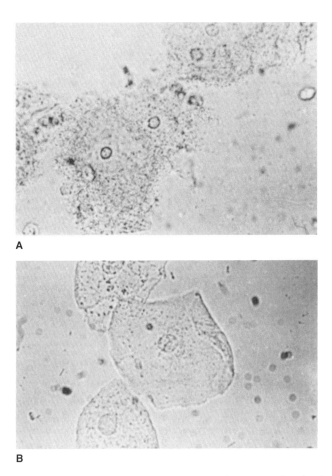

Figure 22–1. Bacterial vaginosis (A) Clue cells, (B) Normal epithelium. (Reproduced with permission, from Kasper DL, Braunwald E, Fauci A, et al. *Harrison's Principles of Internal Medicine,* 16th ed. 2005. Copyright © McGraw Hill LLC. All rights reserved.)

with higher risk and if follow-up is unlikely. The first-line treatment recommendation for gonorrhea is dual antibiotic treatment with ceftriaxone 250 mg intramuscularly and a 1 g oral dose of azithromycin. Per CDC guidelines, all patients with a positive gonorrhea test should be treated for chlamydia as well regardless of chlamydia test results. The recommended treatment for *Chlamydia* infections is azithromycin in a single 1 g oral dose or doxycycline 100 mg orally twice daily for 7 days. Recent sex partners should be treated, and follow-up testing for reinfection in 4 to 6 months can be considered. In pregnancy, a test of cure should be obtained 4 to 6 weeks after treatment.

Pelvic Inflammatory Disease

Pelvic inflammatory disease (PID) is inflammation of the upper genital tract, including pelvic peritonitis, endometritis, salpingitis, and tubo-ovarian abscess, caused by infection with gonorrhea, *Chlamydia*, or vaginal and bowel flora.

Table 22–1 • TREATMENT REGIMENS FOR PELVIC INFLAMMATORY DISEASE
Oral and Intramuscular
• Ceftriaxone 250 mg IM single dose *or* cefoxitin 2 g IM with probenecid 1 g orally given concurrently
• *Plus* doxycycline 100 mg orally twice daily for 14 days
• *With or without* metronidazole 500 mg orally twice daily for 14 days
Parenteral
Regimen A
• Cefotetan 2 g IV every 12 hours *or* cefoxitin 2 g IV every 6 hours
• *Plus* doxycycline 100 mg orally *or* IV every 12 hours
Regimen B
• Clindamycin 900 mg IV every 8 hours
• *Plus* gentamicin 2 mg/kg loading dose (IV or IM) followed by 1.5 mg/kg IV every 8 hours Single daily dosing (3-5 mg/kg) can be substituted

The presence of lower abdominal tenderness with both adnexal and cervical motion tenderness, without other explanation of illness, is enough to diagnose PID. Other criteria that enhance the specificity of the diagnosis include temperature more than 101 °F, abnormal cervical or vaginal discharge, elevated sedimentation rate or C-reactive protein, and cervical infection with gonorrhea or *Chlamydia*. **Because of the clinical similarity between PID and ectopic pregnancy, a serum pregnancy test should be performed on all patients suspected of having PID.**

Determination of appropriate treatment should consider pregnancy status, severity of illness, and compliance. Less severe disease can generally be treated on an outpatient basis. Women who are pregnant, have HIV, or have severe disease generally require inpatient therapy and treatment with parenteral antibiotics. Table 22–1 lists PID treatment regimens.

Patients who have PID need to be aware of potential complications, including the potential for recurrence of disease, the development of tubo-ovarian abscess, chronic abdominal pain, development of pelvic adhesions, infertility, and the increased risk of ectopic pregnancy. All patients with STIs or who are at risk for developing STIs should be counseled on safe sexual practices.

CASE CORRELATION

- See also Case 11 (Adult Female Health Maintenance), Case 16 (Male Genitourinary Conditions), and Case 45 (HIV, AIDS, and Other Sexually Transmitted Infections).

COMPREHENSION QUESTIONS

22.1 A 24-year-old nulliparous woman is noted to have a bothersome vaginal discharge. On examination, she is found to have a homogenous discharge with a fishy odor. Which of the following characteristics is most likely to be noted on examination?

A. Evidence of excoriation of the vulva

B. Vulvar erythema

C. Budding hyphae on KOH examination

D. Many white blood cells on a saline "wet prep"

E. A vaginal pH > 4.5

22.2 A 38-year-old woman complains of new-onset vaginal discharge and irritation. She notes having had a urinary tract infection 10 days previously, with subsequent resolution of her symptoms following treatment. Which of the following is the best empiric therapy for her condition?

A. Oral metronidazole

B. Vaginal metronidazole

C. Oral fluconazole

D. Oral clindamycin

E. Oral estrogen and progestin therapy

22.3 A 24-year-old woman is noted to have lower abdominal tenderness, cervical motion tenderness, and a vaginal discharge. She has a low-grade fever of 100.5 °F (38 °C). Which of the following is the best therapy for her condition?

A. Ceftriaxone intramuscularly and doxycycline orally

B. Ampicillin orally and azithromycin orally

C. Metronidazole orally as a single dose

D. Ciprofloxacin orally as a single dose

ANSWERS

22.1 **E.** This homogenous discharge with a fishy odor is most likely BV associated with an alkaline pH. Partner treatment is not necessary for BV. Oral metronidazole is one treatment. Lower pH, excoriation, inflammation, and budding yeast (answers A, B, and C) and itching are more likely with *Candida*. Answer D (many white blood cells on the slide) is indicative of an inflammatory condition such as trichomoniasis; BV usually does not present with many white blood cells.

22.2 **C.** This patient most likely has *Candida* vulvovaginitis since her discharge appeared after her cystitis, which was likely treated with antibiotics. Treatment for this includes oral fluconazole or topical azole agents such as miconazole. The other answer choices (answer A, oral metronidazole; answer B, vaginal metronidazole; answer D, oral clindamycin; and answer E, oral estrogen and progestin) do have not a predisposition to follow antibiotic use.

22.3 **A.** An option for outpatient therapy of PID is intramuscular ceftriaxone and oral doxycycline. Oral metronidazole as a single dose (answer C) is a treatment for *Trichomonas* vaginitis. Fluoroquinolones (answer D, ciprofloxacin) are not recommended in the United States for the treatment of gonorrhea or associated conditions, such as PID, due to increasing rates of resistance.

CLINICAL PEARLS

► Remember to treat sexual partners when you diagnose an STI and to test for other STIs that may initially be asymptomatic, such as HIV, hepatitis B and C, and syphilis.

► Single-dose therapy is available for many types of infections, including *Trichomonas*, gonococcal and chlamydial cervicitis, and *Candida* vaginitis. Providing single-dose therapy in your office will improve your patient's compliance as well as rates of successful treatment.

► Most women have at least one episode of *Candida* vulvovaginitis during their lifetime. Symptoms include a thick, whitish discharge that has no odor and significant pruritus of the external and internal genitalia.

► The presenting complaint in trichomoniasis is copious amounts of a thin, frothy, green-yellow or gray malodorous vaginal discharge.

► Bacterial vaginosis arises when normal vaginal bacteria are replaced with an overgrowth of anaerobic bacteria and *G. vaginalis*. Although not sexually transmitted, it is associated with having multiple sexual partners. Treatment of BV in pregnant women may reduce the incidence of miscarriage and postpartum endometritis.

► The presence of lower abdominal tenderness with both adnexal and cervical motion tenderness, without other explanation of illness, is enough to diagnose PID.

REFERENCES

Gradison M. Pelvic inflammatory disease. *Am Fam Physician.* 2012;85(8):791-796.

Maier R, Katsufrakis PJ. Sexually transmitted diseases. In: South-Paul JE, Matheny SC, Lewis EL, eds. *CURRENT Diagnosis & Treatment: Family Medicine.* 4th ed. New York, NY: McGraw Hill; 2015: Chap. 14. http://accessmedicine.mhmedical.com/content.aspx?bookid=1415&Sectionid=77055487. Accessed March 2019.

Paladine HL, Desai UA Vaginitis: diagnosis and treatment. *Am Fam Physician.* 2018;97(5):321-329.

Workowski KA, Bolan GA; Centers for Disease Control and Prevention. Sexually transmitted diseases treatment guidelines, 2015. *MMWR Recomm Rep.* 20155;64(RR-03):1-137.

A 62-year-old man presents to your office for a routine evaluation. His only complaint is of fatigue over the past 2 to 3 months despite no changes in diet or lifestyle. On questioning, the patient reports that he has never smoked and admits to an increase in his consumption of alcohol upon retiring, to about two to three beers per day. He has occasional headaches the day after a night of heavier drinking and takes ibuprofen for the headaches. As you talk to the patient and examine his chart, you note no distress and proceed with your examination. Compared to a visit from 6 months ago, you note a 4-lb weight loss and an increase in his pulse. His blood pressure is 129/81 mm Hg. He has pale conjunctivae, but the rest of his general examination is unchanged from the previous examination. You perform a digital rectal examination and find a smooth, normal-size prostate; some soft, reducible protrusions within the internal sphincter; and guaiac-positive stool. You decide on a more direct approach and delve into his drinking, bowel habits, and medication use. His only addition is the occasional production of bloody stools accompanied by some diffuse abdominal discomfort.

▶ What is the most likely diagnosis?
▶ What is your next diagnostic step?
▶ What is the next step in therapy?

ANSWERS TO CASE 23:

Lower Gastrointestinal Bleeding

Summary: A 62-year-old man presents with

- Desire for a routine checkup
- Fatigue for 2 to 3 months
- Increased alcohol intake
- Occasional bloody stools, as well as headaches, for which he takes ibuprofen
- Guaiac-positive stool
- Stable vital signs and pale appearance

Most likely diagnosis: Hemorrhoids.

Next diagnostic step: Complete blood count (CBC) and colonoscopy.

Next step in therapy: Avoid nonsteroidal anti-inflammatory drug (NSAID) use and decrease alcohol consumption.

ANALYSIS

Objectives

1. Know how to recognize the subtle signs and symptoms of lower gastrointestinal (GI) bleeding. (EPA 1)

2. Understand the etiologies of lower GI bleeding. (EPA 2)

3. Understand how to correctly evaluate and treat patients with lower GI bleeding in outpatient settings. (EPA 3, 4)

Considerations

This 62-year-old man presented to your office for a routine examination but is found to have some type of lower GI bleeding that needs further evaluation. During his office visit, there are no signs of hemodynamic instability or active bleeding that require immediate referral to an emergency department or inpatient treatment, so close outpatient follow-up is reasonable. His immediate identifiable and modifiable risk factors for GI bleeding include the regular consumption of alcohol and NSAIDs. This patient should be counseled on both these matters and sent to the laboratory for a CBC, chemistry panel, liver function tests, and coagulation profile prior to his discharge home from your office. Barring any abnormal laboratory values that require emergent management, he should be scheduled for an outpatient colonoscopy later in the week. The differential diagnosis at this time is wide, but the most frequent offenders in his age group should be considered. These include diverticular disease, hemorrhoids, colon and rectal tumors, and ulcerative colitis. For the time being, factors that may contribute to any of these etiologies should be modified while awaiting laboratory results.

APPROACH TO:
Lower Gastrointestinal Bleeding

DEFINITIONS

HEMATOCHEZIA: Bright red blood visible in the stool.

LOWER GASTROINTESTINAL BLEEDING: Bleeding that comes from a source distal to the ligament of Treitz.

MELENA: Dark, sticky feces containing partly digested blood.

CLINICAL APPROACH

Pathophysiology

The most common causes of lower GI bleeding include hemorrhoids (59%), colorectal polyps (38% to 52%), diverticulosis (34% to 51%), colorectal cancer (8%), ulcerative colitis, arteriovenous malformations, and colonic strictures. Percentages vary among age groups, and most serious causes are expected in the elderly.

Hemorrhoids. Hemorrhoids are dilated veins in the hemorrhoidal plexus of the anus. They are defined as "internal" if they arise above the dentate line and "external" if they arise below the dentate line. Both can be the cause of hematochezia. Chronic constipation, straining for bowel movements, pregnancy, and prolonged sitting (eg, truck drivers) are risk factors. Along with bleeding, external hemorrhoids can cause pain, irritation, and a palpable lump. Internal hemorrhoids can cause bleeding and can prolapse through the anus. Conservative treatment with a high-fiber diet, stool softeners, sitz baths, and precautions against prolonged straining are usually successful. When necessary, surgical procedures can be performed for definitive treatment.

Diverticular Disease. **Diverticula** are outpouchings of the colonic mucosa through weakened areas of the colon wall. They occur most often where blood vessels penetrate through the muscles of the colon. They are **most often asymptomatic and found on endoscopy or bowel imaging studies.** They can cause symptomatic, and occasionally massive, bleeding that is usually painless. Diverticular bleeding occurs in 10% to 20% of cases of lower GI bleeding. In diverticular disease, bleeding is often self-limited and ceases approximately 75% of the time; it recurs at a rate of approximately 38%. When the bleeding is extremely heavy or fails to stop, surgical resection of the affected portion of the colon may be necessary. Asymptomatic diverticulosis is managed with dietary modification, primarily a high fiber diet.

Diverticulitis is a painful inflammation and infection of a diverticulum. Diverticulitis frequently causes left lower quadrant abdominal pain along with fever, nausea, diarrhea, and constipation. Perforation of a diverticulum resulting in peritonitis or intra-abdominal abscess formation can be a complication. Diverticulitis is typically treated with bowel rest and antibiotics effective against gut flora. A combination of a quinolone and an agent for anaerobic organisms, such as metronidazole, is one commonly used regimen. In severe cases, recurrent cases, or when perforation occurs, surgery is indicated.

Inflammatory Bowel Disease. Ulcerative colitis and Crohn disease are the two primary diagnoses considered in the category of inflammatory bowel disease (IBD). **Ulcerative colitis causes continuous inflammation of the large bowel,** starting from the rectum and extending proximally. Severe disease can cause pancolitis, affecting the entire colon. **Crohn disease causes areas of focal inflammation, but it can occur anywhere in the GI tract, with healthy colon occurring in between (skip lesions).** Both diseases can cause recurrent episodes of abdominal pain, diarrhea, weight loss, rectal bleeding, fistulas, and abscesses. The definitive etiology of IBD is not known, but these are autoimmune syndromes, and a family history of IBD is a major risk factor. Along with GI symptoms, **numerous extraintestinal manifestations may occur, most frequently arthritis.** Other extraintestinal manifestations include sclerosing cholangitis, cirrhosis, fatty liver, pyoderma gangrenosum, and erythema nodosum. Ulcerative colitis is a significant risk factor for the development of colon cancer. Patients with ulcerative colitis require frequent surveillance colonoscopies. IBD can be managed with symptomatic therapy, such as antidiarrheal medications, along with anti-inflammatory medications (aminosalicylates, corticosteroids) given orally or as enemas, and immunosuppressive medications. Ulcerative colitis can be definitively treated with a total colectomy, which is usually reserved for severe pancolitis, failure to respond to medical therapy, or cases for which the risk of colon cancer is significant (eg, disease present for 10 years). The rate of colectomy has steadily decreased recently due to newer immunomodulator therapy.

Colon Neoplasms. Polyps are benign neoplasms of the colon. Hyperplastic polyps tend to be small, smooth growths found incidentally during endoscopy and are of no prognostic significance. Adenomatous polyps are benign growths that have a potential to become malignant. Listed in order of potential for becoming cancerous (from least to most), the three types of adenomas are tubular adenomas, tubulovillous adenomas, and villous adenomas. Larger polyps have a higher risk of causing bleeding and becoming malignant than smaller polyps. Polyps can be identified and removed during endoscopic procedures.

Colon cancer is the third most common cancer and the second leading cause of cancer deaths in men and women. The risk of colon cancer increases with age, a history of colon polyps, a family history of colon cancer, or a personal history of ulcerative colitis. **Any patient older than age 50 years who has lower GI bleeding or unexplained anemia must be evaluated for the presence of colon cancer.** Because of the presence of premalignant lesions (polyps) that can be identified and removed in asymptomatic patients, colon cancer screening is recommended for all adults older than age 50 and at younger ages for those with increased risks. The treatment and prognosis of colon cancer depends upon the stage in which it is found. The preferred staging system for colon cancer is the TNM classification. The *T* in TNM refers to the primary tumor, which is staged based on the penetration of the tumor through the bowel wall layer. The *N* refers to the number of regional lymph nodes that are positive, and the *M* refers to distant metastasis. Both the stage and the grade of colorectal tumors contribute to prognosis, with the worst prognosis predicted for patients with distant metastasis and histologically high-grade tumors.

Clinical Presentation

The manifestations of GI bleeding depend on the source, rate of bleeding, and underlying or coexisting disease. An older patient or someone with significant comorbidities, such as coronary artery disease, would be at a higher risk of presenting in shock. A younger, healthier individual may present with symptoms such as fatigue or dyspnea on exertion or may complain directly of seeing blood in the stool. Signs and symptoms of anemia are common and include weakness, easy fatigability, pallor of the conjunctivae or skin, chest pain, dizziness, tachycardia, hypotension, and orthostasis.

A history of blood in the stool or finding guaiac-positive stool on examination should prompt further evaluation to determine the source of the bleeding. Depending on a patient's history and hemodynamic status, more immediate and invasive measures may be necessary once GI bleeding is identified. For example, **hematochezia is usually pathognomonic of lower GI bleeding but can also be found in patients with heavy upper GI bleeding.** In this setting, a nasogastric aspirate may help differentiate this small subset of patients. An aspirate that shows bile but not blood will help to confirm that the bleeding is from a lower GI source. **Melena is usually associated with upper GI bleeding, but it may also be associated with a slow-rate lower GI bleed.**

The test of choice for the determination of the source of a lower GI bleeding is colonoscopy. Adequate bowel preparation with an oral sulfate purge to clear the bowel of blood, clots, and stool increases the yield in diagnosing colonic bleeding sites. Angiography and technetium-labeled colloid or red blood cell scans may be of value if colonoscopy cannot be performed or if heavy bleeding prevents adequate visualization of the colon. However, the magnitude of bleeding required to reveal the bleeding site limits their usefulness. Sigmoidoscopy with air contrast barium enema x-rays may be an alternative when colonoscopy is unavailable or if the patient refuses colonoscopy. If the initial sigmoidoscopy is negative, a colonoscopy must be performed. If both of these studies are negative, panendoscopy should be carried out. Capsule endoscopy has a diagnostic yield of 61% to 74% and can be done when a source of bleeding is still elusive after both upper and lower GI endoscopy.

Treatment

Treatment should be based upon the etiology of the GI bleeding. Additionally, modifiable risk factors for GI bleeding (eg, alcohol, NSAID use) should be addressed. Hemodynamically stable patients can be treated as outpatients, pending colonoscopy or other diagnostic measures.

It is critical to transport unstable patients who present with GI bleeding to the emergency department for hospitalization. Instability is indicated by persistent hypotension, tachycardia, and other signs or symptoms of shock. Intensive care unit admission should not be delayed in those with severe bleeding, and a team approach, consisting of a gastroenterologist, a surgeon with expertise in GI surgery, and skilled nursing, should always be anticipated. Major causes of morbidity and mortality in patients with GI bleeding include blood aspiration and shock. To prevent these complications, endotracheal intubation should always be considered to protect the airway of patients with altered mental status. Most cases of lower GI bleeding do not warrant emergency therapy, but be prepared for decompensation in the elderly and in those with borderline normal hemodynamic parameters.

CASE CORRELATION

- See also Case 1 (Adult Male Health Maintenance), Case 9 (Anemia in the Geriatric Patient), and Case 11 (Adult Female Health Maintenance).

COMPREHENSION QUESTIONS

23.1 A 52-year-old man presents with a 2-hour history of acute bright red blood per rectum. In the emergency center, his pulse is 110 beats/min, blood pressure is 90/50 mm Hg, he is cool and clammy appearing, and he has gross blood present on rectal examination. Which of the following is the best initial next step?

A. Colonoscopy

B. Flexible sigmoidoscopy

C. Placement of a nasogastric tube

D. Bolus of intravenous normal saline

E. Transfusion of type O-negative blood

23.2 A 67-year-old man presents to the clinic for a routine checkup. He complains of mild fatigue and occasional dyspnea on exertion. Physical examination is notable for conjunctival pallor. A rectal examination notes no hemorrhoids or masses but guaiac-positive stools. A CBC reveals a hemoglobin of 10 g/dL and a hematocrit of 27%; iron studies are consistent with iron deficiency. What is the most appropriate next step in evaluation and management?

A. Tagged red blood cell scan

B. Iron supplementation

C. Colonoscopy

D. Anoscopy

E. Repeat stool hemoccult in 2 weeks

23.3 A 25-year-old man has a colonoscopy for diagnostic evaluation of abdominal pain, weight loss, diarrhea, and blood in the stool. The colonoscopy shows diffuse mucosal inflammation in the anus and descending colon. Which of the following is the most likely diagnosis?

A. Ulcerative colitis

B. Crohn disease

C. Pseudomembranous colitis

D. Colon cancer

ANSWERS

23.1 **D.** The initial evaluation of this acutely ill patient is "ABC"—airway, breathing, and circulation. As he appears to be in hypovolemic shock, with tachycardia and hypotension, a bolus of an isotonic crystalloid fluid, such as normal saline or lactated Ringer solution, is necessary before proceeding with any of the other evaluations. Further evaluation for this patient should include a CBC, blood transfusion as necessary (answer E), and other evaluation to determine the source of bleeding, such as colonoscopy (answer A), flexible sigmoidoscopy (answer B), or nuclear medicine bleeding scan. Answer C (nasogastric tube) is not indicated since this is a lower GI process and not an upper GI process.

23.2 **C.** Colonoscopy is the most appropriate next step and is an essential evaluation in any older adult with unexplained iron-deficiency anemia. Iron-deficiency anemia can be a common presenting symptom of colon cancer. Tagged red blood cell scans (answer A) have limited indications only in acute, large-volume GI bleeding where colonoscopy is unable to be performed. Anoscopy (answer D) would give some examination of the rectum but does evaluate the colon appropriately. Iron supplementation without evaluating the cause of the iron deficiency (answer B) is inappropriate. A repeat stool occult blood (answer E) is not necessary to confirm the results of a guaiac-positive stool.

23.3 **A.** Ulcerative colitis causes continuous inflammation of the colon anywhere from rectum only to the entire colon, whereas Crohn disease (answer B) causes patchy inflammation with skip areas throughout the alimentary canal but often the ileum and right side of colon. Pseudomembranous colitis (answer C) is a complication of *Clostridium difficile* infection of the colon. Answer D (colon cancer) would not present as diffuse mucosal inflammation and instead would be a tumor or growth.

CLINICAL PEARLS

▶ Lower GI bleeding is usually suspected in lesions or pathology that is distal to the ligament of Treitz. Simple measures like nasogastric lavage can aid in ruling out upper GI bleeding as a cause of hematochezia.

▶ In a patient with acute lower GI bleeding, consider performing colonoscopy. Other diagnostic procedures that may be useful include radionuclide imaging and mesenteric angiography.

▶ Any patient older than age 50 years should be screened for colon cancer. If a patient has a family history of colon cancer, colonoscopy screening should be performed 10 years prior to the age of diagnosis in the relative, or at age 50, whichever comes first.

REFERENCES

Ahmed R, Gearhart SL. Diverticular disease and common anorectal disorders. In: Kasper D, Fauci A, Hauser S, Longo D, Jameson J, Loscalzo J, eds. *Harrison's Principles of Internal Medicine*. 20th ed. New York, NY: McGraw Hill; 2019: Chap. 353. http://accessmedicine.mhmedical.com/content.aspx?bookid=1130&Sectionid=79748127. Accessed January 25, 2019.

Bull-Henry K, Al-Kawas FH. Evaluation of occult gastrointestinal bleeding. *Am Fam Physician*. 2013;87(6):430-436.

Fargo MV, Latimer KM. Evaluation and management of common anorectal conditions. *Am Fam Physician*. 2012;85(6):624-630.

Gralnek IM, Neeman Z, Strate LL. Acute lower gastrointestinal bleeding. *N Engl J Med*. 2017; 376:1054-1063.

A 61-year-old woman presents to the emergency department complaining of a cough for 2 weeks. The cough is productive with green sputum and is associated with sweating, shaking chills, and fever up to 102 °F (38.8 °C). She was exposed to her grandchildren, who were told that they had upper respiratory infections 2 weeks ago but now are fine. Her past medical history is significant for diabetes for 10 years, which is under good control using oral hypoglycemics. She denies tobacco, alcohol, or drug use. On examination, she looks ill and in distress, with continuous coughing and chills. Currently, her blood pressure is 100/80 mm Hg, pulse is 110 beats/min, temperature is 101 °F (38.3 °C), respirations are 24 breaths/min, and oxygen saturation is 97% on room air. Examination of the head and neck is unremarkable. Her lungs have rhonchi and decreased breath sounds, with dullness to percussion in bilateral bases. Her heart is tachycardic but regular. Her extremities are without signs of cyanosis or edema. The remainder of her examination is normal. A complete blood count (CBC) shows a high white blood cell count of 17,000 cells/mm^3, with a differential of 85% neutrophils and 20% lymphocytes. Her blood sugar is 120 mg/dL.

▶ What is the most likely diagnosis?
▶ What is your next diagnostic step?
▶ What is the next step in therapy?
▶ What are potential complications to this condition?

ANSWERS TO CASE 24:

Pneumonia

Summary: This 61-year-old woman presents with

- Fever, chills, and a productive cough with green sputum
- Pulmonary examination revealing rhonchi and decreased breath sounds, with dullness to percussion in bilateral bases
- A high white cell count
- Medical history significant for diabetes mellitus
- Exposure to her grandchildren, who had upper respiratory infections 2 weeks ago

Most likely diagnosis: Community-acquired pneumonia (CAP).

Next diagnostic step: Chest x-ray, sputum Gram stain and culture, and blood cultures.

Next therapeutic step: Determine whether the patient requires inpatient or outpatient therapy and start antibiotics.

Potential complications: Bacteremia, sepsis, parapneumonic pleural effusion, and empyema.

ANALYSIS

Objectives

1. Recognize the differential diagnosis of pneumonia. (EPA 1, 2)
2. Be familiar with widely accepted decision-making strategies for the diagnosis and management of different kinds of pneumonia. (EPA 3, 4)
3. Learn about the treatment and follow-up of pneumonia. (EPA 4, 5, 12)
4. Recognize the effects of comorbid conditions. (EPA 1, 12)

Considerations

This 61-year-old patient presents with a common diagnostic dilemma: productive cough with green sputum and fever. The first priority for the provider is to assess whether the patient is more ill than the complaint would indicate. Helpful clues to the patient's overall condition include a toxic appearance, using accessory muscles to breathe, and low oxygen saturation. Tachycardia, hypotension, and altered mental status are signs of more critical illness. **Cardiopulmonary stabilization must always be addressed.**

Fortunately, this patient does not have those alarming symptoms. If a patient has respiratory distress, the clinician may need to check arterial blood gases. If the patient has low oxygen saturation, give oxygen by nasal cannula and then proceed to your history and physical examination.

The most common etiology of cough is an upper respiratory tract infection. This patient has several features that make pneumonia more likely, including her age, cough with green sputum, fever with chills, and exposure to close contacts with respiratory infections. The gold standard for diagnosis of pneumonia is the presence of an infiltrate on chest x-ray, although a normal x-ray does not exclude the diagnosis. X-rays may be normal early in the course of disease, and a patient who is dehydrated may not demonstrate an infiltrate until adequately rehydrated.

APPROACH TO:
Pneumonia

DEFINITIONS

COMMUNITY-ACQUIRED PNEUMONIA: Pneumonia that occurs in persons who are not hospital inpatients or residents of long-term care facilities.

HEALTH CARE–ASSOCIATED PNEUMONIA: Health care–associated pneumonia (HAP) includes infections that develop in hospitals, nursing homes, skilled nursing facilities, or other long-term care facilities.

PNEUMONIA: Infection of lung parenchyma caused by agents that include bacteria, viruses, fungi, and parasites.

PNEUMONITIS: An inflammation of the lungs from a variety of noninfectious causes, such as chemicals, blood, radiation, and autoimmune processes.

CLINICAL APPROACH

Pathophysiology

Bronchitis and pneumonia represent a continuum of lower respiratory infection. The extent of involvement of adjacent lung parenchyma determines whether there is an infiltrate on x-ray. **Pneumonia is defined as an infection of lung parenchyma** caused by agents that include bacteria, viruses, fungi, and parasites. It should be distinguished from pneumonitis, which is an inflammation of the lungs from a variety of noninfectious causes such as chemicals, blood, radiation, and autoimmune processes. The occurrence and severity of pneumonia depend on both the state of the body's defense mechanism against infection and the characteristics of the infectious agent. The **most common mechanism triggering pneumonia is upper airway colonization** by potentially pathogenic organisms that are subsequently aspirated. The type of organism involved depends, in part, on host characteristics.

Community-Acquired Pneumonia. Community-acquired pneumonias can be either viral or bacterial in etiology, and both can range from a mild-to-severe presentation. Common viral causes of pneumonia include influenza A and B, adenoviruses, respiratory syncytial viruses, and parainfluenza viruses. The most common bacterial cause of CAP is *Streptococcus pneumoniae* (pneumococcus). Other common bacterial etiologies are *Mycoplasma pneumoniae, Haemophilus influenzae,* and *Moraxella catarrhalis.* Pneumococcal pneumonia classically causes an illness of acute onset with cough productive of rust-colored sputum, fever, shaking chills, and a lobar infiltrate on chest x-ray. *Haemophilus influenzae* is often seen in patients with underlying chronic obstructive pulmonary disease.

M. pneumoniae, Chlamydia pneumoniae, and *Legionella pneumophila* are bacteria that cause what is classified as "atypical" pneumonia. Atypical pneumonia is also caused by several different viruses. The **"typical" pneumonia organisms are more common in the very young and in the older patient.** Atypical pneumonias occur more commonly in adolescent or young adult patients. Atypical organisms tend to cause bilateral, diffuse infiltrates rather than focal, lobar infiltrates on x-ray.

Health Care–Associated Pneumonia. HAP is a major source of morbidity, mortality, and prolonged hospitalization. **Risk factors include hospitalization within 90 days, home infusion therapy, dialysis, and being a resident at a nursing home.** The pathogens found in health care facilities may have multidrug resistance, so the recommended treatments include extended-spectrum antibiotics until the sensitivity of the causative organism is found. Risks for drug-resistant organisms include being hospitalized for greater than 5 days, antibiotics within the last 90 days, immunosuppression, and high rates of antibiotic resistance in the community. The causative organisms include the pathogens involved in CAP as well as aerobic gram-negative bacteria (*Pseudomonas, Klebsiella, Acinetobacter*) and gram-positive cocci such as *Staphylococcus aureus.* The incidence of drug-resistant organisms, such as methicillin-resistant *S. aureus* (MRSA), is substantial in most communities. The risk of HAP can be reduced by giving appropriate vaccinations, smoking cessation, good nutrition, avoiding intubation when possible, and using contact precautions (hand hygiene, gloving, and gowning).

Clinical Presentation

History. Patient history in cases of pneumonia commonly includes the symptoms of productive cough, fever, pleuritic chest pain, and dyspnea. The symptoms can be very nonspecific in the very old and very young. In young children, rapid breathing is commonly seen; in the elderly, pneumonia may present as altered mental status. Sometimes, the history may assist in determining the specific organism involved. An abrupt onset or abruptly worsening illness is seen frequently in pneumococcal pneumonia. *Legionella* often causes diarrhea, hyponatremia, and elevated liver enzymes along with pneumonia. *S. aureus* is a common cause of postinfluenza pneumonia.

Physical Examination. Physical examination findings can include fever, tachycardia, tachypnea, hypotension, and reduced oxygen saturation. Auscultation of the lungs may reveal rhonchi or rales. Egophony (E-to-A change) can be a sign of focal lung consolidation, and dullness to percussion may be the result of a pulmonary effusion.

Imaging. **All patients with suspected pneumonia should have a chest x-ray or computed tomography scan.** The presence of an infiltrate can confirm the diagnosis. Absence of an infiltrate on x-ray does not rule out pneumonia as a diagnosis. A chest x-ray can also identify a pleural effusion, which may be a complication of pneumonia (parapneumonic effusion). Outpatient facilities with trained primary care clinicians are using ultrasound to diagnose pneumonia and pleural effusions with excellent sensitivity and specificity.

Specific x-ray findings may also lead to consideration of certain etiologic agents or types of pneumonia. As noted previously, lobar infiltrates are more common with typical infections, and diffuse infiltrates are more likely with atypical infections. A bilateral infiltrate appearing like "ground glass" is associated with *Pneumocystis jiroveci* infections, which are seen most often in patients with AIDS. Apical consolidation may be seen with tuberculosis. Pneumonia caused by the aspiration of gastrointestinal contents commonly is seen in the right lower lobe because of the branching of the bronchial tree.

Laboratory Values. Other testing indicated in patients with pneumonia includes a CBC and a chemistry panel. Specific microbiologic diagnosis is possible with blood or sputum cultures. **Cultures have a low sensitivity** (many false negatives), but a positive culture can help to guide treatment. *Legionella* can be confirmed in suspected cases by urine antigen testing.

Treatment

When pneumonia is diagnosed, the initial decision to be made is whether the patient can be treated safely as an outpatient or whether hospitalization is required. This prediction should be based primarily on mortality and severity prediction scores. **Commonly used prediction scoring systems include the CURB-65 Mortality Prediction Tool for Patients with CAP and the Pneumonia Severity Index (PSI)**, which have approximately 75% sensitivity for need for inpatient care. The PSI tool assigns patients to a risk category based on their age, comorbid illnesses, specific examination, and laboratory findings. High-risk comorbidities include neoplastic disease, liver disease, renal disease, congestive heart failure, and diabetes. Physical examination findings taken into consideration are tachypnea, fever, hypotension, tachycardia, and altered mental status. Laboratory findings include a low pH, low serum sodium, low hematocrit, low oxygen saturation, high glucose, high blood urea nitrogen (BUN), and pleural effusion on x-ray. Based on the patient's demographics and individual findings, a risk class and mortality risk are assigned. Low-risk classes can be safely treated as an outpatient; higher risk classes should be hospitalized with possible admission to the intensive care unit (ICU).

Community-Acquired Pneumonia. The emergence of drug-resistant pneumococci and the development of new antimicrobials have changed the empiric treatment of CAP. In healthy persons suitable for outpatient treatment, a macrolide (clarithromycin or azithromycin) or doxycycline is recommended empiric therapy. If the patient has chronic comorbidities such as diabetes or heart and lung disease, treatments with fluoroquinolones (levofloxacin, moxifloxacin) or the combination of a beta-lactam (high-dose amoxicillin, amoxicillin/clavulanate, cefpodoxime, or cefuroxime) plus a macrolide would be recommended.

For hospitalized patients with CAP who do not require ICU treatment, an intravenous beta-lactam (cefotaxime, ceftriaxone, or ampicillin/sulbactam) and an intravenous macrolide (erythromycin or azithromycin) are recommended. An intravenous fluoroquinolone with activity against *S. pneumoniae* can be substituted. If it is suitable for the patient to begin outpatient treatment, a follow-up visit to the office 3 to 4 days later will help to assess response to therapy. Early follow-up chest x-rays are mandatory in those who fail to show clinical improvement by 5 to 7 days, as bronchogenic carcinoma can present with the picture of a typical pneumonia.

Health Care-Associated Pneumonia. HAPs require broader antibiotic coverage of the likely pathogens, many of which have developed multiple-drug resistance. If *Pseudomonas* is considered a likely cause, such as in a patient with immuno-compromise or recent hospitalization with intubation, treatment with an antipneu-mococcal and antipseudomonal beta-lactam (pipercillin/tazobactam, cefepime, imipenem, or meropenem) plus a fluoroquinolone (levofloxacin, moxifloxacin) and/or an aminoglycoside (amikacin or tobramycin and azithromycin) is advised. MRSA may require treatment with vancomycin or linezolid.

Steroids. As an adjunct, corticosteroids are also used to reduce rates of complica-tions and hospital days. Intravenous steroids (methylprednisolone) used within 36 hours of presentation can reduce the risk of acute respiratory distress syndrome, mechanical ventilation, and mortality.

The duration of the treatment is influenced by the severity of illness, the etiologic agent, the response to therapy, the presence of other medical problems, and com-plications of the infection. CAP therapy lasts from 5 to 10 days or until the patient is afebrile for at least 72 hours. Two to three weeks of therapy is appropriate for hospital-acquired pneumonias caused by *S. aureus*, *Pseudomonas aeruginosa*, *Klebsiella*, anaerobes, *M. pneumoniae*, *C. pneumoniae*, or *Legionella* species.

Complications

Bacteremia occurs in approximately 25% to 30% of patients with pneumococcal pneumonia. Mortality rates for patients with bacteremia range from 20% to 30%, but they can be as high as 60% in the elderly. Parapneumonic pleural effusion devel-ops in 40% of hospitalized patients with pneumococcal pneumonia. Fewer than 5% of cases progress to empyema. If more than a minimal amount of fluid is present, as evidenced by significant blunting of the costophrenic angle on x-ray, it may be necessary to perform a thoracentesis with Gram stain and culture of the pleural fluid. The presence of an empyema usually requires drainage with a chest tube or surgical procedure.

Prevention. **Pneumococcal vaccine** is recommended for all persons age 65 years and older, all adults with chronic cardiopulmonary diseases, cigarette smokers, and all immunocompromised persons. **In addition to the traditional immunization with the 23-valent pneumococcal polysaccharide vaccine for all adults aged 65 and older, the Advisory Committee on Immunization Practices now recommends routine use of the 13-valent pneumococcal conjugate vaccine** in a series with the original 23-valent vaccination. Revaccinate 5 years after the initial dose in patients known to be immunocompromised or without a functioning spleen.

Influenza vaccination is recommended in the late fall and winter months for all individuals aged 6 months and older. The association between influenza virus infection and pneumonia is well recognized. The number of cases of invasive pneu-mococcal disease from influenza peaks in midwinter, when influenza is prevalent. Influenza virus infection can lead to a secondary pneumonia by facilitating bacterial colonization and impairing host defense mechanisms. *S. aureus* is the most com-mon causative organism in these cases. A prospective study of patients 65 years of age and older demonstrated the effectiveness of influenza and pneumococcal vaccination at reducing hospitalizations for pneumonia and preventing invasive pneumococcal disease.

> ### CASE CORRELATION
>
> - See also Case 19 (Upper Respiratory and Ear Infections) and Case 56 (Wheezing and Asthma).

COMPREHENSION QUESTIONS

24.1 A 17-year-old adolescent male presents to the emergency department with a temperature of 101 °F (38.3 °C), a deep nonproductive cough, and generalized malaise for 3 days. He does not recall being around any particular sick contacts but is around many people in his afterschool job and at school. He states that he never had the chicken pox and is unaware of what immunizations he received as a child. He was diagnosed at age 12 with leukemia but has since been healthy. He is worried that his cancer may no longer be in remission. A chest x-ray reveals bilateral, diffuse infiltrates. Which of the following is the most likely cause of illness?

A. Pneumonia caused by *S. pneumonia*

B. Pneumonia caused by *P. jiroveci*

C. Pneumonia caused by *L. pneumophila*

D. Pneumonia caused by *M. pneumonia*

E. Pneumonia caused by *H. influenza*

24.2 A 35-year-old morbidly obese woman patient is being evaluated in the emergency center from an outlying clinic. She was seen 8 days ago for headache, fever of 102 °F, nonproductive cough, and myalgias, for which she was diagnosed with influenza and prescribed oseltamivir for 5 days. She felt better after taking the medication initially but now feels she is getting worse. She is sent to the emergency department for expedited evaluation. She states that she has had night sweats, chills, shortness of breath, and cough productive of yellowish-green sputum for 3 days. Today, her vital signs show a temperature of 104 °F, with a respiratory rate of 30 breaths/min, heart rate of 100 bpm, and pulse oximetry of 93% on room air. Assuming admission for pneumonia, which of the following is the best empiric antibiotic treatment for this patient?

A. Continuation of oseltamivir for another week

B. Azithromycin

C. Penicillin

D. Levofloxacin

E. Ceftriaxone with vancomycin

24.3 A 64-year-old man sees you in the office because of a cough he has had for the past 4 days and a fever that started last night. He is short of breath and has significant malaise. He is a nonsmoker and has no history of lung disease. His medical history is significant for type 2 diabetes mellitus, which is well managed with medications and diet. A physical examination reveals an alert and mildly ill-appearing man who is speaking in complete sentences. His temperature is 38.1 °C (100.6 °F), pulse rate 95 beats/min, respiratory rate 22 breaths/min, blood pressure 115/70 mm Hg, and oxygen saturation 97% on room air. His heart has a regular rhythm, and respirations appear unlabored. He has rhonchi in the left lower lung field but has good air movement overall. A chest radiograph reveals a left lower lobe infiltrate. Which one of the following is the most appropriate setting for the management of this patient's pneumonia?

A. Home with close monitoring

B. An inpatient medical bed without telemetry monitoring

C. An inpatient medical bed with telemetry monitoring

D. An inpatient intensive care bed

ANSWERS

24.1 **D.** Bilateral, diffuse infiltrates are more likely to be seen in patients with pneumonia caused by atypical agents, such as *Mycoplasma*, than in patients with typical pneumonia (answer A, *S. pneumonia*; answer E, *H. influenzae*) or aspiration pneumonia. *Legionella* (answer C), another atypical pneumonia, generally is seen in older patients, and usually affected patients have diarrhea, which this patient did not have. It is more likely that the patient contracted an atypical pneumonia than having a relapse of leukemia with such profound immunodeficiency as to have contracted a *Pneumocystis* infection (answer B) with no prior symptoms.

24.2 **E.** This patient is most likely suffering from postinfluenza pneumonia, which is often a bacterial process superimposed on the influenza. Due to the higher risk of mortality associated with morbid obesity and some vital signs indicating risk of sepsis, this patient should be evaluated quickly for possible admission. If admitted for pneumonia, antibiotic coverage should cover for *Pneumococcus* and *S. aureus*. Levofloxacin (answer D) would be reasonable for CAP but does not provide good coverage for staph infections. Answer A (continue osteltamivir) would not be effective and puts the patient at increased risk for further pulmonary decompensation and possibly death. Answer B (azithromycin) would be effective for a simple CAP in a healthy patient. Answer C (penicillin) is no longer used to treat pneumonia due to the high rate of resistance.

24.3 **A.** In an outpatient setting, clinical decision tools like the Confusion, Urea, Respiration, Blood pressure-65 (CURB-65) score are an easy way to assess risk and should always be used. In this scenario, the patient does not clinically appear markedly ill, and his vital signs and physical examination do not fit any criteria for increased risk. Using the CURB-65, he is not confused (C), we do not have the BUN value (U), respiratory rate is not > 30 breaths/min (R), his systolic blood pressure is higher than 90 mm Hg (B), and his age is not 65 or older (65). With possibly 1 point depending on the BUN value, he can be observed as an outpatient.

CLINICAL PEARLS

▶ Elderly patients often have fewer or less severe symptoms or atypical presentations of pneumonia. Consider pneumonia in the differential diagnosis of altered mental status in the elderly.

▶ Appropriate use of influenza and pneumococcal vaccinations reduce the risk of pneumonia in susceptible populations. Current vaccination guidelines now recommend both the 23-valent and 13-valent pneumococcal vaccines given in series to all patients 65 and older.

▶ Consider the diagnosis of empyema in patients with pneumonia and a pleural effusion, especially if the patients continue to have fever despite appropriate antibiotic therapy.

▶ *S. pneumoniae* is the most common cause of community acquired pneumonia (CAP).

▶ Organisms associated with ventilator associated pneumonia (VAP) include *E. coli*, Pseudomonas, Klebsiella, and MRSA.

REFERENCES

Chesnutt AN, Chesnutt MS, Prendergast NT, Prendergast TJ. Pulmonary disorders. In: Papadakis MA, McPhee SJ, Rabow MW, eds. *Current Medical Diagnosis & Treatment 2019*. New York, NY: McGraw Hill; 2019: Chap. 9.

Kaysin A, Viera A. Community acquired pneumonia in adults: diagnosis and management. *Am Fam Physician*. 2016;94(9):698-706.

Mandell LA, Wunderink RG. Pneumonia. In: Jameson J, Fauci A, Kasper D, Hauser S, Longo D, Loscalzo J, eds. *Harrison's Principles of Internal Medicine*. 20th ed. New York, NY: McGraw Hill; 2018: Chap. 121. https://accessmedicine-mhmedical-com.evms.idm.oclc.org/content.aspx?bookid=2129&sectionid=184041853 Accessed May 9, 2020.

Tomczyk S, Bennett NM, Stoecker C, et al. Use of PCV-13 and PPSV-23 vaccine among adults aged 65 and older: recommendations of the Advisory Committee on Immunization Practices (ACIP). *MMWR Morb Mortal Wkly Rep*. 2014;63(37);822-825.

A 38-year-old woman presents to the office with complaints of weight loss, fatigue, and insomnia of 3 months' duration. She feels tired most of the time and frequently does not want to get out of bed. Conversely, she has been staying up late at night because she cannot fall asleep. She feels she is performing poorly at work as an administrative assistant and states that she has trouble remembering things. She does not enjoy going outdoors or being with friends like she used to and avoids social activities. She denies any recent medication, illicit drug, or alcohol use. She feels intense guilt regarding past relationships, believing that it was her fault they failed. She states she has never thought of suicide but has begun to feel increasingly worthless.

Her vital signs and general physical examination are benign, except she becomes tearful while discussing her symptoms. Her mental status examination is significant for depressed mood, psychomotor slowing, and poor concentration.

▶ What is the most likely diagnosis?
▶ What is your next step?
▶ What are important considerations and potential complications of the likely condition?

ANSWERS TO CASE 25:

Major Depression and Other Mood Disorders

Summary: This 38-year-old woman presents with

- Weight loss, fatigue, and insomnia of 3 months' duration
- Anhedonia and feelings of worthlessness
- Feelings of intense guilt regarding past failed relationships
- Denial of any recent medication, illicit drug, or alcohol use
- Mental status examination significant for depressed mood, psychomotor slowing, and poor concentration

Most likely diagnosis: Major depression.

Next step: Check thyroid-stimulating hormone, basic metabolic panel, and complete blood count.

Important considerations and potential complications: Rule out other medical diagnoses, such as hypothyroidism, anemia, diabetes, and infectious processes that could mimic some symptoms of depression. Review any recent medication changes for agents that may contribute to these symptoms (eg, beta-blockers, steroids, sedatives, chemotherapy agents); verify that no substance use disorder is present. Screen for bipolar disorder and inquire about a family history of mood disorders; investigate and address suicidal ideation.

ANALYSIS

Objectives

1. Recognize common presenting signs and symptoms of major depressive disorder. (EPA 1, 2, 10)

2. Be able to verbalize the multifactorial pathogenesis of depressive disorders. (EPA 12)

3. Describe the treatment of depressive disorders and the sequelae of this condition. (EPA 4, 12)

4. Be familiar with the appropriate follow-up of this condition. (EPA 4, 9)

5. Recognize the need for assessing suicide risk. (EPA 10)

Considerations

The vignette is a common presentation of major depressive disorder. The patient often presents with symptoms of fatigue, insomnia, and mood swings and often does not report mood changes unless specifically asked. The astute clinician will recognize this pattern as depression. Symptoms of depressive disorder, such as poor concentration and impaired working memory, may limit your patient's ability to provide a good history. Close friends and family can help make the diagnosis clearer with the patient's permission.

The diagnosis of major depressive disorder can made because she meets at least five of the *Diagnostic and Statistical Manual of Mental Disorders, Fifth Edition* (*DSM-5*) diagnostic criteria during a 2-week period that represents a change from her previous level of functioning. At least one of the symptoms must be either depressed mood or loss of interest or pleasure.

Treatment is based on severity of symptoms, and the clinician must specifically and directly address the patient's risk of harming self or others. If the patient is actively suicidal, such as describing the desire to hurt him- or herself and having a plan to do so, then hospitalization may be necessary. Similarly, if the patient is unable to perform self-care, hospitalization should be considered. If the patient does not have suicidal ideations, is not assessed as a risk to self or others, and has support at home, then outpatient therapy with close follow-up is usually appropriate, with follow-up generally at 1- to 2-week intervals until stable.

APPROACH TO:
Major Depressive Disorder and Other Mood Disorders

DEFINITION

MAJOR DEPRESSIVE DISORDER (MDD): Symptoms lasting for 2 consecutive weeks and occurring nearly every day. Must have five of the nine diagnostic criteria listed in the *DSM-5*, and one of them must be depressed mood or anhedonia.

DSM-5 criteria:

1. Depressed mood
2. Anhedonia: Diminished interest or pleasure
3. Change in appetite or weight: Decreased appetite, or increased appetite associated with specific food cravings; significant weight loss or weight gain
4. Change in sleep patterns: Insomnia or hypersomnia
5. Change in activity: Psychomotor agitation or retardation
6. Fatigue or loss of energy
7. Feelings of worthlessness or excessive or inappropriate guilt
8. Change in cognition: Diminished ability to think or concentrate; indecisiveness
9. Recurrent thoughts of death, suicidal ideation, suicide attempt, or specific plan

Also,

- Symptoms cause clinically significant distress or impairment of functioning.
- Symptoms are not a result of the direct physiologic effects of a substance or a generalized medical condition.

- There has never been a manic or hypomanic episode.

- Symptoms are not better explained by schizoaffective disorder, schizophrenia, schizophreniform disorder, delusional disorder, or other psychotic disorders.

CLINICAL APPROACH TO DEPRESSIVE DISORDER

Epidemiology

Depression has a lifetime prevalence of 7% to 12% in men and 20% to 25% in women. Risk factors for developing depression are family or personal history of depression, female sex, younger age, traumatic brain injury, chronic medical illnesses, chronic pain, low income, low self-esteem, poor social support, chronic minor daily stress, and being single, divorced, or widowed. Untreated depressive disorder can lead to suicide, and those with depression carry a suicide risk of 0.5% to 4% increase from the general population.

Screening. Screening for depression is recommended by the US Preventive Services Task Force (Grade B) starting at age 12 when there are systems to ensure accurate diagnosis, treatment, and follow-up. Adult screening can be completed using the two-question Patient Health Questionnaires (PHQ2), followed up with the PHQ9 if positive. For older adults who are healthy or have mild-moderate cognitive impairment, the Geriatric Depression Scale or Cornell Scale for depression may be used. The Beck Depression Inventory and Children's Depression Inventory should be used in children, and the PHQ2 and PHQ9 may be used in adolescents. In pregnant and postpartum women, the Edinberg Depression scale can be used. Screening for depression is a Merit Incentive Payment System (MIPS) quality measure.

Pathophysiology

Etiology. The etiology of depressive disorder is likely "part nature, part nurture" due to a complex interaction of genetic, psychosocial, and neurobiologic factors. Adverse life events may trigger those with a genetic risk. Theoretical psychosocial contributors include stressful life events, particularly involving loss of a loved one, early childhood stress, and lack of positive reinforcement. MDD does not require such events, and those with seemingly stable lives may still experience intense suffering from this disease. Depression runs in families without a clear inheritance pattern. Multiple neurotransmitter systems are involved, including the serotoninergic, noradrenergic, and dopaminergic systems. This mechanism is supported by the known action of antidepressant medications, which have demonstrated response and remission of this disease.

Differential Diagnosis. **Bereavement** can be defined as a depressed mood and impaired functioning following the loss of a loved one. Although once considered an exclusion criterion for the diagnosis of depression—as grief is expected following a major loss—patients with significant depressive symptoms during bereavement may be diagnosed with depression based upon the amount of functional impairment the patient is experiencing.

Dysthymic disorder is a low-grade, chronic down mood that may not reach the typical lows of major depression but is long standing, often existing for years.

It is often associated with low self-esteem, chronic stress, poor mood modulation, and poor stress coping techniques.

Morbidity and Mortality. Major depressive disorder causes significant morbidity and mortality in numerous ways. The World Health Organization stated that depression is the fourth leading cause of disability in the world and that it causes more disability and social impairment than diabetes, arthritis, hypertension, or coronary artery disease. Depression is frequently reported in persons with underlying medical conditions, such as stroke, Parkinson disease, traumatic brain injury, diabetes, coronary atherosclerotic disease, and terminal illnesses.

There is a bidirectional finding in that patients with MDD are more likely to develop atherosclerotic coronary artery and cerebrovascular disease, diabetes, and osteoporosis. Depression is a common occurrence following myocardial infarction and stroke. Persons with depression and preexisting cardiac disease have three times greater risk of dying after a heart attack than do patients without depression. Patients with coexisting MDD and diabetes have more microvascular and macrovascular complications. Studies also show that **persons with depression have a greater chance of developing or dying from cardiovascular disease,** even after controlling for other risk factors. Depression also contributes to the disruption of interpersonal relationships, the development of substance abuse, and absenteeism from work and school.

All depressed patients should be screened for suicidal and homicidal ideations. A history of suicide attempts or violence is a significant risk factor for future attempts. MDD plays a role in more than half of all suicide attempts. **Women, especially those younger than age 30 years, attempt suicide more frequently than men, but men are more likely to complete suicide.** Firearms are the most commonly used method in completed suicides. Table 25–1 lists the risk factors for suicide attempts and completed suicides.

Table 25–1 • RISK FACTORS FOR SUICIDE	
Demographic, social, and environmental factors	Males more likely to complete; Females more likely to attempt
	Age > 65 more likely to complete; age < 30 more likely to attempt
	American Indian, Alaska Native, non-Hispanic white
	Social isolation (divorced, widowed, living alone)
	Lesbian, gay, bisexual, or transgender
	Stressful life events
	Access to firearms
Historical factors	Family history of suicide
	History of suicide attempt and lethality of prior attempt
	Concurrent chronic medical illness
Psychiatric and behavioral factors	Major depression, substance abuse (especially alcohol), schizophrenia, panic disorder, borderline personality disorder
	Symptoms: hopelessness, anhedonia, insomnia, severe anxiety, panic attacks, impaired concentration, psychomotor agitation

Data from American Psychiatric Association. Diagnostic and Statistical Manual of Mental Disorders. 5th ed. Washington, DC: American Psychiatric Association Press; 2013; Ebert MH, Loosen PT, Nurcombe B, Leckman JF, eds. CURRENT Diagnosis & Treatment: Psychiatry. 2nd ed. 2008. Copyright © McGraw Hill LLC. All rights reserved; U.S. Preventive Services Task Force. Screening for suicide risk in adolescents, adults, and older adults in primary care: recommendation statement. Am Fam Physician. 2015 Feb 1;91(3):190F-190I.

Clinical Presentation

As alluded to in the opening case, patients often present with fatigue or poor con-centration, and mood symptoms need to be specifically elicited from the patient. **The cardinal symptoms are anhedonia and down mood.** It is important to note that the physical symptoms are manifestations of the disease and should respond to treatment. The mnemonic **SIGECAPS** is helpful in remembering common features and stands for

- Sleep (decreased or increased)
- Interest (decreased/anhedonia)
- Guilt
- Energy (decreased)
- Concentration (reduced)
- Appetite (decreased or increased)
- Psychomotor slowing
- Suicidal ideation

Some typical nonspecific symptoms of depression include headache, neck or back pain, joint pain, abdominal pain, constipation, poor sleep, weakness, and fatigue. The elderly may present with confusion or a general decline in function (pseudodementia). Children and adolescents may present with irritability. **The diagnosis of MDD should be considered in scenarios where a patient presents with multiple unrelated physical symptoms.**

A mental status examination is very important, including mood, affect, appear-ance, behavior, speech, and thought process and content. Those who have more severe symptoms may reveal a decline in grooming or hygiene along with weight changes. Speech may be normal, slow, monotonic, or lacking in content. Pressured speech is suggestive of mania, whereas disorganized speech suggests the need to evaluate for psychosis. The thought content of patients with depression includes feelings of inadequacy, helplessness, hopelessness, or feeling overwhelmed. Psycho-motor retardation can manifest as slowing of movements or reactions, especially in the elderly. The physical examination should include evaluation for possible under-lying causes of depressed mood, and a cognitive examination may be helpful in older adults.

Treatment

Pharmacotherapy with psychotherapy is more effective than either pharmacotherapy or psychotherapy alone; however, either may be pursued alone based on patient comfort and severity of disease. Patients should be encouraged to pursue both ther-apies to improve chances of success. Initial pharmacotherapy should be based on the health care provider's familiarity with medication, anticipated safety and toler-ability, anticipation of adverse effects, and history of prior treatments. The PHQ9 can be used to assess symptom severity and track improvement over time.

Antidepressant agents work by increasing the amount of neurotransmitter available in the synaptic cleft. This is accomplished by (1) enhancing neurotransmitter release, (2) reducing neurotransmitter breakdown, or (3) inhibiting the reuptake of the neurotransmitter by the presynaptic neuron. There are a few effective antidepressants that do not have a fully elucidated mechanism of action.

An adequate trial of an antidepressant requires a minimum of 4 to 6 weeks on an appropriate dose. Up to half of patients do not respond to the first antidepressant they try and will need to be switched to another agent. However, treatment failures typically result from medication nonadherence, inadequate duration of therapy, or inadequate dosing. No class of medication has been proven to be more effective than other classes. Response (in improvement in symptoms) occurs in 63% of patients after 8 to 12 weeks and remission (resolution of symptoms) in 47% of cases.

Maintenance therapy should be pursued based on the number of major depressive episodes, duration of episode, and severity of symptoms. After a first episode of major depression, treatment should continue for at least 4 to 9 months after stability is achieved. For a patient with two or three episodes, 3 years is a reasonable duration of therapy, with consideration of lifelong therapy in a patient with a serious suicide attempt. The need for lifelong therapy increases with each episode of depression. **All antidepressants carry a Food and Drug Administration "black box" warning that they increase the risk of suicidal thoughts and behaviors in children, adolescents, and young adults, especially in the first months of treatment.** Table 25–2 lists the medications used in the treatment of depression.

Selective Serotonin Reuptake Inhibitors. Because of their efficacy and safety, selective serotonin reuptake inhibitors (SSRIs) are frequently used as first-line agents for the treatment of depression. SSRIs are first line for children. Fluoxetine (Prozac), citalopram (Celexa), sertraline (Zoloft), and escitalopram (Lexapro) have been approved for use in children. SSRIs increase the amount

Table 25–2 • MEDICATIONS USED IN THE TREATMENT OF DEPRESSION				
SSRIs	**SNRIs**	**TCAs**	**Atypical**	**MAOIs**
Fluoxetine (Prozac)	Venlafaxine (Effexor)	Amitriptyline (Elavil)	Bupropion (Wellbutrin)	Phenelzine (Nardil)
Paroxetine (Paxil)	Duloxetine (Cymbalta)	Nortriptyline (Pamelor)	Amoxapine (Asendin)	Tranylcypromine (Parnate)
Sertraline (Zoloft)	Mirtazapine (Remeron)	Desipramine (Norpramin)	Trazodone (Desyrel)	Selegiline transdermal (Emsam)
Fluvoxamine (Luvox)	Desvenlafaxine (Pristiq)	Clomipramine (Anafranil)		
Citalopram (Celexa)		Doxepin (Sinequan)		
Escitalopram (Lexapro)		Imipramine (Tofranil)		

SSRI, selective serotonin reuptake inhibitor; SNRI, serotonin-norepinephrine reuptake inhibitor; TCA, tricyclic antidepressant; MAOI, monoamine oxidase inhibitor.

of the neurotransmitter serotonin (5-hydroxytryptamine) available to the post-synaptic neuron by blocking the presynaptic removal of serotonin. Common side effects include sexual dysfunction, weight gain, nausea/gastrointestinal disturbance, insomnia or somnolence, and agitation. When used in combination with another serotonergic agent, the clinician should be aware of the possibility of developing serotonin syndrome.

Serotonin-Norepinephrine Reuptake Inhibitors. Serotonin-norepinephrine reuptake inhibitors (SNRIs) affect both the serotonergic and noradrenergic systems, preventing norepinephrine and serotonin reuptake. Their side effects are similar to SSRIs. They can be used as first-line treatment for depression and, because of their effects on two neurotransmitter systems, may be used as second-line agents in SSRI failure.

Tricyclic Antidepressants. Tricyclic antidepressants (TCAs) are older agents that affect, to varying degrees, the reuptake of norepinephrine and serotonin. They are effective for the treatment of depression, and because they have been in use for many years, they are inexpensive. However, they have numerous side effects, including antimuscarinic effects (dry mouth, blurry vision, constipation, urinary retention, and sinus tachycardia); histamine blockade (sedation, drowsiness, weight gain); and alpha-1-receptor blockade (orthostatic hypotension and sedation). TCAs also carry a significant risk of lethality in an overdose. Because of these side effects and risks, TCAs have largely been replaced by other agents.

Atypical Agents. Atypical agents may have an unknown mechanism of action but likely have similar effects on neurotransmitters as other antidepressants. They are often utilized for their side-effect profile or to alleviate sexual disturbances caused by typical agents. Bupropion is associated with increased risk of seizure at higher doses and is contraindicated in patients with a history of seizure disorders and anorexia. Trazodone carries the risk, although rare, of causing priapism. It is also highly sedating and is frequently used as a sleep aid. Mirtazapine can be a good choice for patients with insomnia or anorexia, as it can improve sleep latency and duration and stimulate appetite.

Monoamine Oxidase Inhibitors. Monoamine oxidase inhibitors (MAOIs) cause increased amounts of serotonin and norepinephrine in the cleft by inhibiting breakdown. MAOIs require a low tyramine diet to reduce the risk of hypertensive crisis and interact with numerous medications, with a significant risk of dangerous complications. Therefore, MAOIs should be restricted to patients who do not respond to other treatments and should only be prescribed by experienced clinicians.

Strategies to consider when there is an inadequate response to initial medication and psychotherapy include optimizing the medication dose, changing medications, or adding an antidepressant from a different pharmacological class (not an MAOI). Patients who are refractory to medications should be referred to a psychiatrist who can consider the following: electroconvulsive therapy (ECT), MAOI therapy, transcranial magnetic stimulation, and lastly, vagus nerve stimulation (for patients who are refractory to at least four adequate treatment trials, including ECT).

CLINICAL APPROACH TO OTHER MOOD DISORDERS

Anxiety Disorders

Anxiety disorders are a group of mood disorders that are characterized by worry and distress. **Patients with anxiety disorders are at high risk for developing comorbid depression.**

- **Generalized Anxiety Disorder (GAD):** Patients with GAD have excessive and difficult-to-control worry and anxiety that causes physical symptoms, including restlessness, irritability, sleep disturbance, and difficulty concentrating.

- **Panic Disorder:** Panic disorder is characterized by recurrent panic attacks, which are defined as periods of intense fear of abrupt onset. They often live in fear of the next episode.

- **Obsessive-Compulsive Disorder (OCD):** OCD manifests as either obsessions (recurrent, intrusive thoughts) or compulsions (repetitive behaviors) that are unreasonable, excessive, and cause much distress to the patient.

- **Posttraumatic Stress Disorder (PTSD):** PTSD is a response to a severe traumatic event in which the patient suffers fear, helplessness, or horror and reliving of the event.

- **Phobia:** A phobia is an irrational fear that causes a conscious avoidance of a situation, subject, or activity. These can become debilitating when this phobia is of commonly encountered subjects.

Bipolar Disorder

Bipolar disorder affects genders equally and often presents in young people. It is characterized by fluctuations ("cycling") between periods of mania and depression. Symptoms of mania include the abrupt onset of elevated or irritable mood, inflated self-esteem, decreased need for sleep, pressured speech, racing thoughts, distractibility, increased goal-directed activity, and engaging in pleasurable activities with potentially painful consequences. Concomitant substance abuse should always be investigated. Episodes of mania must last at least 1 week (or any duration if hospitalization is needed) and occur during a distinct period, not continuously. Continuous behavior of this type suggests personality disorders or schizophrenia. A single episode of mania is sufficient for the diagnosis of bipolar disorder. **All patients diagnosed with depression should be questioned about mania** since the treatments are different and SSRIs can trigger manic episodes. Bipolar disorder is typically treated with mood stabilizers, which include valproate, carbamazepine, and lithium.

CASE CORRELATION

- See also Case 36 (Family Violence), Case 41 (Substance Use Disorder), and Case 59 (Opioid Use Disorder and Chronic Pain Management).

COMPREHENSION QUESTIONS

25.1 A 62-year-old man presents for a follow-up office visit for severe depression. He has been seen for 2 months by his provider. His symptoms have included crying episodes, insomnia, and decreased appetite. He has suicidal ideations and states that he has a gun in his home that he might use. He has had auditory hallucinations, saying he hears a voice telling him that his wife is the devil. His symptoms have not been relieved by maximum doses of sertraline (Zoloft), venlafaxine (Effexor), or citalopram (Celexa). He is currently taking duloxetine (Cymbalta), which has also failed to improve his symptoms. Which of the following would most likely provide the most rapid relief of his symptoms?

A. Electroconvulsive therapy

B. Bupropion (Wellbutrin)

C. Stopping duloxetine and starting on an MAOI

D. Behavioral modification

25.2 A 40-year-old woman sees you in the office for follow-up of treatment for recurrent depression. Her symptoms have improved slightly after 2 months of fluoxetine (Prozac) 10 mg a day and weekly counseling sessions with a psychologist. She states that she is still having feelings of "low energy" and "crying episodes." She is having no medication side effects, and both she and her husband state that she is taking her medication regularly. Which of the following would be the most appropriate next step?

A. Continue with your current plan and give it more time.

B. Increase the fluoxetine dose to 20 mg daily and continue counseling.

C. Discontinue fluoxetine and start paroxetine 10 mg daily.

D. Continue fluoxetine and add bupropion as adjunctive therapy.

E. Discontinue medications and arrange for psychiatric consultation for ECT.

25.3 Three weeks ago, you started a 22-year-old man on sertraline for his first episode of major depressive disorder. Today, you receive a telephone call from his mother stating that he has not slept in days, is speaking very rapidly, and has maxed out his credit card buying electronic equipment. Which of the following is the most likely explanation for this situation?

A. He is having a medication side effect.

B. He is secretly taking too much of his sertraline.

C. The sertraline has unmasked underlying bipolar disorder.

D. The sertraline has precipitated a hyperthyroid state.

ANSWERS

25.1 **A.** This patient has psychotic depression with suicidal ideation and has not responded to maximum doses of several antidepressants. He is more likely to respond to ECT than to counseling (answer D) or a change in medication (answers B and C). Most studies have shown that ECT produces significant response within the first week of therapy and complete remission within 3 to 4 weeks. This is much faster than the 3 to 4 weeks of lag time from anti-depression pharmacological therapy.

25.2 **B.** The most common causes of treatment failure or poor response to therapy are inadequate medication dosing, inadequate length of treatment, or nonadherence. In this setting, where the patient is adherent and has had adequate time for response, increasing the dose of medication from 10 mg (a low starting dose) to 20 mg would be your first step. Typically, antidepressant medication dosages can be increased after 4 weeks of treatment if the response is inadequate. Answer A (continue current plan and give more time) is not necessary since 2 months are an adequate time for response. Answer C (discontinue fluoxetine and start paroxetine) would be an option if the patient had significant side effects, but this patient has no side effects. Adding a second antidepressant (answer D) would be indicated if the patient continued to be symptomatic despite the maximum amount of one agent. Answer E (discontinue medication and start ECT) would be an option if pharmacological therapy were found to be ineffective or if a rapid response were required.

25.3 **C.** In bipolar patients, the use of an SSRI can precipitate a manic state. It is critically important to assess for a history of manic episodes prior to starting antidepressant therapy. In some cases, bipolar disorder may initially present as major depression, so the institution of antidepressant medication may unmask an undiagnosed bipolar condition. Another condition to assess for in this situation is the concomitant use of recreational drugs, such as cocaine or methamphetamine. Sertraline does have some side effects (although much less than the older tricyclic agents), but "mania" is not a typical side effect (answer A). Instead, the typical side effects include sexual dysfunction, dizziness, and nausea.

CLINICAL PEARLS

▶ While working up a diagnosis of depression, other medical diagnoses, such as hypothyroidism, anemia, diabetes, or infectious processes, that could mimic some symptoms of depression must be ruled out.

▶ Always investigate the use of alcohol and drugs when evaluating for mood disorders.

▶ Suicidal and homicidal ideation should always be investigated and thoroughly addressed when evaluating depression.

▶ The addition of any new medication should be investigated to ensure it is not contributing to the patient's symptoms.

REFERENCES

American Psychiatric Association. *Diagnostic and Statistical Manual of Mental Disorders.* 5th ed. Arlington, VA: American Psychiatric Publishing; 2013.

Eisendrath SJ, Cole SA, Christensen JF, Gutnick D, Cole M, Feldman MD. Depression. In: Feldman MD, Christensen JF, Satterfield JM, eds. *Behavioral Medicine: A Guide for Clinical Practice.* 4th ed. New York, NY: McGraw Hill; 2014: Chap. 25. http://accessmedicine.mhmedical.com/content.asp x?bookid=1116&sectionid=62688871. Accessed May 6, 2019.

Kovich H, DeJong A. Common questions about the pharmacologic management of depression in adults. *Am Fam Physician.* 2015;92(2):94-100.

Maurer DM, Raymond TJ, Davis BN. Depression: screening and diagnosis. *Am Fam Physician.* 2018;98(8):508-515.

Shim RS, Primm A. Depression in diverse populations & older adults. In: South-Paul JE, Matheny SC, Lewis EL, eds. *CURRENT Diagnosis & Treatment: Family Medicine.* 4th ed. New York, NY: McGraw Hill; 2015: Chap. 56. http://accessmedicine.mhmedical.com/content.aspx?bookid=1415 &Sectionid=77061063. Accessed May 6, 2019.

A 26-year-old gravida 1, para 1001 (G1P1001) woman presents for her 6-week postpartum visit following the vaginal delivery of a 7-lb baby girl. She had an uncomplicated prenatal course. She went into labor spontaneously at 39 months, 2/7 weeks' gestation. She had a second-degree perineal laceration that was repaired without difficulty. She started breastfeeding her baby immediately after delivery. Her postpartum course was uncomplicated, and she was discharged from the hospital on the second postpartum day. She is exclusively breastfeeding and reports that it is going well. She says that she felt "stressed, sad, and overwhelmed" during her first week at home but that those feelings have resolved. She is now in excellent spirits and has strong support at home from her husband and her mother. On examination, she appears well and has normal vital signs. Her general physical examination is normal. A pelvic examination shows a well-healed laceration repair, no cervical or vaginal discharge, closed cervical os, and no cervical motion tenderness. Her uterus is normal size, firm, and nontender, and there are no adnexal masses. She is interested in birth control, but she is considering another child next year.

▶ What additional tools can be used to assess mood and screen for depression?
▶ If she prefers oral contraception, which type would be most appropriate for this patient?
▶ When can the patient resume sexual activity?
▶ What are the maternal benefits of breastfeeding?

ANSWERS TO CASE 26:

Postpartum Care

Summary: A 26-year-old woman presents with

- Status as a first-time mother presenting for a 6-week postpartum visit
- Normal examination and reports of breastfeeding her baby going well
- A brief period in which she felt sad and overwhelmed, but that has resolved
- A request for contraception counseling

Depression Screening: Mood assessment is one of the most important aspects of the postpartum visit. The nine-question Patient Health Questionnaire (PHQ9) can be used to assess mood in a variety of patients, but the Edinburgh Postnatal Depression Scale has been adjusted to reflect the unique life events of early newborn care such as lack of sleep.

Recommended oral contraception: Estrogen-containing oral contraceptive pills (OCPs) must be avoided in all postpartum women for the first 30 days. In breastfeeding women, the progestin-only "minipill" is recommended, as combined hormonal contraceptives can interfere with milk supply.

Resumption of sexual activity: In general and in the absence of complications, postpartum women may resume sexual activity (vaginal intercourse) after 6 weeks.

Maternal benefits of breastfeeding: Along with benefits to the baby, the maternal benefits include (but are not limited to) a more rapid return of uterine tone with reduced bleeding; a quicker return of the uterus to nonpregnant size; a more rapid return to prepregnancy body weight; a reduced incidence of ovarian and breast cancer; contraceptive effects; the convenience of always having a readily available feeding supply for the baby; lower costs since formula does not need to be purchased.

ANALYSIS

Objectives

1. Be able to discuss the diagnosis and management of common postpartum complications. (EPA 1, 10)

2. Be able to counsel patients on common postpartum issues such as contraception, breastfeeding, and postpartum depression. (EPA 10, 12)

Considerations

The postpartum period is defined as the time starting after the delivery of the placenta and lasting for 6 to 12 weeks. The postpartum period is a time of great change for the woman and her family. There are numerous normal physiologic changes that occur during the transition from the pregnant to the nonpregnant state. Just as important are the many personal, social, and family changes that occur, which can be magnified for first-time parents or when there are unforeseen complications.

The time following discharge from the hospital and the subsequent 6 to 12 weeks usually represents the period of greatest adjustment. There are normal changes that occur, along with many potential medical and emotional complications. Future family planning and contraceptive issues need to be addressed as well. A 6-week postpartum examination is usually scheduled, but many of the issues that can occur during this time frame should be addressed prior to discharge from the hospital. A 2-week postpartum visit mainly to assess mood is becoming the standard of care.

APPROACH TO:
Postpartum Care

DEFINITIONS

ENDOMETRITIS: A polymicrobial infection of the endometrium, myometrium, and parametrial tissues of the uterus, usually caused by ascending infection from the vagina.

LOCHIA: Normal postpartum vaginal discharge that is initially reddish in color and consists of blood, decidua, and epithelial cells and then becomes thicker and yellow-white as leukocytes predominate.

PREECLAMPSIA: A pregnancy complication characterized by high blood pressure and signs of damage to another organ system, most often the kidneys (proteinuria). Preeclampsia usually begins after 20 weeks of pregnancy in women whose blood pressure had been normal. It can present postdelivery, although less commonly.

CLINICAL APPROACH POSTPARTUM WELLNESS

Inpatient Care of the Postpartum Patient

The expected postdelivery hospital stay is 24 to 48 hours for an uncomplicated vaginal delivery and 72 to 96 hours for a cesarean delivery. This time allows for recovery, allows further monitoring for maternal and neonatal complications, and can be used to provide education and support. Only 3% of vaginal deliveries and 9% of cesarean deliveries result in complications that require a prolonged hospital stay. Goals of postpartum care include early ambulation, resuming a regular diet, perineal and bladder care, establishing a bowel regimen, addressing postpartum blues, and providing breastfeeding support.

Common Problems. Typical maternal problems that occur during this time frame include pain, bleeding, lactation difficulties, and urinary problems (infections, incontinence, and retention). Postpartum fever is most often a sign of endometritis (infection of the uterus), but it can also be caused by urinary tract or wound infections, thromboembolic disease, and mastitis. Endometritis and mastitis are the most common postpartum infections and typically will present prior to the 6-week postpartum visit. Preeclampsia can present in the postpartum period, usually within 1 week but up to 4 weeks.

Discharge Instructions. Prior to discharge, women should be instructed on normal physiological changes after delivery, including lochia, diuresis, and milk letdown, as well as what to do in the case of alarming symptoms such as fever, excessive vaginal bleeding, leg pain or swelling, persistent headaches, shortness of breath, and chest pain. Women who are not already immune to rubella should receive the combined measles-mumps-rubella vaccination. A tetanus, diphtheria, and acellular pertussis (Tdap) vaccine is recommended for women who were not vaccinated during their pregnancies. Influenza vaccine is also recommended for women who have not yet been vaccinated. Rh status must also be addressed. If the mother is Rh negative and the infant confirmed to be Rh positive, then the mother should receive Rho(D) immune globulin (RhoGAM) in order to reduce the risk of isoimmunization affecting future pregnancies.

Normal Physiological Changes

Uterine Changes. The uterus increases significantly in size and weight during pregnancy. Immediately after delivery it weighs approximately 1 kg, is the size of a uterus at 20 weeks' gestation (fundus palpable at the umbilicus), and begins the process of involution, the return to its nonpregnant size. Contractions of the uterus, promoted by endogenous oxytocin secretion, improve hemostasis by compressing the uterine blood vessels. Oxytocin release increases during breastfeeding, so early breastfeeding is encouraged to assist involution. Supplemental oxytocin (Pitocin) given by intravenous infusion during or immediately after the third stage of labor also aids in increasing uterine tone. By the end of the first postpartum week, the uterus will be about the size of a 12-week gestation and palpable at the symphysis pubis; in most cases, it will return to normal size (weighing less than 100 g) by the time of the 6-week follow-up visit. If the normal process of involution does not occur, the patient should be evaluated for infection and retained placenta.

Vaginal Bleeding. Vaginal bleeding is usually heaviest in the hours following delivery, then decreases significantly. Brown or blood-tinged lochia occurs for about the next week. This is followed by white or yellow lochia, which continues for approximately 4 to 6 more weeks. **In women who are not breastfeeding, menstruation usually restarts by the third postpartum month.** In women who are breastfeeding, ovulation and menstruation can be suppressed for much longer. Anovulation will persist for longer periods of time in women who exclusively breastfeed their babies. This confers a contraceptive benefit but, by itself, is not as reliable as other methods of contraception.

Breast Changes. Breast engorgement, signaling increased milk production, typically occurs 1 to 4 days after delivery and can cause breast pain, milk leakage, and fever. In breastfeeding women, this is best managed by increased frequency of feedings. In women who are not breastfeeding, the use of ice packs, supportive bras, and nonsteroidal anti-inflammatory drugs (NSAIDs) can reduce discomfort.

CLINICAL APPROACH TO MEDICAL COMPLICATIONS

Hemorrhage

Pathophysiology. Postpartum hemorrhage is defined as loss of more than 500 mL of blood after vaginal delivery and 1000 mL following a cesarean delivery. This occurs in about 4% of vaginal deliveries. Early postpartum hemorrhage occurs within 24 hours of delivery and is most often immediately postpartum. Late postpartum hemorrhage occurs between 24 hours and 12 weeks after delivery and is usually the result of retained tissue or abnormal placental site involution. The causes of most cases of postpartum hemorrhage can be remembered with the mnemonic "The Four Ts" (Table 26–1). Careful examination focused on the likely causes should be performed promptly to identify the source of the bleeding in both early and late postpartum hemorrhage.

Risk Factors and Prevention. Risk factors for postpartum hemorrhage include prolonged third stage of labor, multiple delivery, episiotomy, fetal macrosomia, and history of postpartum hemorrhage, but any patient can develop postpartum hemorrhage, so it is important to prepare for prevention and early management at all deliveries. Active management of the third stage of labor is the best way to prevent postpartum hemorrhage. This involves administration of a uterotonic agent, such as oxytocin or misoprostol, coinciding with delivery of the anterior shoulder, gentle cord traction, and uterine massage.

General Treatment. As with all emergency situations, the **first priority in managing postpartum hemorrhage is assessment of cardiopulmonary stability.** It is important to ensure that adequate intravenous access is available, preferably two large-bore intravenous catheters. Fluid resuscitation with a crystalloid solution (normal saline, lactated Ringer solution) should be given as necessary, and massive hemorrhage may require transfusion with packed red blood cells.

Uterine Atony. **Uterine atony causes approximately 70% of postpartum hemorrhage.** Failure of the uterus to contract adequately results in continued bleeding from uterine vasculature. Risks include prolonged labor, prolonged use of oxytocin during labor, a large baby, and grand multipara (five or more previous children). **Initial management of uterine atony includes initiating bimanual uterine compression and massage and administration of oxytocin, which may be given intravenously or intramuscularly.** Additional options for continued bleeding include methylergonovine (Methergine), carboprost (Hemabate), and misoprostol (Cytotec). Methylergonovine is contraindicated in patients with preeclampsia or hypertension, as it may cause an abrupt increase in blood pressure. Carboprost is contraindicated in

Table 26–1 • THE FOUR Ts OF POSTPARTUM HEMORRHAGE	
Tone	Uterine atony
Trauma	Cervical, vaginal, or perineal lacerations; uterine inversion
Tissue	Retained placenta or membranes
Thrombin	Coagulopathies

women with asthma. Misoprostol has limited use due to high gastrointestinal and other side effects.

Trauma. **Trauma** (lacerations, hemotomas, and inverted uterus) causes approximately 20% of bleeds and is managed procedurally. **Retained placenta** causes approximately 10% of bleeds and is also managed procedurally. **Coagualopathies** cause approximately 1% of bleeds and require clotting factor replacement for management.

Fever

Postpartum Fever. Postpartum fever, especially **if associated with uterine tenderness and foul-smelling lochia, is often a sign of endometritis.** Endometritis complicates approximately 10% of cesarean and 1% to 2% of vaginal deliveries, even with antibiotics given prophylactically. When it does occur, endometritis following vaginal delivery should be treated with broad-spectrum antibiotics that cover vaginal and gastrointestinal flora.

Urinary Tract Infection. Urinary tract infections (UTIs) are another common cause of fever after both vaginal and cesarean deliveries. Urinary frequency, urgency, and burning are typical presenting symptoms. Catheterization of the urinary bladder, which occurs routinely during a cesarean delivery and frequently during vaginal deliveries, raises the risk of introducing bacteria into the normally sterile environment of the bladder.

Mastitis. Breast infections such as mastitis may occur as well. Symptoms include breast engorement, erythema, induration, and tenderness. Prompt treatment with continued breastfeeding or pumping from the affected breast and antibiotics that cover staph infections are helpful in preventing breast abscess development. Mastitis should not result in discontinuation of nursing.

Other Causes. Other causes of fever in the postpartum period, especially in women delivered by cesarean, are identical to causes of fever in other postsurgical patients. These include atelectasis, wound infections, and venous thromboembolic disease.

Postpartum Preeclampsia

Up to 5% of preeclampsia can present in the postpartum period, usually within 1 week but up to 4 weeks after delivery. Symptoms and signs include headaches, right upper quadrant abdominal pain, edema, blurry vision, elevated blood pressure, and proteinuria. These patients should have their blood pressure treated and, if they have severe features, should be sent urgently back to the labor floor for postpartum magnesium treatment.

Mood Disorders

Up to three-fourths of women have some change in mood following the delivery of a child. In most cases, the symptoms are mild and self-limited. However, a small but significant percentage can have a severe reaction requiring medical or psychiatric intervention.

Baby Blues. Approximately 30% to 70% of women develop a temporary state known as the **"baby blues."** This condition **develops within the first week after**

delivery and typically resolves by the 10th postpartum day. Symptoms include tearfulness, sadness, and emotional lability. The etiology is not entirely clear, but may be multifactorial and include hormonal changes following delivery, nutritional deficiencies, stress, sleep deprivation, and adjustment to the new role as a mother.

Postpartum Depression. Postpartum depression occurs in 10% to 20% of women following pregnancy and can occur following gestations of any length—term, preterm, miscarriages, or abortions. The onset is defined by the *Diagnostic and Statistical Manual of Mental Disorders, Fifth Edition (DSM-5)* as occurring within 4 weeks' postpartum, but it may occur as late as 1 year postpartum. Up to 50% of "postpartum" major depressive episodes may actually begin prior to delivery. **The symptoms of postpartum depression are the same as those of major depression** (see Case 25). The severity can vary from mild to severe and suicidal. There is a **high recurrence rate in subsequent pregnancies** and **an increased risk in women with a history of depression unrelated to pregnancy.** Untreated postpartum depression is a significant cause of morbidity. All women should be screened for a history of psychiatric disorders during their prenatal care and should be questioned about symptoms of depression at 2-week and 6-week postpartum visits.

The treatment of postpartum depression is **similar to the treatment of nonpregnancy-related depression.** Women who are a risk to themselves or to others or who are unable to care for themselves should be admitted to the hospital. Selective serotonin reuptake inhibitors (SSRIs) are first-line therapy because of their efficacy and safety. They also are considered safe in breastfeeding. Counseling and general supportive measures at home are also important adjuncts to treatment.

Postpartum Psychosis. Postpartum psychosis is a rare, but potentially devastating, complication following pregnancy. Manic or frankly delusional behaviors may present within a few days to a few weeks of delivery in up to 1 in 1000 postpartum patients. All women with postpartum psychosis should be hospitalized and comanaged with a psychiatrist. Without proper treatment, there is a high risk of suicide and infanticide associated with this diagnosis.

CLINICAL APPROACH TO BREASTFEEDING

Benefits of Breastfeeding. Counseling and encouragement regarding both the maternal and infant benefits of breastfeeding should start during the prenatal period. Neonatal benefits include ideal nutrition, increased resistance to infection, and a reduced risk of gastrointestinal tract infections, food allergies, ear infections, and atopic dermatitis. Maternal benefits include improved mother-child bonding, more rapid uterine involution, quicker return to prepregnant body weight, convenience, decreased costs, and long-term reduced risks of ovarian and breast cancer. Breastfeeding promotion and education can increase the rate of breastfeeding and the duration for which women breastfeed their babies (see Table 26–2).

Initial Feedings. Women should be allowed to nurse their newborns as soon as possible following delivery. During this time, the newborns are often very

Table 26–2 • TEN STEPS FOR SUCCESSFUL BREASTFEEDING
1. Have a written breastfeeding policy that is regularly communicated to all health care staff.
2. Train all staff in skills necessary to implement this policy.
3. Inform all pregnant women about the benefits and management of breastfeeding.
4. Help mothers initiate breastfeeding within an hour of birth.
5. Show mothers how to breastfeed and how to sustain lactation, even if they are separated from their infants.
6. Feed newborn infants nothing but breast milk, unless medically indicated, and under no circumstances provide breast milk substitutes, feeding bottles, or pacifiers free of charge or at low cost.
7. Practice rooming-in, which allows mothers and infants to remain together 24 hours a day.
8. Encourage breastfeeding on demand.
9. Give no artificial pacifiers to breastfeeding infants.
10. Help start breastfeeding support groups and refer mothers to them.

Reproduced with permission, from Cunningham F, Leveno KJ, Bloom SL, et al, eds. Williams Obstetrics. *25th ed. 2018. http://accessmedicine.mhmedical.com. Copyright © McGraw Hill LLC. All rights reserved.*

alert and have strong rooting and sucking reflexes, which promote latching on to the nipple. Initial feedings provide colostrum, a yellow fluid that is rich in immunoglobulin A, minerals, amino acids, and proteins. Breast engorgement and milk letdown commonly occur between the second and fourth postpartum days. Mature milk contains fats, proteins, carbohydrates, vitamins, minerals, and hormones.

Contraindications. There are **few contraindications to breastfeeding**, but they include HIV infection, miliary tuberculosis, acute hepatitis B, herpetic breast lesions, and chemotherapy. Substance use disorders with substances such as cocaine, heroin, PCP (phencyclidine), and alcohol are contraindications. Women who have had breast-reduction surgery with nipple transplantation will be unable to breastfeed.

Complications. Common maternal complications of breastfeeding include sore or cracked nipples and mastitis. Sore nipples can be managed by ensuring proper latch-on, frequent position changes, alternating breasts during feedings, nipple shields, keeping the nipples clean and dry between feedings, and applications of lanolin or the patient's own breast milk as a salve. Vitamin E, herbal rubs, and other creams and topical agents should be avoided because of risk of absorption by the infant.

CLINICAL APPROACH TO FAMILY PLANNING

Most women resume sexual activity by 3 months' postpartum, and pelvic rest is recommended for the first 6 weeks. Numerous options are available to women for contraception and family planning. Discussion of these options ideally should occur in the prenatal period and again before discharge from the hospital.

Hormonal Contraception. OCPs are the most widely used reversible form of contraception. Available OCPs contain both estrogen and progestin or are progestin only. **In breastfeeding women, the progestin-only pills are preferred** because combination OCPs might reduce lactation. Both the American College of Obstetricians and Gynecologists and the World Health Organization recommend waiting for 30 days postpartum to start estrogen-containing OCPs. Progesterone-only pills, injectable long-acting depot medroxyprogesterone (Depo-Provera), progestin-eluting birth control implants, and any intrauterine device (IUD) may be used in the immediate postpartum period by breastfeeding women. IUDs have a significant risk of expulsion if placed prior to 6 weeks' postpartum.

Barrier Contraception. Barrier methods of contraception may also be used regardless of breastfeeding status. While not widely used, **diaphragms and cervical caps must be refitted at the 6-week visit** to ensure an appropriate fit since the cervix has changed in size and shape.

Breastfeeding as Contraception. **Lactation-induced amenorrhea provides a high level of natural contraception in the first 6 months' postpartum.** However, this protection wanes if breastfeeding is reduced or if menses restart. As ovulation precedes the return of menses, this method should not be considered as reliable as other methods. After 6 months, if menses restart or if breastfeeding is reduced, alternate forms of contraception should be used.

CASE CORRELATION

- See also Case 25 (Major Depression and Other Mood Disorders) and Case 28 (Family Planning—Contraceptives).

COMPREHENSION QUESTIONS

26.1 You are on call for your practice and receive a page to speak to a 20-year-old woman who delivered a 6 lb, 9 oz baby boy 3 days ago. When you talk to the patient, she reports passing bright red blood and blood clots, requiring more than two heavy pads per hour over the past 2 days. She is awake and talking but feels dizzy. You arrange for transportation to the hospital. In the emergency center, the patient appears slightly confused but responds to instructions. Her blood pressure is noted to be 90/60 mm Hg, and her pulse is 110 beats/min. Which of the following is your most appropriate initial intervention?

A. Add 20 units of oxytocin (Pitocin) to the intravenous line of 0.45% saline that is currently running at 125 mL/h.

B. Perform bimanual uterine massage.

C. Place a large-bore intravenous line and give a 1-L bolus of 0.9% saline.

D. Give an intramuscular injection of methylergonovine (Methergine).

26.2 For the patient in Question 26.1, what is the most likely cause of the delayed postpartum bleeding?

A. Retained tissue with reduced uterine tone

B. Cervical laceration

C. Unrepaired vaginal laceration

D. Coagulopathy

26.3 A 29-year-old first-time mother comes into your office for her routine 6-week postpartum visit. Her husband, who accompanied her to the visit, reports that his wife is tearful much of the time. She has not been sleeping well, has little energy, and has a reduced appetite. She denies any suicidal thoughts, hallucinations, or feelings that she wants to harm her baby. Which of the following is the most appropriate intervention?

A. Reassurance that these feelings will pass within a week or so

B. Referral to a psychiatrist for outpatient management

C. Institution of SSRI therapy and close follow-up

D. Admission to the hospital and urgent psychiatric consultation

26.4 You see a 30-year-old woman for an acute visit 16 days' postpartum. She has been breastfeeding her baby daughter but has developed a very sore left breast. On examination, the patient has a temperature of 101.3 °F (38.5 °C). The left breast is diffusely tender, primarily in the upper inner quadrant. The skin overlying the area of maximal tenderness is erythematous and warm. There is no nipple discharge, and the remainder of the examination is normal. Which of the following is the best treatment?

A. This condition is self-limited, but she should stop nursing the baby on the left breast until this condition resolves.

B. She may nurse from the unaffected breast but should simply pump and discard the milk from the painful breast.

C. The patient should receive oral dicloxacillin or clindamycin.

D. She should have a fine-needle aspiration.

ANSWERS

26.1 **C.** This patient is symptomatically hypovolemic, with dizziness, hypotension, and tachycardia. As with any resuscitation, supporting the circulatory process is extremely important. With hemorrhagic shock, fluid resuscitation with intravenous isotonic solution must be your first intervention. Once you have started the management of this critical issue, you should turn your attention to identifying and correcting the source of the bleeding and transfuse red blood cells or, if needed, massive transfusion (red cells, fresh frozen plasma, and possibly platelets). Answer A (oxytocin added to intravenous fluids of hypotonic saline) will not fill the intravascular space as effectively since it is hypotonic. Answer B (bimanual massage) may be needed if the etiology is uterine atony. Certainly, if uterine atony is noted to be found, then uterotonic agents (answer D) and bimanual massage are critical to reduce ongoing hemorrhage.

26.2 **A.** While any of the listed options (answer B, cervical laceration; answer C, unrepaired vaginal laceration; and answer D, coagulopathy) could result in this scenario, the most common cause for a delayed postpartum hemorrhage is retained tissue. This interferes with proper contraction of the uterus and leads to delayed uterine atony and increased bleeding.

26.3 **C.** This patient has a classic presentation of postpartum depression, and the best plan would be to start an antidepressant (an SSRI being the most common choice). The symptoms are identical to those of a major depressive episode. The maternity blues is a self-limited condition that starts in the first postpartum week and resolves in the second. Fortunately, this patient does not have signs of postpartum psychosis (mania, hallucinations, and delusions), which would require admission to the hospital (answer D). Appropriate management includes the use of an SSRI, counseling, and close follow-up. Answer A (reassurance and follow-up) is appropriate for postpartum blues or mild symptoms, but this patient requires therapy. Answer B (referral to a psychiatrist) is not appropriate since this patient has a straightforward postpartum depressive disorder without psychosis.

26.4 **C.** Mastitis is a common complication of breastfeeding. It is caused by gland obstruction, and sometimes, as in this case, there also are signs of infection. Treatment is directed at relieving the obstruction, so increased breastfeeding or pumping is helpful. The antibiotics typically used for this complication are considered safe to use while nursing. Empiric staphylococcal coverage is recommended. Dicloxacillin and cephalexin are appropriate for areas with low rates of methicillin-resistant *Staphylococcus aureus* (MRSA). Good choices are clindamycin or sulfamethoxazole-trimethoprim for areas with high rates of MRSA. Answer A (reassurance, stop breastfeeding, and observation) would be indicated with breast engorgement but not mastitis, where antibiotic therapy is needed. With mastitis, breastfeeding does not need to be discontinued (answer B). Answer D (fine-needle aspiration) is indicated to biopsy a breast mass or cyst and is not indicated in this case.

CLINICAL PEARLS

▶ Many of the important postpartum issues—mood problems, contraception, and breastfeeding—are best managed by addressing them in the prenatal course first and then readdressing or reinforcing them in the postpartum period.

▶ Most causes of postpartum hemorrhage can be remembered with the four Ts: tone, trauma, tissue, and thrombin.

▶ Uterine atony causes approximately 70% of postpartum hemorrhage. Initial management includes initiating bimanual uterine compression and massage and administration of oxytocin, which may be given intravenously or intramuscularly.

▶ Baby blues develops within the first week after delivery and typically resolves by the 10th postpartum day.

▶ Postpartum fever, especially if associated with uterine tenderness and foul-smelling lochia, is often a sign of endometritis.

▶ In breastfeeding women, progestin-only pills are preferred because combination OCPs might reduce lactation.

REFERENCES

Blenning CE, Paladine H. An approach to the postpartum office visit. *Am Fam Physician*. 2005; 72(12):2491-2496.

Conti TD, Patel M, Bhat S., et al. Breastfeeding & infant nutrition. In: South-Paul JE, Matheny SC, Lewis EL, eds. *CURRENT Diagnosis & Treatment: Family Medicine*. 4th ed. New York, NY: McGraw Hill; 2015: Chap. 4. http://accessmedicine.mhmedical.com/content.aspx?bookid=1415& Sectionid=77054127. Accessed February 10, 2019.

Evensen A, Anderson JM, Fontaine P. Postpartum hemorrhage: prevention and treatment. *Am Fam Physician*. 2017;95(7):442-449.

Obstetrical hemorrhage. In: Cunningham F, Leveno KJ, Bloom SL, Dashe JS, Hoffman BL, Casey BM, Spong CY, eds. *Williams Obstetrics*. 25th ed. New York, NY: McGraw Hill; 2018: Chap. 41. http://accessmedicine.mhmedical.com/content.aspx?bookid=1918&sectionid=185083809. Accessed May 6, 2019.

Puerperal complications. In: Cunningham F, Leveno KJ, Bloom SL, Dashe JS, Hoffman BL, Casey BM, Spong CY. eds. *Williams Obstetrics* 25th ed. New York, NY: McGraw Hill; 2018: Chap. 37. http://accessmedicine.mhmedical.com/content.aspx?bookid=1918&sectionid=141464707. Accessed May 6, 2019.

The puerperium. In: Cunningham F, Leveno KJ, Bloom SL, Dashe JS, Hoffman BL, Casey BM, Spong CY, eds. *Williams Obstetrics*. 25th ed. New York, NY: McGraw Hill; 2018: Chap. 36. http://accessmedicine.mhmedical.com/content.aspx?bookid=1918&sectionid=138823398. Accessed May 6, 2019.

A 66-year-old woman presents to your office complaining of shortness of breath and bilateral leg edema that have been worsening for 3 months. She emphatically tells you, "I get out of breath when I do housework, and I can't even walk to the corner." She has also noticed difficulty sleeping secondary to a dry cough that wakes her up at night and further exacerbation of her shortness of breath while lying flat. This has forced her to use three pillows for a good night's sleep. She denies any chest pain, wheezing, or febrile illness. She has no past illnesses and takes no medications. She has never smoked and drinks socially. On examination, her blood pressure (BP) is 187/90 mm Hg, her pulse is 97 beats/min, her respiratory rate is 16 breaths/min, her temperature is 98 °F (36.6 °C), and her oxygen saturation is 93% on room air by pulse oximetry. She has a pronounced jugular vein. Cardiac examination reveals a pansystolic murmur. Examination of her lung bases reveals dullness bilaterally. You find 2+ pitting edema of both ankles. An electrocardiogram (ECG) shows a normal sinus rhythm, and a chest x-ray demonstrates mild cardiomegaly with bilateral pleural effusions. You decide she needs further workup, so you call the hospital where you have admitting privileges and arrange for a telemetry bed.

► What is the most likely diagnosis?
► What is the next diagnostic step?
► What is the initial step in therapy?

ANSWERS TO CASE 27:
Heart Failure

Summary: A 66-year-old woman presents with

- Worsening shortness of breath, bilateral leg edema, and three-pillow orthopnea
- No known hypertension, but a current BP of 187/90 mm Hg and O_2 saturation 93% on room air
- Jugular venous distension (JVD), a cardiac murmur, and decreased breath sounds at both lung bases
- Bilateral pleural effusions on chest x-ray

Most likely diagnosis: New-onset heart failure (HF).

Next diagnostic step: ECG; blood work including cardiac enzymes, complete blood count (CBC), electrolytes, liver function tests, thyroid function test, lipid profile, B-type natriuretic protein (BNP), and renal function; echocardiogram.

Initial therapy: Telemetry monitoring, intravenous diuretics, and oxygen.

ANALYSIS

Objectives

1. State the common symptoms and clinical signs of HF. (EPA 1, 2, 3)
2. Describe the pathophysiology of common types of HF. (EPA 12)
3. State the mechanism of action and rationale of the drugs used in the treatment of acute and chronic HF. (EPA 4)
4. Be familiar with the outpatient management of HF and the importance of patient education and care management. (EPA 4)

Considerations

This 66-year-old woman presented with HF. Her most immediate problem is oxygenation and volume overload on her weakened heart. The **first priority is optimizing oxygen exchange** by administering oxygen via nasal cannula, dilating pulmonary vasculature, and decreasing cardiac preload and afterload. The most common causes of HF are coronary artery disease (CAD) and hypertension, so it is imperative to evaluate these patients for CAD. The overload of fluid in the lungs is a common cause of anxiety and distress in patients with acute HF because of the continuous struggle to oxygenate adequately. This anxiety activates sympathetic pathways and mounts catecholamine-induced responses, causing tachycardia and increased peripheral vascular resistance, leading to greater stress on the heart and worsening of symptoms. These triggers can be reduced by the use of an agent such as morphine sulfate, which acts as both an anxiolytic and a vasodilator. Furosemide (Lasix) is the diuretic of choice, not only for its diuretic effect but also for its immediate vasodilatory action on bronchial vasculature. Admitting these patients to the hospital allows for closer management of their fluid balances and evaluation of any underlying condition that may have precipitated the HF. Other medications, including angiotensin-converting enzyme inhibitors (ACEIs), angiotensin receptor blockers (ARBs), and beta-blockers help to control HF symptoms by decreasing preload, afterload, and cardiac remodeling.

APPROACH TO:
Heart Failure

DEFINITIONS

FRAMINGHAM HEART STUDY: Large, prospective cohort study of the epidemiologic factors associated with cardiovascular diseases.

HEART FAILURE: Impairment of the ventricle's ability to fill with or eject blood, which results in inadequate circulation of blood to meet metabolic needs. Some expert organizations define specific left ventricular ejection fraction thresholds.

CLINICAL APPROACH

Epidemiology

Heart failure is **the most common cause of hospitalization and readmission in patients older than 65 years.** Poorer prognosis is seen in patients who are male, older, or have more severe symptoms, CAD and acute coronary syndrome, hypotension, impaired renal function, hyponatremia, and elevated plasma BNP. Sudden cardiac death, often from a ventricular arrhythmia, may account for up to 30% of all deaths.

Pathophysiology

Heart failure can be subdivided into reduced or preserved ejection fraction and right- or left-sided HF, all of which can coexist. **Heart failure with reduced ejection fraction** (HFrEF) exists when there is a dilated ventricle with impaired contractility and, possibly, concomitant valvular disease. **Heart failure with preserved ejection fraction** (HFpEF) occurs with normal or intact left ventricular ejection fraction but impaired ventricular relaxation and filling, frequently with left ventricular hypertrophy and stiffness due to systemic hypertension or valvular disease.

Left HF is a syndrome primarily characterized by pulmonary congestion or edema. **Right HF** is characterized by right ventricular (RV) systolic dysfunction accompanied by RV dilation and tricuspid regurgitation, which cause tissue congestion, including peripheral edema, ascites, and abdominal organ engorgement. **The most common cause of right HF is left HF.**

Etiologies. The most common cause of HF in the developed world is CAD. Other common causes are diabetes, uncontrolled hypertension, and valvular heart disease (see Table 27–1). In the developed world, senile degeneration of the aortic valve is

Table 27–1 • ETIOLOGIES OF HEART FAILURE

Heart Failure With Reduced Ejection Fraction (≤ 40%)

Coronary artery disease	Nonischemic dilated cardiomyopathy
Myocardial infarction[a]	Familial/genetic disorders
Myocardial ischemia[a]	Infiltrative disorders[a]
Chronic pressure overload	Toxic/drug-induced damage
Hypertension[a]	Metabolic disorder[a]
Obstructive valvular disease[a]	Viral etiologies
Chronic volume overload	Chagas disease
Regurgitant valvular disease	Disorders of rate and rhythm
Intracardiac (left-to-right) shunting	Chronic bradyarrhythmias
Extracardiac shunting	Chronic tachyarrhythmias

Heart Failure With Preserved Ejection Fraction (≥ 50%)

Pathologic hypertrophy	Restrictive cardiomyopathy
Primary (hypertrophic cardiomyopathies)	Infiltrative disorders (amyloidosis, sarcoidosis)
Secondary (hypertension)	Storage diseases (hemochromatosis)
Aging	Fibrosis
	Endomyocardial disorders

Pulmonary Heart Disease

Cor pulmonale	
Pulmonary vascular disorders	

High-Output States

Metabolic disorders	Excessive blood flow requirements
Thyrotoxicosis	Systemic arteriovenous shunting
Nutritional disorders (beriberi)	Chronic anemia

[a]Indicates disease process that can lead to HFpEF as well.
Reproduced with permission, from Longo DL, Fauci AS, Kasper DL, et al. Harrison's Principles of Internal Medicine. 18th ed. 2012. http://accessmedicine.mhmedical.com. Copyright © McGraw Hill LLC. All rights reserved.

the most common valvular cause of HF; in the developing world, rheumatic valvular disease is more common. Other contributors to HF include smoking, obesity, lower socioeconomic status, and sedentary life style.

Evaluation. Patients presenting with symptoms suggestive of HF should be evaluated with a history, physical examination, and focused testing. Diagnosis of HF is clinical, and there is no single test that can determine its presence or absence. Testing should be designed to confirm HF (or lead to an alternate diagnosis), identify a cause, and assess the severity of the disease. Initial blood tests should generally include a CBC, serum electrolytes, magnesium, calcium, renal function tests, urinalysis, hepatic function tests, lipid panel, thyroid-stimulating hormone, cardiac enzymes, and BNP. Other initial tests should include radiographic studies, electrocardiography, and echocardiography.

Clinical Presentation

Presentation of Right-Sided Heart Failure. The symptoms and signs that occur are characteristic of the alterations to the normal physiologic function of the heart. Signs and symptoms of right-sided HF stem from increased pressure in the systemic veins, causing hepatic congestion, venous engorgement, and visceral edema. Symptoms include nausea, vomiting, abdominal distension or bloating, diminished appetite, early satiety, and abdominal pain, particularly in the right upper quadrant (due to hepatic congestion and stretching of the liver capsule). Signs of right-sided HF are jugular venous distension, peripheral edema, hepatomegaly, right upper quadrant tenderness, hepatojugular reflux, abdominal ascites, and jaundice.

Presentation of Left-Sided Heart Failure. Left-sided HF manifests with elevated pressure in the pulmonary veins, resulting in symptoms of dyspnea on exertion, paroxysmal nocturnal dyspnea, orthopnea, wheezing, tachypnea, and cough. The signs of pulmonary congestion are bilateral pulmonary rales, S_3 gallop rhythm, Cheyne-Stokes respirations (which are associated with low cardiac output), pleural effusion, and pulmonary edema. **Pulmonary edema is often the first manifestation of HF**, but it can also be caused by a variety of noncardiac conditions.

Presentation of Both Right- and Left-Sided Heart Failure. Dyspnea on exertion is the most sensitive symptom for the diagnosis of HF, but its specificity is much lower. Orthopnea and paroxysmal nocturnal dyspnea are more specific for HF, but they are not as sensitive. Symptoms seen in both right- and left-sided HF include weakness, fatigue, nocturia due to increased cardiac preload and decreased renal vasoconstriction in the recumbent position, memory impairment, insomnia, decreased exercise tolerance, headache, stupor, coma, paroxysmal nocturnal dyspnea, and declining functional status. Signs found in both left- and right-sided HF are tachycardia, displaced point of maximal impulse, systolic murmur (mitral or tricuspid), third heart sound (S_3, ventricular filling gallop) associated with volume overload, fourth heart sound (S_4, atrial gallop) associated with diastolic dysfunction, pulsus alternans, diminished pulse pressure, cyanosis, oliguria, dependent peripheral edema, and cardiac cachexia.

Complete Blood Count. A high white blood cell count can help to identify the presence of an underlying infection, which is a common triggering event of HF. Anemia is another common trigger of HF. In an anemic patient, the oxygen-carrying ability of the blood is reduced, and cardiac output must increase to compensate for this. If the anemia is mild or if the heart is normal, this compensation may occur without producing symptoms; if the anemia is severe or if there is underlying cardiac abnormality (from previous ischemia, hypertension, valvular abnormality, etc), HF may occur. Diabetes and hypo- or hyperthyroidism can also precipitate HF.

Electrolyte Values. Electrolyte abnormalities are common in the presence of HF. Neurohumoral responses to a failing heart result in water and sodium retention and potassium excretion. Hyponatremia is a poor prognostic indicator, signifying activation of the renin-aldosterone-angiotensin system. Medications used by patients with chronic heart disease (diuretics, ACEIs, ARBs, and aldosterone antagonists) also can lead to electrolyte abnormalities. Some electrolyte abnormalities, specifically hypo- or hyperkalemia, hypomagnesemia, and hypocalcemia, can lead to arrhythmias, which could incite HF or cause significant morbidity in HF patients. Increased venous pressure can lead to passive congestion of the liver, resulting in elevated serum transaminases. Severe HF can lead to jaundice as a consequence of impaired hepatic function caused by congestion.

Cardiac Enzymes. Measurement of cardiac enzymes is necessary to evaluate for the presence of acute myocardial infarction as the inciting event. Elevated cardiac enzymes that do not reach levels consistent with acute myocardial infarction are seen in about half of patients with systolic HF and indicate elevated left ventricular filling pressure due to volume overload.

B-Type Natriuretic Peptide Values. One of the neurohumoral responses to the presence of a failing ventricle is release of BNP. BNP and its prohormone (pro-BNP) can be used to assist in the diagnosis of HF as a cause of acute dyspnea. Elevated levels of BNP and pro-BNP are sensitive and specific markers for the diagnosis of HF. However, BNP is not recommended as a screening test or as a method of monitoring progression of HF, as the level can be increased by advancing age, renal failure, cardiac ischemia, and pulmonary embolism and can be decreased by acute pulmonary edema, acute mitral regurgitation, and mitral stenosis.

Electrocardiographic Findings. Electrocardiographic findings in HF are variable but can help determine the cause of HF. An ECG is useful to evaluate for evidence of acute ischemia or arrhythmia as a cause of the HF and can also reveal the presence of ventricular hypertrophy, often seen in chronic hypertension. Left bundle branch block seen in the setting of HF indicates higher 1-year all-cause mortality.

Chest X-ray. Chest x-ray can help to evaluate for other causes of dyspnea, such as pneumonia, chronic obstructive pulmonary disease, pneumothorax, or lung cancer. A chest x-ray showing cardiomegaly, pulmonary venous congestion, pulmonary edema, or pleural effusion increases the likelihood of HF in a dyspneic patient. A cardiothoracic ratio greater than 50% indicates systolic dysfunction. **One of the earliest chest x-ray findings in HF is cephalization of the pulmonary vasculature** (upper lobe pulmonary vein dilation with lower lobe pulmonary vein constriction), which indicates increased preload. As the failure progresses, interstitial pulmonary edema can be seen as perihilar infiltrates, often in a butterfly pattern. Kerley lines, which are spindle-shaped linear opacities in the periphery of the lung bases, appear in later HF as well. Pleural effusions can also be found. Effusions are usually bilateral, but if they are unilateral, they are more often seen on the right hemithorax than the left.

Echocardiography. **Echocardiography is the gold standard diagnostic modality in the presence of HF.** It can evaluate left ventricular ejection fraction, ventricle size, wall thickness, ventricular filling pressures, valve function, wall motion abnormalities due to ischemic heart disease, and cardiomyopathy. It can also find pericardial effusion, pericardial constriction, or tamponade. Echocardiography is useful in identifying valvular stenosis or regurgitation, either of which can lead to HF. These findings aid in the determination of whether the HF has a preserved ejection fraction or reduced ejection fraction, critical distinctions when deciding the appropriate treatment.

Table 27–2 • CLASSIFICATION OF SEVERITY OF CONGESTIVE HEART FAILURE			
American Heart Association	New York Heart Association	Objective Assessment	Patient Symptoms
A	I	None with normal activities; no objective evidence of cardiovascular disease	No limitation of physical activity; ordinary physical activity does not cause undue fatigue, palpitation, dyspnea (shortness of breath)
B	II	Mild symptoms and slight limitation during ordinary activity; comfortable at rest; objective evidence of minimal cardiovascular disease	Slight limitation of physical activity; comfortable at rest; ordinary physical activity results in fatigue, palpitation, dyspnea
C	III	Marked limitation in activity due to symptoms, even during less-than-ordinary activity; comfortable only at rest; objective evidence of moderately severe cardiovascular disease	Marked limitation of physical activity; comfortable at rest; less than ordinary activity causes fatigue, palpitation, or dyspnea
D	IV	Severe limitations; experiences symptoms even while at rest; objective evidence of severe cardiovascular disease	Symptoms of heart failure at rest

Treatment Principles

Classification of Heart Failure. Heart failure severity is characterized by the symptoms a patient has and the degree that the symptoms limit a patient's lifestyle. There are several classification systems in use; two of the most widely used are the New York Heart Association (NYHA) and the American Heart Association (AHA) classifications. Table 27–2 summarizes these systems. The classification of HF is important in determining the appropriate treatment and prognosis for the patient.

Prevention. Prevention is the most important part of managing HF. The AHA classification system helps clinicians identify patients at risk so that preventive strategies may be implemented early. **Aggressive control of hypertension has been shown to reduce incidence of HF by up to 50%.** Treating patients who have CAD or who have had a myocardial infarction with ACEIs, ARBs, beta-blockers, and aldosterone antagonists reduces the risk of progression to symptomatic HF. Treating dyslipidemia with statin therapy can also reduce incidence of HF by 20%.

Controlling other risk factors, such as diabetes mellitus, atherosclerotic vascular disease, and thyroid disease and avoidance of cardiotoxic drugs such as tobacco, alcohol, cocaine, and amphetamines, are important for reducing risk as well. Some patients may need cardiac catheterization if CAD is thought to be a significant contributor to the development of a patient's HF. Revascularization of coronary lesions causing ischemic heart disease has been shown to improve outcomes in patients with HF.

Treatment of Acute Heart Failure

In all cases of acute decompensated HF, **the initial management imperative is the stabilization of the cardiopulmonary system.** Supplemental oxygen, initially 100% via nonrebreather face mask, should be administered. If necessary, ventilation can be assisted with continuous positive airway pressure, bilevel positive airway pressure, or mechanical ventilation. Cardiac and continuous pulse oximetry monitors should be placed and intravenous access obtained. The goals of managing an acute exacerbation of HF are to stabilize hemodynamics, treat reversible underlying conditions contributing to HF, and establish an effective regimen for outpatient therapy.

Treating Volume Overload. Ninety percent of patients admitted to the hospital with decompensated HF are volume overloaded. When volume overload caused by HF (which frequently causes acute pulmonary edema) is diagnosed, the next step in management is the administration of a loop diuretic. Furosemide is generally the treatment of choice, both for its potent diuretic effect and for its rapid bronchial vasculature vasodilation. Volume overload may also be treated acutely with vasodilators to reduce filling pressures. Nitrates, particularly nitroglycerin when given intravenously, reduce myocardial oxygen demand by reducing preload and afterload. Nitroglycerin also can rapidly reduce BP and is the treatment of choice in a patient who has HF and whose BP is elevated. It should be used with caution or avoided in a hypotensive patient.

Intravenous morphine sulfate can be an effective adjunct to therapy. Along with its analgesic and anxiolytic properties, morphine is a venodilator (primary effect) and arterial dilator, resulting in a reduction in preload and an increase in cardiac output. Patients with severely reduced ejection fraction may require short-term use of inotropic agents such as dobutamine or milrinone to improve cardiac output. Vasopressors may also be necessary for hypotension, and dopamine is the preferred agent for HF patients. Hemodialysis for fluid removal may be required in patients with concomitant end-stage renal disease.

Treatment of Chronic Heart Failure

Lifestyle Modification. Patient care management and education are important aspects of care for all patients with HF. All patients should be advised about the importance of dietary sodium and fluid restriction. A normal American diet contains 6 to 10 g of sodium chloride a day, and there is evidence to show that sodium reduction is beneficial in all classes of HF. Fluid restriction of 1.5 to 2 L/d can be considered in patients with class D HF. Patients should be warned to avoid nonsteroidal anti-inflammatory medications, as these can worsen fluid retention and reduce the efficacy of diuretics and ACEIs. Exercise training such as cardiac rehabilitation in patients with HF is associated with improved response to pharmacologic vasodilators, reduced hospitalizations, and improvement in well-being and exercise capacity.

Managing Risk Factors. The importance of strict management of BP and modification of other cardiac risk factors, especially smoking, should be emphasized as well. Sleep apnea is common in patients with systolic HF, and treatment with positive airway pressure therapies has been associated with improved ejection fraction and survival. Daily weights, with medication adjustment based on acute shifts in weight, are used by care management teams to reduce risk for emergent need for hospitalization. Interdisciplinary care management should be instituted for patients deemed at high risk for readmissions.

ACEIs and ARBs. **An ACEI or ARB should be considered first-line therapy in patients with HFrEF.** ACEIs and ARBs reduce preload and afterload, improve cardiac output without increasing heart rate, and inhibit tissue renin-angiotensin systems, which improves myocardial relaxation and compliance. The result of this is improvement in symptoms and reduction in mortality and hospitalization. ACEIs or ARBs can also delay the development of symptomatic HF in asymptomatic patients with a reduced cardiac ejection fraction (AHA stage B or NYHA class I). **Better outcomes are seen at higher doses, so patients should be maintained at the highest tolerable dose.** Consider switching from an ACEI or ARB to sacubitril (prodrug neprilysin inhibitor with valsartan) in patients with symptomatic HF, ejection fraction $\leq$ 35%, and elevated BNP, but be aware of risk for symptomatic hypotension. ACEIs and ARBs are contraindicated in pregnancy, hypotension, hyperkalemia, and bilateral renal artery stenosis and should be used with caution in patients with renal insufficiency.

Beta-Blockers. **The administration of beta-blockers, especially in high doses, in the setting of acute HF can worsen symptoms;** consequently, they should preferentially be started when patients have minimal evidence of fluid retention and few symptoms, and initial doses should be low and titrated up over several weeks. Beta-blockers reduce sympathetic tone and the cardiac muscle remodeling associated with chronic HF. In combination with ACEIs, beta-blockers improve mortality. Contraindications to beta-blocker use include symptomatic bradycardia, atrioventricular block in the absence of a pacemaker, hypotension, severe peripheral vascular disease, and severe bronchospasm.

Diuretics. **Diuretics should be used to reduce volume overload in both the acute and chronic settings.** They are most helpful in symptom management and should be used with ACEIs/ARBs and beta-blockers for long-term reduction in HF exacerbations. Loop diuretics (furosemide, bumetanide, torsemide) can be used in all stages of HF and are useful for pulmonary edema and refractory HF. These are preferred because they can increase sodium excretion by 20% to 25% and increase free water excretion. Thiazide diuretics (hydrochlorothiazide, chlorthalidone, others) only increase sodium excretion by 5% to 10%, and this effect is reduced in renal insufficiency. Their primary role in management of HF is in treatment of hypertension. Diuretic doses can be adjusted based on daily weight measurements by the patient, and patients should be monitored closely for overdiuresis.

Aldosterone Antagonists. The aldosterone antagonists, spironolactone and eplerenone improve symptoms, reduce hospitalizations, and reduce mortality in advanced HF. Elevated aldosterone levels contribute to sodium and water retention, potassium and magnesium loss, myocardial hypertrophy and fibrosis, and endothelial dysfunction. Aldosterone blockade promotes reversal of these effects. It also functions as a potassium-sparing diuretic and should be considered in NYHA class III and IV HF. Patients on this medication must be closely monitored for the development of hyperkalemia, which can become profound and lead to arrhythmia. It should be avoided in patients with renal failure.

Nondihydropyridine Calcium Channel Blockers. Nondihydropyridine calcium channel blockers (diltiazem, verapamil) increase mortality in HFrEF and should be **avoided**. The dihydropyridine calcium channel blocker amlodipine does not increase or decrease mortality, and it can be very effective in treating hypertension. Nondihydropyridine calcium channel blockers may be useful in HFpEF, as they promote increased cardiac output by lowering heart rate, which allows for more ventricular filling time.

Digoxin. Digoxin is only indicated to reduce hospital stays in patients with uncontrolled HF on appropriate medical therapy or for ventricular rate control in patients with known arrhythmias, such as atrial fibrillation. It can improve symptoms and exercise tolerance, and it can slightly improve ejection fraction and cardiac output; however, it has no mortality benefit and has a very narrow therapeutic window with significant adverse effects in overdose. Symptoms of digoxin toxicity include nausea, vomiting, headache, somnolence, altered color vision, and arrhythmias. Benefits of digoxin therapy are greatest in patients with NYHA class IV disease, cardiomegaly, and ejection fraction less than 25%.

Other Medications. The combination of hydralazine with nitrates has been shown to provide increased survival and decreased hospitalizations when used in combination with ACEIs, beta-blockers, and spironolactone in patients with HFrEF who self-identified as African American. Anticoagulation is recommended for HF patients with atrial fibrillation and/or history of cardiac thrombus or history of thromboembolic events.

Cardiac Resynchronization Therapy. Approximately one-third of patients with NYHA class III or IV HF and reduced ejection fraction have ECG evidence of abnormal ventricular conduction (ie, prolonged QRS duration), which causes ventricular dyssynchrony. This results in reductions in ventricular filling, left ventricular contractility, paradoxical septal wall motion, and worsening of mitral regurgitation. These patients can be helped by promoting synchronous contraction of both the right and left ventricles using a biventricular pacemaker. This process, also known as **cardiac resynchronization therapy**, has been shown to reduce mortality and hospitalization in patients with symptomatic HF in spite of maximal medical therapy, as well as improve quality of life, exercise capacity, and left ventricular ejection fraction.

Implantable Cardioverter-Defibrillator. Patients with an ejection fraction less than 35%, NYHA class II or III HF, and a reasonable life expectancy of at least 1 year are recommended to have an implantable cardioverter-defibrillator (ICD) placed for secondary prevention of sudden cardiac death due to ventricular arrhythmias, especially if the patient has a history of cardiac arrest, ventricular fibrillation, or unstable ventricular tachycardia.

CASE CORRELATION

- See also Case 2 (Dyspnea [Chronic Obstructive Pulmonary Disease]) and Case 20 (Chest Pain).

COMPREHENSION QUESTIONS

27.1 A 57-year-old man who has known NYHA class II HF presents to the clinic after becoming dyspneic with significant exertion. On physical examination, his BP is 140/86 mm Hg, pulse is 86 beats/min, and respiratory rate is 20 breaths/min. A 2/6 pansystolic murmur is best heard at the right sternal border. There is no JVD, but 1+ pretibial and pedal edema are noted. He currently takes an ACEI and aspirin. Which one of the following additional medications has been shown to improve longevity in this situation?

A. Warfarin (Coumadin)

B. Digoxin

C. Beta-blocker

D. Nondihydropyridine calcium channel blocker

E. Amiodarone (Cordarone)

27.2 A 52-year-old man with a 25-year history of hypertension presents with gradually increasing shortness of breath and reduced exercise tolerance with pain in his calves that causes him to stop walking after one block. His records indicate that his BPs have fluctuated over the years in the range of 140/90 to 160/105 mm Hg. His medications include enalapril and metoprolol. The physical examination reveals a BP of 140/90 mm Hg, a respiratory rate of 22 breaths/min, and a heart rate of 88 beats/min. The heart examination reveals a normal S_1 and S_2 and no murmurs. Lung examination shows bibasilar rales. There is trace pitting edema bilaterally. Posterior tibial and dorsalis pedis pulses are 1+. Which of the following diagnostic tests is most likely to confirm the diagnosis in this patient?

A. Cardiac magnetic resonance imaging (MRI)

B. 24-hour Holter monitoring

C. Spiral computed tomography (CT) of the chest

D. Two-dimensional echocardiography with Doppler

E. Posteroanterior and lateral chest radiographs

27.3 A 64-year-old man is noted to have HF because of CAD. Over the past 2 days, he has developed progressive dyspnea and orthopnea. On examination, he is found to be in moderate respiratory distress and have JVD, and he has rales on pulmonary examination. He is diagnosed with pulmonary edema. Which of the following agents is most appropriate at this time?

A. Hydrochlorothiazide

B. Furosemide

C. Carvedilol

D. Spironolactone

E. Digitalis

27.4 A 70-year-old African American man with a history of HF sees you in the office for follow-up. He has shortness of breath with minimal exertion such as walking 20 feet on level ground. The patient states he is adherent to his medication regimen, which consists of lisinopril 40 mg twice daily, carvedilol 25 mg twice daily, furosemide 80 mg daily, and spironolactone 25 mg daily. His BP is 100/60 mm Hg, and his pulse rate is 70 beats/min and regular. Lung examination findings reveal a few scattered bibasilar rales. Cardiac examination shows a normal S_1 and S_2 and an S_3 gallop. There is no peripheral edema. An ECG reveals a left bundle branch block, and echocardiography reveals an ejection fraction of 25%. Which of the following is the best next step in the management of this patient?

A. Increase the furosemide dosage to 80 mg twice daily.

B. Refer for coronary angiography.

C. Increase the lisinopril dosage to 80 mg twice daily.

D. Increase the carvedilol dosage to 50 mg twice daily.

E. Refer for cardiac resynchronization therapy.

ANSWERS

27.1 **C.** Beta-blockers are recommended to reduce mortality in symptomatic patients with HF. Digoxin (answer B) is only recommended in patients who are already on maximal medical therapy. Nondihydropyridine calcium channel blockers (answer D) should be used with caution in patients with HF because they can cause peripheral vasodilation, decreased heart rate, decreased cardiac contractility, and decreased cardiac conduction. Anticoagulation with warfarin (answer A) is not indicated, and amiodarone (answer E) is used for treatment of arrhythmias.

27.2 **D.** The most useful diagnostic tool for evaluating patients with HF is two-dimensional echocardiography with Doppler to assess left ventricular ejection fraction, left ventricular size, ventricular compliance, wall thickness, and valve function. It should be performed during the initial evaluation. Chest radiography (answer E) and 12-lead ECG should be performed in all patients

presenting with HF but should not be used as the primary basis for determining which abnormalities are responsible for the HF. Answer A (cardiac
MRI) is much more costly and not considered the first-line measure for the
evaluation of HF. Answer B (24-hour Holter monitoring) is appropriate for
symptoms of arrhythmias or palpitations. Answer C (spiral CT of the chest)
is useful for assessing for possible pulmonary embolism.

27.3 **B.** Furosemide, a loop diuretic, is a first-line agent in HF exacerbation with
pulmonary edema. The other medications listed (answer A, hydrochlorothiazide; answer C, carvedilol; answer D, spironolactone; and answer E, digitalis)
may be used in the management of HF but are not indicated in an acute
exacerbation.

27.4 **E.** This patient is already receiving maximal medical therapy; therefore, the
answer choices A (increase furosemide), C (increase lisinopril), and D
(increase carvedilol) are incorrect. Cardiac resynchronization therapy (which
utilizes a pacemaker to produce a more efficient cardiac output) is recommended for patients in sinus rhythm, particularly efficacious with left bundle
branch block with an EF < 35%, QRS >120 ms, and those who remain symptomatic (NYHA III–IV) despite optimal medical therapy.

CLINICAL PEARLS

▶ Compliance with diet and medications is a fundamental part of the treatment plan of HF patients.

▶ Angiotensin-converting enzyme inhibitors and aldosterone inhibitors
have been shown to improve survival in HF patients by decreasing cardiac remodeling, whereas other agents, such as digoxin and loop diuretics, may help with symptoms but not survival.

▶ Beta-blockers can also help in slowing HF disease progression and
improve survival but should be used cautiously in those with significantly
reduced EF.

▶ The initial hour in the management of a patient with either new-onset HF
or an acute exacerbation is crucial to the patient's outcome.

▶ The most common cause of HF is coronary heart disease.

▶ Simple measures, such as decreasing cardiac preload by sitting the
patient up with their legs on the ground and their arms by their side,
maintaining an airway and giving oxygen, and giving sublingual nitroglycerin, can alleviate HF immediately.

▶ Interdisciplinary care management helps in the care of HF patients and
leads to improved outcomes and better survival.

REFERENCES

Inamdar AA, Inamdar AC. Heart failure: diagnosis, management and utilization. *J Clin Med*. 2016;5(7):62.

King M, Perez O. Heart failure. In: South-Paul JE, Matheny SC, Lewis EL, eds. *CURRENT Diagnosis & Treatment: Family Medicine*. 4th ed. New York, NY: McGraw Hill; 2015. https://accessmedicine-mhmedical-com.evms.idm.oclc.org/content.aspx?bookid=1415&sectionid=77056309

Mann DL, Chakinala M. Heart failure: pathophysiology and diagnosis. In: Kasper D, Fauci A, Hauser S, Longo D, Jameson J, Loscalzo J, eds. *Harrison's Principles of Internal Medicine*. 20th ed. New York, NY: McGraw Hill; 2018: Chap. 279. http://accessmedicine.mhmedical.com/content.aspx?bookid=1130&Sectionid=79742466

Mehra MR. Heart failure: management. In: Kasper D, Fauci A, Hauser S, Longo D, Jameson J, Loscalzo J, eds. *Harrison's Principles of Internal Medicine*. 20 ed. New York, NY: McGraw Hill; 2018: Chap. 280. http://accessmedicine.mhmedical.com/content.aspx?bookid=1130&Sectionid=79742558

Metra M, JR Teerlink. Heart failure. *Seminar*. 2017;390(10106):1981-1995.

Quesada O, Klein L. Heart failure with reduced ejection fraction. In: Crawford MH, ed. *Current Diagnosis & Treatment: Cardiology*. 5th ed. New York, NY: McGraw Hill; 2017: Chap. 27. http://accessmedicine.mhmedical.com.evms.idm.oclc.org/content.aspx?bookid=715&Sectionid=48214560

Yancy CW, Jessup M, Bozkurt B, et al. 2013 ACCF/AHA guideline for the management of heart failure: a report of the American College of Cardiology Foundation/American Heart Association Task Force on Practice Guidelines. *Circulation*. 2013;128(16):e240.

A 30-year-old woman who is a para 3 (P3), divorced executive presents to your clinic for contraceptive advice. She has been in a monogamous relationship with her boyfriend for several months. She denies any drug allergies. She occasionally drinks alcohol and does not smoke. She mentions that she used to take birth control pills without any problems. All three of her children were born via vaginal delivery without complication. She and her partner are free of sexually transmitted infections (STIs) based on their recent checkups. She said that her life is very busy because of work, so she would like something that "she doesn't have to think about" using. She fears any form of surgery and has not excluded having another child. Her only significant medical history is an occasional migraine headache with aura. Her laboratory workup is normal. Her physical examination is normal. She is looking for the "best contraceptive method" for her situation.

▶ What contraceptive options are available to this woman?
▶ What option would be contraindicated because of the history of migraines with aura?

ANSWERS TO CASE 28:
Family Planning—Contraceptives

Summary: A 30-year-old woman presents with

- Parity 3 history
- A current monogamous relationship
- No history of STIs in herself or in her partner
- History of taking birth control pills
- Questions about her contraceptive options
- Dissatisfaction with barrier options
- Statement that she is not ready for permanent sterilization
- Migraine with aura

Available contraceptive options: This patient has a contraindication to estrogen due to migraine with aura, and she prefers something she doesn't have to think about to fit her busy lifestyle. This makes her a good candidate for a long-acting reversible contraception (LARC), such as a progestin implant or intrauterine device (IUD), which have the highest contraceptive success.

Contraindicated contraceptive options for someone with migraine with aura: Combined estrogen/progesterone contraceptives, which can be found as pills, patches, or vaginal rings, are relatively contraindicated in those with migraine headaches due to the increased risk of ischemic stroke. This especially applies to those with migraine headaches with aura (neurological deficits). These are also contraindicated for women with a history of blood clots or uncontrolled hypertension or who are over age 35 and smoke.

ANALYSIS

Objectives

1. Be able to talk about the available methods of contraception. (EPA 4, 12)

2. Be able to discuss contraindications for and side effects of contraceptives. (EPA 4)

Considerations

Choosing a method of contraception is a personal decision based on individual preferences, medical history, and lifestyle. In the United States, approximately 50% of pregnancies are unintended, and approximately 25% of women will have had an abortion by age 45. Eighty percent of women having unprotected sex will become pregnant within a year. All methods of contraception have a number of risks and benefits of which the patient should be aware. The methods also all have a failure rate, defined as inability to prevent pregnancy over a 1-year period. Sometimes, the failure rate is a result of the method or drug interactions, and sometimes it is a result of human error. Each method has possible side effects. Some methods require lifestyle modifications. Patients with certain medical conditions cannot use certain types of contraceptives.

There are numerous contraceptive options available, and recommendations regarding contraceptive use must be individualized. In the case given, there are several important factors that must be considered. Given the patient's fear of surgery and because she is not certain whether she wants to have more children in the future, surgical sterilization via bilateral tubal ligation or hysteroscopic tubal occlusion or division is not a choice. A vasectomy for the partner, although potentially reversible, should be considered permanent sterilization and is not ideal for this patient. Barrier methods could be a viable option, but the patient may feel that these are an inconvenience to her busy lifestyle. Given that both the patient and her boyfriend have no history of STIs and are in a long-term relationship, appropriate methods of contraception for them include LARCs, such as IUDs or progestin implants. IUDs can last 3, 5, or 10 years before replacement, depending on the type used, and implants can last 3 years. LARCs have a very low failure rate and, after insertion, do not require active patient effort for contraceptive success.

APPROACH TO:
Family Planning—Contraceptives

DEFINITIONS

BARRIER CONTRACEPTIVE: Contraceptive method that prevents sperm from entering the upper female reproductive tract.

HORMONAL CONTRACEPTION: Estrogen plus progestin or progestin alone to provide contraception in various methods, including pills, patches, vaginal rings, injections, and implants.

INTRAUTERINE CONTRACEPTIVE DEVICE: Small, T-shaped device placed in the endometrial cavity as a method of long-term contraception.

PERFECT USE EFFECTIVENESS: Efficacy of a method in perfect conditions, when consistent and reliable use occurs.

TYPICAL USE EFFECTIVENESS: Efficacy of a method as it is actually used, when forgetfulness and improper use can occur.

CLINICAL APPROACH

Choosing which contraception agent is best for a patient can be complex. Review of the patient's individual situation, medical problems, and ability to remember to take medication each day are important factors to consider. Table 28–1 summarizes some of the characteristics of various contraceptive agents.

Table 28-1 • CONTRACEPTION AGENTS COMPARED, INCLUDING BEST-SUITED PATIENTS

Category/Agents	Mechanism	Best Suited for	Disadvantages/ Contraindications
Barrier • Diaphragm • Cervical caps • Condoms (male and female)	Mechanical obstruction to sperm	Avoidance of hormones **Decrease risk of STI (condoms)**	Pelvic organ prolapse Patient discomfort with placing devices on genitals Lack of spontaneity Allergies to material Diaphragm may be associated with more UTIs
Combined hormonal (estrogen and progestin) • Combined oral contraceptives • Contraceptive patch • Vaginal ring	Inhibit ovulation Thicken cervical mucus to inhibit sperm penetration Alters tubal transport Thins endometrium	Iron-deficiency anemia Dysmenorrhea Ovarian cysts Endometriosis **OCP**—take pill each day **Patch**—less to remember but may cause more nausea **Ring**—less to remember but may cause vaginal irritation and discharge	Known thrombogenic mutations Active or history of thromboembolic disease Cerebrovascular or coronary artery disease (current or remote) Cigarette smoking (especially over age 35) Uncontrolled hypertension Diabetic retinopathy or nephropathy Peripheral vascular disease Breast or endometrial cancer Unexplained uterine bleeding Migraines with aura Liver tumors (benign or malignant), active liver disease Known or suspected pregnancy Application site reaction (for patches)
Progestin-only oral • Micronor and others	Thickens cervical mucus to inhibit sperm penetration Alters tubal transport Thins endometrium	**Breastfeeding**	Patient needs to remember to take pill at the same time each day

(Continued)

Category/Agents	Mechanism	Best Suited for	Disadvantages/ Contraindications
Table 28–1 • CONTRACEPTION AGENTS COMPARED, INCLUDING BEST-SUITED PATIENTS (continued)			
Injectables • Depo-medroxyprogesterone acetate (Depo-Provera and others)	Inhibits ovulation Thins endometrium Alters cervical mucus to inhibit sperm penetration	Breastfeeding Desire for long-term contraception Iron-deficiency anemia Sickle cell disease Epilepsy Dysmenorrhea Ovarian cysts Endometriosis	Depression Osteopenia/osteoporosis—partially reversible with cessation Appetite stimulation leading to weight gain Unexplained uterine bleeding Breast cancer Active or history of thromboembolic disease Cerebrovascular disease Liver tumors (benign or malignant), active liver disease Known or suspected pregnancy
Implants (subdermal in arm) • Etonogestrel (Implanon, Nexplanon)	Inhibits ovulation Thins endometrium Thickens cervical mucus to inhibit sperm penetration	Breastfeeding Desires long-term, reversible contraception (3 years) Iron-deficiency anemia Dysmenorrhea Ovarian cysts Endometriosis	Active or history of thromboembolic disease (relative contraindication) Liver tumors (benign or malignant), active liver disease Unexplained uterine bleeding Breast cancer Hypersensitivity to any of the components of Etonogestrel implant May lead to irregular vaginal bleeding
IUD • Levonorgestrel secreting (Mirena and others)	Thickens cervical mucus Thins endometrium	Desires long-term, reversible contraception (3 or 5 years) Stable, mutually monogamous relationship Menorrhagia Dysmenorrhea (Note: decreased bleeding)	Current STI or recent PID Unexplained uterine bleeding Untreated cervical or endometrial cancer Breast cancer Anatomic abnormalities or uterine fibroids distorting the uterine cavity

(Continued)

Table 28–1 • CONTRACEPTION AGENTS COMPARED, INCLUDING BEST-SUITED PATIENTS (continued)

Category/Agents	Mechanism	Best Suited for	Disadvantages/ Contraindications
• Copper-T (Paragard)	Inhibits sperm migration and viability Changes transport speed of ovum Damages ovum	Desires long-term, reversible contraception (10 years) Stable, mutually monogamous relationship Contraindication to contraceptive hormones	Current STI Current PID or PID within the past 2 months Unexplained uterine bleeding Malignant gestational trophoblastic disease Untreated cervical or endometrial cancer Breast cancer Anatomic abnormalities or uterine fibroids distorting the uterine cavity Wilson disease May cause more bleeding or dysmenorrhea
Permanent sterilization • Bilateral tubal ligation Vasectomy	Mechanical obstruction of tubes Disruption of vas deferens	Does not desire more children	Contraindications to procedure or surgery May want children in the future

Abbreviations: OCP, oral contraceptive pill; PID, pelvic inflammatory disease; STI, sexually transmitted infection; UTI, urinary tract infection.

Fertility Awareness and Other Methods

Fertility awareness (natural family planning or rhythm method) entails abstinence during the woman's fertile period or using a barrier method during this time period. Fertility awareness has a failure rate of up to 25% with typical use and 3% to 5% with perfect use. Women with irregular cycles have the highest failure rates. This method is dependent on the ability to identify the approximately 10 days in each menstrual cycle that a woman is fertile, which can be accomplished using calendar calculation, basal body temperature charting, cervical mucus monitoring, or the symptothermal method.

Calendar Calculation. The calendar calculation uses the length of past reproductive cycles to predict fertile periods. The beginning of the fertile period is calculated by subtracting 18 days from the shortest of the previous 6 to 12 cycles. The end of the fertile period is calculated by subtracting 11 days from the longest cycle. For a consistent 28-day cycle, the fertile period would occur from days 10 through 17.

Basal Body Temperature. The basal body temperature method is based on the knowledge that a woman's basal temperature increases during the luteal phase of the reproductive cycle. Temperature must be recorded early in the morning at the same time each day. An increase of 0.4 °F from baseline indicates that ovulation has occurred. For this method to be most effective, a woman must either avoid intercourse or use barrier methods from the first day of menses to the third day after the temperature increase.

Cervical Mucus Method. The cervical mucus method, also called the Billings ovulation method, depends on a woman recognizing the changes in cervical mucus that indicate ovulation is occurring or has occurred. The symptothermal method combines all three: calendar, basal body temperature, and cervical mucus methods.

Other Methods. Other methods include coitus interruptus, also known as the withdrawal method; postcoital douching; and lactational amenorrhea. Coitus interruptus involves withdrawing the penis before ejaculation and has a 27% typical use failure rate. Postcoital douching is used to flush semen out of the vagina, but sperm have been found within cervical mucus within 90 seconds of ejaculation, so this method is unreliable. Lactational amenorrhea occurs with suppression of ovulation due to breastfeeding. During the first 6 months following delivery, women who are exclusively breastfeeding have mostly anovulatory menstrual cycles, and pregnancy rates have been found to be approximately 1%.

Barrier Methods

Barrier contraceptive methods include the male condom, female condom, diaphragm, cervical cap, sponge, and spermicides. The diaphragm, cervical cap, sponge, and spermicides are falling out of favor due to high contraception failure rates with typical use and limited protection against STIs. Barrier methods work by keeping the sperm and egg apart. The main possible side effect is an allergic reaction either to the material of the barrier or to the spermicides that should be used with them.

Condoms. Condoms on the market are made of latex rubber, polyurethane, or sheep intestine. Of these types, **only latex and polyurethane condoms are effective in preventing STIs by providing a good barrier to viruses and bacteria.** Polyurethane condoms have a higher rate of breaking or slipping than latex, and thus higher failure rates, but they can be used by patients with a latex allergy. Each condom can only be used once. Condoms have a typical use failure rate of approximately 15%, with most of the failures the result of improper use. Perfect use failure rate is about 2%. For maximal efficacy, a condom must be used with every coital act, it should be in place before contact of the penis with the vagina, withdrawal must occur with the penis still erect, the base of the condom must be held during withdrawal, and an intravaginal spermicide or a condom lubricated with spermicide should be employed. Only water-based lubricants should be used with latex condoms, as oil-based lubricants reduce efficacy.

The female condom consists of a lubricated polyurethane sheath with a flexible polyurethane ring on each end. One ring is inserted into the vagina while the other remains outside, partially covering the labia. The female condom may offer some protection against STIs but is not as effective as the male latex condom due to increased user error. The estimated typical use failure rate is estimated at 21% and perfect use at 5%.

Oral Contraception

Oral contraception is a form of hormonal contraception that temporarily impacts fertility and has the potential for rare but serious side effects. When starting an oral contraceptive pill (OCP), ideally a patient should take the first pill on the first day of the start of menses. Women may choose to start on the Sunday after the start of their menses for convenience. A quick-start method has also been proposed, in which patients start taking the pills as soon as they obtain the prescription (if pregnancy is unlikely), which improves compliance. Both Sunday-start and quick-start methods require an additional backup method to be used for the first week. Per the Centers for Disease Control and Prevention, estrogen-containing OCPs should not be started until 3 weeks following delivery and 6 weeks if at increased risk for thromboembolism. Progestin-only pills (POPs) can be started immediately postpartum. Estrogen-containing OCPs should be avoided in breastfeeding mothers until 6 months postpartum. OCPs can be started the day after an induced or spontaneous abortion.

Efficacy. When properly used, hormonal methods are extremely effective. OCPs include both combination pills, which contain both estrogen and a progestin (a natural or synthetic progesterone), and POPs (commonly known as the "minipill"). When taken as directed, the failure rate for the POP is 1% to 3%; the failure rate of the combination pill is 1% to 2%. Typical use of OCPs has a failure rate of 8% to 10%. The effectiveness of OCPs may be reduced by a few other medications, including some antibiotics, barbiturates, antiepileptics, and antifungal medications.

Combination Pills. Combination pills are the most commonly used contraceptive method. The combination pill suppresses ovulation through inhibition of the hypothalamic-pituitary-ovarian axis, alteration of the cervical mucus, retarding sperm entry, and discouraging ovum implantation by creating an unfavorable endometrium. **Combination OCPs offer significant protection against ovarian cancer, endometrial cancer, iron-deficiency anemia from menstrual blood loss, pelvic inflammatory disease (PID), and fibrocystic breast disease.** Women who take combination pills have a lower risk of functional ovarian cysts.

Progestin-Only Pills. The POP reduces cervical mucus and causes it to thicken. The mucus thickening prevents the sperm from reaching the egg and keeps the uterine lining from thickening, which prevents a fertilized egg from implanting in the uterus. The POP is ideal for breastfeeding mothers because it does not interfere with milk production, which combined OCPs can do.

Contraindications. Women over the age of 35 who smoke cigarettes and women with certain medical conditions should not take the combined OCP. Table 28–2 lists the absolute and relative contraindications to taking the combined OCPs. Minor side effects, which usually subside after a few months of usage, include nausea, headaches, breast swelling, fluid retention, weight gain, irregular bleeding, and depression.

Table 28–2 • CONTRAINDICATIONS TO COMBINED HORMONAL CONTRACEPTION	
Absolute Contraindications	Relative Contraindications
Previous thromboembolic event	Severe vascular headache (classic migraine, cluster)
Cerebral vascular disease	Severe hypertension (if younger than 35-40 years and in good medical control, can elect OCP)
Coronary occlusion	Diabetes mellitus (prevention of pregnancy outweighs the risk of complicating vascular disease in a diabetic who is younger than 35-40 years)
Impaired liver function	Gallbladder disease (may exacerbate emergence of symptoms when gallstones are present)
Known or suspected breast cancer	Obstructive jaundice in pregnancy
Smokers (> 15 cigarettes/day) older than 35 years	Epilepsy (antiepileptic drugs may decrease effectiveness of OCPs)
Congenital hyperlipidemia	Morbid obesity

Other Hormonal Contraception Methods

Transdermal Contraceptive. A transdermal contraceptive patch (Ortho Evra and others) is a combined hormone patch containing norelgestromin and ethinyl estradiol. The treatment regimen for each cycle is three consecutive 7-day patches followed by one patch-free week, so that withdrawal bleeding can occur. It can be started in a similar fashion to combined OCPs. If the Sunday-start or quick-start methods are used, a backup method of contraception is needed for 7 days. The patch may be placed on the buttocks, lower abdomen, upper outer arm, and upper torso, except for the breasts. If a patch becomes detached, it should be replaced as soon as possible. If the patch is detached for more than 24 hours, it should be replaced and a backup method of contraception used for the next 7 days. **The patch's efficacy and side effects are comparable to that of combined OCPs,** although there may be an increased risk of vascular thrombosis with use of the patch. Women who weigh more than 90 kg may be at increased risk of pregnancy with patch use.

Intravaginal Ring Contraceptive. The etonogestrel/ethinyl estradiol vaginal ring (Amneal, NuvaRing) is a flexible, transparent ring about 5 cm in diameter that delivers etonogestrel and ethinyl estradiol. **A woman inserts the etonogestrel/ethinyl estradiol vaginal ring herself, wears it for 3 weeks, then removes and discards the device.** After one ring-free week, during which withdrawal bleeding occurs, a new ring is inserted. It does not need to be fitted by a health professional and does not need to be removed during intercourse. If a patient or her partner experiences problems with the ring during intercourse, it may be removed, but it should be replaced within 3 hours. If it is out for more than 3 hours, ovulation may occur. The manufacturer recommends using backup birth control for the first 7 days after placement if not switching from another hormonal contraceptive. Rarely, the etonogestrel/ethinyl estradiol vaginal ring can slip out of the vagina, and it is recommended to check the position of the ring before and after intercourse. The efficacy and side effects of etonogestrel/ethinyl estradiol vaginal ring are similar to those of combined OCPs, although vaginitis, discomfort, and foreign body sensation are also commonly reported.

Medroxyprogesterone Injection. Medroxyprogesterone acetate (Depo-Provera, depo-subQ provera 104) is an injectable form of a progestin. Medroxyprogesterone acetate has a failure rate of only 0.3% with perfect use and 3% with typical use. **Each injection provides contraceptive protection for 13 weeks, but it can last for up to 4 months.** It is injected every 3 months (90 days) into the gluteus or deltoid muscle. The first dose should be given within 5 days of the onset of menses, so that no backup contraception is needed. Its side effects include irregular menses, weight gain, acne, reversible bone loss, and injection site reactions. Irregular bleeding and spotting are more significant during the first few months and then are followed by periods of amenorrhea. About half of women develop amenorrhea after a year of medroxyprogesterone acetate use. **There may be a prolonged period of time prior to the return of fertility after discontinuing medroxyprogesterone acetate injections, up to 18 months in a small proportion of women.**

Contraceptive Subdermal Implant. The contraceptive etonorgestrel subdermal implant (Nexplanon) is inserted subdermally in an in-office minor surgical procedure and may be removed with another minor procedure. Placement should be timed during the menstrual cycle or during the hormone-free week if using a combined hormonal contraceptive method. The implant contains the progestin etonorgestrel and is effective for 3 years. At the end of 3 years, when the device is removed, a new device may be placed in the same site. The failure rate is less than 1% for women who weigh less than 70 kg. The potential side effects of the implant include irregular menstrual bleeding, which is the most common reason for discontinuation; headaches; depression; acne; breast tenderness; abdominal pain; and weight gain.

Intrauterine Devices

The IUDs are small, plastic, flexible devices that are inserted into the uterus through the cervix by a trained clinician. Several IUDs are presently marketed in the United States:

- Cooper T IUD (ParaGard T380A) is a T-shaped plastic device partially covered by copper that is effective for 10 years.

- Levonorgestrel IUD (Mirena) is also a T-shaped plastic device, but it contains levonorgestrel (a progestin) released over a 5-year period. Smaller levonorgestrel IUDs (Skyla and Kyleen) are designed for the nulliparous uterus and release slightly less levonorgestrel. They last for 3 and 5 years, respectively.

Efficacy. All IUDs are very effective: The copper-T IUD has a 0.6% to 0.8% failure rate, and the levonorgestrel IUDs have failure rates of 0.2% to 0.9%. An IUD alters the uterine and tubal fluids, particularly in the case of copper-bearing IUDs, inhibiting the transport of sperm through the cervical mucus and uterus. Progesterone-containing IUDs also thin the uterine lining. Timing of placement should occur during the menstrual cycle due to ease of insertion and greater certainty that the patient is not pregnant.

Contraindications. Manufacturer contraindications for IUDs include current or suspected pregnancy; current or recent acute PID or mucopurulent cervicitis; postpartum endometritis or infected abortion in the past 3 months; anatomically distorted uterine cavity; known or suspected uterine or cervical malignancy; or unexplained uterine bleeding. The copper IUD is contraindicated in Wilson disease. Levonorgestrel IUDs are contraindicated in acute liver disease or with liver tumors, breast cancer, and prior ectopic pregnancy. A history of STIs is not a contraindication to IUD placement, but if a woman has a known STI, it is recommended to delay insertion for 3 months following resolution of the infection.

Side Effects. Side effects of IUDs include irregular bleeding patterns during the first few months of use, headache, nausea, hair loss, acne, depression, decreased libido, ovarian cysts, and mastalgia. Many patients will become amenorrheic or oligomenorrheic with a levonorgestrel IUD in place, so it can be used to treat patients with menorrhagia. The copper IUD may actually cause heavy, irregular bleeding. Women may also experience some short-term side effects, such as cramping and dizziness (due to stimulation of the vagal nerve) at the time of insertion; bleeding, cramps, and backache may continue for a few days after the insertion.

Complications. Complications include expulsion, perforation of the uterus, and ectopic pregnancy. Approximately 5% of women expel their IUD within the first year. The patient should check that the strings are palpable once a month, and if she cannot find the strings, she should see a health care provider. The absolute rate of ectopic pregnancy is reduced with the IUD because of its high contraceptive efficacy. However, when accidental pregnancy does occur, there is increased likelihood of ectopic pregnancy.

Surgical Sterilization

Tubal ligation seals a woman's fallopian tubes so that an egg cannot travel to the uterus. Vasectomy involves closing off a man's vas deferens so that sperm will not be carried to the penis. Vasectomy is a minor surgical procedure, most often performed in a doctor's office under local anesthesia. Tubal ligation is an operating room procedure performed under general anesthesia. Major complications, which are rare in female sterilization, include infection, hemorrhage, and problems associated with the use of general anesthesia. The failure rate is less than 1%. Although there has been some success in reopening the fallopian tubes or the vas deferens, the success rate is low, and **sterilization should be considered irreversible.**

Emergency Contraception

All female patients of reproductive age should be made aware of postcoital contraception, some types of which are available over the counter. It is well documented that knowledge of emergency contraception does not increase the likelihood of high-risk sexual behavior.

Hormonal methods of emergency contraception prevent release of oocytes but do not affect eggs that have already been fertilized or that are already released into the tube. The Yuzpe method consists of taking high-dose combined OCPs for emergency contraception and can decrease the risk of pregnancy by about 75%. **This method can be used up to 5 days after unprotected intercourse but is most effective when used within 72 hours.** Consider prescribing an antiemetic to be used 1 hour before each dose, as nausea and vomiting are common side effects.

Progestin-only emergency contraception is available without a prescription. One or two oral doses of levonorgestrel (Plan B) 0.75 mg, with 12 hours between doses, are more effective than the Yuzpe method, are better tolerated, and work best within 72 hours of intercourse. Preven, a convenient emergency contraception kit, includes two doses of medication and a pregnancy test.

A single dose of mifepristone (RU-486), a progesterone antagonist, is the most effective emergency contraceptive and has few side effects. A selective progesterone receptor modulator, known as ullipristal acetate (Ella), is taken in a single dose up to 5 days after unprotected intercourse. Placing a copper-containing IUD within 5 days after unprotected sex is the most effective form of emergency contraception and also provides another 10 years of birth control. In the setting of emergency contraception, the copper IUD likely works by preventing implantation. Copper IUDs should be avoided in those at significant risk for STIs or ectopic pregnancy or if long-term contraception is not desired.

> ## CASE CORRELATION
> - See also Case 16 (Male Genitourinary Conditions), Case 22 (Vaginitis and Other Vaginal Infections), and Case 26 (Postpartum Care).

COMPREHENSION QUESTIONS

28.1 While working in the clinic of the county jail you see a gravida 5, para 2032 (G5P2032) for a well-woman examination. She openly tells you that she was arrested for a history of prostitution. On arrest, she was found to be HIV positive. She is to be released next week and would like contraception. Which of the following agents is most appropriate for this patient?

   A. Oral contraceptive agent

   B. Depot medroxyprogesterone

   C. Intrauterine contraceptive device

   D. Condoms

28.2 An 18-year-old woman reported having intercourse with her boyfriend 20 hours ago. She was concerned because the condom broke. She used no other form of contraception. The patient reported a history since age 14 of regular periods of heavy flow that usually last for longer than 7 days. Her body mass index (BMI) is 25 kg/m². She plays as a forward on her high school basketball team and is worried about becoming pregnant. Which of the following is the most appropriate method of "emergency contraception"?

    A. Yuzpe method

    B. Plan B method

    C. Insertion of a copper IUD

    D. Intramuscular methotrexate

28.3 A 16-year-old young woman presents to your clinic for a wellness check. She has been having regular periods for over 2 years, does not drink or smoke, gets straight. As on her report cards, and is in the 75th percentile for height and weight. She is Tanner stage 5 for both breast and pubic hair development. During your interview, she reveals that she is sexually active and not using contraception. If she continues to have unprotected intercourse, what is the likelihood that she will become pregnant over the course of the next year?

    A. 20%

    B. 40%

    C. 80%

    D. 100%

28.4 A 36-year-old woman is seeking contraception. She delivered her baby 8 weeks ago and is breastfeeding. She undergoes a history and physical examination and is counseled regarding the various options. She is healthy, drinks an occasional glass of wine per month, does not smoke, and plans to have another child in a year or two. Her blood pressure is 114/70 mm Hg. The patient would like to initiate birth control at this visit. Which method is the most appropriate in her case?

    A. Laparoscopic sterilization

    B. Natural family planning

    C. The minipill

    D. Combination oral contraception pills

    E. Coitus interruptus

28.5 Which one of the following is an absolute contraindication to combined oral contraceptives in a 40-year-old woman?

    A. Obesity (BMI 32 kg/m²)

    B. Smoking 1 pack of cigarettes/day

    C. Sickle cell disease

    D. A family history of ovarian cancer

    E. Varicose veins

ANSWERS

28.1 **D.** Protection from STIs for this patient and prevention from transmitting HIV to her future partners are of utmost concern. Condoms are the most effective agents to prevent the transmission of an STI. A history of STIs is not an absolute contraindication for IUD use, but with this patient's history of high-risk behavior, IUDs (answer C) probably should be avoided. The patient should be counseled extensively on the need to protect sex partners from contracting HIV, but other forms of contraception should not be withheld given the benefits of preventing unwanted pregnancy and vertical transmission. The provider should also be on the alert that this patient may be a victim of sex trafficking and use a nonjudgmental and supportive manner in querying. Use of nonbarrier contraception (answer A, oral contraceptive agent, and answer B, depot medroxyprogesterone) is unlikely to increase the patient's high-risk sexual behaviors, and reliable birth control will have a positive impact on her life.

28.2 **B.** Emergency contraception may include combination hormonal therapy, ideally used within 72 hours, but it can cause significant nausea and vomiting. Plan B is levonorgestrel and is more effective than the combined OCPs (such as Yuzpe method, answer A) for postcoital contraception without the prominent side effect of nausea. Placing a copper IUD (answer C) can cause heavy and irregular vaginal bleeding and would not be a good choice for a patient who already experiences these symptoms. Intramuscular methotrexate (answer D) is not used for emergency contraception.

28.3 **C.** Eighty percent of women having unprotected intercourse will be pregnant in 1 year. The other percentages (answer A, 20%; answer B, 40%; answer D, 100%) are not correct.

28.4 **C.** The POP minipill is the most effective form of birth control in the postpartum period for women desiring to breastfeed. Natural family planning (answer B) and coitus interruptus (withdrawal method, answer E) have high rates of user error, leading to failure. Laparoscopic tubal ligation (answer A) is a permanent method of birth control. Combination OCPs (answer D) can affect a woman's milk supply and have varying safety in lactation.

28.5 **B.** In a woman 35 years or older, cigarette use poses an unacceptable risk with combined oral contraceptives. Women with nonmorbid obesity (answer A) are at greater risk for deep vein thrombosis, but the advantages of oral contraceptives often outweigh the disadvantages in these patients. A BMI of 35 kg/m² or greater is a relative contraindication. A patient with sickle cell disease (answer C) is at a higher risk of adverse events from an unintended pregnancy than from the use of combined oral contraceptives. Combined oral contraceptives lower the risk of ovarian cancer (answer D). Patients with varicose veins (answer E) are not at increased risk for deep vein thrombosis.

CLINICAL PEARLS

▶ The male latex condom remains the best shield against HIV and other STIs.

▶ Barrier methods, which work by keeping the sperm and egg apart, usually have only minor side effects.

▶ Combination oral contraceptives offer protection against ovarian cancer, endometrial cancer, anemia due to blood loss, PID, and fibrocystic breast disease.

▶ To reduce barriers to providing oral hormonal contraception, it is recommended that pelvic examination not be required and a year's worth of prescription be provided.

▶ Noncontraceptive benefits of combination oral contraceptives include decreased incidence of benign breast disease, relief from menstrual disorders (dysmenorrhea and menorrhagia), reduced risk of uterine leiomyomata, protection against ovarian cysts, reduction of acne, improvement of bone mineral density, and a reduced risk of colorectal cancer.

▶ Intrauterine and implantable contraceptives are also extremely effective and reduce the contribution of user error to the failure rate.

▶ Surgical sterilization must be considered permanent. Vasectomy is considered safer than tubal ligation.

REFERENCES

Barrows-nees E, Landy K. Hormonal contraceptives in women who are overweight or obese. *Am Fam Physician.* 2017;95(11):732.

Brunsell SC. Contraception. In: South-Paul JE, Matheny SC, Lewis EL, eds. *CURRENT Diagnosis & Treatment: Family Medicine.* 4th ed. New York, NY: McGraw Hill; 2015. http://accessmedicine.mhmedical.com.evms.idm.oclc.org/content.aspx?bookid=1415&sectionid=77056012. Accessed May 9, 2020.

Burkman RT, Brzezinski A. Contraception & Family Planning. In: DeCherney AH, Nathan L, Laufer N, Roman AS, eds. *CURRENT Diagnosis & Treatment: Obstetrics & Gynecology,* 12th ed. New York, NY: McGraw Hill; Chapter 60. http://accessmedicine.mhmedical.com.evms.idm.oclc.org/content.aspx?bookid=2559&sectionid=206968141. Accessed May 9, 2020.

Hardeman J, Weiss BD. Intrauterine devices: an update. *Am Fam Physician.* 2014;89(6):445-450.

Klein DA, Arnold JJ, Reese ES. Provision of contraception: key recommendations from the CDC. *Am Fam Physician.* 2015;91(9):625-633.

Lesnewski R, Prine L. Initiating hormonal contraception. *Am Fam Physician.* 2006;74(1):105-112.

Smoley BA, Robinson CM. Natural family planning. *Am Fam Physician.* 2012;86(10):924-928.

Wieslander CK, Hadnott TN, Bukowski K. Therapeutic Gynecologic Procedures. In: DeCherney AH, Nathan L, Laufer N, Roman AS, eds. *CURRENT Diagnosis & Treatment: Obstetrics & Gynecology.* 12th ed. New York, NY: McGraw Hill; Chap. 48. http://accessmedicine.mhmedical.com.evms.idm.oclc.org/content.aspx?bookid=2559&sectionid=206966408. Accessed May 9, 2020.

Wieslander CK, Wong KS. Therapeutic gynecologic procedures. In: DeCherney AH, Nathan L, Laufer N, Roman AS, eds. *CURRENT Diagnosis & Treatment: Obstetrics & Gynecology*. 11th ed. New York, NY: McGraw Hill; 2013: Chap. 46. http://accessmedicine.mhmedical.com.evms.idm .oclc.org/content.aspx?bookid=498&Sectionid=41008638. Accessed May 9, 2020.

A 16-year-old young woman presents for a routine wellness examination. She is a junior in high school and has no significant medical history. She plays on the school softball team and requests that you complete a preparticipation clearance form. She is accompanied by her mother, who wants to know if her daughter needs a routine gynecologic examination. While she is up to date on her immunizations, her mother has questions about the human papillomavirus (HPV) vaccine. There is no significant medical history in her nuclear family, but one of her cousins died at the age of 21 years of a sudden cardiac death. When interviewed without her mother in the room, the patient reports that she is generally happy, gets As and Bs in school, and has an active social life. She has never been sexually active and denies tobacco or illicit drug use. She reports that she has a "drink or two" at parties with her friends once a month. On examination, her vital signs are within normal limits. On cardiac auscultation, you hear a 2/6 systolic murmur that gets louder when you have her perform a Valsalva maneuver. Peripheral pulses are strong and symmetric, and there is brisk capillary refill. The remainder of the physical examination is unremarkable.

- What immunizations should be recommended at this visit?
- At what age is it recommended to start routine cervical cancer screening?
- What is the most common cause of sudden cardiac death in young athletes?
- What is the best strategy to address sexual activity and gender identity in adolescents?

ANSWERS TO CASE 29:

Adolescent Health Maintenance

Summary: A healthy 16-year-old adolescent female presents with

- Desire for a routine checkup and sports preparticipation examination
- A 2/6 systolic murmur that gets louder when you have her perform a Valsalva maneuver
- No significant medical history in her nuclear family, but a cousin who died at the age of 21 years of a sudden cardiac death
- Denial of sexual activity or tobacco or illicit drug use
- Report of having a drink or two at parties with her friends once a month

Recommended immunizations: Review of current immunization record and if not up to date: tetanus-diphtheria-acellular pertussis (Tdap) vaccination, meningococcal vaccination, HPV vaccine series, and annual influenza vaccine (seasonal).

Recommended age to start cervical cancer screening: The United States Preventive Services Task Force (USPSTF) and American College of Obstetrics and Gynecology recommend initial screening at age 21 years.

Most common cause of sudden cardiac death in young athletes: Hypertrophic cardiomyopathy (HCM).

Best strategy to discuss sexual activity and gender identity: Discuss with adolescent alone after excusing parent(s); use open-ended questions and active listening.

ANALYSIS

Objectives

1. Know the evidence-based guidelines for screening and disease prevention in adolescents. (EPA 3, 12)

2. List the immunizations routinely recommended for adolescents. (EPA 12)

3. Describe the components of sports preparticipation examinations. (EPA 12)

4. State the acceptable terminology for gender identity and how to address this issue in adolescents. (EPA 5, 12)

Considerations

This is a healthy adolescent female who presents for a sports preparticipation physical examination. Required preparticipation examinations provide an excellent opportunity for recommended health maintenance, including immunizations, age-appropriate screening, risk reduction counseling, and general health education. Her medical history is unremarkable, and she has a 2/6 systolic murmur that increases with Valsalva. The focus should be to identify potential conditions that can lead to sudden cardiac death. The hallmark physical examination finding in

HCM is a systolic murmur that *decreases* in intensity with the athlete in the supine position (increased ventricular filling, decreased obstruction). This contrasts with functional outflow murmurs common in athletes that *increase* in intensity upon lying down. The murmur of HCM increases with the Valsalva maneuver (decreased ventricular filling, increased obstruction). Marfan syndrome is associated with aortic root dilation or dissection, hence stigmata of Marfan and family history are also important. Any athlete with a new-onset murmur or any other murmur that the examiner finds suspicious—such as this one—should be held from participation and referred to a cardiologist for evaluation. Most athletes with HCM are asymptomatic.

APPROACH TO:
Adolescent Health Maintenance

DEFINITIONS

CISGENDER: A person whose gender identity matches sex assigned at birth.

GENDER IDENTITY: A person's internal sense of maleness or femaleness, which may or may not conflict with sex assigned at birth. A person's gender identity should not be confused with their gender expression, which is the external manifestation of their gender. It is important to recognize that in addition to male and female identities, a variety of nonbinary (eg, not strictly masculine or feminine) genders are also recognized, as well as gender fluidity, in which an individual identifies with different gender categories over time.

HUMAN PAPILLOMAVIRUS VACCINE: The nine-valent vaccine protects against high-risk and common types of HPV to protect against cervical, vaginal, vulvar, anal, and penile cancers as well as reduces the incidence of genital warts. The vaccine is now recommended for females and males ages 9 to 45 years, including high-risk males (men who have sex with men, immunocompromised males). It is recommended to begin the series at ages 11 to 12, but can be started as early as age 9. Two-dose and three-dose schedules are offered depending upon age of initiation of the series.

TRANSGENDER: A person whose gender identity conflicts with the sex assigned at birth.

TRANSMAN/TRANS BOY: A person assigned female at birth who identifies as a man.

TRANSWOMAN/TRANS GIRL: A person assigned male at birth who identifies as a woman.

CLINICAL APPROACH TO ADOLESCENT HEALTH MAINTENANCE

Adolescence is a time of physical, emotional, cognitive, and psychosocial changes. It is also a time of experimentation and, frequently, risk taking. For most, adolescence is also a time of relatively good health. The choices made during adolescence often impact both the short-term and the long-term health of the patient. Addressing the unique health care needs of adolescents can be challenging, as they may be more likely to present to the clinician for acute illness rather than for health maintenance. Adolescents rarely seek advice from health care providers regarding prevention of morbidity and mortality in their age group. During health maintenance visits, providers should discuss risks and interventions surrounding issues such as unintended pregnancy, sexually transmitted infections (STIs), unintentional injuries, depression, and suicide.

Confidentiality. Concerns about confidentiality can be a barrier to providing effective care to adolescent patients. Many adolescents believe that clinicians share any information provided with their parent(s) and may not volunteer information such as sexual activity, gender identity, and use of tobacco, alcohol, and/or illicit drugs. It is recommended that health care providers take a history with the parent in the room to allow the parent to present any concerns, then interview the adolescent alone to allow the patient to speak confidentially with the provider. Policies to ensure provider-patient confidentiality while balancing the parent's right to be involved should be discussed with and agreed upon by the patient and parent in advance to promote an honest, trusting, and therapeutic relationship.

In most states, adolescents can consent independently to STI testing and contraceptive services. Laws regarding abortion services vary from state to state and often require parental consent. Clinicians must consider maturity and age of the adolescent patient when contemplating breaking confidentiality. In cases of abuse or harm to the adolescent or to other persons, clinicians are required to break provider-patient confidentiality.

Screening

Various organizations have created and revised guidelines for preventive services for adolescents, including *Guidelines for Adolescent Preventive Services (GAPS)*, the USPSTF, American Academy of Pediatrics Bright Futures, and the Advisory Committee on Immunization Practices. Most insurance payers cover annual examinations, and current recommendations support at least three complete physical examinations: early adolescence (age 11-14), middle adolescence (age 15-17), and late adolescence to early adulthood (18-21).

The Society for Adolescent Medicine compiles similarities among guidelines for preventive services. All adolescents should be screened for hypertension; obesity; eating disorders; hyperlipidemia if indicated (in individuals at above-average risk based on a personal history of comorbid conditions or a family history of hyperlipidemia, coronary artery disease, or other vascular diseases); tuberculosis (TB) if at risk (having lived in a homeless shelter or an area with a high prevalence of TB, having been incarcerated or exposed to active TB, or working in a health care setting); physical or emotional abuse; learning or school problems; substance abuse; depression; and suicide.

Sexually Transmitted Infection Screening. The USPSTF recommends **chlamydia and gonorrhea screening** in all sexually active women under age 25 years (Grade B)

Table 29-1 • ANTICIPATORY GUIDANCE TOPICS FOR ADOLESCENTS
Growth and development parameters
Healthy dietary habits
Exercise
Oral health
Injury prevention
Sleep hygiene
Sun protection
Responsible sexual behaviors
Avoidance of alcohol, tobacco, illicit drugs, and anabolic steroids
Safe practices of social media
Strategies to cope with bullying

with insufficient evidence to recommend for or against such screening in men (Grade I). HIV testing is recommended for all adolescents and adults age 15 to 65 (Grade A), although the interval for screening is not certain. Screening for hepatitis B and syphilis is recommended for those at risk.

Depression Screening. The USPSTF recommends screening for major depressive disorder in adolescents aged 12 to 18 years, with adequate systems in place to ensure accurate diagnosis, effective treatment, and appropriate follow-up (Grade B).

Anticipatory Guidance

As with younger children, anticipatory guidance is a key component of adolescent care. At minimum, adolescents and their parents should be counseled on a variety of topics (see Table 29–1).

Gender Diversity

Childhood and adolescence are common times for children to explore and develop their gender identities. Current estimates suggest that approximately 1 in 200 people in the United States is transgender or gender nonconforming. With increased recognition of gender diversity, demand for gender-affirming services is increasing. Providers should ask adolescents about preferred pronouns (ie, she/he/they) as well as preferred names, and these should be documented in the medical record for future encounters. It should be made clear to patients that being gender diverse is not a mental illness. Care should be taken to avoid implicit rejection of the child's identity via "watchful waiting" (deeming the experience a phase), redirection toward cisgender norms, or attempts to convert the child to being cisgender.

Immunizations

The adolescent health maintenance examination allows for immunization history review and interval administration. In those who have received the recommended primary series, Tdap is recommended at ages 11 to 12 years. Routine meningococcal vaccination with conjugate vaccine (MCV) is recommended in a two-dose series at ages 11 to 12 years and again at age 16. If the booster at age 16 is not administered, it should be given before entering college dormitories or the military barracks. MCV is also recommended for travelers to endemic areas or if patients are functionally/anatomically asplenic. Catch-up vaccines for adolescents who did not receive vaccinations on the childhood schedule can be offered for varicella; measles, mumps, and rubella; and hepatitis B. The hepatitis A vaccine can be offered to males who have sex with males as well as to those who live in areas with high infection rates, travel to high-risk areas, have chronic liver disease, or inject intravenous drugs.

HPV is recommended during adolescence. The nine-valent vaccine protects against high-risk and common types of HPV that cause 90% of cervical, vaginal, vulvar, anal, and penile cancers. The vaccine also reduces the incidence of strains causing genital warts. The vaccine is now recommended for all females and males ages 9 to 45 years. It is given as a two-dose series for those under age 16 and three doses for those age 16 and up or anyone who is immunocompromised.

CLINICAL APPROACH TO SPORTS PREPARTICIPATION EXAMINATION

A common reason for healthy adolescents to present to primary care providers is for a preparticipation examination as a requirement to play a sport in school. The goal of these examinations is to identify conditions that may place a young athlete at risk during athletic participation. These conditions are primarily cardiac and orthopedic, but they are not limited to these systems. **A preparticipation examination allows the provider to perform a focused history and physical examination to clear the patient for safe participation in sports.** These encounters also serve to meet legal and insurance requirements of the school or school system.

Sudden Cardiac Death

The rate of sudden cardiac death in athletes is very low. Congenital cardiac anomalies are the most common etiology, with HCM accounting for about one-third and anomalous coronary arteries for about one-fifth of cardiac anomalies. All adolescents and their parents should be asked about personal history of exertional chest pain, dyspnea, syncope, and heart murmurs; they should also be queried about family history of HCM, other congenital cardiac abnormalities, or premature cardiac deaths. Other important historical information includes history of asthma or other pulmonary disorders, orthopedic injuries, heat-related illness, and absence of one of a paired organ (eg, single kidney, testicle, ovary, etc).

Eating Disorder Screening

It is important to screen for eating disorders, as well as for a desire to change body weight, either for body image or for athletic purposes (eg, "weight cutting" for wrestlers). Eating disorders are more common in cisgender females than males and are more common still among sexual orientation and gender minority populations with highest rates for the transgender population. Female patients should be questioned about menstrual irregularities, as amenorrhea could signal anorexia, and amenorrheic female athletes could be at risk for osteoporosis.

Cardiovascular Examination

Blood pressure should be measured and compared with age- and gender-appropriate norms. General appearance, specifically looking for signs of Marfan syndrome, should be noted. These signs, which include arachnodactyly, an arm span greater than height, pectus excavatum, tall-thin habitus, high-arched palate, and ocular lens subluxations, should prompt further evaluation, as persons with Marfan syndrome can have aortic abnormalities that predispose to rupture during sports. Auscultation of the heart should be performed, at minimum, in both the lying and the standing positions. **The murmur of HCM, while not always present, is best heard along the left sternal border and accentuates with activities that decrease cardiac preload and end-diastolic volume of the left ventricle.** Therefore, standing or straining with a Valsalva maneuver would increase the murmur; conversely, squatting would be expected to decrease the murmur. **Any adolescent with stigmata of Marfan syndrome, a murmur suggestive of HCM, with a grade 3/6 or louder systolic murmur, or any diastolic murmur should undergo an echocardiogram and be evaluated by a cardiologist prior to clearance for athletic participation.**

Contraindications

No specific screening tests are recommended for universal screening of all athletes, although specific tests may be indicated based upon history or physical examination findings. Participation in athletics or exercise should be encouraged. **Absolute contraindications to all athletic participation are rare;** more commonly, clearance to participate may be delayed for further evaluation of a suspected condition, rehabilitation of an injury, or recovery from an acute illness.

CASE CORRELATION

- See also Case 5 (Well-Child Care) and Case 28 (Family Planning—Contraceptives).

COMPREHENSION QUESTIONS

29.1 A 16-year-old high school student is being evaluated for a sports preparticipation examination. The student is currently asymptomatic and desires to participate on the basketball team. Which of the following should prompt a referral to a cardiologist prior to clearance to participate in high school sports?

    A. Grade 2/6 systolic murmur in an asymptomatic 16-year-old adolescent girl

    B. Grade 1/6 diastolic murmur heard at the apex in a 17-year-old adolescent girl

    C. Grade 2/6 systolic murmur in a 17-year-old adolescent boy that is heard while lying down and that gets softer when standing

    D. An asymptomatic 16-year-old whose grandfather died of a heart attack at age 72

29.2 A 15-year-old girl presents to your office with her mother for a preparticipation sports physical. She would also like to discuss the addition of birth control. When her mother leaves the room, you learn that the girl is not sexually active but wants to start oral contraceptives because she heard they help improve acne. She does not smoke, drink alcohol, or use illicit drugs; is in honors classes in ninth grade; and plays on the junior varsity softball team. Vital signs are within normal limits, and she has a body mass index (BMI) in the 97th percentile for her age. Physical examination is unremarkable. Which of the following should be performed at this time?

A. Perform routine Papanicolaou (Pap) smear before offering contraception
B. Periodic screening for drug use with a urine drug toxicology test
C. Cholesterol testing
D. Refer to obesity clinic or weight loss program

29.3 A mother brings her 12-year-old child to the clinic for a routine health maintenance examination. She mentions that the child, who was assigned male gender at birth, has shown interest in presenting in a traditionally feminine fashion, including wearing makeup and dresses. The child recently asked to be referred to as "she" and to go by a female name. The mother requests guidance on how to respond. Which of the following is the best response?

A. Advise the mother that gender exploration is common in adolescence, but that it is usually a self-limited phase that will resolve spontaneously.
B. Advise the mother that gender exploration is common in adolescence, but that it is important to affirm the child's gender identity with the correct name and pronouns and respect their gender expression.
C. Refer the patient to a psychiatrist for evaluation of mental illness.
D. Encourage the mother to use male pronouns and encourage traditionally masculine activities such as sports.

ANSWERS

29.1 **B.** This answer choice is a 16-year-old female adolescent student with a diastolic murmur. Any patient with a diastolic murmur, grade 3/6 or louder systolic murmur, murmur suggestive of HCM, or signs of Marfan syndrome should be evaluated by a cardiologist prior to clearance to participate in athletics. The murmur of HCM typically gets louder with maneuvers that reduce preload, such as the Valsalva maneuver or when standing. The patients in answers A and C have systolic murmurs, but these murmurs were both 2/6 and did not meet the threshold of 3/6 for referral to a cardiologist.

29.2 **D.** Per the USPSTF, BMI should be calculated annually for adolescent patients. If BMI is greater than the 95th percentile, it is recommended to refer patients to a weight loss program or obesity clinic. Further counseling by the provider on dietary advice and physical activity should also be done at this time. Pap smears for cervical cancer screening (answer A) are recommended to start at age 21 regardless of sexual activity and are not indicated for this patient, who is 16. Lipid screening (answer C) should be targeted to those who are at high risk based on personal or family history; while obesity is a risk factor for hyperlipidemia, there is not consensus regarding cholesterol screening in the absence of other risk factors. Routine toxicology screening (answer B) in adolescents is not recommended.

29.3 **B.** An affirming approach is important for the transgender adolescent, who is at risk of social stigma and for whom supportive family structures are predictive of better health outcomes. While gender exploration is common in childhood and adolescence, patients' gender identities should be treated as real and not questioned or refuted (answer D). While psychiatry referral is often required prior to initiation of hormone therapy or gender-affirming surgery, it should not be communicated to the parent or child that the child has a mental illness (answer C). A referral to psychiatry is, however, warranted if the child manifests signs of anxiety, depression, or suicidal ideation. Answer A (advise that gender exploration is common in adolescence but is usually self-limited and will resolve spontaneously) is not necessarily accurate and should not be communicated; by the time adolescence is reached, playtime and imagination are less common.

CLINICAL PEARLS

▶ Adolescents may see health care providers irregularly. Take the time at each visit to ensure that age-appropriate provisions of screening are up to date.

▶ Review the immunization history and current guidelines with each adolescent at every visit, ensuring adequate opportunity for education and shared decision-making.

▶ True contraindications to participation in sports are rare. Almost everyone should be able to participate in some form of athletic activity.

▶ Providers should ask adolescents about preferred pronouns (ie, she/he/they) as well as preferred names, and these should be documented in the medical record for future encounters.

▶ All adolescents and their parents should be asked about personal history of exertional chest pain, dyspnea, syncope, and heart murmurs, and about family history of HCM.

REFERENCES

American Medical Association. *Guidelines for Adolescent Preventive Services (GAPS): Recommendations Monograph.* Chicago, IL: American Medical Association; 1997.

Centers for Disease Control and Prevention. FDA licensure of quadrivalent human papillomavirus vaccine (HPV4, Gardasil) for use in males and guidance from the Advisory Committee on Immunization Practices (ACIP). *MMWR Morb Mortal Wkly Rep.* 2010;59(20):630-632.

Centers for Disease Control and Prevention. Prevention and control of meningococcal disease: recommendations of the Advisory Committee on Immunization Practices (ACIP). *MMWR Morb Mortal Wkly Rep.* 2013;62(RR-02):1-22.

Centers for Disease Control and Prevention. Vaccines and immunizations. http://www.cdc.gov/vaccines/. Accessed January 8, 2019.

Crissman HP, Berger MB, Graham LF, Dalton VK. Transgender demographics: a household probability sample of US adults, 2014. *Am J Pub Hlth.* 2017;107(2):213-215.

Hagan JF, Shaw JS, Duncan PM, eds. Bright Futures: Guidelines for Health Supervision of Infants, Children, and Adolescents [pocket guide]. 4th ed. Elk Grove Village, IL: American Academy of Pediatrics; 2017.

Ham P, Allen C. Adolescent health screening and counseling. *Am Fam Physician.* 2012;86(12):1109-1116.

Mirabelli MH, Devine MJ, Singh J, Mendoza M. The pre-participation sports evaluation. *Am Fam Physician.* 2015;92(5):371-376.

Olson J, Forbes C, Belzer M. Management of the transgender adolescent. *Arch Pediatr Adolesc Med.* 2011;165(2):171-176.

United States Preventive Services Task Force. Chlamydia and Gonorrhea Screening. https://www.uspreventiveservicestaskforce.org/uspstf/recommendation/chlamydia-and-gonorrhea-screening. Accessed May 15, 2020.

A 47-year-old African American man presents to your office for a follow-up visit. He was seen 3 weeks ago for an upper respiratory infection and noted incidentally to have a blood pressure (BP) of 164/98 mm Hg. He vaguely remembers being told in the past that his BP was "borderline." He feels fine and has no complaints, and his review of systems is entirely negative. He does not smoke cigarettes, drinks "a few beers on the weekends," and does not exercise regularly. He has a sedentary job. His father died of a stroke at the age of 79 years. His mother is alive and in good health at the age of 72 years. He has two siblings and is not aware of any chronic medical issues that they have. In the office today, his BP is 156/96 mm Hg in his left arm and 152/98 mm Hg in the right arm. He is afebrile, his pulse is 78 beats/min, and his respiratory rate is 14 breaths/min. He is 70 inches tall and weighs 210 lb (body mass index [BMI] 30.1 kg/m^2). A general physical examination is normal.

▶ What diagnosis (or diagnoses) can you make today?
▶ What further evaluation needs to be performed?
▶ What nonpharmacologic intervention(s) may be beneficial?
▶ What is the recommended initial medication management?

ANSWERS TO CASE 30:

Hypertension

Summary: A 47-year-old African American man presents with

- An elevated BP reading when seen for an unrelated problem visit and another elevated BP on a follow-up visit
- Obesity and a sedentary lifestyle but no other high risks based on his personal or family history
- No history of smoking and statement that he drinks "a couple of beers on the weekends"
- Normal general examination

Diagnoses: Hypertension and obesity.

Necessary further evaluation: Blood glucose; serum potassium, fasting cholesterol panel, estimated glomerular filtration rate (GFR), creatinine, and calcium levels; hematocrit; urinalysis; electrocardiogram (ECG).

Nonpharmacologic interventions: DASH (Dietary Approaches to Stop Hypertension) diet; alcohol limitation to no more than two drinks per day; increased physical activity; weight reduction.

Recommended initial medication: Thiazide diuretic or calcium channel blocker.

ANALYSIS

Objectives

1. State the diagnostic criteria for hypertension. (EPA 1, 2, 3)

2. Be able to state the recommended initial evaluation of persons found with an elevated BP. (EPA 3)

3. State the medication and lifestyle modifications that can help to control BP. (EPA 4)

4. Be able to report the complications and risks of uncontrolled hypertension. (EPA 10, 12)

Considerations

The patient presented here is typical of one seen every day in primary care offices and represents the most common presentation of hypertension. Most hypertensive patients do not have any symptoms of their disease. They are typically seen for another reason and noted to have a high BP reading. Untreated hypertension significantly raises an individual's risk of myocardial infarction, cerebrovascular accident, and renal failure, among other conditions. **The risk of cardiovascular disease doubles with each increase in BP of 20/10 mm Hg above 115/75 mm Hg.** Because of the high prevalence of the problem, the lack of symptoms, and the demonstrated efficacy of treatment in reducing the risk of complications, the United States Preventive Services Task Force recommends screening adults aged 18 and older for hypertension by measuring their BP. For patients aged 18 to 39 without increased risk, the interval for screening is every 3 to 5 years. The recommended screening is annually in low-risk patients age 40 and older and for all adults with increased risk for hypertension, such as high normal (> 130/85 mm Hg) BP measures and in overweight/obese patients. Most practitioners will check the BP of every adult patient at every office visit.

APPROACH TO:
Hypertension

DEFINITIONS

AMERICAN HEART ASSOCIATION/AMERICAN COLLEGE OF CARDIOLOGY (AHA/ACC) CONSENSUS STATEMENT: 2018 guidelines that recommend pharmacologic BP management based on 10-year risk estimates, such as the atherosclerotic cardiovascular disease (ASCVD) risk calculator (see Case 35).

JNC 8: The eighth report of the Joint National Committee on Prevention, Detection, Evaluation, and Treatment of High Blood Pressure. A comprehensive, evidence-based review of the diagnosis, evaluation, and management of hypertension published in 2013.

CLINICAL APPROACH

Epidemiology

Hypertension is the most common primary diagnosis at office visits in the United States. **Approximately 32% to 46% of American adults have hypertension, with 30% being unaware of the problem.** The prevalence is higher in African Americans and in older patients. National Health and Nutritional Examination Surveys (NHANES) data suggest that hypertension is responsible for approximately one-third of heart attacks, one-half of heart failure, and one-fourth of premature deaths. Most patients with end-stage kidney disease are hypertensive. Hypertensive nephrosclerosis is responsible for approximately one-fourth of end-stage kidney disease. **The risk of complications is directly related to the elevation of the BP—the higher the BP, the higher the risk.**

Pathophysiology

The diagnosis of hypertension relies on accurate measurement of BP. The appropriate technique is to allow the patient to sit quietly in a chair (not on the examination table) with a supported back and feet on the floor for 5 minutes prior to making the measurement. Allowing patients to empty their bladder prior to BP measurement can also reduce the chance of a falsely elevated reading. The BP should be measured at least twice, using a calibrated sphygmomanometer and an appropriate size cuff for the patient. The BP cuff should encircle at least 80% of the patient's arm; a cuff that is too small can result in a falsely elevated reading. The diagnosis of hypertension is made based on the average of two properly taken BP measurements at two or more office visits.

Evaluation. When hypertension is diagnosed, an evaluation consisting of a history, physical examination, and focused diagnostic studies should be performed, with the goals of assessing overall cardiovascular risks, identifying possible secondary causes of hypertension, and determining the presence of any end-organ damage. Secondary causes should be considered, especially in patients with difficult-to-control BP. The most common secondary causes include obstructive sleep apnea, hyperaldosterone states, drugs (recreational, prescription, or over-the-counter like caffeine and nonsteroidal anti-inflammatory drugs), and renovascular or renal disease. Less common secondary causes include coarctation of the aorta, Cushing disease, hyperthyroidism, hyperparathyroidism, and pheochromocytoma. Historical information should include personal and family medical histories, an assessment of diet and activity levels, and specific questioning regarding tobacco, alcohol, recreational drug, and medication (both prescription and nonprescription) use. Patients should be questioned about cardiovascular, cerebrovascular, and peripheral arterial disease symptoms.

Physical Examination. Along with BP in both arms, examination should include all other vital signs and a measurement of BMI. Other specific components of the examination should include a fundoscopic examination for signs of retinopathy; oropharynx and neck for signs of obstructive sleep apnea; palpation of the thyroid; auscultation for carotid, femoral, and renal bruits; palpation of peripheral pulses; abdominal palpation for signs of organomegaly or aortic aneurysm; and a complete cardiopulmonary examination.

Testing. Initial testing should include measurement of serum potassium, creatinine (with GFR calculation), calcium, blood glucose, fasting lipids, and hematocrit. A urinalysis should be done to look for proteinuria or cellular components suggestive of renal disease. An ECG should be performed to evaluate for changes consistent with coronary artery disease and to screen for left ventricular hypertrophy.

Treatment

Elevated systolic BP is a greater risk for cardiovascular disease complications than elevated diastolic pressure. Control of systolic BP tends to be more difficult to achieve, and when it is achieved, the diastolic BP usually comes under control as well. JNC 8, the American College of Physicians, and the American Academy of Family Physicians recommend the goal of treatment of lowering the BP to less than 140/90 mm Hg in adults up to age 59 and 150/90 mm Hg in patients age 60 and above. For persons with diabetes or kidney disease, the goal is to achieve a BP of less than 140/90 mm Hg. The AHA/ACC consensus statement's recommendations are for target BPs of less than 130/80 mm Hg.

Nonpharmacologic Management. Once the diagnosis of hypertension is made, patients should be advised of specific lifestyle modifications that can both reduce their BP and reduce their overall cardiac risk factors. These should include efforts to lose weight if overweight or obese, increase physical activity, and reduce consumption of alcohol. Men should consume no more than two alcoholic beverages a day and women no more than one. Any smoker should be counseled to quit. A DASH diet that is rich in potassium, calcium, magnesium, fiber, and protein; low in saturated and trans fats; and lower in sodium reduces BP in an amount comparable to single-agent drug therapy. An informational brochure detailing the DASH diet is available from the National Heart, Lung, and Blood Institute. Combining the various lifestyle modifications provides additive benefits, and these efforts should continue even when the decision is made to start medications.

Pharmacologic Management. Lowering BP reduces the risk of adverse outcomes such as strokes and heart attacks. In the primary treatment of hypertension in African American patients, thiazide diuretics or calcium channel blockers are the recommended first-line therapy. In non–African American patients, according to the JNC 8, the first-line pharmacologic treatment can be diuretics, calcium channel blockers, angiotensin-converting enzyme (ACE) inhibitors, or angiotensin receptor blockers (ARBs), with a goal of < 140/90 mm Hg in those under age 60 and < 150/90 mm Hg if age 60 or older. Patients with hypertension that is inadequately controlled with nonpharmacologic interventions alone should be started on the agents described unless there is a compelling reason to start another class of medication (Table 30–1). The goal of therapy is to attain and maintain goal BP. If goal BP is not reached with one agent after 1 month, then the provider can either increase the dose of the initial agent or add a second drug.

Table 30–1 • JNC 8 RECOMMENDATIONS FOR STARTING SPECIFIC CLASSES OF ANTIHYPERTENSIVE MEDICATION	
Indication	Class of Medication
Black patients	Calcium channel blocker Thiazide diuretic
Nonblack patients younger than 60 years	Angiotensin-converting enzyme inhibitor Angiotensin receptor blocker Thiazide diuretics Calcium channel blockers
Nonblack patients 60 years or older	Calcium channel blocker Thiazide diuretic Angiotensin-converting enzyme inhibitor Angiotensin receptor blocker
Patients with chronic kidney disease	Angiotensin-converting enzyme inhibitor Angiotensin receptor blocker initial or add on for goal of blood pressure < 140/90 mm Hg
Patints with history of coronary artery disease	Beta-blocker (especially if reduced systolic function) Angiotensin-converting enzyme inhibitor Angiotensin receptor blocker

(Continued)

Table 30–1 • JNC 8 RECOMMENDATIONS FOR STARTING SPECIFIC CLASSES OF ANTIHYPERTENSIVE MEDICATION (continued)	
Indication	Class of Medication
Patients with diabetes mellitus without kidney disease	Nonblack: Angiotensin-converting enzyme inhibitor Angiotensin receptor blocker Thiazide diuretic Calcium channel blocker patients Black: Thiazide diuretics Calcium channel blockers
Patients with heart failure	Angiotensin-converting enzyme inhibitor Angiotensin receptor blocker Beta-blocker Spironolactone
Prevention of recurrent cerebrovascular accident	Angiotensin-converting enzyme inhibitor Angiotensin receptor blocker Calcium channel blockers Thiazide diuretics

---

CASE CORRELATION

- See also Case 33 (Obesity) and Case 35 (Hyperlipidemia).

COMPREHENSION QUESTIONS

30.1 A 62-year-old woman presents for a routine physical examination. She is asymptomatic and is not taking any medications. Her BP is found to be 145/85 mm Hg on two readings, and her BMI is 29 kg/m². Review of her chart reveals that her BP was 143/84 mm Hg on a visit 4 months ago for a urinary tract infection. Which of the following is the most accurate statement regarding her BP?

A. Her BP is normal, and she is at average risk for developing hypertension.

B. She is at risk for needing pharmacologic treatment for hypertension.

C. She has hypertension and should be started on a thiazide diuretic.

D. She has hypertension and should be started on multidrug therapy.

30.2 A 66-year-old Caucasian woman has an average BP of 155/70 mm Hg despite appropriate lifestyle modification efforts. Her only other medical problems are osteopenia, kidney stones, and mild depression. Her last lipid panel revealed a total cholesterol of 160 mg/dL, high-density lipoprotein of 40 mg/dL, and low-density lipoprotein of 90 mg/dL. Which of the following would be the most appropriate treatment at this time?

A. Lisinopril (Prinivil, Zestril)

B. Propranolol (Inderal)

C. Amlodipine (Norvasc)

D. Chlorthalidone

E. Losartan (Cozaar)

30.3 A 48-year-old Caucasian man with type 2 diabetes has had persistent BP readings of 150/95 mm Hg for the past 6 months. Current medications include glyburide and metformin. His last hemoglobin A_{1c} was 7.9%, and the patient has a BMI of 24 kg/m². On physical examination, position sense is intact but a peripheral neuropathy is detected in a stocking-and-glove pattern. Vibratory sensation is decreased bilaterally on both lower extremities. Eye examination shows mild papilledema but no cotton wool spots. When questioned, he says that he still occasionally sneaks a cookie after dinner and drinks alcohol nightly. Which of the following is the most appropriate treatment for him?

A. DASH diet and recheck BP in 3 months

B. Thiazide diuretic alone

C. ACE inhibitor alone

D. Combination of ACE inhibitor and thiazide diuretic

30.4 At a routine checkup, a 6-year-old boy is found to have a BP of 150/90 mm Hg. Repeated BP readings are consistently elevated. The child was delivered at 36 weeks by normal spontaneous vaginal delivery with no complications. All major milestones were met on time, and he currently is enrolled in first grade. The child has been healthy up until this point. Which of the following are the most appropriate diagnosis and therapeutic step?

A. The child has essential hypertension and should be started on the DASH diet.

B. The child most likely has hyperthyroidism, should be started on a beta-blocker, and should have thyroid studies performed.

C. The child most likely has renal parenchymal disease and should have a urinalysis and renal ultrasound ordered.

D. The child most likely has "white coat" hypertension; follow up in 3 months if there is no family history of hypertension.

E. The child most likely has a pheochromocytoma and should start a 24-hour urine collection for metanephrines.

ANSWERS

30.1 **B.** This patient's BP falls within the definition of hypertension (it is not normal, as answer A states) but outside the need for immediate pharmacologic intervention. The first treatment is to implement lifestyle modifications, such as the DASH diet and exercise. The AHA/ACC consensus statement recommends that, if the patient has maximized lifestyle therapy and her 10-year risk is > 10%, she should start antihypertensive medications (answers C and D).

30.2 **D.** In the JNC 8 guidelines, calcium channel blockers, thiazides, ARBs and ACE inhibitors are first-line treatments in nonblack patients over age 60. In this case, beta-blockers (answer B) may worsen the depression. Thiazide diuretics such as chlorthalidone may improve osteoporosis and reduce hypercalciuria, which can reduce nephrolithiasis. Nevertheless, both lisinopril (answer A) and losartan (answer E) would be effective as first-line agents but would not have the secondary goal of helping with the osteopenia. Answer C (Amlodipine), a calcium channel blocking agent, may be considered a first-line agent as well and especially may be helpful in black patients; however, calcium channel blocking agents again do not have a secondary added benefit of helping with osteopenia.

30.3 **C.** Because of his diabetes, the BP goal for this patient is less than 140/90 mm Hg. He is above the BP goal, so an ACE inhibitor or ARB is first-line therapy regardless of BMI or hemoglobin A_{1c}. The dose of the medication can be maximized if BP is not controlled after 1 month or another agent can be added (answer D). A DASH diet (answer A) may be considered, although a diabetic diet is likely more important; nevertheless, beginning pharmacological therapy is important to prevent cardiovascular complications. Answer B (thiazide diuretic alone) is not preferable since these agents would likely elevate the blood sugar.

30.4 **C.** The most common cause of hypertension is renal parenchymal disease, and a urinalysis, urine culture, and renal ultrasonography should be ordered for all children presenting with hypertension. Essential hypertension (answer A) is rarely found in children less than 10 years of age and should be a diagnosis of exclusion. Hyperthyroidism (answer B) or pheochromocytoma (answer E) is possible in children but is more common in adults, and there are no findings in the scenario suggesting either condition. A BP of 150 systolic in a child is markedly elevated and outside of the range of white coat hypertension (answer D).

CLINICAL PEARLS

▶ Patients with BPs > 160/90 mm Hg will most likely need two or more agents to achieve JNC 8 recommended control.

▶ Thiazide diuretics or calcium channel blockers should be the first-line drug treatment in black patients with hypertension.

▶ Diuretics, calcium channel blockers, ACE inhibitors, or ARBs are the first-line agents for nonblack patients. Choice of first-line medication can be tailored to mitigate other comorbidities.

▶ Goal BP for patients greater than age 60 is < 150/90 mm Hg if they do not have diabetes or kidney disease. Patients under the age of 60 or patients of any age with diabetes and/or chronic kidney disease have a BP goal of < 140/90 mm Hg.

▶ All patients with chronic kidney disease should have ACE inhibitors or ARBs as first-line agents or add-on treatment.

▶ All patients with hypertension are at risk for cardiovascular and cerebrovascular disease. Be sure to address their other significant risks for these diseases, including lipids, smoking, diabetes, and obesity.

REFERENCES

James P, Opani S, Carter BL, et al. 2014 evidence-based guideline for the management of high blood pressure in adults: report from the panel members appointed to the Eighth Joint National Committee (JNC 8). *JAMA*. 2014;311(5):507-520.

Kotchen TA. Hypertensive vascular disease. In: Kasper D, Fauci A, Hauser S, Longo D, Jameson J, Loscalzo J, eds. *Harrison's Principles of Internal Medicine*., 20th ed. New York, NY: McGraw Hill; 2018: Chap. 298. http://accessmedicine.mhmedical.com/content.aspx?bookid=1130&Sectionid=79743947

Langan R, Jones, K. Common questions about the initial management of hypertension. *Am Fam Physician*. 2015;91(3):172-177.

Riley M, Bluhm B. High blood pressure in children and adolescents. *Am Fam Physician*. 2012; 85(7):693-700.

Whelton PK, Carey RM, Aronow WS, Casey DE Jr, et al. 2017 ACC/AHA/AAPA/ABC/ACPM/AGS/APhA/ASH/ASPC/NMA/PCNA guideline for the prevention, detection, evaluation, and management of high blood pressure in adults: a report of the American College of Cardiology/American Heart Association Task Force on Clinical Practice Guidelines. *Hypertension*. 2018; 71(6):e13-e115.

The mother of a 12-month-old infant boy calls at midnight stating that her son has been crying incessantly for the last 6 hours. His bouts of crying last for about 20 minutes, then completely disappear for 15 minutes at a time. Since early afternoon, the child has not been eating much, and he has started to vomit the small amounts of juice and milk he had ingested. She decided to call you because the vomitus is now green, and the bouts of crying seem to be getting worse. The mother is advised to bring the child to the emergency department.

In the emergency department, you recall that the patient does not have any significant past medical history, was born at term without complications, and is up to date on immunizations. On examination, his temperature is 100 °F (37.7 °C), his respiratory rate is 40 breaths/min, his pulse is 155 beats/min, his blood pressure is 109/60 mm Hg, and his weight is 22 lb. He cries inconsolably for 15 minutes, drawing his legs up to his chest, and then becomes quiet. You notice he still produces tears, and his mucosae are moist. Heart and lung examinations are normal; abdominal examination reveals markedly decreased bowel sounds with generalized tenderness to palpation. You feel a sausage-like mass in the right side of the abdomen. His diaper holds some amount of bloody stool mixed with mucus. The rest of the examination is normal.

▶ What is the most likely diagnosis?
▶ What is the next diagnostic step?
▶ What are the possible complications?

ANSWERS TO CASE 31:
Abdominal Pain and Vomiting in a Child

Summary: A 12-month-old infant boy presents with

- Sudden onset of intermittent crying that progressed with the day, each bout lasting about 20 minutes
- Vomiting that later became bilious
- No signs of hypovolemia, sepsis, or shock
- Generalized tenderness of the abdomen and a sausage-like mass on the right side
- A small amount of bloody-mucus stool

Most likely diagnosis: Intestinal obstruction caused by intussusception.

Next diagnostic step: Abdominal plain x-rays to rule out perforation.

Possible complications: If perforation occurs, rapid deterioration as a consequence of shock/sepsis.

ANALYSIS

Objectives

1. Be able to state the most likely causes of intestinal obstruction in the pediatric population. (EPA 1, 2)

2. State the differentiating features between life-threatening abdominal emergencies and urgent conditions. (EPA 1, 10)

3. Explain the diagnostic approach to the pediatric patient presenting with abdominal pain and vomiting. (EPA 3)

Considerations

This 12-month-old infant boy presented with vomiting and intermittent abdominal pain. His vomitus was initially the gastric contents of what he had ingested, but later became bilious, which is suggestive of intestinal obstruction. The description of his abdominal pain reveals the pathophysiologic nature of intussusception. The intermittency and "pain-free" intervals correlate with the gradual and slow telescoping of the intussusceptum (proximal or leading part of the intestine) into the intussuscipiens (distal or receiving end of the intestine). As the "telescoping" progresses, the portions of bowel that are trapped within the lumen of the intestine become edematous, which will ultimately lead to obstruction, ischemia, and perforation of the bowel wall. The sausage-shaped mass felt on examination will not be present in all cases. It represents the portions of bowel that are involved and have become edematous. "Currant jelly" stools are basically a mixture of blood and mucus that has sloughed from the affected bowel wall. While common, this is not present in all cases.

Before proceeding to diagnostics, the patient should be stabilized with intravenous fluid hydration, and surgery consultation should not be delayed. A nasogastric tube may need to be placed if obstruction is suspected. A plain film of the abdomen is done to rule out perforation. If perforation has occurred, surgical intervention is required. If no perforation is evidenced, an ultrasound of the abdomen may reveal a "target" lesion or "donut sign" that reflects the layers of intestine within the lumen of a different portion of intestine. Fluoroscopic guided air contrast enema is the first-line treatment and may be both diagnostic and therapeutic. The therapeutic value of the enema is a result of the constant application of hydrostatic pressure on the bowel, mechanically forcing it to telescope back. Air reduction may also be achieved. Air reduction is effective in 75% to 90% of cases, after which a 12- to 24-hour observation period is needed until bowel function is adequate and a bowel movement has been produced. The risk of recurrence in this patient with idiopathic intussusception is approximately 10%.

APPROACH TO:
Pediatric Abdominal Pain With Vomiting

DEFINITIONS

HYPERTROPHIC PYLORIC STENOSIS: Condition of hypertrophy of the pylorus leading to gastric outlet obstruction, commonly manifesting in infants at about 1 month of age.

INTUSSUSCEPTION: A telescoping of the intestine within itself, leading to abdominal pain, fever, vomiting, and ultimately bowel necrosis if not resolved.

MALROTATION WITH VOLVULUS: Condition in which the small bowel twists around the superior mesenteric artery and results in vascular compromise to large portions of the midgut, commonly before 1 month of age.

CLINICAL APPROACH

Pathophysiology

The most important aspect of a diagnostic approach in these cases is to differentiate between emergent and nonemergent causes. Although the case presented is that of the most common cause of intestinal obstruction in children, it is by no means the only cause. **Among the diagnoses that have to be entertained are hypertrophic pyloric stenosis, malrotation with volvulus/obstruction, foreign-body ingestion, and poisoning.**

Intussusception

As described, intussusception will present with intermittent, severe abdominal pain, associated with vomiting that becomes bilious as obstruction sets in. The finding of an elongated mass along the right abdomen is very suggestive of this diagnosis.

This right-sided location occurs because most idiopathic intussusceptions occur at the ileocecal junction; however, intussusceptions may be entirely in the jejunum, between the jejunum and ileum, or entirely colonic. Currant jelly stool is most often used to describe the finding in this condition, and it correlates with the ongoing bowel ischemia as the intussusception and edema progress.

Hypertrophic Pyloric Stenosis

Hypertrophic pyloric stenosis is **the most common cause of gastrointestinal (GI) obstruction in infants.** It occurs in approximately 3 in 1000 live births, with a male-to-female ratio of 4:1. The usual presenting age is 3 to 6 weeks old and is often described as a "hungry baby" with projectile vomiting. Vomiting is nonbilious and occurs immediately after meals. The infant will demand to be refed immediately. On examination, there may be an **olive-shaped mass felt in the right upper quadrant, and peristaltic waves may be seen across the upper abdomen moments before emesis occurs.** Ultrasonography shows the thickened pyloric muscles that are causing a gastric outlet obstruction. An upper GI contrast study usually reveals an elongated pyloric canal and a "double-track sign," which is explained by two thin tracks of barium that are created by compressed pyloric mucosa. Once the diagnosis is made, surgical referral is indicated, as it is the definitive management. Because of the early age and dramatic nature of the symptoms, parents will usually seek help before the infant becomes severely ill from not eating.

Malrotation

Malrotation occurs in about 1 in 500 live births, but it becomes symptomatic in only 1 in 6000 live births. Approximately **60% of patients will be younger than 1 month of age,** with approximately 10% presenting after 1 year of age, even into adulthood. Because it is primarily a defect that occurs during embryogenesis, the mesentery that is formed will have an abnormally narrow base, which allows the small bowel to move more freely than normal. This creates a problem when the intestinal attachment to the mesentery twists around itself, creating a volvulus. Once obstruction occurs, the **child will present with bilious vomiting and abdominal pain.**

If diagnosis is delayed, the involved segments of bowel will eventually become necrotic, leading to fluid losses and sepsis. The diagnostic approach in such cases will depend on the stability of the patient. If the patient is hemodynamically stable, imaging may be performed to confirm the diagnosis. In 75% of patients, the diagnosis will be clearly seen on an upper GI series. Diagnostic findings on an upper GI series are an obviously misplaced duodenum or a duodenal obstruction with the classic "beak-like" appearance of the contrast medium caused by a volvulus. If the patient is hypovolemic or hypotensive, has GI blood loss, or has signs of peritonitis, immediate surgical intervention is necessary, and surgery is the only definitive treatment. Volvulus may recur in up to 8% of cases, even after surgical intervention. Malrotation can go undiagnosed if a patient never experiences symptoms, and older children may present with intermittent vomiting, episodes of abdominal pain, failure to thrive, or syndromes of malabsorption.

Foreign Body Ingestion

Foreign body ingestion may also present with abdominal pain and vomiting in a pediatric patient. **Only 10% of patients who ingest a foreign body will need an intervention,** either to relieve an obstruction or to prevent GI complications. Approximately 90% of patients will pass a foreign body spontaneously, and parents need only check the stool within 24 hours to confirm passage. Sometimes, if an object can be seen on plain radiographs, a repeat x-ray within 24 hours can be done. **Among objects that require immediate intervention are flat disk, or "button," batteries in the esophagus.** These batteries will conduct electricity when both poles are in contact with the esophageal wall, which may lead to perforation. Sharp objects and multiple magnets also need to be removed. As a general rule, any foreign body in the esophagus needs to be removed in less than 24 hours by upper endoscopy. If a sharp or elongated object (> 6 cm) has already passed through the stomach and duodenum, daily x-rays should be done to follow the progress of the object. Those that do not advance within 3 days will require surgical intervention for removal.

Toxic Ingestion

Toxic ingestion **must also be included in the differential diagnosis in the evaluation of a child with vomiting and abdominal pain.** Ingestion of over-the-counter analgesic drugs, cold remedies, insecticides, pesticides, personal care products, and fume inhalation are commonly associated with hospital visits. Ingestion of nicotine or insecticides may cause a cholinergic syndrome, characterized by salivation, lacrimation, diarrhea, vomiting, diaphoresis, intestinal cramps, and seizures. Antihistamines or tricyclic antidepressants produce anticholinergic symptoms, with dry skin, dry mucosae, urinary retention, and decreased bowel sounds. Some medications and substances are radiopaque, such as iron tablets, mercury, lithium, tricyclic antidepressants, Play-Doh, and enteric-coated aspirin. Finding the likely agent of poisoning will mostly depend on the history given. Poison control should be consulted for all patients with suspected toxic ingestion.

Treatment

Initial management in all pediatric patients presenting with nausea and vomiting should include assessment of volume status with appropriate supportive care and stabilization. This should include appropriate intravenous fluid resuscitation when necessary. In cases of intestinal obstruction, a nasogastric tube is recommended. Surgical intervention will almost always be necessary if an anatomical/mechanical defect of the GI tract is present.

CASE CORRELATION

- See also Case 5 (Well-Child Care) and Case 17 (Electrolyte Disorders).

COMPREHENSION QUESTIONS

Match the following etiologies (A-F) to the clinical vignette (31.1-31.6):

   A. Malrotation with intermittent volvulus
   B. Intussusception
   C. Insecticide ingestion
   D. Esophageal foreign body
   E. Pyloric stenosis
   F. Volvulus

31.1 A 6-year-old boy left alone for 10 hours, now with hematemesis and pneumo-mediastinum on chest x-ray.

31.2 A 3-week-old male infant with 2 days of projectile, nonbilious vomiting, and constant feeding.

31.3 A 7-year-old boy with three episodes of severe abdominal pain and vomiting in the last month, previously diagnosed with failure to thrive.

31.4 An 8-month-old girl with bilious vomiting, constant abdominal pain for 12 hours, and upper GI study showing beak-like appearance of contrast.

31.5 An 11-month-old boy with sudden-onset intermittent bouts of crying, non-bilious vomiting, and currant jelly stools. A small, elongated mass is felt on the right side of his abdomen.

31.6 A 4-year-old girl with profuse vomiting, sweating, lacrimation, and diarrhea, who seizes in the emergency department.

31.7 A 30-month-old girl is brought to your urgent care clinic with the acute onset of diffuse abdominal pain that began approximately 6 hours ago. She has also had two episodes of bilious emesis in the last hour. The parents report decreased appetite earlier in the day but no fever, weight loss, diarrhea, or bloody stools. On examination, the patient's height and weight are in the 50th percentile for age, blood pressure is normal, heart rate is 115 beats/min, and temperature is 36.9 °C (98.4 °F). Heart and lung examinations are normal. On examination, the abdomen is significant for slightly hypoactive bowel sounds and diffuse tenderness to palpation without rebound, guarding, or rigidity. A urine dip is unremarkable. Which one of the following is the most appropriate next step for the abdominal pain in this patient?

   A. Send home with antiemetics and oral rehydration solutions
   B. Send to the emergency department for abdominal ultrasonography
   C. Send to the emergency department for abdominal and pelvic computed tomography (CT)
   D. Send to the emergency department for an upper GI series

ANSWERS

31.1 **D.** The presence of blood in the vomitus and a pneumomediastinum point to an esophageal perforation, most likely from a foreign body in the esophagus.

31.2 **E.** The young age and presence of projectile, nonbilious vomiting after feeding are the keys to this diagnosis. The diagnosis of pyloric stenosis is much more common in males than females.

31.3 **A.** This is the presentation of a malrotation that did not cause enough symptoms at a younger age to lead to a diagnosis.

31.4 **F.** An infant with bilious vomiting and abdominal pain has a volvulus until proven otherwise. The upper GI study is diagnostic of this condition.

31.5 **B.** The intermittent nature of the symptoms, currant jelly stool, and palpable mass are highly suggestive of intussusception. The currant jelly stool especially is a classic finding.

31.6 **C.** These symptoms (hypermotility of intestines, increased sweating, and lacrimation) are characteristic of a cholinergic syndrome, possibly caused by insecticide or nicotine poisoning.

31.7 **D.** In young children with bilious emesis, anorexia, and lack of fever, the most likely diagnosis is intestinal malrotation with volvulus. The child should be sent to the emergency department for further evaluation. Abdominal ultrasonography (answer B) is less sensitive and specific for malrotation than an upper GI series, so an upper GI series should be ordered initially if volvulus is suspected. If appendicitis were suspected, ultrasonography would be preferred. CT (answer C) is not a good choice because of the amount of radiation it delivers, especially given efforts to decrease the use of CT in children unless absolutely necessary.

CLINICAL PEARLS

▶ When a child appears critically ill, do not delay resuscitative efforts or surgical consultation while waiting for laboratory tests and imaging results.

▶ Surgical intervention may be required for mechanical intestinal defects such as intussusception, malrotation, and volvulus.

▶ For the pediatric patient presenting with abdominal pain, nausea, and vomiting, the differential diagnosis should include intussusception, malrotation, volvulus, pyloric stenosis, foreign body ingestion, and toxic ingestion.

REFERENCES

Hoffenberg EJ, Furuta GT, Kobak G, Walker T, Soden J, Kramer RE, Brumbaugh D. Gastrointestinal Tract. In: Hay, Jr. WW, Levin MJ, Deterding RR, Abzug MJ. eds. *Current Diagnosis & Treatment: Pediatrics, 24e* New York, NY: McGraw Hill. http://accessmedicine.mhmedical.com/content.aspx?bookid=2390&sectionid=189079593. Accessed May 19, 2020.

Maclin J. Acute abdominal pain. In: Rudolph C, Rudolph A, eds. *Rudolph's Pediatrics.* New York, NY: McGraw Hill; 2018: Chap. 378.

Reust CE, William A. Acute abdominal pain in children. *Am Fam Physician.* 2016;93(10):830-837.

An 83-year-old woman is brought to the clinic by her husband, who is concerned with his wife's memory problems. He noticed some memory decline a few years ago, but the onset was subtle and did not interfere with her day-to-day activities. The patient's husband reports that she has some difficulty remembering details. She often repeats herself and seems forgetful. The patient's family reports these problems have gradually gotten worse over the past year. She is unable to remember her appointments and relies heavily on written notes and appointments books. Recently, she got lost while driving and was found by her family 10 hours later. She was unable to use her cell phone and was unsure about her home address and phone number. She has also become more reclusive. She does not enjoy her church activities anymore and prefers to stay at home most of the time. She does not want to cook and is less attentive to her housework. She is insistent that she is not having any issues with her memory. Her medical history is significant for well-controlled hypertension and a history of mastectomy secondary to breast cancer diagnosed 20 years ago. She has no significant history of tobacco or alcohol use. She is independent with all activities of daily living but needs assistance with medication administration, banking, and transportation. She is up to date with her health maintenance and immunizations. Her vital signs and general physical examination are normal.

▶ What is the most likely diagnosis?
▶ What office testing can help to determine a diagnosis?
▶ What laboratory testing and imaging studies are indicated at this time?

ANSWERS TO CASE 32:

Dementia

Summary: An 83-year-old woman presents with

- Her family noting that she is having increasing memory difficulties at home
- Forgetfulness, repeating questions, and not remembering conversations
- A very significant episode of getting lost in her hometown
- Being seemingly unaware that there is a problem that is slowly and progressively worsening
- Normal vital signs and general examination

Most likely diagnosis: Dementia of Alzheimer type.

Office-based testing: Folstein Mini-Mental State Examination (MMSE) is the most widely used instrument. Others available include the clock test, the Short Portable Mental Status Questionnaire, the Mini-Cog Test, and the Montreal Cognitive Assessment (MoCA). In addition, a screening test for depression should be performed.

Laboratory testing and imaging studies: Blood count, electrolytes, glucose, calcium, liver function tests, folate, vitamin B_{12}, and thyroid-stimulating hormone (TSH). Consider HIV, syphilis, and Lyme disease screening if there is a risk factor or evidence of prior infection or if the patient lives in an area of high incidence. Noncontrast magnetic resonance imaging (MRI) (preferred by expert opinion) or noncontrast computed tomography (CT) of the head can be used.

ANALYSIS

Objectives

1. Develop a differential diagnosis for dementia. (EPA 1, 2)
2. Describe how to appropriately evaluate a complaint of memory loss. (EPA 1, 3)
3. List treatments for Alzheimer dementia, the most common specific diagnosis of dementia. (EPA 4)

Considerations

This 83-year-old woman is noted by her family to have a progressive decrease in cognitive function. She is forgetful and gets lost easily, and her condition has been slowly but steadily worsening. The most likely diagnosis is dementia; however, other conditions should be considered in the differential diagnosis, such as medications, stroke, thyroid disorders, chronic syphilis, or other metabolic conditions. Depression can also present as dementia at times. The workup for this patient includes a careful history and physical examination, imaging of the brain, and selective laboratory tests such as TSH, vitamin B_{12} level, complete blood count (CBC), and comprehensive metabolic panel. Screening for syphilis should also be considered.

APPROACH TO:
Dementia

DEFINITIONS

EXECUTIVE FUNCTIONS: High-level cognitive abilities that control other, more basic, abilities. Executive functions include the ability to start and stop behaviors, alter behaviors to fit circumstances, and adapt behaviors to new situations.

CLINICAL APPROACH TO DEMENTIA

Pathophysiology

The essential features of the diagnosis of dementia are memory loss and impairment of executive function. Dementia is a clinical diagnosis that can go unrecognized until it is in an advanced stage. Patients rarely report memory loss; the informants are usually their family members. However, relatives may fail to recognize signs and symptoms of dementia because many have a tendency to think that memory loss can be a part of normal aging. Studies of aging have showed that nonverbal creative thinking and new problem-solving strategies may decline with age, but information, skills learned with experience, and memory retention remain intact.

Differential Diagnosis. Depression in the elderly **can present with symptoms of memory disturbance.** This is known as "pseudodementia." As depression is common and treatable, a screening test for depression should be performed when dementia is evaluated. Similarly, hypothyroidism and vitamin B_{12} deficiency are common and treatable conditions that can cause cognitive problems. TSH and vitamin B_{12} levels should be performed as a routine part of the workup. Neurosyphilis could present in this fashion but is such an uncommon diagnosis that routine screening would not be recommended. Evaluation for neurosyphilis would be warranted if there were identified high-risk factors or history of the disease, or if the patient lived in an area with a high prevalence of syphilis. Neuroimaging with either a noncontrast CT scan or an MRI of the brain is recommended to rule out other confounding diagnoses. Other testing, such as positron emission tomography, genetic testing, and spinal fluid analysis, is not routinely recommended. Referral to neurology is appropriate when a diagnosis is uncertain.

Clinical Presentation

Clinicians should assess cognitive function whenever cognitive impairment or deterioration is suspected. These concerns may be based upon direct observation, patient report, or concerns raised by family members, friends, or caretakers. Patients with dementia may have difficulty with one or more of the following:

- Learning and retaining new information (rely on lists, calendars)
- Handling complex tasks (banking, bills, payments)
- Reasoning (adapting to unexpected situations, unfamiliar environments)
- Spatial ability and orientation (getting lost driving or walking, wandering)

- Language (word finding, repetition, confabulation)
- Behavior (agitation, confusion, paranoia)

Evaluation. The evaluation of a patient with suspected dementia should include a mental status examination. The **Folstein MMSE** is one of the most widely used tool in the screening for dementia. The sensitivity of the MMSE for dementia is as high as 87%, and the specificity is as high as 82%. The interpretation of the score depends on the patient's education level. It is most accurate in those with at least a high school education.

Another valuable test that can be used in a busy primary care setting is the **clock drawing test.** The patient is asked to draw a clock with a specific time. The patient must then accurately draw the clock face with the "big hand" and "small hand" in the correct positions. It is quick, easy to administer, and evaluates executive function in multiple cognitive domains. Other brief cognitive screening tests, such as the Short Portable Mental Status Questionnaire, modified MMSE, MoCA, and Mini-Cog (three-item recall combined with clock drawing) can be used. In the outpatient setting, the Mini-Cog and the MoCA are widely used.

In the evaluation of dementia, it is necessary to obtain information from people who know the patient well. Useful information can be obtained from informant-based functional tests, such as the functional activities questionnaire (FAQ), the instrumental activities of daily living (IADL), and caregiver burden assessments. This information can be important for providers and families in making plans for long-term care. See Case 18 for more on functional assessment.

Vascular Dementia

Vascular dementia, or multi-infarct dementia, is the second most common cause of dementia. In vascular dementia, there is neuronal loss as a consequence of one or more strokes. The **symptoms are related to the amount and location of the neuronal loss.** Vascular dementia can exist along with Alzheimer disease or other causes of dementia, resulting in a mixed-dementia syndrome. Unlike Alzheimer disease, which is a gradually progressive process, **vascular dementia often has a sudden onset and progresses in a stepwise fashion.** Patients tend to function at a certain level and then show an acute deterioration when the initial, or subsequent, infarcts occur. The risk factors include those for cerebrovascular disease (hypertension, tobacco use, diabetes, etc). There are no controlled trials showing medication effectiveness in vascular dementia, so the treatment is aimed at reducing the risk of further neurologic damage.

Lewy Body Dementia

Lewy body dementia is the third most common form of dementia. This dementia presents early on with **vivid hallucinations, fluctuation in cognition, and often parkinsonian extrapyramidal signs and postural instability.** Tremor is less apparent, and levodopa is not very effective in these patients. Daytime drowsiness and sleeping, staring into space for prolonged periods of time, and episodes of disorganized speech can further distinguish Lewy body dementia from Alzheimer disease. Therapies are similar to those for Alzheimer disease.

Frontotemporal Lobe Dementia

Frontotemporal lobe dementia is the fourth most common form of dementia, and due to the behavior disturbances associated with this dementia, it can be very distressing for the patient's family. In this form of dementia, a patient's personalities can significantly change, becoming antisocial or disinhibited from social norms with poor impulse control. Patients can develop apathy; emotional blunting; perseveration behaviors, including echolalia; and stereotypical behaviors, such as toe tapping and repetitive motor activity. There are few pharmacologic therapies with significant evidence for efficacy. Counseling and support of the family can mitigate the stress of caring for these patients.

Other Illnesses Associated With Dementia

Numerous other conditions may present with dementia or have dementia as a prominent symptom. **Parkinson disease** commonly has an associated dementia, especially as the overall disease advances. **Huntington disease** is an autosomal dominant disorder that presents with progressive dementia, depression, and choreiform movements. Dementia can be a complication of **chronic alcohol abuse,** reinforcing the need for a complete history of substance use. Potentially reversible forms of dementia include **normal-pressure hydrocephalus** (presents with the triad of dementia, gait disturbance, and urinary incontinence); **chronic subdural hematoma; repeated head trauma;** and **depression.** Many **prescription and over-the-counter medications** can cause memory disturbances. Chief among these are anticholinergic medications, sedatives (benzodiazepines), sleeping pills, and narcotic pain medications. **Metabolic abnormalities,** such as hyponatremia or abnormal calcium levels, and infections, such as **HIV,** can present with signs and symptoms similar to dementia.

Delirium

Delirium is an **acute change in mental status that is characterized by fluctuations in levels of consciousness.** It is usually caused by an acute medical illness, the use of a medication, or the withdrawal from a drug or alcohol. Delirium affects 10% to 30% of hospitalized patients, with a higher incidence in the elderly, in those with an underlying dementia, and in those with multiple underlying medical conditions. **The treatment of delirium consists of addressing the condition that precipitated it.** Delirium is often reversible if the underlying cause can be found and aggressively managed. Patients with delirium have significantly longer hospital stays and increased mortality rates.

CLINICAL APPROACH TO ALZHEIMER DISEASE

Pathophysiology

Alzheimer disease is the most common cause of dementia. Although a definitive diagnosis can only be made by the presence of senile plaques and neurofibrillary tangles detected on autopsy, clinical diagnostic criteria have been developed. **Common diagnostic criteria include the gradual onset and progression of cognitive dysfunction in more than one area of mental functioning that is not caused by**

another disorder. These areas of mental functioning include learning and memory, language, executive function, complex attention, perceptual-motor skills, and social cognition.

Clinical Presentation

The initial evaluation includes a detailed history from both the patient and another informant (usually a spouse, child, or other close contact) and complete physical and neurologic examinations to evaluate for any focal neurologic deficit that may be suggestive of a focal neurologic lesion. **A validated test, such as the MMSE, should be used to confirm the presence of dementia.** The results of this test can also be used to follow the clinical course, as a reduction in score over time is consistent with worsening dementia.

A focused evaluation to rule out other causes of dementia must be performed as well. The physical examination should focus upon neurologic deficits consistent with prior strokes, signs of Parkinson disease (eg, cogwheel rigidity and/or tremors), gait abnormalities or slowing, and eye movements. Patients with Alzheimer disease generally have no motor deficits at presentation.

Treatment

When the diagnosis of Alzheimer disease is made, a comprehensive care plan should be initiated. **The management of Alzheimer disease must be directed toward both the patient and the patient's family or caregivers.** The goals of therapy are to maximize cognition, delay functional decline, and prevent or improve behavioral disturbances.

Table 32–1 lists the medications that are primarily used in the treatment of Alzheimer disease. Family members should understand that the **medications may delay the progression of the disease but may not reverse any decline that has already**

Table 32–1 • MEDICATIONS USED IN THE TREATMENT OF ALZHEIMER DEMENTIA		
Medications	Indications	Side Effects/Comments
Cholinesterase Inhibitors		
Donepezil (Aricept)	Mild-moderate Alzheimer dementia	Common: nausea, vomiting, diarrhea, dizziness, headaches
Galantamine (Razadyne)	Mild-moderate Alzheimer dementia	Common: nausea, vomiting. Uncommon and severe: arrhythmias, dementia bradycardia, urinary obstruction
Rivastigmine (Exelon)	Mild-moderate Alzheimer dementia	Common: nausea, vomiting, diarrhea, weight loss, tremor, fatigue, falls
N-Methyl-D-aspartate (NMDA) antagonist		
Memantine (Namenda)	Moderate-severe Alzheimer dementia	Side-effect profile comparable to placebo; can be used in combination with cholinesterase inhibitors

occurred. For that reason, the medications may be more beneficial if started earlier in the course of the disease.

Antipsychotic medications have also been used to control hallucinations and agitation in patients with Alzheimer disease. However, this is an "off-label" use of medication, and data show a higher death rate associated with the use of the newer antipsychotics. The Food and Drug Administration has placed a black box warning against the use of typical and atypical antipsychotic medications for dementia-related psychosis due to the increased risk of deaths. Herbal medications such as gingko biloba and huperzine A have inconsistent evidence for efficacy, but appear to be safe alternatives. These should not be used with prescription medications due to potential interactions.

Behavioral interventions also may be beneficial. These can include scheduled toileting in an effort to reduce episodes of incontinence, writing reminder notes, keeping familiar objects around, providing adequate lighting, and making duplicates of important objects (eg, keys) in case they are lost. Caregivers also need support and may benefit from appropriate training, support groups, and periodic respite care.

Unfortunately, even with the best of care, Alzheimer disease is relentless and progressive. Families may have significant difficulties and conflicts regarding issues surrounding end-of-life care and placement in assisted living or nursing homes. Resources such as local chapters of the Alzheimer Association (https://www.alz.org) may provide valuable services, information, and support.

CASE CORRELATION

- See Case 18 (Geriatric Health Maintenance and End-of-Life Issues).

COMPREHENSION QUESTIONS

32.1 A 63-year-old man is brought in by his family because of memory loss. They have noted a worsening of his symptoms over several months. They also report that he has had multiple falls, hitting his head on one occasion, and has had frequent urinary incontinence. On examination, a gait apraxia (slow shuffling steps) is noted. Which of the following is the most likely diagnosis?

A. Alzheimer disease

B. Normal pressure hydrocephalus

C. Dementia with Lewy bodies

D. Delirium

32.2 An 82-year-old woman is admitted to the hospital for altered mental status. Her family says that she has been confused, falling asleep frequently, and hallucinating—talking to people who are not in the room. Her family reports that prior to this illness, the patient was independent and "sharp as a tack." On urine analysis, she is found to have a urinary tract infection. Which of the following is the most appropriate treatment?

A. Start rivastigmine (Exelon) for worsening of Alzheimer dementia.

B. Start an alerting agent such as modafinil (Provigil) for symptomatic treatment of her hypersomnia.

C. Start an antibiotic for treatment of her infection and optimize management of any other medical conditions.

D. Give her a dose of ziprasidone (Geodon) for her hallucinations.

32.3 A 77-year-old man is brought to your office by his wife, who states that he has been having mental difficulties in recent months, such as not being able to balance their checkbook or organize the paperwork for his annual visit with the accountant. She also tells you that he has reported seeing animals in the room with him and that he can describe them vividly. He takes frequent naps and stares blankly for long periods of time. He seems almost normal at times, but then he randomly appears very confused at other times. He has also been dreaming a lot and has fallen down more than once recently. He currently takes aspirin, 81 mg/d. On examination, the patient walks slowly with a stooped posture and almost falls when turning around. He has only minimal facial expressiveness. No tremor is noted, and the remainder of the examination is normal. He is able to recall three words out of three, but clock drawing is abnormal. Laboratory studies are normal, and CT of the brain shows changes of aging. What type of dementia does this patient most likely have?

A. Dementia with Lewy bodies

B. Alzheimer disease

C. Frontotemporal dementia

D. Vascular dementia

E. Dementia of Parkinson disease

32.4 A 66-year-old woman is brought in to the office by her family because of difficulty with memory and being disoriented. These mental status changes have worsened over the past 6 months. A careful history and physical examination is performed, which confirms cognitive impairment but no focal neurological findings. Which of the following tests is most appropriate next diagnostic step in this patient?

A. Head CT or MRI

B. Lumbar puncture

C. Rapid plasma reagin

D. Electroencephalogram

ANSWERS

32.1 **B.** Normal-pressure hydrocephalus classically causes the triad of dementia, incontinence, and gait disturbance. All of the other listed conditions (answer A, Alzheimer disease; answer C, dementia with Lewy bodies; and answer D, delirium) may cause memory disturbance, but the constellation of these three symptoms is most consistent with normal-pressure hydrocephalus. Also, delirium is usually of acute onset and not over months.

32.2 **C.** Treat the underlying infection. This scenario is one that is commonly seen in elderly patients and is consistent with delirium. The patient is elderly and has an infection, causing both an acute change in her mental status and a fluctuating level of consciousness. The main cause of sepsis in an older patient is urinary tract infection. The treatment is to address the underlying infection and any associated medical conditions. Dementia (answer A) does not likely explain the patient's mental status since this is an abrupt change. Answer D (ziprasidone) for hallucinations may be indicated, but it is not as important as addressing a possibly life-threatening condition of urinary tract infection.

32.3 **A.** This patient has dementia with Lewy bodies, which is the third most common type after Alzheimer disease and vascular dementia. He demonstrates typical signs and symptoms, including well-formed hallucinations, fluctuating cognition, sleep disorder with periods of daytime sleeping, frequent falls, deficits in visuospatial ability (abnormal clock drawing), and REM (rapid eye movement) sleep disorder (vivid dreams). In Alzheimer disease (answer B), the predominant early symptom is memory impairment without the other symptoms found in this patient. In dementia of Parkinson disease (answer E), extrapyramidal symptoms such as tremor, bradykinesia, and rigidity precede the onset of memory impairment by more than 1 year. Hallucinations are not as common with Parkinson disease. Frontotemporal dementia (answer C) presents with behavioral changes, including disinhibition, or language problems, such as aphasia.

32.4 **A.** This 66-year-old woman has a 6 month history of progressive cognitive decline consistent with dementia. A noncontrast head CT or MRI is recommended by the American Academy of Neurology for the routine evaluation of dementia. All of the other tests (answer B, lumbar puncture; answer C, rapid plasma reagin; and answer D, electroencephalogram) may be appropriate if there is a finding on the history or examination that calls for further testing (an exposure to syphilis, episodes suggestive of seizures, or symptoms of normal-pressure hydrocephalus for which a spinal tap may be performed).

CLINICAL PEARLS

▶ Consider a broad differential diagnosis in patients who present with "memory problems" and be sure to perform a thorough history and physical examination, cognitive testing, laboratory studies, and imaging diagnostic workup.

▶ The presentation of acutely altered mental status (delirium) should prompt an aggressive workup for an underlying cause, as treatment may result in correction of the mental status.

▶ Alzheimer disease is a disease of the family, not just the individual. It is critical to treat the patient while giving support to the caregivers.

REFERENCES

Alzheimer's Association. Home page: https://www.alz.org

American Geriatric Society website: https://www.americangeriatrics.org

American Psychiatric Association. *Diagnostic and Statistical Manual of Mental Disorders*, 5th ed. Arlington, VA: American Psychiatric Association; 2013.

Cardarelli E, Kertesz A, Knebl JA. Frontotemporal dementia: a review for primary care physicians. *Am Fam Physician.* 2010;82(11):1372-1377.

Falk N, Cole A, Meredith TJ. Evaluation of suspected dementia. *Am Fam Physician.* 2018;97(6):398-405.

Neef D, Walling AD. Dementia with Lewy bodies: an emerging disease. *Am Fam Physician.* 2006;73(7):1223-1230.

Seeley WW, Miller BL. Alzheimer's Disease. In: Jameson J, Fauci AS, Kasper DL, Hauser SL, Longo DL, Loscalzo J. eds. *Harrison's Principles of Internal Medicine,* 20e New York, NY: McGraw Hill. http://accessmedicine.mhmedical.com/content.aspx?bookid=2129&sectionid=192532255. Accessed May 19, 2020.

A 20-year-old woman comes to clinic for an annual physical examination. She has no complaints. She has no significant medical or surgical history. She is currently taking oral contraceptive pills because of irregular menstrual cycles. She attained menarche at age 13 years and has had irregular cycles since. She has never been sexually active. Her family history is positive for hypertension, diabetes, and obesity in her parents. On examination, her blood pressure is 120/85 mm Hg, her pulse is 78 beats/min, and her respiratory rate is 14 breaths/min. Her weight is 188 lb, and she is 63 inches tall. Her physical examination is unremarkable except for a brownish/black, velvety thickening of the skin on the back of her neck, hirsutism, and abdominal obesity. Her laboratory test results included total cholesterol of 202 mg/dL, high-density lipoprotein (HDL) cholesterol of 35 mg/dL, low-density lipoprotein (LDL) cholesterol of 120 mg/dL, and triglycerides of 172 mg/dL. Her fasting glucose was 104 mg/dL, and she had normal renal and liver function tests.

▶ What are the clinical issues that need to be addressed during this preventive visit?
▶ What is your next step in the evaluation of this patient?
▶ What are the therapeutic options available for this patient?

ANSWERS TO CASE 33:

Obesity

Summary: A 20-year-old woman presents with

- Obesity—body mass index (BMI) of 33.5 kg/m²
- History of menarche at age 13 years and irregular cycles since then
- Acanthosis nigricans and hirsutism
- Total cholesterol of 202 mg/dL, HDL cholesterol of 35 mg/dL, LDL cholesterol of 120 mg/dL, triglycerides of 172 mg/dL, and fasting glucose of 104 mg/dL
- Family history of hypertension, diabetes, and obesity in her parents

Clinical issues to address: Obesity and possible polycystic ovarian disease.

Next step in evaluation: Calculate a BMI, measure waist circumference, and repeat blood pressure evaluation. Order laboratory testing to measure thyroid-stimulating hormone (TSH).

Therapeutic options: Ask about her interest in losing weight. Advise on the health benefits of weight loss, address other risk factors, and collaborate with the patient to devise weight-loss goals; advise on diet and physical activity to achieve these goals. Assess her ability and desire to follow the plan developed together and explore options to achieve goals. Arrange follow-up. At subsequent visits, you can consider adding pharmacotherapy as an adjunct to diet and exercise.

ANALYSIS

Objectives

1. Be able state the etiology and pathogenesis of obesity. (EPA 12)
2. Be able to state other comorbid conditions associated with obesity. (EPA 12)
3. Be able to state the diagnostic criteria for obesity and metabolic syndrome. (EPA 3)
4. Be able to state the therapeutic options available for the management of obesity. (EPA 4)

Considerations

Obesity is a chronic and stigmatizing disease that begins early in life. Increased caloric intake, types of foods consumed, decreased physical exertion, and genetic predisposition are common causes of obesity. Routine physical examination visits serve as a good platform to address issues related to obesity and its associated comorbid conditions. This visit should be taken as an opportunity to address obesity, metabolic risk, and its management.

Increased body weight is a major risk factor for the development of disease and for premature death. Metabolic syndrome is an important risk factor for the subsequent development of type 2 diabetes and cardiovascular disease (CVD).

Metabolic syndrome is more common in overweight and obese patients and has a higher prevalence in those age $\geq$ 60. It is a worldwide health issue and is present in approximately one-third of Americans age 18 and over. This patient has metabolic syndrome based on her abdominal circumference, increased triglycerides, low HDL, and mildly elevated LDL cholesterol levels. She may also need further investigation for the presence of polycystic ovary syndrome (PCOS) because of her obesity, hirsutism, and history of irregular cycles. PCOS should be a consideration in patients with chronic anovulation, ovarian cysts, and evidence of hyperandrogenism. Both metabolic syndrome and PCOS are very closely associated with obesity and insulin resistance.

Based on the provided information, in this situation, the key clinical implication of these diagnoses is identification of a patient needing aggressive lifestyle modification focused on weight reduction and increased physical activity.

APPROACH TO:
Obesity

DEFINITIONS

BODY MASS INDEX: A measurement of the relative composition of lean body mass and body fat; calculated as (Weight in kilograms)/(Height in meters)^2.

METABOLIC SYNDROME (SYNDROME X, INSULIN RESISTANCE SYNDROME): A constellation of metabolic abnormalities that confer increased risk of CVD and diabetes mellitus. Major features include central obesity, hypertriglyceridemia, low HDL cholesterol, hyperglycemia, and hypertension.

OBESITY: A state of excess adipose tissue mass. Defined by most authorities as BMI of $\geq$ 30 kg/m^2. Morbid obesity is defined as a BMI $\geq$ 40 kg/m^2. Super obesity is defined as a BMI $\geq$ 50 kg/m^2.

OVERWEIGHT: Defined as BMI $\geq$ 25 kg/m^2, the point at which all-cause, metabolic, cancer, and cardiovascular morbidity begin to rise.

SATIATION: Level of fullness during a meal.

SATIETY: Level of fullness/satisfaction (lack of hunger) after a meal.

CLINICAL APPROACH

Epidemiology

Obesity is a chronic and easily diagnosed disease that is associated with life-threatening morbidity and mortality. Data from the National Health and Nutrition Examination Surveys (NHANES) show that in 2015 to 2016, obesity affected 18.5% of 2- to 19-year-olds and 39.8% of adults aged 20 years or older. The prevalence of obesity was higher in middle-aged adults (42.8%) compared to young adults (35.7%).

Table 33–1 • DIAGNOSTIC CRITERIA FOR METABOLIC SYNDROME	
Three of more of the following:	
Waist circumference	> 102 cm (male) or > 88 cm (female)
Hypertriglyceridemia	Triglycerides ≥ 150 mg/dL or specific medication
Low HDL cholesterol	< 40 mg/dL (male) or < 50 mg/dL (female) or specific medication
Hypertension	≥ 130 mm systolic or ≥ 85 mm diastolic or specific medication
Fasting plasma glucose	≥ 100 mg/dL or specific medication or previously diagnosed type 2 diabetes

HDL, high-density lipoprotein.

Metabolic Syndrome. Current minimum estimates are that the prevalence of metabolic syndrome in the United States is at least 34.5% using the National Cholesterol Education Program's 3rd Adult Treatment Panel (ATP III) criteria (Table 33–1). Metabolic syndrome is an important risk factor for subsequent development of type 2 diabetes and CVD. Thus, the key clinical implication of a diagnosis of metabolic syndrome is identification of a patient needing aggressive lifestyle modification focused on weight reduction and increased physical activity.

Pathophysiology

Energy balance is the relationship of energy intake to energy expenditure. When more energy is expended than taken in, weight loss ensues. When the intake of energy exceeds the amount expended, weight gain occurs. Thus, **obesity is caused by positive caloric balance and quality of food ingested, and it is relative to the amount of energy expended through physical activity.** Risk of obesity is affected by genetic, physiologic, and environmental factors. A positive energy imbalance results in weight gain and obesity, but the possible causes of positive energy imbalance are not well understood and are likely different for different people.

It has been **estimated that genetic background can explain 40% or more of the variance in body mass in humans.** The genetic component is complex and involves the interaction of multiple genes. However, the marked increase in obesity cannot be completely attributed to genetics. Social factors such as lower education level, lower socioeconomic class, and diet composition are all associated with a high risk of obesity. Likewise, physiologic factors such as various gut hormones, level of spontaneous physical activity (fidgeting), and age-related decline in energy expenditure are key determinants in regulation of food intake and energy expenditure. An **increase in energy consumption with a decrease in physical activity is thought to be the main contributor to the current obesity epidemic.** Additionally, the availability of convenience foods and the increase in palatability and serving size, compounded with industrialization leading to a sedentary lifestyle, have led to an altered energy balance.

Screening. The US Preventive Services Task Force recommends screening all adult patients for overweight and obese statuses by measuring height and weight and calculating BMI as part of the routine physical examination. BMI is used as

Table 33–2 • DEFINITION OF OBESITY BASED ON BMI		
	BMI (kg/m^2)	Obesity Class
Underweight	< 18.5	
Normal	18.5-24.9	
Overweight	25.0-29.9	
Obesity	30.0-34.9	I
	35.0-39.9	II
Extreme obesity (also called morbid or severe obesity)	> 40	III
Super obesity	> 50	III

a measure of weight status and as a tool to predict risk of disease, as it generally correlates well as an estimate of total body fat. However, **BMI is not as accurate a measure of being overweight/obese in patients with heart failure, pregnant women, bodybuilders, professional athletes, elderly patients, and certain ethnic groups.** Moreover, abdominal obesity is associated with increased risk for hypertension, heart disease, dyslipidemia, and diabetes. Additional measurements, like waist circumference and waist-to-hip ratio, need to be used to accurately identify the population at risk. Direct measurement of percentage of body fat may also provide additional information. Table 33–2 lists the classification of overweight/obese statuses based on BMI.

Along with the measurements mentioned, a health history, physical examination, and focused laboratory workup should be performed to look for complications and comorbid conditions. Any previous weight-loss efforts, recent smoking cessation, daily physical activity levels, and eating habits should be assessed to identify factors that might be contributing to weight gain and obesity.

Laboratory Workup. A **fasting glucose and glycosylated hemoglobin** level should be measured to evaluate for diabetes mellitus and impaired glucose tolerance. The presence of acanthosis nigricans—a velvety, hyperpigmented thickening of the skin commonly found on the neck and axillary regions—may also be a sign of insulin resistance. **Fasting lipids** should also be measured, both to evaluate for the presence of metabolic syndrome and for the assessment of the patient's risk for CVD. **TSH** should be measured to screen for hypothyroidism. **Liver enzymes** should be requested, as abnormal results may indicate the development of a fatty liver.

Treatment

The goal of therapy is to prevent, treat, or reverse the complications of obesity and improve quality of life. Treatment of obesity should begin in patients with a BMI greater than 25 kg/m^2 or who have visceral obesity, documented by increased waist circumference greater than 40 inches in men and greater than 35 inches in women, or a waist-to-hip ratio greater than 0.9 in men and greater than 0.85 in women. Weight loss of as little as 5 pounds (2.3 kilos) reduces the risk of developing comorbid conditions. Developing a **treatment plan** for obesity is complex and should use a **combination of dietary/caloric modifications, increased physical activity, and behavior therapy** as a gold standard.

Dietary Changes. Dietary intervention is the cornerstone of weight-loss therapy. Most diets work in two principal dimensions: energy content and nutrient composition. The National Heart, Lung, and Blood Institute recommends initiating treatment with a calorie deficit of 500 to 1000 kcal/d compared with the patient's habitual diet. This reduction produces a weight loss of 1 to 2 lb/wk (0.45 to 0.91 kg/wk). **Loss of more than 5% of initial body weight can improve CVD risk.** There are different kinds of specific dietary modifications recommended, but they all work based on caloric expenditure greater than intake through portion control. The selection of a diet should be based upon patient preferences to promote optimal dietary adherence, a key determinant of weight loss irrespective of the type and nutrient composition of the diet. Portion control should not compromise the nutrient content of the diet; patients should still aim for a balanced meal. Most diets (both low carbohydrate and low fat) have good short-term results but limited long-term efficacy, with patients typically losing 5% of body weight over the first 6 months, then returning to the initial weight by 12 to 24 months. A "Mediterranean" diet or low-carbohydrate diet may be more effective for modest long-term weight loss compared to a low-fat diet.

Physical Activity. The addition of exercise training to a diet program can add to the weight loss. **Physical activity alone is not an effective method for achieving weight loss,** although it is very important for long-term weight management and cardiovascular health benefits. Physical activity can improve insulin sensitivity and glycemic control, decrease abdominal fat, and reduce cardiovascular risk. Patients should engage in moderate-to-vigorous physical activity for at least 30 min/d, 5 to 7 d/wk, both to maintain weight loss and for the independent health benefits of exercising.

Other Lifestyle Modifications. The purpose of behavior modification therapy is to help patients identify and make long-term changes in their eating and physical activity habits that contribute to obesity. The targets of behavior modification are avoiding triggers, maintaining dietary diaries, using portion-controlled plates, slowing the rate of eating to enhance satiation, avoidance of high-risk situations, increasing physical activity, and breaking repetitive behaviors, such as watching TV while eating.

Pharmacotherapy. Table 33–3 lists the medications commonly used in the treatment of obesity. Pharmacologic therapy may be offered to those with a BMI greater than 30 kg/m² or BMI of 27 to 30 kg/m² with comorbid conditions. Orlistat, lorcaserinphenteramine/topiramate, naltrexone ER (extended release)/bupropion ER and liraglutide are US Food and Drug Administration (FDA) approved for long-term weight-loss management. All of these approved medications have generally been found to have modest weight loss over placebo and often are limited in efficacy due to side effects and/or cost.

With the exception of orlistat, which inhibits the absorption of dietary fat by inhibiting pancreatic lipases, all medications approved for obesity act as anorexiants. Anorexiant medications increase satiation, satiety, or both. Increasing satiation results in a reduction in the amount of food eaten, and increasing satiety reduces the frequency of eating. FDA-approved medications are generally recommended to be used as short-term adjuncts to diet, exercise, and behavioral modification. Their use should be tapered off after prolonged use or if there is lack of efficacy.

Table 33–3 • MEDICATIONS USED IN THE TREATMENT OF OBESITY

Drug Name (Trade Name)	Mechanism of Action	Notes
Bupropion-naltrexone (Contrave)	Antidepressant and opioid antagonist	Not recommended as first line. Can be used in obese smokers who want to quit. Full cardiovascular effects are unknown, but this should not be used with uncontrolled hypertension. Warn about suicidal ideation in young adults.
Dextroamphetamine (Dexedrine, Dextrostat)	Sympathomimetic (increased norepinephrine release)	Numerous drug interactions; stimulant side effects include insomnia, agitation, tachycardia, hypertension; additive effects with other stimulants (caffeine, cold medications, etc); can be addicting; avoid with monoamine oxidase (MAO) inhibitors; all indicated for short-term (generally interpreted as up to 12 weeks) use only.
Phendimetrazine (Bontril)	Sympathomimetic (increased norepinephrine release)	
Diethylpropion (Tenuate)	Sympathomimetic (increased norepinephrine release)	
Phentermine (Fastin, Pro-Fast, Ionamin, Adipex-P)	Sympathomimetic (increased norepinephrine release)	
Phentermine-topiramate (Qsymia)	Sympathomimetic (increased norepinephrine release) and anticonvulsant	Significant side effects of topiramate include paresthesias, somnolence, and difficulty concentrating. Topiramate has also been associated with metabolic acidosis.
Lorcaserin (Belviq)	Serotonin receptor agonist	Selective serotonin 2C receptor agonist (less cardiac side effects than nonselective serotonin agonists).
Orlistat (Xenical, Alli)	Selective inhibitor of pancreatic lipase, results in reduced intestinal digestion of fat and increased fecal fat excretion	Recommended as first-line pharmacotherapy along with behavioral and dietary changes. Gastrointestinal side effects common: diarrhea, fecal incontinence, bloating, cramps, gas, oily stools; must follow low-fat diet to reduce side effects; may give vitamin supplements for decreased absorption of fat-soluble vitamins (A, D, E) and beta-carotene; indicated for short- or long-term use.
Liraglutide (Saxenda)	Glucagon-like peptide-1 (GLP-1) agonist causing appetite suppression	3-mg subcutaneous injection once daily (after 4-week escalation); inform patient of unconfirmed risk of thyroid tumors; risk of pancreatitis. Common side effects include nausea, vomiting, diarrhea, and increased heart rate.

Metformin and glucagon-like peptide-1 (GLP-1) receptor agonists (medications approved for treatment of type 2 diabetes mellitus) may be a useful adjunct for weight loss in patients with comorbid obesity. Metformin can also help with weight loss in patients with PCOS.

Many previously approved medications for weight loss have been removed from the market due to significant risks greater than benefits. Over-the-counter weight-loss medications and supplements have similar risk-benefit profiles or have limited research for safety and efficacy.

Bariatric Surgery. **Patients with a BMI greater than 40 kg/m² who have failed diet and exercise (with or without drug therapy), or greater than 35 kg/m² with serious comorbid conditions, are potential candidates for surgical treatment of obesity.** Weight-loss surgeries fall into one of two categories: restrictive and restrictive-malabsorptive. Restrictive surgeries, such as laparoscopic adjustable gastric banding, limit the amount of food the stomach can hold and slow the rate of gastric emptying. Restrictive-malabsorptive bypass procedures, such as the Roux-en-Y gastric bypass, combine the elements of gastric restriction and selective malabsorption.

The two most common surgeries done are Roux-en-Y gastric bypass and laparoscopic adjustable gastric banding, or "lap banding." The Roux-en-Y procedure involves the construction of a small (10- to 30-mL) gastric pouch that empties into a segment of jejunum. With the small pouch and the small outlet to limit caloric intake, the Roux-en-Y is mostly a restrictive procedure with some degree of associated malabsorption. The surgical mortality rate from bariatric surgery is generally < 1% but varies with the procedure, patient's age and comorbid conditions, and experience of the surgical team. The most common surgical complications include stomal stenosis or marginal ulcers (occurring in 5% to 15% of patients) that present as prolonged nausea and vomiting after eating or inability to advance the diet to solid foods.

In lap banding, an adjustable silicone gastric band is laparoscopically placed around the upper stomach just distal to the gastroesophageal junction. The band has a balloon connected to a subcutaneously implanted port, which can be inflated or deflated to reduce the circumference of the band. Complications of the banding procedure are less common and less severe than in gastric bypass, but the long-term weight loss may also be less. The adjustable band allows for the flexibility of addressing various nutritional demands after the surgery. For example, the band can be adjusted to have the stoma widened to accommodate a greater demand for caloric and fluid intake when a patient becomes pregnant.

Complications

Obesity is a risk factor for the development of diabetes and CVD, as well as numerous other medical conditions (Table 33–4). In general, greater BMI is associated with more health complications, and grade II or higher obesity is associated with greater risk of mortality. Also, the more complications that develop, the more difficult it becomes to manage the underlying obesity. For example, a person with degenerative arthritis and heart disease may have significant symptoms during exercise, impairing his or her ability to expend more energy in an effort to lose weight.

Table 33–4 • COMMON MEDICAL COMPLICATIONS OF OBESITY
Cardiovascular disease
Cerebrovascular disease
Cholelithiasis
Chronic kidney disease
Degenerative joint disease
Eating disorders
Hyperlipidemia
Hypertension
Infertility/reduced fertility
Malignancies
Menstrual cycle irregularities
Mood disorders
Nonalcoholic fatty liver disease/nonalcoholic steatohepatitis
Polycystic ovary syndrome
Psychosocial dysfunction
Sleep apnea
Type 2 diabetes mellitus

CASE CORRELATION

- See also Case 15 (Thyroid Disorders), Case 35 (Hyperlipidemia), and Case 50 (Menstrual Cycle Irregularity).

COMPREHENSION QUESTIONS

33.1 A 35-year-old man presents to the clinic stating that he has been experiencing chest pain and shortness of breath and is having increased episodes of asthma exacerbation. He is 5 ft 10 inches and weighs 399 lb. An electrocardiogram in the office shows a normal sinus rhythm. He performs very little physical activity due to his weight. He has friends but has some esteem issues because of his weight issue. He has tried to lose weight but has not been successful in many attempts at dieting. He asks about who would be candidates for bariatric surgery. Which of the following patients has the best evidence to be a candidate for bariatric surgery as initial treatment for obesity?

A. A man with a BMI of 32 kg/m^2 and arthritis of the knees.

B. A woman with a BMI of 33 kg/m^2 and type 2 diabetes.

C. A woman with a BMI of 42 kg/m^2 but no identifiable complications.

D. Any obese patient who desires bariatric surgery should have it offered.

33.2 A patient with a BMI of 35 kg/m² whom you have been seeing for 10 years recently lost his job as a truck driver due to uncontrolled obstructive sleep apnea and need for insulin to control his diabetes. He states that he does not really think that he is "fat." For which of the following patients is a BMI measurement most likely to be an accurate assessment of obesity?

A. A bodybuilder with a BMI of 38 kg/m²

B. A pregnant woman with a BMI of 31 kg/m² in her 37th week of gestation

C. A man with congestive heart failure, pitting edema, and a BMI of 30 kg/m²

D. A hypertensive woman with a BMI of 32 kg/m²

33.3 A 34-year-old woman comes to your clinic to discuss weight management. She is currently 5 ft 2 inches and 265 lb. She says she always had a hard time managing her weight as a child, but she let things get out of control when she was living on her own in college. She has had two children in the past 5 years. With her first child, she gained 50 lb during the pregnancy and lost 30 lb after delivery. With the second child, she gained 35 lb and lost 10 lb. She has tried many diets where she initially loses weight but eventually gains the weight back. She exercises some but is limited by osteoarthritis of the knees. She has thought about gastric bypass but is fearful of undergoing a surgical procedure. Which of the following medications is the best option for the long-term management of her obesity?

A. Orlistat

B. Phendimetrazine

C. Dextroamphetamine

D. Phentermine

ANSWERS

33.1 **C.** The best evidence for bariatric surgery is for people with a BMI of greater than 40 kg/m² who have failed diet and exercise (with or without drug therapy), or those with a BMI of greater than 35 kg/m² and obesity-related complications. Answer A (BMI of 32 kg/m² and knee arthritis) is not an indication since the BMI is not > 35 kg/m². Patients with grade I obesity with diabetes mellitus (answer B) or significant medical conditions can be considered for bariatric surgery, but the evidence of benefit over risk is less robust. Bariatric surgery can be effective but carries significant risks and should not automatically be offered to all obese patients who request it (answer D).

33.2 **D.** A BMI reading will not accurately assess the ratio of lean body mass to body fat in highly muscled persons such as weightlifters and athletes (answer A), persons with decreased muscle mass such as the elderly population, pregnant women because of the enlarged uterus and fetus (answer B), and patients with symptomatic congestive heart failure due to the pedal edema (answer C).

33.3 **A.** Orlistat is indicated for the long-term treatment of obesity. The mechanisms of this agent are as a lipase inhibitor and decreasing fat absorption. Orlistat promotes weight loss and leads to about a 2- to 3-kg loss over a year. All of the pure stimulant medications (answer B, phendimetrazine; answer C, dextroamphetamine; and answer D, phentermine) should be for short-term use only.

CLINICAL PEARLS

▶ Obesity is a chronic disease that is reaching epidemic status in the United States and worldwide.

▶ Body mass index is a common tool used to grade obesity, but in certain cases it may be inadequate.

▶ Obesity treatment should always include dietary modifications and portion control, increased activity, and behavioral modifications.

▶ Even 5% to 15% weight loss can significantly reduce the complications associated with obesity.

REFERENCES

Curry SJ, Krist AH, Owens DK, et al. US Preventive Services Task Force. Behavioral weight loss interventions to prevent obesity-related morbidity and mortality in adults: US Preventive Services Task Force recommendation statement. *JAMA*. 2018;320(11):1163-1171. doi:10.1001/jama.2018.13022.

Flier JS, Maratos-Flier E. Pathobiology of Obesity. In: Jameson J, Fauci AS, Kasper DL, Hauser SL, Longo DL, Loscalzo J. eds. *Harrison's Principles of Internal Medicine, 20th ed.* New York, NY: McGraw Hill. http://accessmedicine.mhmedical.com/content.aspx?bookid=2129&sectionid=192288213. Accessed May 21, 2020.

Garvey WT, Mechanick JI, Brett EM, et al; American Association of Clinical Endocrinologists/American College of Endocrinology (AACE/ACE) Comprehensive Clinical Practice Guidelines for Medical Care of Patients with Obesity. *Endocr Pract*. 2016.

Hales CM, Carroll MD, Fryar CD, Ogden CL. *Prevalence of Obesity Among Adults and Youth: United States, 2015–2016*. Hyattsville, MD: National Center for Health Statistics; 2017. NCHS data brief, no 288.

Moore JX, Chaudhary N, Akinyemiju T. Metabolic syndrome prevalence by race/ethnicity and sex in the United States, National Health and Nutrition Examination Survey, 1988–2012. *Prev Chronic Dis*. 2017;14:160287.

Moyer VA; US Preventive Services Task Force. Screening for and management of obesity in adults: US Preventive Services Task Force recommendation statement. *Ann Intern Med*. 2012;157(5):373-378.

Via MA, Mechanick JI. Chapter 26. Metabolic Syndrome. In: Fuster V, Harrington RA, Narula J, Eapin ZJ. eds. *Hurst's The Heart, 14th ed.* New York, NY: McGraw Hill; 2017.

A 33-year-old woman presents with a complaint of headaches. She has had headaches since she was a teenager, but they have become more debilitating recently. The episodes occur once or twice each month and last for up to 2 days. The pain begins in the right temple or at the back of the right eye and spreads to the entire scalp over a few hours. She describes the pain as a sharp, throbbing sensation that gradually worsens and is associated with severe nausea. Several factors aggravate the pain, including loud noises and movement. She has taken several over-the-counter (OTC) medications for the pain, but the only thing that works is going to sleep in a quiet, darkened room. A thorough history reveals that her mother suffers from migraine headaches. Her vital signs, general physical examination, and a thorough neurologic examination are all within normal limits.

► What is the most likely diagnosis?
► What imaging study is most appropriate at this time?
► What are the most appropriate therapy?

ANSWERS TO CASE 34:
Migraine and Other Headache Syndromes

Summary: A 33-year-old woman presents with

- Headaches that have occurred since she was a teenager and have progressively worsened
- Right-sided, throbbing headaches and nausea that worsen with loud noises and movement and are relieved by sleeping in a dark, quiet room
- No relief from headaches from OTC preparations
- Family history of migraines in mother
- Vital signs, general physical examination, and thorough neurologic examination that are all within normal limits

Most likely diagnosis: Migraine without aura.

Most appropriate imaging study: No imaging is indicated at this time since there are no "red flag" symptoms or signs.

Most appropriate therapy: A "triptan" medication given in a means that does not have to be swallowed (subcutaneous, intranasal, or orally dissolving tablet).

ANALYSIS

Objectives

1. State a differential diagnosis for chronic headaches. (EPA 2)

2. List the red flag symptoms and signs that should prompt rapid, specific diagnostic and treatment interventions. (EPA 1, 10)

3. Describe the management of common headache syndromes. (EPA 4)

Considerations

The patient described in the case has symptoms that are very characteristic of migraine without aura. Her headaches are unilateral, throbbing in nature, and have been progressively worsening. Migraines typically cause recurrent episodes of headache, nausea, and vomiting. They can also be associated with other neurologic symptoms, such as photophobia, lightheadedness, paresthesias, vertigo, and visual disturbances. In the patient described in this case, the history and lack of physical findings can reasonably lead to the diagnosis of migraine headaches without aura ("common migraine"), the most frequently occurring form. Other classifications of migraines include migraine with aura ("classic migraine"), ophthalmoplegic migraine, retinal migraine, and childhood periodic syndromes that may be precursors to or associated with migraines. During the evaluation of this patient, the focus should be on determining the etiology of the headache, assessing for any red flags that may indicate worse pathologic causes, identifying triggers, and determining appropriate therapy for the condition.

According to the International Headache Society, symptoms diagnostic of migraine headache include moderate-to-severe headache with a pulsating quality; unilateral location; nausea and/or vomiting; photophobia; phonophobia; worsening with activity; multiple attacks lasting from 4 hours to 3 days; and absence of history or physical examination findings that would make it likely that the headache is the result of another cause.

APPROACH TO:
Migraine and Other Headache Syndromes

DEFINITIONS

CHRONIC DAILY HEADACHE: Experiencing headache on 15 days or more per month. Chronic daily headache (CDH) is not a single entity; it can encompass a number of headache syndromes, including chronic tension headaches, migraines, infection, inflammation, trauma, and medication overuse.

CLUSTER HEADACHE: Unilateral headaches that may have a high male predominance; can be located in the orbital, supraorbital, or temporal region. Pain is generally described as deep and excruciating, lasting from 15 minutes to 3 hours. These headaches are usually episodic; however, a small subset may have chronic headaches.

MIGRAINE HEADACHES: Vascular headaches typically throbbing and unilateral in character; may be present with or without an aura. There is a high female predominance.

PRIMARY HEADACHE SYNDROME: Syndrome in which headache and associated features occur in the absence of any exogenous cause. The most common are migraine, tension-type headache, and cluster headache.

TENSION HEADACHE: The most common primary headache syndrome, typically presenting with pericranial muscle tenderness and a description of a bilateral band-like distribution of the pain.

CLINICAL APPROACH TO MIGRAINES

Pathophysiology

Headaches are an extremely common complaint in primary care, urgent care, and emergency settings. The vast majority of adults have at least one headache each year, although most do not present for medical care. Migraine headaches are the most common headaches of vascular origin and the second most common cause of headaches overall. Migraines are a member of a group of primary headache syndromes differentiated by their associated features. Diagnostic criteria for migraine headaches are listed in Table 34–1.

Table 34–1 • SIMPLIFIED DIAGNOSTIC CRITERIA FOR MIGRAINE	
Repeated attacks of headache lasting 4-72 h in patients with a normal physical examination, no other reasonable cause for the headache, and	
At Least 2 of the Following Features:	**Plus at Least 1 of the Following Features:**
Unilateral pain	Nausea/vomiting
Throbbing pain	Photophobia and phonophobia
Aggravation by movement	
Moderate or severe intensity	

Adapted from the International Headache Society Classification (Headache Classification Committee of the International Headache Society, 2004).

Functional limitations during headaches will determine the categorization of the migraine and the choice of treatment (see Table 34–2). Clinicians should stratify treatment based on severity rather than using stepped care.

The role of the practitioner is to attempt to accurately diagnose the cause of the headache, rule out secondary causes of headaches ("red flags") that may signify a serious underlying pathology, provide appropriate acute management, and assist with headache prevention when needed. It is important that each individual headache be evaluated in the context of the patient's prior headaches. The clinician should remain alert to the possibility of a secondary cause for the headache. Migraine headaches do not preclude the presence of underlying pathology.

Clinical Presentation

History. The medical history in a patient with headaches should focus on several important areas. The quality and characteristics of the headache and its specific location and radiation should be identified. The presence and extent of associated symptoms, especially neurologic symptoms that may suggest the presence of a focal neurologic lesion or increased intracranial pressure, must be documented. The age at which the patient first developed the headaches, the frequency and duration of the headaches, and the amount of disability and distress that is caused to the patient should be explored. It is also important to note what the patient has done to try to treat the headaches in the past, including as much detail as possible regarding medication usage (both prescription and OTC).

Physical Examination. The examination should include both a general examination and a detailed neurologic examination. A fundoscopic examination revealing papilledema may be supportive of the presence of increased intracranial pressure.

Table 34–2 • MIGRAINE SEVERITY LEVELS	
Mild	Patient is aware of a headache but able to continue daily routine.
Moderate	The headache inhibits daily activities but is not incapacitating.
Severe	The headache is incapacitating.
Status	A severe headache that has lasted more than 72 h.

Table 34–3 • "RED FLAG" SYMPTOMS AND SIGNS IN THE EVALUATION OF HEADACHES

Red Flag	Differential Diagnosis	Workup Studies
Sudden-onset maximum severity "worst headache" or new and different headache	Subarachnoid hemorrhage, pituitary apoplexy, hemorrhage into a mass lesion or vascular malformation, mass lesion	Neuroimaging first; lumbar puncture if neuroimaging negative
Headaches increasing in severity and frequency, brought on by Valsalva or physical exertion	Mass lesion, subdural hematoma, medication overuse	Neuroimaging, drug screen
Headache beginning after age 50, especially if jaw pain on chewing (jaw claudication)	Temporal arteritis, mass lesion	Neuroimaging, erythrocyte sedimentation rate level
New-onset headache in patient with risk factors for HIV infection or cancer	Meningitis, brain abscess (including toxoplasmosis), metastasis	Neuroimaging first; lumbar puncture if neuroimaging negative
Headache with signs of systemic illness (fever, stiff neck, rash)	Meningitis, encephalitis, Lyme disease, systemic infection, collagen vascular disease	Neuroimaging, lumbar puncture, serology
Focal neurologic signs or symptoms of disease (other than typical aura)	Mass lesion, vascular malformation, stroke, collagen vascular disease	Neuroimaging, collagen vascular evaluation (including antiphospholipid antibodies)
Papilledema	Mass lesion, pseudotumor cerebri, meningitis	Neuroimaging, lumbar puncture
Headache subsequent to head trauma	Intracranial hemorrhage, subdural hematoma, epidural hematoma, posttraumatic headache	Neuroimaging of brain, skull, and cervical spine

Data from South-Paul JE, Matheny SC, Lewis EL, et al. Current Diagnosis and Treatment in Family Medicine. *2004.* Copyright © McGraw Hill LLC. All rights reserved.

Identifying a focal neurologic deficit increases the likelihood of finding a significant central nervous system pathology as the cause of the headache.

Imaging. A patient with symptoms and signs consistent with migraine who does not have any red flag findings (see Table 34–3) does not require any further testing prior to instituting treatment. Neuroimaging should be performed if there is an unexplained neurologic abnormality on examination or if the headache syndrome is not typical of either migraines or some other primary headache disorder. The **presence of rapidly increasing headache frequency or a history of lack of coordination, focal neurologic symptom, or headache awakening the patient from sleep raises the likelihood of finding an abnormality on an imaging test.** Magnetic resonance imaging may be more sensitive than computed tomography (CT) scanning for the identification of abnormalities, but it may not be more sensitive at identifying *significant* abnormalities. CT scan would be the initial imaging for "thunderclap" headaches where intracranial bleeds are considered. Other testing (eg, blood tests, electroencephalogram) should only be performed for diagnostic purposes if there is a suspicion based on the history or physical examination.

Treatment

The treatment of headache is best individualized based on a thorough history, physical examination, and the interpretation of any additional study results.

Nonpharmacologic Treatment. Migraines can often be managed to some degree by a variety of nonpharmacologic approaches. Nonpharmacologic treatment can include patient education, bed rest in a dark room, and removal of known triggers. Most patients benefit from simple avoidance of specific headache triggers. Lifestyle modifications may be helpful. These could include diet changes, regular exercise, regular sleep patterns, avoidance of excess caffeine and alcohol, and avoidance of acute changes in stress levels. Migraine patients do not encounter more stress or triggers than the general population; however, they may have overresponsiveness to these triggers.

First-line Medications. First-line therapies for mild-to-moderate migraines include oral nonsteroidal anti-inflammatory drugs (NSAIDs) and acetaminophen. Triptans are used as a first-line agent for moderate-to-severe migraines. Triptans come in a variety of forms (oral, sublingual, subcutaneous), and patients may demonstrate responsiveness to one triptan but not to others.

Second-line Medications. Second-line therapies for migraines include intranasal dihydroergotamine and opioids. Antiemetics, such as prochlorperazine or metaclopramide, can also be used. For refractory migraines, intravenous dihydroergotamine can be used as long as a triptan was not administered in the preceding 24 hours. Intravenous magnesium, valproic acid, and dexamethasone are other alternatives.

Treating Children and Pregnant Women. Pregnant women with migraines can use a combination of acetaminophen and metoclopramide (which are the only safe options in pregnancy). In children who experience migraines, ibuprofen and acetaminophen can be used. Certain triptans (rizatriptan, sumatriptan, and almotriptan) can be considered in children as well.

Chronic migraines (more than two or three migraines per week) may require daily prophylaxis with beta-blockers, calcium channel blockers, amitriptyline, or topiramate. Options for pharmacologic treatment and prophylaxis of migraines are listed in Tables 34–4 and 34–5, respectively.

CLINICAL APPROACH TO OTHER HEADACHE SYNDROMES

Tension-Type Headache

Clinical Presentation. Tension headache is the **most prevalent form of primary headache disorder,** typically presenting with pericranial muscle tenderness and a description of a bilateral band like distribution of the pain. Headaches can last from 30 minutes to 7 days, and there is no aggravation by routine physical activity. There is no associated nausea or vomiting. Photophobia and phonophobia are both absent, or one, but not the other, is present. They can be either episodic (< 180 days/year) or chronic (> 180 days/year).

Table 34–4 • TREATMENT OF ACUTE MIGRAINE

Drug	Trade Name	Dosage
I. Simple Analgesics		
Acetaminophen, aspirin, caffeine	Excedrin Migraine	Two tablets or caplets every 6 h (max 8 per day)
II. NSAIDs		
Naproxen	Aleve, Anaprox, generic	220-550 mg orally twice daily
Ibuprofen	Advil, Motrin, Nuprin, generic	400 mg orally every 3-4 h
Tolfenamic acid	Clotam Rapid	200 mg orally; may repeat ×1 after 1-2 h
Diclofenac potassium	Cambia	50 mg orally (powder packet mixed with water)
III. 5-HT$_1$ Receptor Agonists		
• Oral		
Ergotamine 1 mg, caffeine 100 mg	Cafergot	One or two tablets at onset, then one tablet every ½ h (max 6 per day, 10 per week)
Naratriptan	Amerge	2.5-mg tablet at onset; may repeat once after 4 h
Rizatriptan	Maxalt Maxalt-MLT	5- to 10-mg tablet at onset; may repeat after 2 h (max 30 mg/d)
Sumatriptan	Imitrex	50- to 100-mg tablet at onset; may repeat after 2 h (max 200 mg/d)
Frovatriptan	Frova	2.5-mg tablet at onset; may repeat after 2 h (max 5 mg/d)
Almotriptan	Axert	12.5-mg tablet at onset; may repeat after 2 h (max 25 mg/d)
Eletriptan	Relpax	40 or 80 mg
Zolmitriptan	Zomig Zomig Rapimelt	2.5-mg tablet at onset; may repeat after 2 h (max 10 mg/d)
• Nasal		
Dihydroergotamine	Migranal Nasal Spray	Prior to nasal spray, the pump must be primed 4 times; 1 spray (0.5 mg) is administered, followed in 15 min by a second spray
Sumatriptan	Imitrex Nasal Spray	5-20 mg intranasal spray as 4 sprays of 5 mg or a single 20-mg spray (may repeat once after 2 h, not to exceed a dose of 40 mg/d)
Zolmitriptan	Zomig	5-mg intranasal spray as 1 spray (may repeat once after 2 h, not to exceed a dose of 10 mg/d)

(Continued)

Table 34–4 • TREATMENT OF ACUTE MIGRAINE (continued)		
Drug	Trade Name	Dosage
III. 5-HT₁ Receptor Agonists (Cont.)		
• Parenteral		
Dihydroergotamine	DHE-45	1 mg IV, IM, or SC at onset and every 1 h (max 3 mg/d, 6 mg per week)
Sumatriptan	Imitrex Injection Alsuma Sumavel DosePro	6 mg SC at onset (may repeat once after 1 h for max of 2 doses in 24 h)
IV. Dopamine Receptor Antagonists		
• Oral		
Metoclopramide	Reglan,ᵃ genericᵃ	5-10 mg/d
Prochlorperazine	Compazine,ᵃ genericᵃ	1-25 mg/d
• Parenteral		
Chlorpromazine	Genericᵃ	0.1 mg/kg IV at 2 mg/min; max 35 mg/d
Metoclopramide	Reglan,ᵃ generic	10 mg IV
Prochlorperazine	Compazine,ᵃ genericᵃ	10 mg IV
V. Other		
• Oral		
Acetaminophen, 325 mg, *plus* dichloralphenazone, 100 mg, *plus* isometheptene, 65 mg	Midrin, generic	Two capsules at onset followed by 1 capsule every 1 h (max 5 capsules)
• Nasal		
Butorphanol	Generic	1 mg (1 spray in 1 nostril), may repeat if necessary in 1-2 h
• Parenteral		
Opioids	Genericᵃ	Multiple preparations and dosages

Abbreviations: 5-HT, 5-hydroxytryptamine; IV, intravenous; IM, intramuscular; max, maximum; NSAIDs, nonsteroidal anti-inflammatory drugs; SC, subcutaneous.
Note: Antiemetics (eg, domperidone 10 mg or ondansetron 4 or 8 mg) or prokinetics (eg, metoclopramide 10 mg) are sometimes useful adjuncts.
ᵃNot all drugs are specifically indicated by the FDA for migraine. Local regulations and guidelines should be consulted.
Reproduced with permission, from Kasper D, Fauci A, Hauser S, et al, eds. Harrison's Principles of Internal Medicine. 19th ed. 2015. Copyright © McGraw Hill LLC. All rights reserved.

Treatment. Initial medical therapy of episodic tension-type headache includes aspirin, acetaminophen, and NSAIDs. Combination analgesics containing caffeine are second-line options. Use of analgesics for more than 15 days a month may paradoxically lead to a "rebound" or medication overuse headache. Measures to minimize risk of medication overuse headaches include limiting use of drugs to treat acute headache to two to three days/week, avoiding opioids and sedative hypnotics, and monitoring medication intake.

The general management principles for the treatment of migraine headaches can also be applied to the treatment of chronic tension-type headaches. In frequent

Table 34–5 • PREVENTIVE TREATMENTS IN MIGRAINE[a]		
Drug	Dose	Selected Side Effects
Pizotifen[b]	0.5-2 mg daily	Weight gain Drowsiness
Beta-blockers		
Propranolol	40-120 mg twice daily	Reduced energy
Metoprolol	25-100 mg twice daily	Tiredness Postural symptoms Contraindicated in asthma
Antidepressants		
Amitriptyline	10-75 mg at night	Drowsiness
Dosulepin	25-75 mg at night	
Nortriptyline	25-75 mg at night	*Note:* Some patients may only need a total dose of 10 mg, although generally 1-1.5 mg/kg body weight is required
Venlafaxine	75-150 mg daily	
Anticonvulsants		
Topiramate	25-200 mg daily	Paresthesias Cognitive symptoms Weight loss Glaucoma Caution with nephrolithiasis
Valproate	400-600 mg twice daily	Drowsiness Weight gain Tremor Hair loss Fetal abnormalities Hematologic or liver abnormalities
Serotonergic drugs		
Methysergide[c]	1-4 mg daily	Drowsiness Leg cramps Hair loss Retroperitoneal fibrosis (1-mo drug holiday is required every 6 mo)
Other classes		
Flunarizine[b]	5-15 mg daily	Drowsiness Weight gain Depression Parkinsonism
Candesartan	16 mg daily	Dizziness

(Continued)

Table 34–5 • PREVENTIVE TREATMENTS IN MIGRAINE[a] (continued)		
Drug	Dose	Selected Side Effects
Chronic migraine		
Onabotulinum toxin type A	155 U	Loss of brow furrow
No convincing evidence from controlled trials		
Verapamil		
Controlled trials demonstrate *no effect*		
Nimodipine		
Clonidine		
Selective serotonin reuptake inhibitors: fluoxetine		

[a]Commonly used preventives are listed with typical doses and common side effects. Not all listed medicines are approved by the US Food and Drug Administration; local regulations and guidelines should be consulted.
[b]Not available in the United States.
[c]Not currently available worldwide.
Reproduced with permission, from Kasper D, Fauci A, Hauser S, et al, eds. Harrison's Principles of Internal Medicine. 19th ed. 2015. Copyright © McGraw Hill LLC. All rights reserved.

headache sufferers, the combination of antidepressant medications and stress management therapy reduces headache activity significantly. Other prophylactic treatments of chronic tension-type headaches include electromyographic biofeedback, acupuncture, cognitive behavioral therapy, and relaxation training. Pharmacologic therapies for prophylaxis include amitriptyline as a first line, mirtazapine, venlafaxine, calcium channel blockers, and beta-blockers.

Cluster Headache

Clinical Presentation. **Cluster headache** is strictly unilateral in location and can be located in the orbital, supraorbital, or temporal region. It is generally described as a deep, excruciating pain lasting from 15 minutes to 3 hours. The frequency can vary from one every other day to eight attacks per day. Cluster headaches are associated with ipsilateral autonomic signs and symptoms (conjunctivitis and rhinorrhea) and have a much greater prevalence in men. Compared to migraine sufferers, who often desire sleep and a quiet, dark environment during their headache, individuals with cluster headache pace around, unable to find a comfortable position.

Treatment. **The first-line treatment of cluster headache includes the use of 100% oxygen and triptans.** Second-line treatment for acute attacks includes intranasal lidocaine, dihydroergotamine, prednisone, octreotide, corticosteroids, and somatostatin. Verapamil, lithium, melatonin, and antiepileptics may be used for prophylactic treatment. Because of side effects related to chronic use, ergotamine and corticosteroids need to be used with caution.

Chronic Medical Conditions

Patients with certain underlying medical conditions have a greater incidence of having an organic cause of their headache. Patients with cancer may develop headaches as a consequence of metastases. Someone with uncontrolled hypertension (with diastolic pressures > 110 mm Hg) may present with the chief complaint of headache. Patients with HIV infection or AIDS may present with central nervous system metastases, lymphoma, toxoplasmosis, or meningitis as the cause of their headache. It is always important to evaluate each headache in context and consider secondary causes.

Medication-Related Headache

Numerous medications have headache as a reported adverse effect. Medication-overuse headache (formerly drug-induced or "rebound" headache) may occur following frequent use of any analgesic or headache medication. This includes both nonprescription (eg, acetaminophen, NSAIDs) and prescription medications. Caffeine use, whether as a component of an analgesic or a beverage, is another culprit in this category. The duration and severity of the withdrawal headache following discontinuation of the medication vary depending on the medication(s) involved. Any contributing, underlying psychological conditions that may lead to medication overuse may make discontinuation of the medication difficult and should be addressed.

CASE CORRELATION

- See also Case 30 (Hypertension) and Case 44 (Cerebrovascular Accident/ Transient Ischemic Attack).

COMPREHENSION QUESTIONS

34.1 A 28-year-old man presents for evaluation of headaches that have been going on for the past several days. He describes them as unilateral throbbing headaches that last 8 to 12 hours and occur once or twice day. When the headaches occur, he gets nauseated and just wants to go to bed. Usually, the headaches improve after he lies down in a dark, quiet room for the remainder of the day. He is missing significant work time due to the headaches. He has a normal examination today. Which of the following statements is the most appropriate next step for this patient?

A. Schedule a CT scan of his head.

B. Instruct the patient to breathe in 100% oxygen and use a triptan medication with next headache.

C. Recommend stress reduction and aspirin orally every 4 hours as needed.

D. Prescribe an injectable or nasal spray triptan.

34.2 A 52-year-old woman presents to your office for a severe headache of 2 hours' duration that began earlier that day. She says that the headache came on suddenly and is the worst headache she has ever had. She denies any head trauma. She has had migraines since she was an early adult. The pain is described as "stabbing" and is more severe on the left side. She takes no medications and recently stopped taking oral contraceptive pills after going through menopause. Her blood pressure is elevated at 145/95 mm Hg, but otherwise she has no focal neurologic abnormalities on examination. She is alert and oriented to person, place, time, and situation. Which of the following is the most appropriate management at this time?

A. Prescribe a triptan medication.

B. Schedule a noncontrast head CT scan for tomorrow morning.

C. Call 911 and transfer the patient to an emergency center.

D. Prescribe an antihypertensive medication and follow up in 2 weeks.

34.3 A 43-year-old man presents to the office for daily headaches that he has had now for several months. Every morning at work, usually between 9 and 10 AM, he develops a headache that is bilateral from his forehead to his neck area. He has to take 650 mg of acetaminophen to relieve the headache, and he says he takes the acetaminophen at 8 AM to try to prevent the headache. This has been going on for the past 3 months, and he is at the point of looking for a new job, as he thinks that job stress is the cause of his symptoms. His examination is normal. Which of the following is the most appropriate advice for him?

A. He should continue with the as-needed acetaminophen and find a less stressful career.

B. He should start an antidepressant for headache prophylaxis.

C. His headaches are most likely to improve if he stops taking the acetaminophen.

D. A triptan is an appropriate treatment for him.

ANSWERS

34.1 **D.** This patient gives a history very consistent with common migraine headaches. The best treatment is triptan medications (abortive therapy). There are no red flags found on history or examination that would be suggestive of an intracranial process such as neurological symptoms or rapidly progressive headaches, so no further testing such at CT imaging of the head (answer A) is necessary at this point. As he has significant nausea, he may benefit from something other than an oral medication. A triptan delivered by injection or nasal spray is a reasonable starting point for him. Answer B (100% oxygen) can be helpful with cluster headaches; often nasal congestion or drainage is found with this condition. Answer C (aspirin and stress relief) is somewhat reasonable in that the stress relief recommendation may be helpful, though this advice may be most useful for tension headaches.

34.2 **C.** The acute onset of the most severe headache in a patient's life is concerning for the presence of a subarachnoid hemorrhage (SAH). This is a medical emergency, and delay in diagnosis and treatment can lead to death. This patient should be transported by emergency medical services to the nearest emergency facility for stabilization and management. Scheduling imaging for the next day (answer B) or following up in 2 weeks (answer D) will be too long an interval in the case of SAH.

34.3 **C.** This patient very well could have the recently described "medication overuse headache," in which the daily use of medication such as acetaminophen or aspirin or other agents can exacerbate primary headaches (migraines, tension, or cluster). This patient likely has tension headaches, which may be due to the daily use of acetaminophen. If the headaches resolve when he stops the acetaminophen, then the diagnosis is confirmed and treatment enacted. While finding a new, less-stressful job (answer A) may be beneficial, the problem will not resolve until he discontinues the daily use of his OTC analgesic. Answer D (triptan medication) is useful for migraine headaches, which would usually present as a unilateral, throbbing headache.

CLINICAL PEARLS

▶ Migraine headaches can occur in children and adolescents as well as adults.

▶ Most patients presenting for the evaluation of headaches do not need diagnostic testing beyond the history and physical. However, the presence of focal neurologic deficits or other red flag symptoms/signs should prompt an immediate workup or referral.

▶ Tension headache is the most prevalent form of primary headache disorder, typically presenting with pericranial muscle tenderness and a description of a bilateral band-like distribution of the pain.

▶ Cluster headache is strictly unilateral in location and can be located in the orbital, supraorbital, or temporal region.

▶ An individual who complains of the worst headache of their life may have a subarachnoid hemorrhage, which is a life-threatening condition.

REFERENCES

Clinch C. Evaluation & management of headache. In: South-Paul JE, Matheny SC, Lewis EL, eds. *CURRENT Diagnosis & Treatment: Family Medicine.* 4th ed. New York, NY: McGraw Hill; 2015: Chap. 29. http://accessmedicine.mhmedical.com/content.aspx?bookid=1415&sectionid=77057346. Accessed May 7, 2019.

Goadsby PJ, Raskin NH. Migraine and other primary headache disorders. In: Kasper D, Fauci A, Hauser S, Longo D, Jameson J, Loscalzo J, eds. *Harrison's Principles of Internal Medicine.* 20 ed. New York, NY: McGraw Hill; 2018: Chap. 447. http://accessmedicine.mhmedical.com/content .aspx?bookid=1130&Sectionid=79755453. Accessed Jan 25, 2019.

Hainer BL, Matheson EM. Approach to acute headache in adults. *Am Fam Physician.* 2013;87(10):682-687.

Headache Classification Committee of the International Headache Society (IHS). The international classification of headache disorders, 3rd edition. *Cephalalgia.* 2018;38(1):1-211. doi:10.1177/0333102417738202.

Myans L, Walling A. Acute migraine headache: treatment strategies. *Am Fam Physician.* 2018; 97(4):243-251.

A 56-year-old man comes in for a routine health maintenance visit. He is new to your practice and has no specific complaints today. He has hypertension, for which he takes hydrochlorothiazide. He has no other significant medical history. He does not smoke cigarettes, occasionally drinks alcohol, and does not exercise. His father died of a heart attack at age 60 years, and his mother died at age 72 years of cancer. He has two younger sisters who are in good health. On examination, his blood pressure is 130/80 mm Hg, and his pulse is 75 beats/min. He is 6 ft tall and weighs 200 lb (body mass index [BMI] 27.1 kg/m²). His complete physical examination is normal. You order a fasting lipid panel, which subsequently returns with the following results: total cholesterol 242 mg/dL; triglycerides 138 mg/dL; high-density lipoprotein (HDL) cholesterol 48 mg/dL; and calculated low-density lipoprotein cholesterol (LDL-C) 166 mg/dL.

▶ What are the recommendations for providing statin therapy?
▶ What other laboratory testing is indicated at this time?
▶ What is the recommended management at this point?

ANSWERS TO CASE 35:

Hyperlipidemia

Summary: A 56-year-old man presents with

- Well-controlled hypertension
- Elevated cholesterol on a screening blood test as part of a physical examination
- No known history of coronary artery disease or of any coronary artery disease risk equivalent
- Family history of his father dying of a heart attack at age 60 years and his mother dying at age 72 years of cancer

Recommendations for statin treatment: American College of Cardiology/American Heart Association (ACC/AHA) and National Institute for Health and Care Excellence (NICE) guidelines recommend treatment with statins based on calculated risk using validated prediction rules.

Other laboratory testing at this time: Blood glucose, creatinine, liver function tests, and thyroid- stimulating hormone (TSH) to rule out secondary causes of hypercholesterolemia.

Recommended management: Therapeutic lifestyle changes (TLCs) with consideration for implementation of statin therapy.

ANALYSIS

Objectives

1. State the risk factors for cardiovascular disease (CVD). (EPA 12)

2. Be able to discuss the basic differences between the ACC/AHA, US Preventive Services Task Force (USPSTF), and NICE recommendations for prevention of CVD. (EPA 4)

3. Be able to counsel patients on TLCs to lower their cholesterol levels. (EPA 4, 12)

Considerations

This case illustrates a 56-year-old man with well-controlled hypertension and total cholesterol of 242 mg/dL; triglycerides of 138 mg/dL; HDL cholesterol of 48 mg/dL; and a calculated LDL-C of 166 mg/dL. Based on the pooled cohort risk equation, his 10-year risk of atherosclerotic CVD (ASCVD) is 9.3% (based on his age, race, nonsmoking status, controlled hypertension, total cholesterol, and HDL level). Whether medication for cholesterol levels is initiated at this time is based on the current recommendations you follow; however, any medication regimen should be accompanied by TLCs such as weight loss, exercise, and diet.

APPROACH TO:
Hyperlipidemia

DEFINITIONS

ACC/AHA: American College of Cardiology and American Heart Association, which made joint recommendations for cholesterol management based on risk assessment, updated in 2018.

HDL CHOLESTEROL: High-density lipoprotein cholesterol, also known as the "good cholesterol" and helps to decrease the serum LDL fraction by transporting the latter to the liver.

LDL CHOLESTEROL: Low-density lipoprotein cholesterol, also known as the "bad cholesterol", makes up most of the body's cholesterol, and increases the cardiovascular disease risk.

NICE: National Institute for Health and Care Excellence, which is based in the United Kingdom and made recommendations in 2014 for cholesterol management based on risk assessment.

STATIN: Medication in the beta-hydroxy-beta-methylglutaryl-coenzyme A (HMG-CoA)–reductase inhibitor class. These are the most widely used medications for lowering LDL cholesterol.

USPSTF: United States Preventive Services Task Force, which made recommendations in 2016 for cholesterol management based on risk assessment.

CLINICAL APPROACH

Pathophysiology

It is important to remember that cholesterol is not a disease. High cholesterol is a risk factor for coronary heart disease (CHD). As such, **an individual's cholesterol levels must be interpreted in the context of the individual's overall risks for CHD.**

When high blood cholesterol is identified, an investigation should be performed to evaluate for **secondary causes of dyslipidemia.** Included among these causes are **diabetes, hypothyroidism, obstructive liver disease, and chronic renal failure.** Consequently, a reasonable laboratory workup includes fasting blood glucose, TSH, liver enzymes, and a creatinine level. Certain medications, including progestins, anabolic steroids, and corticosteroids, also can result in elevated cholesterol. Consideration should be given to changing or discontinuing these when possible.

Statin Therapy Guidelines

In someone with known CHD, statin therapy is recommended in all guidelines. **The first-line pharmacotherapy for LDL-C reduction is a statin.** Statins not only reduce LDL-C but also reduce the rates of coronary events, strokes, cardiac death, and all-cause mortality.

Statin treatment for lipids is generally recommended for those with known ASCVD or diabetes mellitus type 2 as secondary prevention. Similarly, statin therapy is generally recommended for primary prevention in patients with no known ASCVD but a calculated high risk. Guidelines developed by the ACC/AHA in 2013 and updated in 2018, the USPSTF in 2016, and NICE in 2014 vary in their recommendations for primary prevention initiation and intensity of treatment with statins. Like many areas of medicine, the current guidelines for treatment of cholesterol are actively changing, and providers, in collaboration with their patients, have the opportunity to decide which recommendations to use.

The recommended intensity of the statin medication should be proportionate to the risk of CHD: the higher one's risk, the higher intensity the statin therapy should be. It also is important to note that for patients who do not tolerate high-intensity statins, using a lower intensity statin would still provide some cardiovascular benefit if the lower intensity statin can be tolerated. Assessment scores can overestimate or underestimate risk in certain groups, so use of the appropriate assessment tool for the patient is important. There are insufficient data to support one assessment tool over another for predicting cardiovascular risk. Comparison of ACC/AHA, USPSTF, and NICE guidelines is provided in Table 35–1.

ACC/AHA Guidelines. The ACC/AHA guidelines recommend statin therapy for all persons age 20 and up in the following four additional groups:

- **Patients ≤ 75 years old with clinical CVD**

- **Patients with LDL-C ≥ 190 mg/dL**

- **Patients age 40 to 75 years with diabetes and LDL-C ≥ 70 mg/dL**

- **Patients age 40 to 75 years with 10-year CVD risk ≥ 7.5% and LDL-C ≥ 70 mg/dL**

The risk assessment is based on the pooled cohort equations, which can be accessed online (http://static.heart.org/riskcalc/app/index.html#!/baseline-risk). The USPSTF also recommends using the pooled cohort equations for risk calculation.

NICE Guidelines. The NICE recommendations for the primary prevention of CVD use the QRISK®2 risk assessment tool, which includes renal disease in its calculation (https://www.qrisk.org). Statin therapy for adults should begin with a ≥ 10% ten-year risk. Statin therapy should begin with a focus on high intensity and low cost. NICE recommends offering atorvastatin 20 mg for primary prevention if 10-year risk ≥ 10% and to people age 85 years or older. If a statin is contraindicated or not tolerated, ezetimibe can be offered. For patients with known CHD, treatment should be started with atorvastatin 80 mg. NICE recommends against use of fibrates, nicotinic acid, anion exchange resins, or omega-3 fatty acids for primary or secondary prevention.

American Academy of Family Physicians Guidelines. The American Academy of Family Physicians (AAFP) released its clinical practice guideline with endorsement of the AHA/ACC recommendations, with qualifications, in June 2014. The key recommendations are listed in Table 35–2. The qualifications listed by the AAFP were that the CVD risk assessment tool has not been validated and may overestimate risk, and a cutoff of 7.5%, rather than 10%, will significantly increase the

Table 35–1 • ACC/AHA, NICE, AND USPSTF GUIDELINES FOR TREATING CHOLESTEROL

ACC/AHA Guidelines

Risk Category	Statin Therapy Recommended If	Reasonable to Consider Statin Therapy If
Clinical atherosclerotic cardiovascular disease	Age 20-75 years	Age > 75 years
LDL-C ≥ 190 mg/dL	Age ≥ 20 years	Not applicable
Diabetes plus LDL-C 70-189 mg/dL	Age 40-75 years	Age 21-40 years or > 75 years
Age 40-75 years plus LDL-C 70-189 mg/dL	Estimated 10-year risk of atherosclerotic cardiovascular disease ≥ 7.5%	Estimated 10-year risk of atherosclerotic cardiovascular disease 5% to < 7.5%
Age 20-39 years plus LDL-C ≥ 160 mg/dL	Not applicable	Early ASCVD in family history
Age 0-19 with lifestyle management	Familial severe hypercholesterolemia and premature ASCVD in family	Age 10, a LDL-C ≥ 190 or ≥ 160 with strong early family history

NICE Guidelines

Risk Category	Drug Recommendations
Existing cardiovascular disease (secondary prevention)	Atorvastatin 80 mg/d for all adults with cardiovascular disease Do not delay statin treatment in patients with acute coronary syndrome
10-year cardiovascular disease risk > 10%	Atorvastatin 20 mg/d
10-year cardiovascular disease risk < 10%	Optimize all other modifiable cardiovascular risk factors Statin not recommended

USPSTF Guidelines for Primary Prevention

Risk Category	Statin Therapy Recommended If	Statin Therapy
LDL > 190 mg/dL	No recommendation	
Age 40-75	Estimated 10-year risk of atherosclerotic cardiovascular disease < 10% and 1 or more risk factors	Consider low- to moderate-intensity statin
Age 40-75 years	Estimated 10-year risk of atherosclerotic cardiovascular disease ≥ 10% and 1 or more risk factors	Initiate low- to moderate-intensity statin
Age > 75 years	No recommendation	Insufficient evidence to recommend

Data from Dynamed, NICE, USPSTF, and ACC/AHA guidelines.

Table 35–2 • AAFP CLINICAL PRACTICE GUIDELINES KEY RECOMMENDATIONS FOR CHOLESTEROL MANAGEMENT

Individuals with LDL-C ≥ 190 mg/dL or triglycerides ≥ 500 mg/dL should be evaluated for secondary causes of hyperlipidemia.

Adults ≥ 21 years of age with a primary LDL-C ≥ 190 mg/dL should be treated with high-intensity statin therapy unless contraindicated.

Adults 40-75 years of age with an LDL-C 70-189 mg/dL without clinical ASCVD or diabetes and an estimated 10-year ASCVD risk ≥ 7.5% should be treated with moderate- to high-intensity statin therapy.

Adults 40-75 years of age with diabetes mellitus and an LDL-C 70-189 mg/dL should be treated with moderate-intensity statin therapy.

Individuals ≤ 75 years of age who have clinical ASCVD should be treated with high-intensity statin therapy unless contraindicated.

There is not enough evidence to recommend for or against treating blood cholesterol to target levels.

There is not enough evidence to recommend the use of nonstatin medication combined with statin therapy to further reduce ASCVD events.

Adapted from AAFP Clinical Practice Guideline on Cholesterol.

number of patients on statins. Also, many of the recommendations were based on expert opinion, although some points were evidence based, and 7 out of 15 members of the guideline panel had conflicts of interest. Nevertheless, it is indisputable that statin agents decrease mortality in patients with elevated LDL-C.

Other Forms of Treatment

Therapeutic lifestyle changes are the cornerstone of all treatments for hyperlipidemia. All patients should be educated on healthier living, including dietary modifications, increased physical activity, and smoking cessation. Weight reduction should be encouraged.

Specific dietary recommendations include limiting trans-fatty acid intake to < 1% of total calories, limiting saturated fats to < 7% of total calories, replacing saturated fats with polyunsaturated fats, and having a total intake of < 200 mg/d of cholesterol. Total dietary fat should be kept to no more than 35% of total calories, with < 10% polyunsaturated fat. AHA diet and lifestyle modifications include

- Balancing calorie intake and physical activity to achieve or maintain healthy body weight
- Consuming a diet rich in vegetables and fruits
- Choosing whole-grain, high-fiber foods
- Consuming fish, especially oily fish, at least twice a week
- Minimizing added sugars and sugary beverages
- Choosing low-salt foods
- Consuming alcohol in moderation

The addition of dietary soluble fiber and plant stanols/sterols can be beneficial as well. Soluble fiber (10 to 25 g) and plant stanols/sterols (2 g) can be added to reduce CVD and CHD risk. Referral to a dietician may be helpful as well. When TLC is instituted, regular follow-up must be arranged.

Therapeutic lifestyle changes should continue to be reinforced and encouraged even when starting medications. Ezetimibe is recommended as the second therapy for patients who cannot tolerate any level statin or have contraindications. A list of medications available for treatment of hyperlipidemia is included in Table 35–3.

Cholesterol treatment is an example of how recommendations can create controversy in the management of chronic disease. The recommendations for evaluation, treatment, and ongoing management of high cholesterol have changed

Table 35–3 • MEDICATIONS USED TO LOWER CHOLESTEROL

Drug Class/ Medication	Effects	Side Effects	Contraindications
Statin • Lovastatin • Pravastatin • Fluvastatin • Atorvastatin • Rosuvastatin • Simvastatin	LDL ↓18% to 55%; HDL ↑5% to 15%; triglytrides (TG) ↓7% to 30%	Myopathy, myalgia, increased liver enzymes	Active or chronic liver disease; relative contraindication with cytochrome P-450 inhibitors, cyclosporine, macrolides, antifungals
Bile acid sequestrants • Cholestyramine • Colestipol • Colesevelam	LDL ↓15% to 30%; HDL ↑3% to 5%; TG no change; or increase	Gastrointestinal distress, constipation, decreased absorption of other medications	Dysbetalipoprotein-emia; TG > 400
Nicotinic acids • Immediate-release, sustained-release, or extended-release nicotinic acid	LDL ↓5% to 25%; HDL ↑15% to 35%; TG ↓20% to 50%	Flushing, hyperglycemia, hyperuricemia, upper GI distress, hepatotoxicity	Absolute: chronic liver disease, severe gout Relative: diabetes, hyperuricemia, peptic ulcer disease
Fibric acids • Gemfibrozil • Fenofibrate	LDL ↓5% to 20%; HDL ↑10% to 20%; TG ↓20% to 50%	Dyspepsia, gallstones, myopathy, unexplained non-CHD deaths in a World Health Organization study	Severe renal disease, severe hepatic disease
Cholesterol absorption blocker • Ezetimibe	LDL ↓13% to 25%; HDL ↑3% to 5%; TG ↓5% to 14%	Abdominal pain, diarrhea	Hepatic insufficiency/ active liver disease
Monoclonal antibody, PCSK9 inhibitors • Evolocumab • Alirocumab	LDL ↓50% 82.3% LDL < 70	Nasopharyngitis, upper respiratory tract infection, influenza, back pain	Cost prohibitive

Abbreviation: PCSK9: Proprotein convertase subtilisin/kexin type 9.
Data from ATP III report, ezetimibe product information, and Sullivan et al.

significantly over recent years, with a focus on risk assessment. New development of treatments will also lend to ongoing changes in the future.

> ## CASE CORRELATION
> - See also Case 20 (Chest Pain) and Case 33 (Obesity).

COMPREHENSION QUESTIONS

35.1 A 62-year-old man is being seen in the office for establishment of care. He reports that he had an acute myocardial infarction (MI) 1 year previously and lost his insurance and has not been able to take any medications since his heart attack. He smokes half a pack a day, which is less than the 1 pack per day previously. On examination, his blood pressure is 110/60 mm Hg. The cardiac examination is normal, and there is no jugular vein distension or pedal edema. His LDL-C is 105 mg/dL, HDL cholesterol is 28 mg/dL, and total cholesterol is 170 mg/dL. According to the NICE guidelines, what medication therapy should be initiated at this time?

A. Ezetimibe

B. Atorvastatin

C. Niacin

D. Gemfibrozil

35.2 A 55-year-old woman presents to your office for follow-up. She was discharged from the hospital 1 week ago following an acute MI. She has quit smoking since that time and vows to stay off cigarettes forever. Her lipid levels are total cholesterol 240 mg/dL, HDL 50 mg/dL, LDL-C 160 mg/dL, and triglycerides 150 mg/dL. In addition to initiation of TLCs, which of the following is the most appropriate management at this time?

A. Nothing further

B. Start on a statin

C. Start on nicotinic acid

D. Start on a statin and nicotinic acid

35.3 A 48-year-old man is being seen for follow-up from an elevated cholesterol level at a health screening, which is recorded as 250 mg/dL. He denies significant medical history and has no symptoms. Which of the following tests is the most important further evaluation of this patient's condition?

A. Electrocardiogram (ECG)

B. Stress test

C. Complete blood count (CBC)

D. Thyroid-stimulating hormone level

ANSWERS

35.1 **B.** This patient has known CHD (prior acute MI) and should be started on statin therapy. A high-intensity statin dose should be initiated for secondary prevention of CVD. Other lipid agents (answer A, ezetimibe; answer C, niacin; and answer D, gemfibrozil) do not have as much efficacy in lowering mortality. Other agents that reduce mortality after an acute MI include baby aspirin and beta-blocking agents.

35.2 **B.** This patient has known CHD, documented by her recent MI. All guidelines recommend therapeutic life changes as an integral part of care. With known CHD, statin therapy is also indicated and has been shown to decrease mortality. Therefore, neither lifestyle changes alone (answer A) nor nicotinic therapy alone (answer C) are the best choice for this patient. ACC/AHA guidelines would recommend high-intensity statin therapy. Also, combined therapy with a statin agent and nicotinic agent (answer D) is not indicated unless the lipid levels are not controlled with maximal monotherapy.

35.3 **D.** Hypothyroidism is a potential cause of secondary dyslipidemia. A TSH level is a reasonable test to perform in this setting in a patient with an elevated cholesterol level. There is no indication to screen for CHD with an ECG (answer A) or stress test (answer B) in this asymptomatic person, who has no findings of CHD, stroke, or peripheral arterial disease. Other tests to perform could include fasting blood glucose, liver enzymes, and a measurement of renal function. A CBC (answer C) is often used as a screening test but would not be used to further diagnose hyperlipidemia.

CLINICAL PEARLS

▶ Lipid levels must always be interpreted in the context of the individual's overall risk factors for CHD.

▶ Statins have the best data to support improvement in outcomes that are clinically significant, such as heart attacks, strokes, and death. Unless there is a contraindication, a statin should be the first medication used for cholesterol reduction.

▶ Pharmacotherapy may be considered in patients with ASCVD risk above 7.5% according to ACC/AHA guidelines and 10% according to NICE and USPSTF guidelines.

▶ Remind patients who are taking lipid-lowering medications that lifestyle modifications are still necessary. Medications are not a substitute for a healthy lifestyle.

REFERENCES

2016 ACC expert consensus decision pathway on the role of non-statin therapies for LDL-cholesterol lowering in the management of atherosclerotic cardiovascular disease risk. *J Am Coll Cardiol.* 2016;68(1):92-125.

2017 focused update of the 2016 ACC expert consensus decision pathway on the role of non-statin therapies for LDL-cholesterol lowering in the management of atherosclerotic cardiovascular disease risk. *J Am Coll Cardiol.* 2017;70(14):1785-1822.

Grundy SM, Stone NJ, Bailey AL, Beam C, et al. 2018 AHA/ACC/AACVPR/AAPA/ABC/ACPM/ ADA/AGS/APhA/ASPC/NLA/PCNA guideline on the management of blood cholesterol: executive summary. *J Am Coll Cardiol.* 2019;73(24). doi:10.1016/j.jacc.2018.11.002

Last AR, Ference JD, Menzel ER. Hyperlipidemia: drugs for cardiovascular risk reduction in adults. *Am Fam Physician.* 2017;95(2):78-87.

National Cholesterol Education Program. The third report of the NCEP Expert Panel on the detection, evaluation and treatment of high blood cholesterol in adults. Item no: 02-5215; 2002.

National Institute for Health and Care Excellence (NICE). Lipid modification: cardiovascular risk assessment and the modification of blood lipids for the primary and secondary prevention of cardiovascular disease. *BMJ.* 2014;349:g4356.

Nayor M, Ramachandran VS. Recent update to the US cholesterol treatment guidelines: a comparison with international guidelines. *Circulation.* 2016;133:1795-1806.

Rader DJ, Kathiresan S. Disorders of lipoprotein metabolism. In: Kasper D, Fauci A, Hauser S, Longo D, Jameson J, Loscalzo J, eds. *Harrison's Principles of Internal Medicine.* 20th ed. New York, NY: McGraw Hill; 2018.

Sullivan D, Olsson AG, Scott R, Xue A, Gebski V, Wasserman SM, Stein EA. Effect of a monoclonal antibody to PCSK9 on low-density lipoprotein cholesterol levels in statin-intolerant patients: the GAUSS randomized trial. *JAMA.* 2012;308(23):2497-2506. doi:10.1001/jama.2012.25790

US Preventive Services Task Force. Statin use for the primary prevention of cardiovascular disease in adults: US Preventive Services Task Force recommendation statement. *JAMA.* 2016;316(19): 1997-2007. doi:10.1001/jama.2016.15450

A 20-month-old girl who is new to your practice is brought in by her mother because the child has been crying and not walking for the past day. Her mother reports that the child is "very clumsy and falls a lot." She says that the little girl may have injured her leg by falling off the sofa because, she repeats, "She really is clumsy and falls a lot." Upon review with the mother, she states that the child has no significant medical history and takes no medications regularly. There are two older children in the family, ages 4 and 6 years, who are in good health but also are "clumsy and forever hurting themselves." The husband lives in the home. Without any questioning or prompting, the mother states that her husband is "a good man but he's under a lot of stress." You ask the mother to undress the child for an examination, and she quickly replies, "Do you really have to undress her? She's very shy." You politely, but firmly, say that you need to examine her, and she removes the child's pants. You see that her right knee is visibly swollen and tender to palpation on the medial bony prominences. You also note numerous bruises of the buttocks and posterior thighs, which appear to be of different ages. There are also several small, circular scars on the legs, each about a centimeter in size. "See how clumsy she is?" the mother says, pointing to her bruises. An x-ray of the child's knee shows a corner fracture of the distal femoral metaphysis.

▶ What is the likely mechanism of this child's injuries?
▶ What further evaluation is necessary at this time?
▶ What legal obligation must a health care provider fulfill in this circumstance?

ANSWERS TO CASE 36:

Family Violence

Summary: A 20-month-old girl presents with

- Crying and not walking
- Multiple bruises at different stages of healing and circular wounds that are suspicious for cigarette burns
- Knee x-ray that shows a metaphyseal corner fracture, an injury that is inconsistent with the stated history of "falling off the sofa"
- Reports from her mother that the child is "clumsy and falls a lot"

Most likely mechanism of injuries: Inflicted injuries, including leg injury from forceful pulling, bruising from hitting the child's legs, and cigarette burns.

Further evaluation at this time: Complete, unclothed physical examination of the child (including ophthalmoscopic and neurologic examinations); radiographic skeletal survey.

Legal obligation: Report suspected child abuse to the appropriate child protective services organization.

ANALYSIS

Objectives

1. Be able to state the symptoms and signs suggestive of child maltreatment and abuse. (EPA 1, 2)

2. Be able to state the situations in which the risk of family violence increases. (EPA 12)

3. Be able to state the medicolegal requirements involved in situations of family violence. (EPA 5, 9, 12)

Considerations

Family violence can occur in families of any socioeconomic class and in households of any composition. The term *family violence* **includes child abuse, intimate partner violence (IPV), and elder abuse.** The abuse that occurs can be physical, sexual, emotional, psychological, or economic. It can take the forms of battering, raping, threatening, intimidating, isolating from friends and family, stealing, and preventing the earning of money, among many others.

In the case presented here, there are several signs of intentionally inflicted injuries to the child. The presence of **numerous bruises of varying ages**, especially on relatively protected areas such as the buttocks and upper posterior thighs, should raise suspicion. Finding injuries inconsistent with the reported history also can be a clue. Certain types of fractures, such as **metaphyseal corner fractures** (caused by forceful jerking or twisting of the leg), are usually a result of abuse. The identification of wounds consistent with cigarette burns is highly specific for abuse.

Clinicians often find dealing with these situations extremely difficult and uncomfortable. They may feel caught between two partners—both of whom are patients—who give conflicting stories. They may have concerns about the legal implications of their findings and fear legal actions if they make reports to authorities. They may have frustrations in dealing with a person who will not leave an abusive spouse and may feel ill-trained to deal with many of these situations. By becoming familiar with situations in which family violence is more likely to occur, knowing the laws regarding disclosure and reporting, and learning to recognize the signs of family violence, clinicians can be better prepared to address these situations when they occur.

APPROACH TO:
Family Violence

DEFINITIONS

CHILD MALTREATMENT: An inclusive term covering physical abuse; sexual abuse; emotional abuse; parental substance abuse; physical, nutritional, and emotional neglect; supervisional neglect; and Munchausen syndrome by proxy.

ELDER MISTREATMENT: Intentional or neglectful acts by a caregiver or trusted individual that harm a vulnerable older person.

NEGLECT: Failure to provide the needs required for functioning or for the avoidance of harm.

PHYSICAL ABUSE (BATTERY): Intentional physical actions (eg, biting, kicking, punching) that can cause injury or pain to another person.

CLINICAL APPROACH

Screening

Family violence is a pattern of abusive behavior in any relationship in which one individual gains or maintains power or control over another individual. This abuse can take the form of physical violence (battery), sexual violence, intimidation, emotional and psychological abuse, economic control, neglect, threats, and isolation from others. During screening, evaluation, and intervention related to cases of domestic and family violence, it is important to consider cultural influences and the unique dynamics of special populations (eg, lesbian, gay, bisexual, transgender, older couples, and immigrant populations).

Numerous professional organizations, such as the American Medical Association, the American Academy of Family Physicians, and the American College of Obstetricians and Gynecologists, advocate for the routine screening of women for abuse by direct and nonjudgmental questioning. Many tools exist for screening, from simple questioning to more formal inventory tools. The simple question, "Do you feel safe in your home?" has a sensitivity of 8.8% and a specificity of 91.2%, so more formal testing may be necessary in some cases. Since 2013, the United States Preventive Services Task Force (USPSTF) has recommended (Grade B) that clinicians regularly screen women of childbearing age for IPV. It also found insufficient evidence to assess the balance of benefits and harms of screening all elderly or vulnerable adults for abuse and neglect and found insufficient evidence to recommend routine IPV screening. The USPSTF does recommend that **all clinicians should be alert to physical and behavioral signs and symptoms associated with abuse and neglect and that direct questions about abuse are justifiable** due to high levels of undetected abuse in women and the potential value of helping these patients. Multiple studies have shown that screening does not result in harm to participants. Recommendations regarding interactions with victims of abuse include exhibiting compassionate, nonjudgmental, supportive care in a private, secure environment.

Human Trafficking

Human trafficking is a form of modern day slavery in which victims are forced or coerced into performing sexual acts or work against their will. About 90% of victims will seek health care at some point when they are trafficked; therefore, clinicians have an important role to identify and free these individuals. Some red flags may include

- Stated age older than appearance
- Accompanying individuals refuse to leave examination room
- Tattoos or marks indicating ownership
- Delay in seeking medical care
- Scripted or mechanically recited history
- Evidence of physical violence

Intimate Partner Violence

Although it is common to think of IPV as a man abusing a woman, abuse can occur in both homosexual and heterosexual relationships with a male or a female victim. **It is estimated that greater than one in five women and nearly one in seven men have experienced severe violence by an intimate partner.** Abuse can occur in any relationship or in any socioeconomic class. Certain situations increase the likelihood, or escalate the occurrences, of abuse. These situations include changes in family life (eg, pregnancy, illnesses, deaths); economic stresses; and substance abuse. Personal and family histories of abuse also increase the likelihood of family violence. Most women do not disclose abuse to their health care providers.

Clinical Presentation. Victims of abuse can present with varied symptoms and signs suggestive of the problem. Direct physical findings can include obvious traumatic injuries, such as contusions, fractures, "black eyes," concussions, and internal bleeding. Genital, anal, or pharyngeal trauma; sexually transmitted infections; and unintended pregnancy may be signs of sexual assault. Depression, anxiety, panic, somatoform and posttraumatic stress disorders, and suicide attempts can also result from abusive relationships.

Some signs and symptoms may be less obvious and may require numerous encounters until the finding of family violence is made. Victims of abuse may present to doctors frequently for health complaints or have physical symptoms that cannot otherwise be explained. Delays in treatment for physical injuries may be a sign of IPV. Chronic pain, frequently abdominal or pelvic pain, is commonly a sign of a history of abuse. The development of substance abuse or eating disorders may prompt inquiry into family violence as well. Children of women abused often directly witness the abuse of their mother. Children and adolescents of abused women can exhibit aggression, anxiety, bed-wetting, and depression.

Assessing Home Safety. When abuse is identified, an initial priority is to assess the safety of the home situation. Direct questioning regarding increasing levels of violence, the presence of weapons in the home, and a plan for safety for the victim and others at home (children, elders) are critical. Resources and support, such as shelters, community-based treatment, and advocacy programs, should be provided. It may be helpful to allow the patient to contact a shelter, law enforcement, family members, or friends while still in the health care provider's office. Multidisciplinary interventions, including family, medical, legal, mental health, and law enforcement, are often necessary.

The **laws regarding clinician reporting of partner violence vary from state to state.** It is important to know the statutes in your locality. Many states do not require contacting legal authorities if the victim of the abuse is a competent adult.

Child Abuse

Epidemiology. Approximately 1 million cases of child abuse, with more than 1000 deaths, are reported each year in the United States; the number of unreported cases makes the overall prevalence much higher. **Child abuse is the third leading cause of death in children between 1 and 4 years of age**, and almost 20% of child homicide victims have contact with health care professionals within a month of their death.

The situations that increase the risk of child abuse are similar to those that increase the likelihood of other family violence. These include parental depression and previous history of abuse, substance abuse, social isolation, and increased stress. Societal factors include dangerous neighborhoods and poor access to recreational resources. Children who are chronically ill or who have physical or developmental disorders may be at even higher risk. Protective factors include family support from the community or relatives, parental ability to ask for help, and access to mental health resources. Identification of at-risk families and home visitation interventions have been shown to significantly reduce child abuse. Short- and long-term physical, psychological, and social consequences are often seen in the victims of child abuse.

Clinical Presentation. Certain history and physical examination findings raise the suspicion for child abuse. Several presenting history and behavioral features may be associated with increased risk of maltreatment or abuse (Table 36–1). **Injuries that are inconsistent with the stated history or a history that repeatedly changes** with questioning should raise the suspicion of abuse. Children who are taken to multiple health care providers or emergency departments, or who are brought in repeatedly

Table 36–1 • CONCERNING FEATURES THAT MAY BE ASSOCIATED WITH CHILD ABUSE
Evolving or absent history about injury
Delay in seeking care for concerning condition
Unusual interactions between child and parent
Overly compliant child with painful medical procedures
Overly affectionate behavior from child to medical staff
Overly protective parent
Parental substance abuse or intoxication
Poor self-esteem in parent
History of abuse in parent's childhood
History of domestic abuse
Loss of control of parent triggered by child's behavior

Data from Tintinalli JE, Ma O, Yealy DM, et al, eds. Tintinalli's Emergency Medicine: A Comprehensive Study Guide, 9th ed. 2020. Copyright © McGraw Hill LLC. All rights reserved.

with traumatic injuries, may be victims. Delay in seeking medical care for an injury may also be a clue to abuse. **Any serious injury in a child < 5 years old, especially in the absence of a witnessed event, should be viewed with suspicion.**

Children frequently have bruises, fractures, and other injuries that occur accidentally, and it can be difficult to distinguish with certainty whether an injury is accidental or intentional. However, **certain types of injuries are uncommon as accidents** (Table 36–2). The presence of these injuries is highly suggestive of child abuse. **Neglect is also a form of child abuse.** An injury or illness that occurred because of lack of appropriate supervision may be a sign of neglect. Failure to provide for basic nutritional, health care, or safety needs are other forms of neglect.

Evaluation. When an injury suspicious for child abuse is identified, attention should initially focus on treatment and protection from further injury. A complete examination should be performed and all injuries documented with drawings or photographs. An x-ray skeletal survey can be performed to look for evidence of current or previous bony injuries. **Skeletal survey is typically recommended for all cases of suspected abuse in children younger than 2 years.** Ophthalmologic examination should be performed to look for retinal hemorrhages. Other imaging, such as computed tomography (CT) of the head, nuclear medicine imaging, or positron emission tomography, may be indicated depending on patient circumstance. Laboratory studies can be useful both in identifying disorders that might explain observed findings and in discovering occult or more severe injury not evident on examination. Testing for sexually transmitted infections may be necessary as well. The clinical findings, pertinent history, and results of evaluation should be documented carefully and legibly.

All 50 states require reporting of suspected child abuse to child protective services or other appropriate authorities (refer to local laws to determine the appropriate authority). Communication to parents should be in a neutral, nonaccusatory manner. They should be informed that a report is going to be made and educated

Table 36–2 • INJURIES SUGGESTIVE OF CHILD ABUSE
Stocking-and-glove burns of the extremities (immersion in scalding water)
Burns of the buttock and groin that spare the intertriginous areas (immersion in scalding water)
Centimeter-size circular burns (cigarettes)
Multiple bruises of differing ages (most common manifestation of child abuse)
Epiphyseal separations
Multiple fractures and/or fractures in different stages of healing
Unexplained injury to buttocks, thighs, ears, or neck
Bite marks
Bruises in the shape of a hand, belt buckle, or loops of a cord
Retinal hemorrhages ("shaken baby syndrome")
Corner or "bucket-handle" fractures of metaphysis of long bones
Spiral fracture of femur or humerus
Rib fractures, especially posteriomedial fractures
Vertebral body fractures and subluxations
Digital fractures
Scapular fractures
Spinous process fractures
Sternal fractures
Complex, bilateral, or wide skull fractures
Injury to external genitalia
Sexually transmitted infections, genital warts
Circumferential hematoma of anus (forced penetration)

Data from Tintinalli JE, Ma O, Yealy DM, et al, eds. Tintinalli's Emergency Medicine: A Comprehensive Study Guide, *9th ed. 2020. Copyright © McGraw Hill LLC. All rights reserved.*

regarding the process that is likely to occur after the report is made. Your role as an advocate for the child's health and safety should be explained. Consideration must also be given to the possibility that there are other victims of abuse in the home (spouse, other children, elders). **Any health care provider who makes a good-faith report of suspected abuse or neglect is immune from any legal action, even if the investigation reveals that no abuse occurred.** Providers may be held liable for failure to report child abuse.

Elder Abuse

Epidemiology. Many types of elder abuse may occur, including physical, sexual, and psychological abuse; neglect; and financial exploitation. The **estimated prevalence of elder abuse ranges from 2% to 10%,** and out of the 1 in 10 elders that may experience abuse, only 1 in 5 incidents are reported. Along with the other risks for domestic violence, several factors unique to the care of elders may play a role. The majority of abusers are family members. Caregiver frustrations and burnout are commonly heard excuses for abuse. Abusers often have histories of mental health problems or substance abuse and have little insight into the fact that they are abusing the patient. Women older than 75 years are statistically the most abused group.

Persons who are older, are more cognitively and physically debilitated, and have less access to resources are more likely to be abused or exploited.

Evaluation. A history of abuse may be difficult to obtain, as the patient may fear worsening of the abuse or may not have the cognitive ability to make an accurate report. If feasible, it is **helpful to interview the patient without the presence of the caregiver.** Screening the caregiver for stress, in private, with referral for community resources may prevent abuse in the elderly. The physical examination, like in child abuse, should carefully document any injuries that are found. Suspicions of dehydration or malnutrition should be confirmed with appropriate laboratory testing, and radiographs should be performed as necessary.

By law, elder abuse should be reported to the appropriate adult protective services, but the reporting requirements vary by state. A multidisciplinary approach involving medical providers, social workers, legal authorities, and families is usually necessary to address the issues involved.

> ## CASE CORRELATION
> - See also Case 5 (Well-Child Care), Case 18 (Geriatric Health Maintenance and End-of-Life Issues), and Case 37 (Limping in Children).

COMPREHENSION QUESTIONS

36.1 A 42-year-old woman presents to your office for evaluation of chronic abdominal pain. She has seen you multiple times for this complaint, but the workup has always been negative. On examination, her abdomen is soft, and there are no peritoneal signs. She has no rash, but she does have a purpuric lesion lateral to her left eye orbit. Which of the following is the best next step in the management of this patient?

A. Ask the patient about physical abuse and report suspicions to the local police.

B. Ask the patient about physical abuse and provide information about local support services.

C. Exclude a bleeding diathesis before inquiring about abuse.

D. Order an abdominal x-ray.

E. Refer to psychiatry.

36.2 A 7-month-old boy is brought to the emergency department by his father after a 1-day history of intractable vomiting. On examination, the child is lethargic. The anterior fontanel is closed. An abdominal x-ray shows a non-specific bowel gas pattern and incidentally reveals a midshaft fracture of the right femur. When confronted about the fracture, the father states that the child climbed onto a chair and jumped off yesterday. Which of the following is the most appropriate next step in management?

A. Outpatient radiographic bone survey

B. Consulting a child abuse specialist

C. Social services consult

D. Disclosing to the parent the intention of contacting child protection services

E. Inpatient noncontrast CT of the head

36.3 Which of the following injuries is most likely to be caused by abuse in a toddler?

A. Three or four bruises on the shins and knees

B. Spiral fracture of the tibia

C. A displaced posterior rib fracture

D. A forehead laceration

36.4 An 80-year-old man who resides in a local nursing home is seen in your office for unexplained scratches on his arms and band-like bruises on his wrists and ankles consistent with restraint use. The patient is mildly demented and appears scared. There is no family to contact. Examination and laboratory results show no medical reason for easy bruising. Which of the following should be your next step?

A. Refer to nursing home social worker.

B. Contact nursing home ombudsmen program.

C. Have the patient observed by nursing home staff.

D. Contact nursing home vice president for nursing care.

E. Send the patient back to the nursing home.

ANSWERS

36.1 **B.** It is appropriate to discuss your concerns in a nonaccusatory, nonjudg-mental fashion with your patient. Waiting for her to bring up the subject may result in her suffering further abuse. The reporting of the abuse (answer A) of competent adults (not elders) is not mandated by law in most states. You should offer assistance, evaluate her safety, and provide her with information regarding available services in the area. There is no reason to exclude a bleed-ing diathesis (answer C) before approaching the subject of abuse. Answer D (abdominal x-ray) is not needed since there are no abdominal complaints.

Answer E (refer to psychiatry) is not indicated since there is no evidence of depressive disorder.

36.2 **E.** This child has injuries consistent with physical abuse. Although the findings and further investigation for abuse are important, the most important primary concern is (a) assessment for a life-threatening injury, which in this case is possibly a head injury; and (b) protection of the child from possible further injury. For this reason, CT of the head is of primary importance. In children younger than 1 year of age, 75% of fractures are due to abuse. Moreover, the shape of a fracture—spiral, transverse, or other—is less important in suspected abuse than the age of the child and location of the fracture. The purported history of fall is inconsistent with the developmental abilities of a 7-month-old child. The child has intractable vomiting and is lethargic on examination. These findings are worrisome for neurologic damage. An inpatient evaluation with CT of the head should be ordered to exclude intracranial bleed since this disorder may lead to irreversible brain damage or even death if not identified quickly; additionally, the child is protected from further abuse while workup is being completed. Of note, the anterior fontanel closes between 4 and 26 months of age (average 13.8 months). It may bulge in conditions such as meningitis or intracranial hemorrhage that increase intracranial pressure. Outpatient management with close follow-up and referral to child protective services is appropriate if caregivers are not suspected of being the abusers. While a radiographic bone survey (answer A) is indicated in all children younger than 2 years of age with suspected abuse, it should be done after excluding more urgent conditions. If you are concerned that the child may be at further risk of abuse and that notifying the parents of your concerns would put the child at immediate danger, it is not necessary to notify the parents of your report to law enforcement or child protective services (answer D). However, in most cases, the parents should have the opportunity to discuss these concerns with you.

36.3 **C.** A posterior rib fracture is often the result of grabbing and squeezing the chest violently. It is very suspicious for abuse. A spiral fracture of the tibia (answer B) is known as a "toddler's fracture" and is a common injury that is often confused with abuse, but not often caused by abuse. Bruises on the anterior and over bony prominences, such as the shins and knees (answer A), and forehead injuries (answer D) are common from falls while learning to walk. Well-padded areas that are bruised such as the thigh, buttock, and cheeks increase the likelihood of abuse.

36.4 **B.** Clinicians have a legal duty to report possible elder abuse to adult protective services in their community. If the patient is living in a nursing care facility, each state has nursing home ombudsmen who can investigate. The Ombudsman Program is mandated by the Federal Older Americans Act. If you feel that this patient is in immediate danger, he can be admitted for evaluation of bruising while the ombudsman and local adult protective services investigate for substandard care or abuse at the nursing care facility. Social worker referral (answer A) may be indicated once there is an investigation to ensure that the patient is not being abused. Observation by nursing home staff (answer C) would not determine whether there is abuse. Contacting the nursing home vice president (answer D) often leads to administrative and legal correspondences rather than safeguarding the patient. Sending the patient back to the nursing home (answer E) is the worse option, since the patient may very well be in a harmful environment.

CLINICAL PEARLS

▶ Suspected child and elder abuse must be reported to either child or adult protective services, respectively. Good-faith reports of suspected abuse are a shield to lawsuits; failure to report can result in legal action against the clinician.

▶ When a patient presents with an injury, there should be a nonjudgmental and nonthreatening method of gathering information to try to reconcile the reported mechanism of injury and the physical findings.

▶ Injuries that are inconsistent with reported activity, delayed seeking medical care, and multiple injuries over time are suspicious for abuse.

▶ Clinicians are in a unique position to identify victims of human traffickers.

▶ When seeing a suspected abuse victim, always consider the possibility that there could be other abuse victims in the household.

REFERENCES

Breiding MJ, Basile KC, Smith SG, Black MC, Mahendra RR. *Intimate Partner Violence Surveillance: Uniform Definitions and Recommended Data Elements.* Version 2.0. Atlanta, GA: National Center for Injury Prevention and Control, Centers for Disease Control and Prevention; 2015.

Colbourne M, Clarke M. Child abuse and neglect. In: Tintinalli JE, Ma O, Yealy DM, Meckler GD, Stapczynski J, Cline DM, Thomas SH. eds. *Tintinalli's Emergency Medicine: A Comprehensive Study Guide,* 9e New York, NY: McGraw Hill; http://accessmedicine.mhmedical.com/content.aspx?bookid= 2353&sectionid=220291943. Accessed May 21, 2020.

Dicola D, Spaar E. Intimate partner violence. *Am Fam Physician.* 2016;94(8):646-651.

Glauser J, Hustey FM. Abuse of the elderly and impaired. In: Tintinalli JE, Stapczynski J, Ma O, Yealy DM, Meckler GD, Cline DM, eds. *Tintinalli's Emergency Medicine: A Comprehensive Study Guide.* 8th ed. New York, NY: McGraw Hill; 2016: Chap. 295.

Hancock M. Intimate partner violence and abuse. In: Tintinalli JE, Stapczynski J, Ma O, Yealy DM, Meckle GD, Cline DM, Meckler GD, eds. *Tintinalli's Emergency Medicine: A Comprehensive Study Guide.* 8th ed. New York, NY: McGraw Hill; 2016: Chap. 294.

Hoover R, Polson M. Detecting elder abuse and neglect: assessment and intervention. *Am Fam Physician.* 2014;89(6):453-460.

Kodner C, Wetherton A. Diagnosis and management of physical abuse in children. *Am Fam Physician.* 2013;88(10):669-675.

A 12-year-old boy is brought to the office with right thigh pain and a limp. His mother has noticed him limping for the past week or so. He denies any injury to his leg but says that it hurts some when he plays basketball with his friends. He denies fever, weight loss, back pain, hip pain, or ankle pain. He occasionally gets some pain in the right knee but does not have any swelling or bruising. He has no significant medical history, does not take any medications regularly, and otherwise feels fine. On examination, he is a well-appearing, overweight adolescent with normal vital signs and initial physical examination. When you have him walk, he has a prominent limp. You note that he seems to keep his weight on his left leg for a greater proportion of his gait cycle than he does on the right leg. Examination of his back reveals a full range of motion, no tenderness, and no muscle spasm. He gets pain in the right hip when it is passively internally rotated. When the hip is passively flexed, there is a noticeable external rotation. His right knee and the remainder of his orthopedic examination are normal.

▶ What is the most likely diagnosis?
▶ What is the most appropriate test to order first for this patient?
▶ What complication could occur if this problem is not diagnosed and treated?

ANSWERS TO CASE 37:
Limping in Children

Summary: A 12-year-old boy presents with

- A limp and right knee pain
- External rotation of the hip when passively flexed and pain on internal rotation of the hip
- No history of injury or trauma
- Bearing weight more on his left leg than his right while walking
- Overweight but well-appearing presentation

Most likely diagnosis: Stable slipped capital femoral epiphysis (SCFE).

Most appropriate test to order: Right hip x-ray with anteroposterior and frog leg lateral views.

Complication that could occur: Avascular necrosis of the hip.

ANALYSIS

Objectives

1. Be able take a history and perform a physical examination for children with leg pain and limping. (EPA 1, 2)

2. Be able to list common causes of leg pain and limping in children of different ages. (EPA 2)

3. Be able to describe appropriate examination, laboratory, and radiologic evaluation for the limping child. (EPA 3)

Considerations

Leg pain is a common complaint in childhood. The **most common causes of leg pain in children are acute trauma** (sprains, strains, contusions) or **overuse injuries.** However, leg pain and limping can be a sign of a more serious, even life-threatening, pathology. Learning an approach to the evaluation and the common diagnoses involved may help in the identification of these problems earlier, when a better outcome is more likely.

In the specific case presented, there are several symptoms and signs that make the diagnosis of SCFE likely. The absence of a specific injury is significant, as SCFE is the most common nontraumatic hip pathology in adolescents. The initial complaint of thigh pain may lead to other considerations, but **hip pathology will frequently present with pain in the groin, thigh, or even the knee.** The patient's age and body habitus are typical for SCFE, which is classically described as occurring most often in overweight adolescent males. Pain with internal rotation of the hip and the finding of external rotation on passive flexion of the affected hip are also suggestive of SCFE.

APPROACH TO:

Limping in Children

DEFINITIONS

AVASCULAR NECROSIS: Death of living bone tissue caused by disruption of blood flow.

DYSPLASIA: Abnormal growth or development.

CLINICAL APPROACH

Pathophysiology

There are many causes of limp with pain in children (Table 37–1). Some of the more common causes may be broadly categorized as being primarily orthopedic, reactive, infectious, rheumatologic, or neoplastic. The prevalence of the specific diagnoses also varies by age. Limp without pain is usually due to congenital orthopedic anomalies or neuromuscular disorders.

Table 37–1 • COMMON CAUSES OF LIMP WITH PAIN IN CHILDREN
Orthopedic • Fracture • Stress fracture • Pathologic fracture through tumor or cyst • Sprain/strain/contusion • Slipped capital femoral epiphysis • Early Legg-Calvé-Perthes disease
Reactive • Toxic synovitis • Transient synovitis following viral infection • Rheumatic fever
Infectious • Septic arthritis • Osteomyelitis • Cellulitis • Diskitis • Gonococcal arthritis
Rheumatologic • Juvenile rheumatoid arthritis • Systemic lupus erythematosus
Tumor • Benign tumors (osteoid osteoma, osteoblastoma) • Ewing sarcoma • Osteosarcoma
Other • "Growing pains"

To understand a limp, it is first important to understand the normal gait. Gait is composed of two phases: the "swing" and the "stance" phases. The stance phase is the weight-bearing phase. The swing phase is the non–weight-bearing phase, when the foot lifts off the ground and is propelled forward. The **antalgic gait occurs when the stance phase of gait is shortened on the side of pain, usually because of pain during weight-bearing.** Antalgic gait is the most common type of limp and is the type of gait described in this case.

Septic arthritis, fractures, neuromuscular disorders, and neoplasms can cause a limp in children of all ages. Night sweats, anorexia, weight loss, and pain that awakens the child at night are suspicious for malignancy. "Growing pains" is a diagnosis of exclusion. It should be considered if the pain is only at night, is bilateral, is not present during the day, and if no other pathology is found.

Clinical Presentation

As always, the initial approach should include a good focused history and physical. The clinician should ask questions about recent trauma; onset and duration of limp; and recent illnesses (viral, pharyngitis, rashes, tick bites, diarrhea, urethritis). Past medical history, previous levels of function, and family history of musculoskeletal disorders can help with diagnosis. Associated symptoms of **fever, weight loss, anorexia, or pain** are especially important.

Assessing Pain. A key characteristic in the evaluation of the child with a limp is assessing whether there is pain or no pain. In an **antalgic gait**, the cause of the **pain may range from the back to the foot.** Therefore, unless there is an obvious source of pain, the examination should include assessment of the back, pelvis, buttock, leg, and foot. In the child who clings to the parent, separating the child from the parent will allow the clinician to observe the child's gait when they walk back to the parent. The child who walks stiffly may be avoiding moving the spine, indicating a possible diskitis. Those with nonantalgic gait abnormalities (Trendelenburg gait [hip drop], inability to dorsiflex the foot, locked knees, toe walking) can have congenital, neurologic, or limb length disorders. Inspecting the feet may show clawing of the toes or cavus deformity, which are signs of neuromuscular conditions.

Hip Evaluation. Because hip pathology often presents with vague pain and hip conditions are likely to need emergent treatment, **evaluation of the hip may be the most important part of the examination of a patient in whom the site of pathology is not immediately obvious.** Restricted internal rotation appears to be the most sensitive marker of hip pathology in children, followed by a lack of abduction. Internal rotation of the hip increases the intracapsular pressure within the acetabulum. Pain during a leg roll and limited internal rotation of less than 30 degrees may indicate infectious or orthopedic hip pathology. A leg roll is performed by having the child supine with the hip and knee extended, and then one examiner stabilizes the pelvis while another rolls the leg internally and externally. The FABER test (*flexion, abduction, external rotation*—the ipsilateral ankle placed on the contralateral knee and mild downward pressure placed on the ipsilateral knee) can find pathology located in the sacroiliac joint, which is often seen in rheumatologic disorders. Bone pain or point tenderness can indicate osteomyelitis or malignancy. Limps from overuse injuries of the foot (eg, Sever disease) and knee disorders (eg, Osgood-Schlatter) can occur.

Imaging and Laboratory Values. X-rays should be obtained when the differential indicates a likelihood of bony abnormalities. An ultrasound of the hip is more sensitive for an effusion of the hip and can be considered. In nonverbal children, x-rays from hip to feet can find a fracture in a significant number of children with limp. A complete blood count (CBC) should be drawn if there is concern of an infection, inflammatory arthritis, or malignancy. Erythrocyte sedimentation rate (ESR) and C-reactive protein (CRP) levels should be considered in evaluating infectious and rheumatologic etiologies. Consider **Lyme disease** in endemic areas, as this can mimic both infectious and rheumatologic causes of hip disorders. If there was recent pharyngitis, consider antistreptolysin titers. In teens with a history of urethritis or febrile diarrhea, consider urine chlamydial antigens or stool cultures for possible Reiter syndrome. Any joint where septic arthritis is considered should have a joint aspiration and evaluation of synovial fluid. **Fever greater than 99.5 °F and ESR greater than 20 mm/hr is 97% sensitive for septic hip joint.** Testing of the fluid should include culture for gonorrhea in teens who are sexually active.

Limping Without Pain. The evaluation of limping without pain (Table 37–2) should include measurements for **leg length discrepancies** (measure anterior superior iliac spine or umbilicus to medial malleolus) and observation for muscular atrophy or limb deformity. Barlow (hip and knee flexed 90 degrees, hold the knee and attempt to displace the thigh posterior), Ortolani (guided abduction), and Galeazzi (knee height discrepancy when patient lies supine with ankles to buttocks and hips and knees flexed) tests can be used to assess for congenital hip abnormalities and femoral length discrepancies.

Infants and Toddlers

Common causes of limping in children in the infant and toddler age group are septic arthritis, fractures, and complications of congenital hip dysplasia. **Septic arthritis** is usually monoarticular and associated with systemic signs such as fever. In young infants, the symptoms may be less obvious, such as crying, irritability, and poor feeding. Children who are ambulatory (crawlers or walkers) will often refuse to do anything that puts weight on the affected joint because of pain. Infection of a joint

Table 37–2 • COMMON ORTHOPEDIC CAUSES OF LIMP WITHOUT PAIN IN CHILDREN
Congenital dislocation (developmental dysplasia) of the hip
Spastic hemiplegia (cerebral palsy)
Legg-Calvé-Perthes (subacute and chronic)
Leg-length discrepancy
Proximal focal femoral dysplasia
Congenital short femur
Congenital bowing of the tibia

Data from Hay WW, Levin MJ, Sondheimer JM, et al, eds. Current Pediatric Diagnosis and Treatment. *15th ed. 2001. Copyright © McGraw Hill LLC. All rights reserved; Leet AI, Skaggs DL. Evaluation of the acutely limping child. Am Fam Physician. 2000;61:1011–1018; and Rudolph CD, Rudolph AM, Hostetter MK, eds.* Rudolph's Pediatrics. *21st ed. 2003. Copyright © McGraw Hill LLC. All rights reserved.*

causes a septic effusion, which raises the pressure inside of the joint capsule. **Children with a septic hip joint will often lay with their hip flexed, abducted, and externally rotated,** which helps to reduce the pain, and they will have significant pain with any internal rotation or extension of the joint. Children with a septic joint will usually have an elevated white blood cell (WBC) count, ESR, and CRP. Definitive diagnosis comes from joint aspiration. **Any suspected septic joint must be aspirated.** In younger infants (4 months or younger), group B *Streptococcus* and *Staphylococcus aureus* are the most common pathogens involved. In older infants and children under the age of 5 years, *S. aureus* and *Streptococcus pyogenes* are the usual causes. Treatment is urgent surgical irrigation and debridement, along with antibiotics.

Unsuspected **fractures**—either stress fractures or traumatic fractures—can present with pain and limping. Abuse must be suspected if the injury is inconsistent with the history presented, if the history changes with repeated questioning, if the child is said to have performed an act outside of his or her developmental ability, or if a fracture usually associated with abuse is found (see Case 36). However, the **history may not reveal the source of the injury,** as a child may fall outside of the view of the parent (see Table 37–3). **A traumatic injury may not result in limping or in complete immobility, but it may cause a change in how the child ambulates.** For example, a child who previously walked and now refuses to walk but will crawl may have an injury of the lower leg or foot.

A **toddler's fracture** is one example of an unsuspected fracture that may present primarily as a limp or a refusal to walk. This fracture is a **spiral fracture of the tibia that results from twisting while the foot is planted.** The diagnosis may be suspected in the setting of an acute limp or change in ambulation, a normal examination of the knee and upper leg, and tenderness of the tibia. It can be confirmed with a plain film x-ray.

Undiagnosed **developmental dysplasia of the hip may present as a painless limp that is present from the time that the child learns to walk.** The American Academy of Pediatrics recommends that newborns and infants up to age 12 months should have their hips examined for instability or dislocation at well-child visits. If undiagnosed, contractures may form that limit movement of the hip. When the child learns to walk, the child will have a painless limp. The diagnosis may be confirmed by x-rays showing abnormal hip alignment. If the problem is found in the first few weeks of life, the child can be treated with splinting of the hip, and normal development usually follows. If diagnosed late, the treatment is often surgical.

Table 37–3 • RED FLAGS REQUIRING IMMEDIATE THOROUGH INVESTIGATION IN A CHILD WITH NONTRAUMATIC LIMP
Child < 3 years old
Child unable to bear weight
Fever in child with limp
Child with comorbid systemic illness
Child > 9 years old with pain or restricted hip movements

Data from Perry DC, Bruce C. Evaluating the child who presents with an acute limp. BMJ. 2010;341:c4250. doi:10.1136/bmj.c4250

Young Children

Transient synovitis is a self-limited inflammatory response that is a common cause of hip pain in children. It occurs typically in children ages 3 to 10 years, is more common in boys than in girls, and **often follows a viral infection.** It is frequently seen as gradually increasing hip pain that results in a limp or refusal to walk. These children have a low-grade or no fever, a normal WBC count, and a normal ESR. On examination, there is pain with internal rotation of the hip, and the overall range of motion is limited by pain. X-rays either are normal or show some nonspecific swelling.

In a situation where the patient is afebrile; has pain-free rotation of the hip greater than 30 degrees; has a normal WBC count, normal ESR and CRP; and short-term follow-up can be ensured, the patient can be followed clinically and should improve in a few days. If these conditions are not met and the diagnosis of a septic joint is considered or if a patient followed expectantly continues to worsen, an aspiration should be done. Kocher criteria are often utilized to assess risk for septic arthritis in children. The four criteria are fever > 101.3 °F (38.5 °C), non–weight-bearing status, ESR > 40 mm/hr, and WBC count > 12,000 cells/mm^3. Zero criteria present equals < 0.2% risk, one criteria is 3%, two criteria present is 40%, three criteria present is 93%, and four criteria present is almost a 100% chance of septic arthritis. **A septic joint will have a purulent aspirate with a WBC count greater than 50,000 cells/mm^3; transient synovitis will have a yellow/clear aspirate with a lower WBC count (< 10,000 cells/mm^3).**

Legg-Calvé-Perthes (LCP) disease is an **avascular necrosis of the femoral head** that typically occurs in children ages 4 to 8 years. It is much more common in boys than in girls. Any disruption of blood flow to the femoral capital epiphysis, such as trauma or infection, may cause avascular necrosis. In LCP, the etiology of the disruption of blood flow is unknown. Children typically have a gradual onset of hip, thigh, or knee pain and limping over a few months. Early in the course, x-rays of the hip may appear normal. Later radiographic findings include collapse, flattening, and widening of the femoral head. Bone scans or magnetic resonance imaging (MRI) may be necessary to confirm the diagnosis. The **treatment is usually conservative,** with protection of the joint and efforts to maintain range of motion. Children who develop more severe necrosis or who develop the disease at older ages may have a worse outcome and a higher risk of developing degenerative arthritis.

Adolescents

The capital femoral epiphysis is the growth plate that connects the metaphysis (femoral head) to the diaphysis (shaft of the femur). A **SCFE** is a separation of this growth plate, which results in the femoral head being medially and posteriorly displaced. This may be caused by an acute injury, but more often is not. It is most often seen in overweight adolescent boys and presents as pain in the hip, thigh, or knee along with a limp. Examination reveals **limited internal rotation** and obligate **external rotation when the hip is passively flexed.** Early x-rays may show only widening of the epiphysis; later x-rays can show the slippage of the femoral head in relation to the femoral neck. The treatment is surgical single-screw pinning of the femoral head. These patients must be closely followed, as up to 50% will develop SCFE in the contralateral hip. Unstable SCFE separations (unable to bear weight on presentation) have a 20% to 50% rate of avascular necrosis developing.

Other causes of limb pain are common in adolescents. Sprains, strains, and overuse injuries are the most common cause of limb pain in this population and are usually readily diagnosed on history and examination (see Case 12). Sexually active adolescents or teens are at risk for sexually transmitted infections (STIs) and their complications, including gonococcal arthritis. In this population, an appropriate history, sexual history, and review of systems are necessary.

CASE CORRELATION

- See Case 12 (Musculoskeletal Injuries) and Case 36 (Family Violence).

COMPREHENSION QUESTIONS

37.1 A 6-year-old boy is brought in for evaluation of a painful right hip. He has been limping and not wanting to walk for the past 2 days. He has had no obvious injury. He feels a little better if he is given some ibuprofen. He has not had a fever and does not have any other current symptoms, although he had "the flu" last week. On examination, his vital signs are normal, including a temperature of 98.8 °F. His right hip has some pain with internal rotation, but there is full range of motion. He walks with a pronounced limp. Which of the following statements is most appropriate?

   A. Send patient home with instructions to take ibuprofen

   B. Complete blood count and ESR

   C. Aspiration of his hip in the office

   D. X-ray of both hips

37.2 An 18-month-old girl is brought into your office because she has been crying and stopped walking today. She will crawl, however. Her mother denies any injury to the child. On examination, she is crying but consolable in her mother's arms. She has bruising and swelling just proximal to the left ankle. An x-ray reveals a spiral fracture of the tibia. Which of the following best describes your advice to the mother of the patient?

   A. You are going to report this to child protective services (CPS) as suspected abuse.

   B. You are going to refer the child for a bone biopsy because this is a pathologic fracture that may represent a neoplasm.

   C. This is a common fracture resulting from twisting on a planted foot.

   D. You will draw blood to evaluate for sickle cell disease, which may cause infarction of the bone.

SECTION II: CLINICAL CASES

37.3 A 2-year-old boy is brought into the emergency center for fever and poor feeding. He started getting sick yesterday and has worsened significantly today. He has had no recent illnesses or injuries and no known ill contacts. On examination, his temperature is 101 °F (38.3 °C), he is tachycardic, and he appears ill. He is lying on his back with his left leg flexed and abducted at the hip. A head, ears, eyes, nose, and throat (HEENT) examination is normal, the heart is tachycardic but regular, and the lungs are clear. The abdomen is nontender, and there are normal bowel sounds. He screams in pain when you move his left leg from its resting position. Blood work reveals an elevated WBC count of 15,000 cells/mm³ and an ESR of 45 mm/h (normal 0-10). An x-ray of his left hip shows a widened joint space but no fractures. Which of the following is your next step at this point?

A. Oral antibiotic and follow-up in 1 day

B. MRI of the hip and referral to an orthopedist

C. Anti-inflammatory medication and close follow-up

D. Hip joint aspiration

37.4 A 6-year-old boy is being seen in the office for a 2-month history of a slight limp. He has no significant past medical history and takes no medications. He has normal vital signs, including a temperature of 98.7 °F. The child is noted to have antalgic gait and decreased range of motion in the left hip (internal rotation more limited). He has mild pain on palpation of the anterior capsule on the left side. X-ray shows fragmentation of the femoral head. Which of the following is the most likely diagnosis?

A. Toxic synovitis of hip

B. Avascular necrosis of hip (LCP)

C. Slipped capital femoral epiphysis

D. Femoral shaft fracture

ANSWERS

37.1 **B.** The case presented is suspicious for transient synovitis following a viral illness. Blood should be drawn for CBC and ESR evaluation. If the CBC and ESR are normal and follow-up can be ensured, this child could be treated expectantly with an oral nonsteroidal anti-inflammatory drug and an expected recovery in a few days (answer A). Although the most common condition is transient synovitis, septic arthritis must be identified and treated or the patient may lose function of the joint or even die. The lack of fever, redness or swelling of the joint, and good range of motion speak against septic joint; nevertheless, the CBC is useful to further assess for possible bacterial infection. If septic joint were suspected, joint aspiration should be performed (answer C). Likewise, SCFE must be identified or avascular necrosis of the hip may ensue. In a child less than age 5, the risk of SCFE is very low, and an x-ray does not need to be performed (answer D), assuming that the range of motion is normal.

37.2 **C.** The case presented (isolated tibial spiral fracture) is classic for a toddler's fracture, which is an accidental fracture due to tripping or falling. Spiral fractures of other long bones (femur, humerus) are more suspicious for abuse. Orthopedic referral is appropriate for management, but a bone biopsy (answer B) or further workup (answer D) is not necessary at this time. Answer A (report to CPS) would be indicated for injuries that would be more suspicious for child abuse, behavior of the child that may indicate abuse, or presence of other injuries, especially in different stages of healing.

37.3 **D.** The child in this case has all of the symptoms and signs of a septic hip joint with the fever, severe joint pain, and x-ray showing increased hip joint space. This situation demands a joint aspiration to confirm the diagnosis. If it is confirmed, he should be promptly referred for urgent surgical management. The reason is that an untreated infected joint will lead to joint destruction and/or sepsis, which may be life threatening. Answer A (oral antibiotics) is insufficient treatment. Answer B (MRI of joint and referral to orthopedist) is somewhat reasonable, but the MRI would delay the management of the patient; nevertheless, prompt referral to an orthopedist, meaning the surgeon would come to the patient's bedside emergently, is an option. Answer C (anti-inflammatory medication and close follow-up) may lead to a fatal consequence.

37.4 **B.** This child is in the correct gender and age group with signs, symptoms, and radiologic findings associated with LCP disease, an avascular necrosis of the femoral head. It is often a self-healing disorder. Treatment is focused on limiting pain and avoiding functional loss. Depending on severity and age, treatment may include watchful waiting, physical therapy, casting, and surgery. The radiological findings are inconsistent with the other conditions listed (answer A, toxic synovitis of hip; answer B, slipped capital femoral epiphysis; and answer D, femoral shaft fracture).

CLINICAL PEARLS

▶ The child with a limp is a common complaint, and the most common cause is transient synovitis.

▶ The septic hip joint must be immediately recognized and treated to avoid permanent joint destruction and/or sepsis.

▶ Hip pathology may not cause hip pain; it may cause groin, thigh, or knee pain instead.

▶ Because of the high risk of bilateral disease, follow-up in SCFE cases should include examination and x-rays of the unaffected hip until the growth plate closes.

▶ A limp that is nonantalgic usually does not need urgent evaluation.

REFERENCES

Dormans JP. Section 16: the musculoskeletal system. In: Rudolph CD, Rudolph AM, Lister G, et al, eds. *Rudolph's Pediatrics*. 23rd ed. New York, NY: McGraw Hill; 2018:931-1038.

Peck DM, Voss LM, Voss TT. Slipped capital femoral epiphysis: diagnosis and management. *Am Fam Physician*. 2017;95(12):779-784.

Perry DC, Bruce C. Evaluating the child who presents with an acute limp. *BMJ*. 2010;341:c4250. doi:10.1136/bmj.c4250

A 70-year-old man comes to the office for his posthospitalization transition of care (TOC) visit following a 2-day hospitalization for an uncomplicated laparoscopic appendectomy that was done under spinal anesthesia by a local surgeon. Last night, on his fourth postoperative day, the patient suddenly developed a temperature of 102.5 °F (39.1 °C) accompanied by chills and vomiting. Just before surgery, a urethral catheter had been placed, which was removed 24 hours later, only to be replaced when he was unable to urinate on his own on the second postoperative day. He was sent home with planned follow up with the surgeon in 1 week, the urologist in 2 weeks, and a TOC visit with you in 48 hours. He has a history of hypertension and benign prostatic hyperplasia (BPH). Physical examination is unremarkable except for costovertebral angle tenderness and suprapubic tenderness. He has no abdominal guarding or rebound tenderness.

► What is the most likely cause of postoperative fever?
► What is the next diagnostic step?
► What is the most appropriate treatment at this time?

ANSWERS TO CASE 38:

Postoperative Fever

Summary: A 70-year-old man presents with

- A history of hypertension and BPH
- Presentation for TOC appointment after laparoscopic appendectomy
- Development of fever, chills, and vomiting on the fourth postoperative day
- Physical examination showing costovertebral tenderness and suprapubic tenderness
- A urethral catheter in place because of a problem in voiding

Most likely cause of postoperative fever: Urinary tract infection (UTI) with probable pyelonephritis.

Next diagnostic step: Urinalysis (UA) and urine culture; possible imaging to rule out intra-abdominal abscess.

Treatment: Readmission and intravenous antibiotics.

ANALYSIS

Objectives

1. Identify the different causes of postoperative fever based on the timing of onset, nature of surgery, and patient's risk factors. (EPA 1, 2)

2. Understand the different clinical presentations that point to the etiology of postoperative fever. (EPA 1, 2)

Considerations

Transition of care posthospital visits are evidence-based interventions to reduce readmissions to hospitals. Hospitals with high readmission rates have lower reimbursement and have readmission rates publicly seen on the Internet (https://www.medicare.gov/hospitalcompare/search.html?). If patients are contacted within 2 business days and seen within 7 days in the outpatient primary care setting, not only are there fewer preventable readmissions, but there is also increased reimbursement for primary care providers.

This 70-year-old man with history of hypertension and BPH is at high risk for a UTI because he recently underwent a pelvic procedure under spinal anesthesia and because he has urinary retention secondary to BPH. Also, the use of a urethral catheter poses an additional risk for bacterial seeding of the urinary bladder. Suprapubic pain and costovertebral tenderness are physical findings suggestive of UTI, most likely acute pyelonephritis. For those without a urethral catheter, symptoms such as dysuria, urgency, and frequency are common.

A UTI is high on the list of causes of fever in the fourth postoperative day, although it could also occur any time during the postoperative period. Less likely could be intra-abdominal abscess, which is more common in laparoscopic appendectomies. UA may detect the presence of bacteriuria, pyuria, nitrites, and leukocyte esterase. Urine culture would determine the type of offending organism, the most common of which are *Escherichia coli, Proteus, Klebsiella, Staphylococcus epidermidis, Pseudomonas,* and *Candida.*

In this patient, the urethral catheter needs to be changed now and discontinued as soon as he is able to void on his own. Symptomatic patients and those who are at high risk for infection are usually treated with appropriate intravenous antibiotics according to the most likely pathogens. The antibiotics subsequently can be adjusted based on culture results. Blood cultures should be ordered if sepsis from a urinary tract source is suspected. Most importantly, it is crucial to address and treat the cause of urinary retention (eg, BPH, kidney stone) to prevent recurrence and avoid complications.

APPROACH TO:
Postoperative Fever

DEFINITIONS

DRUG FEVER: Fever that coincides with the administration of a particular drug and cannot otherwise be explained by clinical and laboratory findings. Resolution of the fever occurs with discontinuation of the suspected drug. Drugs that are usually implicated are beta-lactams, sulfa derivatives, anticonvulsants, allopurinol, heparin, and amphotericin B.

SURGICAL SITE INFECTION (SSI): A concept introduced by the Centers for Disease Control and Prevention and various consensus panels to replace the term *surgical wound infection.* This refers to any infection that occurs in the site of surgery within 30 days of an operative procedure or within 1 year with implants. SSIs are classified as superficial, deep, or organ/space infections. An SSI is a common nosocomial infection.

CLINICAL APPROACH

Pathophysiology

Fever (defined as a temperature > 38 °C or 100.4 °F) is the most common postoperative complication, occurring in 50% of major surgeries in the immediate postoperative period. Tissue trauma during surgery stimulates an inflammatory response that leads to release of pyrogenic cytokines (ie, interleukin, tumor necrosis factor, interferons) from the tissues. In general, more extensive surgical procedures are associated with more tissue trauma and a greater degree of fever response. Elevated levels of bacterial endotoxins and exotoxins that are released from the endogenous gut flora of the colon as a result of surgical complications also elicit the same inflammatory response. This reaction leads to elevation of the thermoregulatory set point and production of fever. This explains why suppression of cytokine release by nonsteroidal anti-inflammatory drugs, steroids, or acetaminophen may alleviate fever and enhance patient comfort.

Table 38–1 • STRATEGIES TO REDUCE THE RISK OF POSTOPERATIVE FEVER
Preoperative Interventions
• Optimize nutritional status.
• Advise patient to stop smoking.
• Treat any existing active infections.
• Optimize management of existing medical conditions (eg, diabetes).
• Reduce dosage of immunosuppressive therapies (when indicated).
Perioperative Interventions
• Administer perioperative antibiotics.
• Use noninvasive ventilation.
• If intubation necessary, use pneumonia prevention protocols.
• Remove catheters, intravenous lines, tubes, and drains as soon as safe.
• Change lines after 72-96 h if they are still needed.
• DVT prophylaxis using early mobilization, sequential compression devices, subcutaneous heparin, or low-molecular-weight heparin.

Abbreviation: DVT, deep venous thrombosis.

As an integral part of informed consent prior to surgery, patients need to be made aware by the physician of the possibility of experiencing postoperative febrile episodes. In addition, adequate preoperative evaluation, which includes performing a history and physical examination to identify risk factors, medications, nutritional status, and comorbid conditions, is imperative to avoid possible life-threatening situations during the perioperative period. Preoperative and perioperative strategies can be used to reduce the risk of developing a postoperative fever (Table 38–1). Fortunately, postoperative fever typically resolves spontaneously and most of the time does not necessarily indicate the presence of infection.

The etiology of postoperative fever could be infectious or noninfectious (Tables 38–2 and 38–3). Most postoperative fevers are not infectious, but all cases of fever require a thorough history and physical to rule out infectious causes. The mnemonic **"5 Ws"** helps in remembering the most common causes of postoperative fever in roughly the order of frequency: **wind** (pneumonia), **water** (UTI), **wound** (SSI), **walking** (deep venous thrombosis [DVT]), and **wonder drugs** (drug fever). When a surgical patient develops fever, the differential diagnosis and investigative methods are directed by the timing of the fever, the type of surgery performed, the preexisting clinical conditions, and the presenting symptoms. Comorbid conditions that increase the risk for infectious postoperative fevers include increasing age, frailty, smoking, diabetes, and immunosuppression. A thorough physical examination should be initiated, followed by inspection of the surgical site, a review of all medications, and a consideration of hospital-related causes (intravenous lines and catheters). In the absence of significant risk factors and clear lack of clinical and physical signs of infection, laboratory tests may not be required.

Fever Within 36 Hours Postsurgery

There are few causes of fever in the immediate postoperative period. Medications and blood products are commonly associated with fevers immediately postoperative.

Table 38–2 • COMMON CAUSES OF POSTOPERATIVE FEVER

Approximate Onset of Fever	Infectious	Noninfectious
Intraoperative up to 24 h after surgery	Preexisting infection Bacteremia from urologic procedures Intraperitoneal leak (up to 36 h) Invasive soft-tissue infection Toxic shock syndrome	Surgical trauma Medications Blood products (at time of transfusion) Malignant hyperthermia
1 d to 1 wk from surgery	UTI (often with indwelling urethral catheters or following genitourinary procedures) Pneumonia (eg, ventilator-associated or aspiration) SSI Catheter-related infection Preexisting infection Cellulitis Viral upper respiratory tract infection	Acute myocardial infarction Alcohol/drug withdrawal Gout Pancreatitis Pulmonary embolism Superficial vein thrombophlebitis (often at intravenous line site) Benign postoperative fever (diagnosis of exclusion)
1 to 4 wk after surgery	SSI Pseudomembranous colitis Antibiotic-associated diarrhea (ie, *Clostridium difficile*) Catheter-related infection (ie, central venous catheters) Device-related infections Abscess	Medication toxicity DVT Pulmonary embolism Thrombophlebitis (particularly in those with impaired mobility)
> 1 mo after surgery	Blood transfusion viral and parasitic infections (ie, hepatitis, CMV, HIV, toxoplasmosis, *Plasmodium malariae*, babesiosis) Infective endocarditis Postpericardiotomy syndrome (following cardiac surgery) SSI Device-related infections Vascular graft infection	Postpericardiotomy syndrome

Abbreviations: *CMV, cytomegalovirus; DVT, deep venous thrombosis; SSI, surgical site infection; UTI, urinary tract infection.*

A rare but dangerous cause in this period is **malignant hyperthermia,** which is an inherited disorder characterized by markedly elevated temperature, up to 104 °F (40 °C), typically within 30 minutes after induction of an inhalational anesthesia (ie, halothane) or depolarizing muscle relaxant (ie, succinylcholine). A more common cause of immediate postoperative fever is **bacteremia,** which occurs more commonly in urologic procedures that involve instrumentation, such as transurethral resection of the prostate. Gram-negative bacteria are the most common pathogen.

Table 38–3 • OTHER CAUSES OF POSTOPERATIVE FEVER WITH VARIABLE TIMING OF ONSET	
Infectious	Noninfectious
Abscess	Withdrawal reaction from drugs/alcohol
Sinusitis	Subarachnoid hemorrhage
Otitis media	Bowel infarction
Parotitis	Pancreatitis
Meningitis	Hyperthyroidism/thyroid storm
Acalculous cholecystitis	Dehydration
Osteomyelitis	Acute hepatic necrosis
Bacteremia	Hypoadrenalism/Addisonian crisis/acute adrenal insufficiency
Empyema	Neoplastic fever
Fungal sepsis	Suture reaction
Hepatitis	Systemic inflammatory response syndrome (SIRS)
Decubitus ulcers	Pheochromocytoma
Perineal infections	Lymphoma
Peritonitis	Hematoma
Pharyngitis	Seroma
Tracheobronchitis	Myocardial infarction/stroke
	Gout/pseudogout
	Transfusion reaction
	Organ transplant–related infection
	Neuroleptic malignant syndrome

Within 30 to 45 minutes, the patient develops chills and a temperature that could exceed 104 °F (40 °C). Accompanying symptoms such as tachycardia, tachypnea, oliguria, and hypotension are common.

If fever occurs within 36 hours postlaparotomy, there are two important infectious etiologies to keep in mind—**bowel injury with leakage of gastrointestinal contents into the peritoneum** and **invasive soft-tissue wound infection** caused by beta-hemolytic streptococci or *Clostridium* species. The former is accompanied by hemodynamic instability. Much less common in this setting is **toxic shock syndrome** caused by *Staphylococcus aureus*.

Atelectasis, Pneumonia, and UTI

Within the first 48 to 72 postoperative hours, **atelectasis** (partial collapse of peripheral alveoli) causes 90% of pulmonary complications of surgery, particularly following abdominal and thoracoabdominal procedures. Contrary to popular belief, its close association with early postoperative fever is probably coincidental. The alveolar collapse is compounded by the loss of functional residual capacity in almost all patients and 50% reduction of vital capacity intraoperatively. Chest x-ray may reveal discoid infiltrate and an elevated hemidiaphragm. Although fever is not likely a consideration, hypoxemia, pneumonia, and scarring that can lead to bronchiectasis can be a consequence of atelectasis.

Postoperative Pneumonia. Instructing the patient on deep inspiration and coughing, the use of incentive spirometry, and the provision of adequate pain control can facilitate the opening of the alveoli. Without resolution of atelectasis, **pneumonia** may ensue. Patients who are on mechanical ventilators are at highest risk for pneumonia (ventilator-associated pneumonia). Fever associated with productive cough, pulmonary crackles, worsening oxygenation, elevation of white blood cells (WBCs), positive sputum culture, and new infiltrates in chest x-ray are the usual indicators of pulmonary infection. Postoperative pneumonia is typically polymicrobial. Enterobacteriaceae and *S. aureus* or Enterobacteriaceae and streptococci are common bacterial combinations. Appropriate use of broad-spectrum intravenous antibiotic therapy is the treatment.

Aspiration Pneumonia. **Aspiration** as the possible cause of pneumonia should be suspected in the elderly, those who reside in a nursing home, and those with neurologic dysphagia, compromised cough reflex, altered mentation, endotracheal intubation, and gastroesophageal reflux disease. Antibiotics are typically given following a witnessed aspiration and discontinued after 48 to 72 hours with no development of infiltrates. **Gram-negative coverage is required for aspiration pneumonia,** with the current agents of choice being piperacillin/tazobactam, meropenem, or cefipime, often with additional gram-negative coverage if there are higher rates of antibiotic resistance or additional risk factors. Vancomycin can be considered to cover for methicillin-resistant *S. aureus* (MRSA).

Urinary Tract Infection. It is also around this time that a **UTI** should be entertained as part of the differential diagnosis. Mild UTIs can be treated with similar agents or with a third-generation cephalosporin or fluoroquinolone. The patient with persistent fever 5 to 7 days after surgery needs to have a thorough examination of the operative site to check for signs of infection, which include erythema, pain, local edema, and purulent discharge.

Surgical Site Infections

Surgical site infections have markedly decreased through wide practice of aseptic technique and team-based perioperative management protocols. Patients at high risk of wound infection are those who underwent lengthy surgical procedure, received blood transfusion, are malnourished, are immunosuppressed, and have diabetes mellitus. Prophylactic antibiotics should be given within 1 hour before surgery and discontinued within 24 hours after surgery to lower the risk of SSIs. Skin site infections may be treated with oxacillin or with vancomycin if MRSA is common in the institution or environment. Deep abdominal infections are often treated with a cephalosporin, such as cefoxitin, or a combination of fluoroquinolone plus metronidazole to cover anaerobic, enterococci, and enteric gram-negative bacilli infections.

Drug Fevers

Drug fevers are often associated with rash and/or lupus-like syndromes. They also may have renal, liver, lung, joint, or hematologic dysfunction associated with the drug toxicity. The risk of developing drug fever correlates with the number of drugs prescribed. Antimicrobial agents account for roughly one-third of all cases.

Common antimicrobial agents associated with drug fever include minocycline, cephalosporins, fluoroquinolones, sulfonamides, and penicillins. Unfractionated heparin, which is common in the hospital setting for DVT prophylaxis, is another medication associated with drug fever. Drug fever typically resolves within 72 to 96 hours after discontinuation of the offending agent.

Abscess

Purulent drainage and fluctuant appearance indicate the presence of an abscess, which requires incision and drainage. When cellulitis is confirmed, treatment with an antibiotic is warranted. Gram-positive bacteria, such as *S. aureus, S. epidermidis* (especially with implants or devices), *Streptococcus pyogenes,* and *Enterococcus,* are important pathogens. Fungal etiology should not be ruled out in patients with severe comorbid conditions. On rare occasions, deep abscesses produce fever 10 to 15 days after surgery. A high level of suspicion leads to diagnostic imaging, such as computed tomographic (CT) scan of the body region most likely to be infected, which depends on the location of the surgery. Interventional radiology specialists can be called upon for radiologically guided drainage of the abscess, which is the definitive treatment. Antibiotics should include coverage for gram-negative enteric bacilli and anaerobes, especially when intra-abdominal or pelvic infections are suspected. Gallium scans may be helpful in finding sites of infection in patients without localizing symptoms and workup.

Line-Associated Infection

An **intravascular catheter or line-associated infection** needs to be entertained when the patient has had intravenous devices for 3 days or more, even when the site appears clean. Any unnecessary lines should be discontinued, as they are potential sites of infection. The catheter tip should be cultured to reveal an offending organism that would direct treatment.

Deep Venous Thrombosis

Fever caused by a DVT usually occurs 1 to 4 weeks postoperatively. Half of the time, patients with DVT are asymptomatic. Common complaints are unilateral leg swelling, tenderness, pain, and warmth. The **Homan sign** (pain in the calf on foot dorsiflexion) is demonstrated in some cases. When possible, surgical patients are encouraged to ambulate early; otherwise, subcutaneous heparin or low-molecular-weight heparin are useful prophylactic measures. If the patient is at high risk for bleeding, intermittent pneumatic compression devices can help. Diagnosis is made by risk stratification, laboratory testing, and duplex ultrasound. Patients who develop **pulmonary embolism** (PE) usually have a concomitant DVT. The treatment of DVTs and PE is initiated with low-molecular-weight heparin or unfractionated heparin, followed by oral anticoagulation.

Types of Surgery and Associated Complications

The type of surgery provides a clue regarding the associated risks of fever-associated surgical morbidity. In general, due to less tissue trauma, laparoscopic surgery comparatively causes fewer cases of fever than open surgery. Pleural effusion develops in all patients undergoing cardiothoracic surgery, and 5% of those patients acquire pneumonia. Particularly unique to abdominal surgery is deep abdominal abscess and pancreatitis. Obstetric and gynecologic surgery could be complicated by postpartum endometritis/deep pelvic abscess, necrotizing fasciitis, and pelvic thrombophlebitis. SSI is the most common infectious cause of fever in orthopedic surgery. Prostatic and perinephric abscesses are more commonly seen in urologic procedures. Arterial embolization, or "blue toe" syndrome due to emboli from an infected vascular graft, can occur following vascular surgery, especially in grafts involving the groin and the legs. Endovascular aortic aneurysm repair may be complicated by "postimplantation syndrome" characterized by self-limited fever, elevated C-reactive protein levels, leukocytosis, and negative blood cultures. Patients undergoing genitourinary procedure are at greater risk of having a UTI. Meningitis is a common cause of fever following a neurosurgical procedure. Neurosurgery patients, who are usually immobilized and less aggressively anticoagulated to avoid brain hemorrhage, have the highest incidence of DVT.

CASE CORRELATION

- See Case 24 (Pneumonia), Case 44 (Cerebrovascular Accident/Transient Ischemic Attack), and Case 48 (Fever and Rash).

COMPREHENSION QUESTIONS

38.1 A 60-year-old man with a diagnosis of adenocarcinoma of the colon underwent a left hemicolectomy with primary anastomosis. Thirty hours after surgery, he was found to have a fever of 102 °F (38.8 °C), blood pressure of 90/60 mm Hg, heart rate of 140 beats/min, respiratory rate of 24 breaths/min, and low urine output. Physical examination showed diffuse abdominal tenderness. The surgical site is clean and without redness. UA was negative, and the complete blood count showed a WBC count of 11,000 cells/mm^3. Which of the following is the most likely cause of this patient's fever?

A. Pneumonia

B. Intraperitoneal leak from bowel injury

C. Surgical site infection

D. Deep tissue abscess

38.2 An 84-year-old nursing home resident underwent emergency open chole-cystectomy under general anesthesia. She has advanced Parkinson disease, hypertension, and diabetes and has been receiving nutrition via nasogas-tric tube (NGT) since the surgery. On the second postoperative day, she was noted to be coughing and vomiting. Four days later, she has a tem-perature of 102 °F (38.8 °C), heart rate of 90 beats/min, respiratory rate of 25 breaths/min, blood pressure of 120/70 mm Hg, and oxygen saturation of 87% on room air. She has a productive cough with what the nursing staff described as "putrid smelling and appearing sputum." Lung ausculta-tion shows crackles on the right, and a chest radiograph reveals a patchy infiltrate in the right lung. Which of the following is the most appropriate next step in management?

A. Obtain an expectorated sputum sample for culture.

B. Treat empirically with antibiotics.

C. Insert percutaneous endoscopic gastrostomy (PEG) tube for long-term feeding.

D. Treat with a proton pump inhibitor (PPI).

38.3 A 42-year-old man underwent open reduction and internal fixation of a comminuted fracture of the right femur, which he suffered from a motor vehicle collision. He was recovering satisfactorily until today, the fifth post-operative day, when he complained of pleuritic chest pain. He currently has a fever of 101 °F (38.3 °C), heart rate of 118 beats/min, respiratory rate of 30 breaths/min, blood pressure of 130/85 mm Hg, and oxygen satura-tion of 85% on room air. His left ankle and calf are found to be edematous, warm, and tender. Which of the following is the most significant risk factor for his condition?

A. Having an intravenous line in his arm for more than 3 days

B. Failure to adequately use his incentive spirometer

C. Urinary bladder catheterization

D. Prolonged immobility

38.4 A 50-year-old woman with diabetes was recuperating from left inguinal hernia repair. Her glycosylated hemoglobin (HbA_{1c}) prior to surgery was 10%. During postoperative follow-up a week after surgery, the surgical site was markedly erythematous, warm, and tender with pus. Which of the fol-lowing is the next step in treatment?

A. Apply topical antibiotic to the surgical site

B. Use warm compresses alone, which will relieve the inflammation

C. Open the surgical site and drain the infected material

D. Send the patient home with prescription for oral antibiotics for 7 days

ANSWERS

38.1 **B.** In the presence of severe hemodynamic changes and diffuse abdominal tenderness, anastomosis bowel leak is the most common cause of fever in the first 36 hours after laparotomy. The incidence varies between 5% and 19%, and risk factors include age, male gender, poor nutrition status, left-sided surgery, and low anastomosis location. Answer A (pneumonia) would be likely with productive cough and fever and usually occurs between 3 and 7 days after surgery. Answer C (SSI) and answer D (deep tissue abscess) would be unlikely so soon after surgery and usually occur about 5 to 7 days after surgery; they present with a red and tender incision (SSI) or fever and localized abdominal tenderness with deep infection.

38.2 **B.** This patient likely has aspiration pneumonia. She has risk factors that include her age, functional status, recent general anesthesia, and advanced neurologic disease. The right lower lung area is commonly affected. She requires treatment with antibiotics that cover anaerobic bacteria. Expectorated sputum (answer A) is unreliable for anaerobic cultures because of likely contamination by oral flora. Answer C (PEG tube placement) is not indicated and does not have a lower risk of aspiration pneumonia than an NG tube. Answer D (PPI) may help to prevent pneumonitis and other future problems but would not help with the acute situation.

38.3 **D.** Based on the findings of a red and tender lower extremity, this patient probably has a venous thromboembolic (VTE) disease or DVT of the left leg, with likely embolization of the thrombus with clinical findings of PE. The presentation of pleuritic chest pain, dyspnea, tachypnea, and low oxygen saturation are consistent with PE. Risk factors for VTE include prolonged immobility, vascular damage, and hypercoagulability. Answer A (intravenous line in the arm for longer than 3 days) can lead to a superficial thrombophlebitis but not a DVT. Answer B (failure to use incentive spirometry) can lead to atelectasis of the lung zones, but not DVT. Answer C (urinary bladder catheterization) can predispose to UTI.

38.4 **C.** An incision and drainage procedure is the most important therapy for SSI. Answer A (topical antibiotics) will not be effective in treating the patient. Answer D (oral antibiotics alone) will not resolve the infection; use of incision and drainage is a mandatory part of the management due to the devitalized tissue and lack of blood supply to tissue in the surgical site. Answer B (warm compresses) will be ineffective and can be used for mild pain of an incision not related to infection.

CLINICAL PEARLS

▶ Postoperative fevers in the first few days after surgery are common and usually resolve on their own.

▶ A thorough risk assessment, history, and physical examination are needed to determine if laboratory testing and antibiotics are warranted.

▶ The timing of the fever is useful in creating an effective differential diagnosis for postoperative fever.

▶ All unnecessary medication, catheters, lines, and tubes should be discontinued in the postoperative febrile patient.

REFERENCES

Beilman G, Dunn D. Surgical infections. In: Brunicardi FC, Anderson DK, Billiar TR, eds. *Schwartz's Principles of Surgery*. 10 ed. New York, NY: McGraw Hill; 2015:135-160.

Hsu V. Prevention of health care-associated infections. *Am Fam Physician*. 2014;90(6):377-382.

Narayan M, Medinilla S. Fever in the post-operative patient. *Emerg Med Clin North Am*. 2013; 31(4):1045-1058.

You are busy seeing patients in your outpatient clinic when you hear a commotion coming from the waiting room. You go to check and find a very frantic mother and her 2-year-old son, who is clutching his throat, coughing, drooling, and visibly struggling to breathe. The mother endorses that just a few minutes ago, the child was running around while eating grapes when she suddenly heard him gagging and wheezing. Her son has an appointment for a well-child examination, and he has apparently been doing well, with no significant history of respiratory illness. The toddler is still conscious but unable to talk, and his cough is becoming weaker. Breath sounds are decreased bilaterally. There are audible wheezing and stridor. You try to ventilate the patient with the chin-lift maneuver, but the chest fails to rise. You open the mouth but are unable to see any foreign object.

▶ What is the most likely diagnosis?
▶ What is the next step in the management of this patient?

ANSWERS TO CASE 39:

Acute Causes of Wheezing and Stridor in Children

Summary: A 2-year-old boy presents with

- Acute onset of coughing, choking, drooling, and wheezing while eating grapes
- Inability to speak and a cough that is weak
- A good state of health prior to the incident and no history of respiratory illness
- Decreased breath sounds, wheezing, and stridor
- No chest rise on ventilation attempt
- No foreign object seen in his mouth

Most likely diagnosis: Foreign body airway obstruction (FBAO).

Next step in management: Heimlich maneuver (subdiaphragmatic abdominal thrusts).

ANALYSIS

Objectives

1. Identify the illnesses, other than asthma, that cause acute wheezing in children. (EPA 1, 2)
2. Understand the steps in the diagnosis and management of a wheezing child. (EPA 3, 4)

Considerations

Acute onset of wheezing in an otherwise healthy child similar to the above case should raise the suspicion for **foreign body airway obstruction.** Witnessed swallowing followed by choking is not necessary for diagnosis, but as much information as possible should be gathered surrounding the onset of symptoms. FBAO is common among children aged 6 months to 3 years old, accounting for approximately 70% of cases. Small toys and objects, balloons, and food (eg, nuts, grapes, and candies) are high-risk objects for aspiration. Older children may be able to identify the object they swallowed and assume the posture of clutching their neck with their hand, which is the **universal choking sign.** One should not attempt to remove the foreign object from a child who is actively coughing and able to vocalize. Blind finger sweep is not recommended because of the danger of further obstruction or injury.

APPROACH TO:
Wheezing and Stridor

DEFINITIONS

HEIMLICH MANEUVER: Performed in children greater than 1 year of age and in adults by standing or sitting behind the person who is choking and placing the thumb side of one fist between the navel and the xiphoid process. The other hand grasps the fisted hand and a series of upward abdominal thrusts are delivered to create an "artificial cough" in a choking victim in an effort to dislodge the object blocking the airway.

STRIDOR: Wheezing coming from obstruction of the large airway that has a constant pitch and intensity throughout the entire inspiratory effort.

WHEEZING: A musical sound heard on pulmonary auscultation produced by the oscillating walls of airways narrowed by mucus, inflammation, and so on.

CLINICAL APPROACH

Among the many causes of wheezing in children, asthma and viral infections are most common. Worldwide studies showed that approximately 10% to 15% of infants wheeze in the first 12 months of life. The diagnosis of wheezing hinges on accurate history, physical examination, laboratory tests, and even response to treatments. It is also important to gather information regarding the age of onset, exposure to cigarette smoke, presence of allergic signs and symptoms, frequency of wheezing, association with vomiting or feeding, and other accompanying symptoms.

The etiology of **acute wheezing** in children could be infectious (eg, bronchiolitis) or mechanical obstruction (eg, FBAO). **Recurrent wheezing,** on the other hand, encompasses anomalies of the tracheobronchial tree (eg, bronchomalacia), cardiovascular disease (eg, vascular rings and slings), gastroesophageal reflux, and immunologic disorders (eg, bronchopulmonary dysplasia, cystic fibrosis). This case concentrates on acute onset of wheezing other than asthma in children (Case 56 provides a more detailed discussion of asthma).

Foreign Body Airway Obstruction

As in the case presented above, symptoms of FBAO include weak cough, inability to speak or cry, high-pitched sounds or no sounds during inhalation, cyanosis, choking, vomiting, drooling, wheezing, blood-streaked saliva, and respiratory distress. Suspected FBAO requires emergent intervention. Physical findings of **unilateral wheezing, unequal or decreased breath sounds, and stridor are common.** In children, the foreign body could lodge on either side of the airway. Eight out of ten times, the foreign body lodges in one the bronchi. If the foreign body lodges in the esophagus, acute wheezing is still possible when the obstruction compresses on the airways.

If a child older than 1 year is no longer able to cough, vocalize, or breathe, a series of abdominal thrusts (Heimlich maneuver) should be the next step to try to expel the foreign body. In children younger than 1 year of age, instead of abdominal thrust, a series of five back blows alternating with chest thrusts is performed. If the child continues to deteriorate even after 1 minute of resuscitative efforts and these maneuvers fail to expel the foreign object, the emergency medical services system should be activated while continuing cardiopulmonary resuscitation.

In the hospital setting, a bronchoscopic procedure is the treatment of choice. **Chest x-ray is often normal**, but in some cases it shows a radiopaque foreign object or identifies localized hyperinflation and/or atelectasis. Most deaths from FBAO occur in children younger than 5 years of age; 65% of the children are infants.

Bronchiolitis

Pathophysiology. **Bronchiolitis** affects more than one-third of children under 2 years of age and is the most common acute cause of wheezing, especially in infants who are 1 to 3 months old. Infants younger than 6 months, premature infants, and infants with preexisting cardiopulmonary conditions are most severely affected, owing to smaller, more easily obstructed airways and a decreased ability to clear secretions. Bronchiolitis is a viral infection causing nonspecific inflammation of the small airways and usually occurs during the winter months. **Respiratory syncytial virus (RSV) accounts for 50% to 80% of cases;** the rest are caused by parainfluenza, adenovirus, influenza, *Mycoplasma pneumoniae*, *Chlamydia pneumoniae*, and human metapneumovirus. These viruses and atypical bacteria elicit inflammatory and immune responses that produce mucus, edema, and cellular debris that block the small airways. Influenza vaccinations in infants and toddlers have reduced the incidence of bronchiolitis caused by the flu virus.

Clinical Presentation. Initially, the child develops nasal congestion and rhinorrhea for 1 to 2 days, followed by low-grade fever, wheezing, cough, irritability, and varying degrees of dyspnea. Affected children may have poor oral intake and possibly dehydration. Symptoms reach a peak in 2 to 5 days and gradually resolve in 1 to 2 weeks. Physical examination may reveal wheezing, fine crackles, prolonged expiratory phase, tachypnea, and increased work of breathing, as evidenced by nasal flaring, intercostal retraction, and even apnea. Other physical findings may include otitis media, irritability, and hypothermia or hyperthermia.

Diagnosis. The diagnosis of bronchiolitis is based on clinical presentation, the patient's age, seasonal occurrence, and findings from the physical examination. Tests are typically used to exclude other diagnoses, such as bacterial pneumonia, sepsis, or heart failure, or to confirm a viral etiology and determine required infection control for patients admitted to the hospital. Current literature does not support the routine use of laboratory tests, as they do not alter clinical outcomes unless the child is less than 3 months (90 days) of age with the need to rule out secondary bacterial infection. If the diagnosis is doubtful or the clinical presentation is concerning for other diagnoses, one may request a chest x-ray. Radiologic findings in individuals with bronchiolitis are variable and may include bronchial wall thickening, tiny nodules, linear opacities, and patchy atelectasis. Infiltrates and lobar consolidation are more consistent with pneumonia.

Management. RSV bronchiolitis is a self-limited disease and can be safely managed in an outpatient setting. However, disease manifestation can be variable, and risk factors for severe disease include preexisting cardiac or pulmonary disease, premature birth, very young age (< 2-3 months), nosocomial RSV infection, and, in some studies, low socioeconomic status. Patients who are in severe respiratory distress; those younger than 3 months old or premature; those with comorbid conditions, lethargy, hypoxemia, or hypercarbia; and those with atelectasis or consolidation in chest radiograph need to be hospitalized. **The single best indicator of severity is low pulse oximetry.** Indicators of mild disease include good oral intake, age greater than 2 months, oxygen saturation greater than or equal to 94%, and normal age-based respiratory rate (< 45 breaths/min for 0-2 months old, < 43 breaths/min for 2-6 months old, and < 40 breaths/min for 6-24 months old).

Supportive Care. The Agency for Healthcare Research and Quality, in collaboration with the American Academy of Family Physicians and the American Academy of Pediatrics, recommends **supplemental oxygen if SpO$_2$ (oxygen saturation measured by pulse oximetry) is < 90% and supportive care as the modes of treatment with clear evidence of effectiveness in RSV bronchiolitis.** Supportive care should consist of supplemental humidified oxygen, fluids, and the suctioning of nasal and pharyngeal secretions; the most important therapy is humidified oxygen. Medications have a limited role in the management of bronchiolitis.

Pharmacological Interventions. Several drugs are commonly used, but little or inconclusive evidence supports the routine use of any drug in the management of bronchiolitis. Nebulized bronchodilators, cool mist, steroids, antibiotics, and ribavirin have insufficient evidence or have not been shown to help in previously healthy children. **Passive immunoprophylaxis** (RSV immunoglobulin or palivizumab) just before the beginning of RSV season has been proven to be an effective preventive therapy for children younger than 2 years with increased risks from chronic lung disease or history of prematurity (less than 35-week gestation), or for children younger than 4 years with acyanotic congenital heart disease.

Croup

Pathophysiology. **Croup** is a very common cause of airway obstruction in children aged 6 months to 6 years, and it is a leading cause of hospitalization for children younger than 4 years. It is a **viral infection that causes inflammation of the subglottic region** of the larynx that produces the characteristic barking cough, hoarseness, stridor, and different degrees of respiratory distress that are more severe at night. The croup syndrome encompasses laryngotracheitis, laryngotracheobronchitis, laryngotracheobronchopneumonitis, and spasmodic croup.

Croup usually occurs during fall and winter. The parainfluenza viruses (I, II, III) are responsible for up to 80% of croup cases, with parainfluenza I accounting for most episodes and hospitalizations. Other pathogens include enterovirus, human bocavirus, influenza virus A and B, RSV, rhinovirus, and adenovirus in approximate order of frequency. In communities with low measles immunization rates, measles should be listed as a rare but possible cause. Influenza A has been implicated in children with severe respiratory compromise.

Clinical Presentation. The prodrome is characterized by 12 to 72 hours of runny nose and low-grade fever, followed by a **barking cough** and variable levels of respiratory distress, usually at night. Hypoxia only occurs in severe cases. These symptoms peak from 1 to 2 days and, in most cases, resolve in 1 week.

Evaluation. Diagnosis is made through clinical presentation. However, imaging studies may confirm the diagnoses. **Frontal neck x-rays show the "steeple sign,"** which is indicative of **subglottic narrowing** of the tracheal lumen. When the diagnosis is uncertain, computed tomography (CT) scan of the neck offers a more sensitive evaluation, but it is rarely indicated. Treatment is geared toward the severity of the croup (the level of respiratory distress). The most reliable clinical features to test severity are resting stridor and chest wall retractions. Use of pulse oximetry can also help assess severity.

Emergency Treatment. Emergency management of croup should begin with assessment of airway obstruction; oxygen should be used liberally. Chest radiographs rarely are of use but can be an option if other pulmonary conditions are strongly considered. Lateral neck films can be considered if there is concern for epiglottitis or bacterial tracheitis. There is no proof that humidified air is of value, and mist tents should be avoided. Hospitalization is appropriate if severe croup is clinically apparent. Severe croup is exemplified by cyanosis, decreased level of consciousness, progressive stridor, severe stridor, severe retractions, markedly decreased air movement, toxic appearance, severe dehydration, and social factors limiting adequacy of outpatient monitoring. Children who are hospitalized with croup should be monitored closely, and frequent physical examinations need to be performed.

Pharmacological Management. The current cornerstones of treatment are **glucocorticoids and nebulized epinephrine. Steroids** have proven beneficial in severe, moderate, and even mild croup. Dexamethasone 0.6 mg/kg by mouth or parenterally as a single dose is beneficial because of its long half-life and anti-inflammatory action, which decreases laryngeal mucosal edema. It also decreases the need for salvage nebulized epinephrine. Nebulized racemic (mixture of d-isomers and l-isomers) or L-epinephrine is typically reserved for patients in moderate-to-severe distress. It works by adrenergic stimulation, which causes constriction of the precapillary arterioles, thereby leading to fluid resorption from the interstitium and improvement in the laryngeal mucosal edema. Its beta-2-adrenergic activity leads to bronchial smooth muscle relaxation and bronchodilation. The following medications should be avoided: sedatives, opiates, expectorants, and antihistamines.

Epiglottitis

Pathophysiology. Epiglottitis is a **bacterial infection of the supraglottic tissue** and surrounding areas that causes rapidly progressive airway obstruction. It usually affects children younger than 5 years old and is most commonly caused by bacteria such as *Streptococcus pyogenes* (group A beta-hemolytic *Streptococcus*) and *Haemophilus influenzae*. With the introduction of the *H. influenzae* type b (Hib) vaccine, there has been a 10-fold decrease in cases of childhood epiglottitis, with group A strep now the leading infectious etiology.

Clinical Presentation. Within 24 hours, the patient with epiglottitis will appear "toxic" and develop fever, severe sore throat, muffled speech ("hot potato voice"), drooling, and dysphagia. The child usually is noticeably anxious and assumes the sitting position, leaning forward on outstretched arms with chin thrust forward and neck hyperextended (tripod position) to increase the airway diameter.

With progression of airway obstruction, the patient may begin to have wheezing and stridor. **Epiglottitis is a medical emergency, and visualization to confirm the presence of severely erythematous epiglottis is preferably done in the operating room with an experienced surgeon or anesthesiologist.** Mortality rates as high as 10% can occur in children whose airways are not protected by endotracheal intubation. With endotracheal intubation, mortality is less than 1%.

The radiographic finding that is characteristic of epiglottitis is the "thumb sign" or protrusion of the enlarged epiglottis from the anterior wall of the hypopharynx; it is seen on lateral neck x-ray. Blood tests should be avoided unless there is the ability to immediately intubate, since the blood draw can provoke anxiety and worsen the respiratory status.

A complete blood count usually shows leukocytosis, neutrophilia, and bandemia.

Treatment. Medical treatment begins by evaluating airway, breathing, and circulation. The patient should be kept in a calm environment to prevent sudden airway obstruction due to patient distress. Supplemental oxygen administration, a nonthreatening initial step, is easily accomplished with blow-by oxygen administered by a parent. Equipment needed for emergent airway management should be placed at the bedside, and the patient should be kept in view at all times. The clinician should **avoid oral and throat examinations,** which can provoke anxiety and acute obstruction.

If acute respiratory arrest occurs, ventilate the child with 100% supplemental oxygen, using a bag-valve-mask device, and arrange for intubation. When a child has a respiratory arrest and appropriate surgical personnel are unavailable, the attending physician may attempt intubation. Alternative methods to gain immediate control of the airway, such as needle cricothyrotomy, are considered temporary until a more permanent procedure (eg, tracheostomy) can be performed. The best setting for an endotracheal intubation is in an operating room with the patient under general anesthesia.

Treatment consists of appropriate antibiotics (second- or third-generation cephalosporins or ampicillin/sulbactam) and airway management, usually in an intensive care unit setting with a team ready to respond for intubation or tracheostomy.

Bacterial Tracheitis

Bacterial tracheitis is an uncommon life-threatening infection most often seen in 5- to 8-year olds. It often follows an upper respiratory infection that suddenly worsens with high fever, stridor, and cough. Patients appear toxic. Secretions are so thick that they threaten to obstruct the upper airway. Patients should be treated similarly to those with epiglottitis, with the patient ideally going to the operating room for sedation, intubation, and bronchoscopy for cultures and suctioning of thick secretions. X-rays can be done, but airway stabilization takes priority. If x-rays are performed, a steeple sign, much like croup, may be seen. *Staphylococcus aureus* is most commonly isolated. *S. pyogenes, Moraxella catarrhalis, H. influenzae*, and anaerobes are also seen. Ampicillin/sulbactam and third-generation cephalosporins with clindamycin cover most likely causative organisms. Vancomycin should be considered in communities with high rates of methicillin-resistant *S. aureus*.

Abscesses

Deep abscesses of the neck are less common causes of acute wheezing, but they have the potential to be very serious. They are located in the peritonsillar, retropharyngeal, and pharyngomaxillary spaces.

Retropharyngeal abscess affects children 2 to 4 years old. The abscess is usually caused by extension of pharyngeal infection, penetrating trauma, iatrogenic instrumentation, or a foreign body. Children with this condition present with fever, drooling, dysphagia, odynophagia, stridor, and respiratory distress. Physical examination may reveal tender, enlarged cervical lymphadenopathy, cervical spine range-of-motion limitation, possibly stridor, and wheezing. Diagnosis is made by lateral neck films, which show bulging in the posterior pharynx (prevertebral soft tissue more abundant in children during expiration). Treatment utilizes antibiotics such as cephalosporins or antistaphylococcal penicillins. Incision and drainage treatment is also an option.

Peritonsillar abscess is an infection of the superior pole of the tonsils and is more common in young teenagers. Fever, severe sore throat, muffled voice, drooling, trismus, and neck pain are typical symptoms. Enlarged tonsils with abscess, cervical adenopathy, and deviation of the uvula may be obvious on physical examination. **CT scan of the neck is the most helpful diagnostic modality for identifying deep neck abscesses.** The predominant pathogens are *S. pyogenes, S. aureus*, and anaerobes. The administration of ampicillin-sulbactam or clindamycin (if penicillin allergic) for 14 days is appropriate treatment. Drainage of the abscess is indicated as first-line treatment or when antimicrobial agents fail to produce an adequate result. Serious complications from deep abscesses result from airway obstruction, septicemia, aspiration, jugular vein thrombosis/thrombophlebitis, carotid artery rupture, and mediastinitis.

CASE CORRELATION

- See Case 56 (Wheezing and Asthma).

COMPREHENSION QUESTIONS

39.1 A 7-month-old infant is brought by her mother to an outpatient clinic because of a 2-day history of fever, copious nasal secretions, and wheezing. The mother volunteers that the baby has been healthy and has not had these symptoms in the past. The infant's temperature is noted to be 100.7 °F (38.1 °C), her respiratory rate is 50 breaths/min, and her pulse oximetry is 95% on room air. Physical examination reveals no signs of dehydration, but wheezing is heard on bilateral lung fields on auscultation. The infant shows no improvement after three treatments with nebulized albuterol. Which of the following is the recommended treatment?

   A. Continued nebulized albuterol every 4 hours

   B. Antihistamines and decongestants

   C. Antibiotics for 7 days

   D. Initiate palivizumab

   E. Supportive care with hydration and humidified oxygen

39.2 A 9-year-old girl is being seen in your office with fever and difficulty breathing. You are concerned about the diagnosis of epiglottitis. Which of the following is the most accurate statement regarding epiglottitis?

   A. The child usually prefers to be in a prone position.

   B. The radiographic finding of steeple sign will be present.

   C. Every effort should be made to visualize the epiglottis in the office to confirm the diagnosis.

   D. Its diagnosis is decreasing in incidence.

39.3 A 5-year-old child is brought into the office due to the mother's concern about difficulty breathing. On examination, the child appears toxic and has a high fever, cough productive of thick mucopurulent expectorant, and stridor with wheezing. The child is up to date regarding immunizations. Which of the following are the most likely condition and causative organism requiring antibiotic therapy?

   A. Epiglottitis due to *H. influenzae*

   B. Tracheitis due to *S. aureus*

   C. Epiglottitis due to *S. pyogenes* (beta-hemolytic streptococcus group A)

   D. Tracheitis due to *S. pyogenes* (beta-hemolytic streptococcus group A)

   E. Retropharyngeal abscess due to *S. aureus*

39.4 A 12-year-old girl is brought to the emergency department because of a severe sore throat, muffled voice, drooling, and fatigue. She has been sick for the past 3 days and is unable to eat because of painful swallowing. The parents deny any history of recurrent pharyngitis. The patient still manages to open her mouth, and you are able to see an abscess at the upper pole of the right tonsil with deviation of the uvula toward the midline. Examination of the neck reveals enlarged and tender lymph nodes. Which of the following is the most appropriate management?

A. Analgesics for pain

B. Oral antibiotics

C. Nebulized racemic epinephrine

D. Incision and drainage of the abscess

E. Tonsillectomy and adenoidectomy

ANSWERS

39.1 **E.** Bronchiolitis is the most likely diagnosis in this case. There is no established treatment for bronchiolitis except for supportive management of the patient's symptoms. Because the infant did not respond to an albuterol trial (answer A), there is no justification for continuing its use. Antihistamines and decongestants (answer B), as well as antibiotics (answer C), are not effective. Palivizumab (answer D) is not helpful in the acute setting.

39.2 **D.** The incidence of epiglottitis has markedly reduced since the introduction of the Hib vaccine. Children with epiglottitis are more likely to be in the tripod position than prone (answer A). The steeple sign (answer B) is seen in croup; the thumb sign is seen in epiglottitis. Visualization of the epiglottis should preferentially occur in an operating room (not in the office, as in answer C), where immediate intubation or tracheostomy can occur.

39.3 **B.** Tracheitis matches the symptom description and is usually caused by *S. aureus*. Group A streptococci (answer C) is now the leading cause of epiglottitis, but the symptom constellation is more likely due to tracheitis; a patient with epiglottitis is usually sitting still and drooling. Because of *H. influenzae* type B immunizations, this organism is now a rare cause of epiglottitis (answer A). Retropharyngeal abscess (answer E) usually presents insidiously with neck pain with swelling, fever, dysphagia, and drooling.

39.4 **D.** This patient is suffering from peritonsillar abscess, which is a surgical emergency since the upper airway can be compromised. Of the choices listed, treatment with incision and drainage is the most appropriate. Tonsillectomy (answer E) is only indicated if there are confirmed cases of **recurrent** pharyngitis and peritonsillar abscess. Answer A (analgesics for pain) is an important consideration but secondary to treatment of the abscess. Answer C (nebulized racemic epinephrine) is useful for conditions such as croup (bronchiolitis). Oral antibiotics (answer B) is not appropriate for peritonsillar abscess.

CLINICAL PEARLS

▶ Sufficient airflow is required for the airway to produce a wheezing sound.

▶ Disappearance of wheezing in a patient who initially presents with wheezing is an ominous sign that suggests complete blockage of the airway or imminent respiratory failure.

▶ Bronchiolitis is the most common lower respiratory disease of infants and the most common reason for hospitalization for infants younger than 1 year.

▶ Never perform a blind finger sweep of a foreign object aspirated in any patient, and especially in an infant or child, since this maneuver can push the object further down the airway.

▶ Epiglottitis and tracheitis are medical emergencies that require the ability to rapidly secure airways.

REFERENCES

Mapelli E. Sabhaney V. Stridor and drooling in infants and children. In: Tintinalli JE, Stapczynski S, Ma OJ, Cline DM, Cydulka RK, Meckler GD, eds. *Tintinalli's Emergency Medicine: A Comprehensive Study Guide.* 8th ed. New York, NY: McGraw Hill; 2016: Chap. 123 [e-version].

Smith DK, McDermott AJ, Sullivan JF. Croup: diagnosis and management. *Am Fam Physician.* 2018;97(9):575-580.

Smith DK, Seales S, Budzik C. Respiratory syncytial virus bronchiolitis in children. *Am Fam Physician.* 2017;95(2):94-99.

A 28-year-old woman presents to your office with a chief complaint of abdominal discomfort, bloating, and constipation intermittently over the last 10 years. While her symptoms have waxed and waned, they have never worsened. She describes her abdominal pain as diffuse, dull, and crampy, and she often finds relief after a bowel movement. She denies radiation of pain, nausea, vomiting, fever, chills, weight loss, heartburn, hematemesis, hematochezia, or melena. Over the last 3 months, she reports abdominal cramping 12 to 15 times per month and has a hard bowel movement every 2 to 3 days with a sensation of incomplete evacuation. She has tried over-the-counter stool softeners and laxatives, with only minimal improvement. She has no significant past medical history and denies tobacco, alcohol, or illicit drugs. Her family history is negative for gastrointestinal (GI) disease, and she reports that her parents and siblings are healthy. She is currently engaged and reports moderate stress in preparing for the wedding. Her vital signs and general physical examination are unremarkable. Her abdomen has normal bowel sounds and mild tenderness on diffuse palpation without rebound, rigidity, or guarding. There is no hepatomegaly and no palpable masses. Pelvic examination is unremarkable, and anorectal examination reveals normal sphincter tone, no masses, and guaiac-negative stool.

▶ What is the most likely diagnosis?
▶ What is the first step in diagnostic evaluation?
▶ What are the recommended treatments for this condition?

ANSWERS TO CASE 40:

Irritable Bowel Syndrome

Summary: A 28-year-old woman presents with

- A several-year history of intermittent crampy abdominal pain and constipation
- Denial of any constitutional symptoms or bloody stools
- Unremarkable past medical history and family history
- Unremarkable physical examination, including abdominal and pelvic examinations

Most likely diagnosis: Irritable bowel syndrome, constipation predominant subtype (IBS-C).

First step in diagnostic evaluation: After conducting a thorough history and physical, in the absence of "alarm signs or symptoms," no diagnostic testing needs to be performed.

Recommended treatments: Education; reassurance; lifestyle modifications, including tracking of IBS symptoms with a food diary, an elimination diet, regular exercise, minimizing environmental and psychosocial stressors; appropriate pharmacotherapy.

ANALYSIS

Objectives

1. Describe the epidemiology, clinical manifestations, and pathophysiology of IBS. (EPA 1, 12)

2. Learn the diagnostic approach to IBS and rationale for ordering diagnostic studies based on symptom subtype and presence or absence of alarm features. (EPA 3)

3. Review current therapeutic strategies in the patient with IBS. (EPA 4)

Considerations

This is a young woman with a long-standing history of crampy abdominal pain and constipation. She denies any "alarm features," including fever, weight loss, bloody stools, or severe abdominal pain, and she denies recent antibiotic use. She has no family history of GI disorders and no physical examination findings of concern. The chronicity, lack of alarm symptoms, and lack of worsening of symptoms coupled with her age suggests a functional gastrointestinal disorder (FGID), such as IBS. Education about IBS, reassurance about lack of organic pathology, guidance on dietary modifications and physical activity, strategies to reduced psychosocial stressors, and options for pharmacotherapy should be discussed.

APPROACH TO:
Irritable Bowel Syndrome

DEFINITIONS

FUNCTIONAL GASTROINTESTINAL DISORDER: Poorly understood and often misdiagnosed GI conditions with varied mechanisms of pathophysiology, clinical presentations, and provisions of management with an absence of identifiable organic function.

IRRITABLE BOWEL SYNDROME: An FGID characterized by chronic abdominal pain and change in form and frequency of stool.

ROME IV: The Rome Foundation is a worldwide organization of scientists and clinicians that classifies and critically appraises the science of GI function and dysfunction. Rome IV criteria are current guidelines for the diagnosis and treatment of FGIDs.

CLINICAL APPROACH

Pathophysiology

The prevalence of IBS is approximately 5% to 20% of the North American population, accounting for a large proportion of GI complaints seen by both primary care providers and gastroenterologists. IBS affects women 1.5 to 3 times more often than men and has a peak incidence from age 20 to 39 years, although any age group can be affected.

Several models to explain the pathophysiology of IBS have been proposed, as **IBS appears to be associated with a combination of host and environmental factors.** Host factors include alterations in GI motility, microbial flora, and gut mucosal barriers; visceral hypersensitivity; dysregulation of the brain-gut axis; and increased reactivity to stressors. Environmental factors include a history of enteric infections and/or antibiotic use, a history of physical or sexual abuse, or other psychosocial stressors.

The Rome IV criteria were developed to aid clinicians in accurate and appropriate diagnosis of IBS in the absence of organic pathology (Table 40–1). Clinicians

Table 40–1 • ROME IV DIAGNOSTIC CRITERIA FOR IRRITABLE BOWEL SYNDROME
Recurrent abdominal pain, on average, at least 1 d/wk in the last 3 months, associated with two or more of the following criteria: • Related to defecation • Associated with a change in the frequency of stool • Associated with a change in form (appearance) of stool Criteria fulfilled for the last 3 months with symptom onset at least 6 months prior to diagnosis

Data from Drossman, DA, ed. Rome IV: Functional Gastrointestinal Disorders, 4th ed. 2016. Copyright © The Rome Foundation. All rights reserved.

Table 40–2 • ALARM FEATURES/RED FLAGS WARRANTING FURTHER WORKUP
Abdominal or rectal mass
Blood in the stool or rectal bleeding
Change in symptom quality
Family history of colon or ovarian cancer, inflammatory bowel disease, or celiac disease
Fever
New onset of symptoms at age 50 or older
Nighttime symptoms that awake the individual
Markers of inflammatory bowel disease
Markers of celiac disease
Recent use of antibiotics
Unexplained anemia
Unintentional or unexplained weight loss

are encouraged to use judicious, cost-effective diagnostic testing when appropriate and to minimize unnecessary testing.

Irritable bowel syndrome may coincide with other functional disorders, including fibromyalgia, chronic fatigue, interstitial cystitis, chronic pelvic pain, and chronic headaches. Conflicting studies suggest that patients with IBS may have higher rates of depression, anxiety, and posttraumatic stress disorder.

The differential diagnosis of IBS includes celiac disease, GI infection, lactose intolerance, diverticular disease, inflammatory bowel disease (IBD), colorectal cancer, ischemic colitis, carcinoid tumor, and adverse effects of various drug classes, including opiates, antidepressants, and calcium channel blockers. Patients should be asked for the presence of alarm symptoms that may suggest an **underlying organic etiology** and warrant further workup or referral to gastroenterology (Table 40–2).

Clinical Presentation

Patients with IBS may complain of recurrent and episodic nonlocalized abdominal pain with a predominant pattern of **constipation (IBS-C), diarrhea (IBS-D),** or **mixed symptoms** of constipation alternating with diarrhea (IBS-M). The pain often has variable intensity and may be worsened by emotional stress. Patients often report crampy abdominal pain that does not awaken them from sleep and can fluctuate over time but is not described as progressive. Other GI symptoms seen in IBS include the passage of mucus with stool, bowel urgency, abdominal distention or bloating, or the sensation of incomplete stool evacuation. Up to 50% of patients with IBS also experience upper GI symptoms, including dyspepsia, nausea, gastroesophageal reflux, dysphagia, early satiety, and noncardiac chest pain.

A thorough history should be obtained using open-ended, nonjudgmental questions that include review of symptoms outside of GI symptoms and psychosocial components. The physical examination should focus on ruling out organic pathologic processes that are inconsistent with IBS. Importance should be paid to all medications, dietary habits, and environmental stressors that may worsen the symptoms of IBS.

Treatment

Treatment of IBS is aimed at **improving symptoms and quality of life.** Treatment options can be challenging due to the recurrent nature of symptoms and because some symptoms may be refractory to treatment. As with all functional disorders, the cornerstone of management is a therapeutic relationship between the provider and the patient. Clinicians should spend time establishing rapport, listening attentively, and explaining pathophysiology, natural history, and prognosis, including the chronic nature of IBS. **Providers should spend time validating patient concerns and answering questions**, especially at the initial visit. Setting realistic goals for functional improvement, not cure, is helpful for creating structured and purposeful visits for patients.

Initial Therapy. Having patients create a food diary may be useful in associating certain foods to IBS symptoms. A **low FODMAP** (fermentable oligosaccharide, disaccharide, monosaccharide, and polyols) is an elimination diet that may provide some symptomatic improvement. Soluble fiber supplementation (eg, psyllium) may provide some symptomatic improvement in patients with IBS-C, but it also may cause bloating. Exercise, stress reduction, psychological treatment, and relaxation may also be useful in improving IBS symptoms.

Pharmacologic Therapy. Medications for IBS-C and IBS-D can be found in Table 40–3.

For abdominal pain, the following medications may be considered:

1. Antispasmodics (eg, dicyclomine, hyoscyamine) are anticholinergic agents that have demonstrated improvement in IBS-related global symptoms and abdominal pain. These may be used on an as-needed basis, especially when pain is mild and infrequent. Side effects include dry mouth, blurred vision, and dizziness.

2. Tricyclic antidepressants (TCAs) have demonstrated modest improvement in abdominal pain and global relief and can be considered when pain is more frequent and severe. TCAs can cause a sedation effect and should be used with caution in patients with prolonged QT intervals.

3. Probiotics and enteric-coated peppermint oil may be helpful for some individuals in improving bowel symptoms and reducing visceral pain.

4. Selective serotonin reuptake inhibitors (SSRIs) have not been shown to improve global symptoms or abdominal pain in patients with IBS alone, but they may be beneficial when depression or anxiety disorders are comorbid with IBS.

Table 40–3 • MEDICATIONS USED FOR IRRITABLE BOWEL SYNDROME		
Drug Name	Mechanism of Action	Comments
Medications for constipation-predominant IBS (IBS-C)		
Polyethylene glycol (PEG)	Osmotic laxative that improves symptoms of constipation by increasing stool frequency	Limited evidence for global symptom improvement
Linaclotide (Linzess)	Stimulates cGMP production to increase intestinal motility and fluid secretion	Modest improvement in abdominal pain and complete spontaneous bowel movements, improvement in global symptoms of IBS
Lubiprostone (Amitiza)	Selectively activates intestinal chloride channels to increase fluid secretions, increase motility, and promote spontaneous bowel movements	Demonstrated global symptom relief
Plecanatide (Trulance)	Guanylate cyclase-C agonist that increases intestinal fluid transit, increases stool frequency, and decreases visceral pain	
Medications for diarrhea-predominant IBS (IBS-D)		
Loperamide (Imodium)	Opioid receptor agonist that decreases activity of the myenteric plexus, which reduces the frequency of loose stools	Also decreases bowel urgency
Rifaximin (Xifaxan)	Nonsystemic antibiotic used in the treatment of traveler's diarrhea	Has shown improvement in abdominal pain, bloating, stool consistency, and IBS-related global symptoms
Alosetron (Lotronex)	Serotonin antagonist that slows fecal movement through the GI tract, decreasing volume and water content of stool	Demonstrated improvement in abdominal pain and IBS-related global symptoms; currently FDA approved for women with IBS-D
Eluxadoline (Viberzi)	Mixed opioid receptor agonist/ antagonist that reduces visceral hypersensitivity and decreases GI motility	

cGMP, cyclic guanosine monophosphate; FDA, Food and Drug Administration, GI, gastrointestinal.

> **CASE CORRELATION**
>
> - See Case 23 (Lower Gastrointestinal Bleeding) and Case 31 (Abdominal Pain and Vomiting in a Child).

COMPREHENSION QUESTIONS

40.1 A 65-year-old man reports a lifelong history of IBS with alternating bouts of constipation and diarrhea. He denies blood in the stool, unintentional weight loss, fevers, or nighttime symptoms that awaken him. He now reports that his symptoms have worsened over the last several months. He has never had a colonoscopy. Which of the following is the recommend initial step in management?

    A. Esophagogastroduodenoscopy (EGD)

    B. Trial of polyethylene glycol

    C. Explore possible underlying psychiatric symptoms

    D. Colonoscopy

    E. Increase in fiber intake

40.2 A 47-year-old woman reports a 10-year history of intermittent abdominal pain and constipation alternating with diarrhea. She has no weight loss, fever, or alarm features on history or examination. Which of the following agents can be used for treatment of mild-to-moderate abdominal pain associated with IBS?

    A. Amitriptyline

    B. Lubiprostone

    C. Dicyclomine

    D. Fluoxetine

40.3 A 27-year-old man in graduate school is evaluated for intermittent abdominal pain and frequent loose stools. He has no fevers, weight loss, bloody stools, or symptoms that wake him up at night. His family history is negative for colorectal cancer and IBD. He is diagnosed with IBS-D and asks about getting a colonoscopy to support his diagnosis. Although not indicated as part of his workup, a colonoscopy in this patient would likely show which of the following?

    A. Focal ulcerations adjacent to normal mucosa

    B. Normal colonic mucosa

    C. Pseudopolyps and mucosal inflammation

    D. Intestinal villous atrophy

40.4 A 22-year-old woman is a college student who has been increasingly stressed with coursework this semester. She has been using over-the-counter antacids more days out of the week than not for an upset stomach. She typically has two to three bowel movements per week but recently has only been having one or two hard bowel movements a week. She reports no blood in the stool. She feels immediate relief after passage of stool and flatulence, but she often feels like her bowel movements are incomplete. She has tried several diets eliminating foods that create GI symptoms and has increased her exercise regimen from once a week to daily without improvement. Which of the following therapies is recommended in IBS-C to improve motility, abdominal pain, spontaneous bowel movements, and IBS-related global function?

A. Hyoscyamine

B. Fluoxetine

C. Linaclotide

D. Loperamide

40.5 A 35-year-old woman comes to your office worried that she might have IBS, which she heard about from her colleagues at work. She reports abdominal pain and diarrhea for 3 months. She also reports observing several bloody stools. She is worried about the impact that frequently having to use the bathroom is having on her job as an attorney. Her physical examination is unremarkable except for a guaiac-positive test after a rectal examination. When reviewing her medical records, you notice that she has lost 15 pounds since she last saw you 4 months ago. Which of the following is an appropriate next step?

A. Refer her for cognitive behavioral therapy.

B. Offer her symptomatic relief with loperamide.

C. Recommend that she take fiber for better bowel regulation.

D. Obtain a colonoscopy.

E. Recommend that she keep a food diary and follow up in 1 month.

ANSWERS

40.1 **D.** Age-appropriate colorectal cancer screening (eg, colonoscopy) is indicated, even in the setting of an established diagnosis of IBS. Dietary modifications, fiber supplementation (answer E), and addressing psychiatric contributions to GI symptoms (answer C) should be considered after colorectal cancer screening is performed. EGD (answer A) is not part of routine screening for colon cancer or workup for IBS. Answer B (polyethylene glycol) is an osmotic laxative and would likely worsen the patient's symptoms.

40.2 **C.** Dicyclomine, an antispasmodic anticholinergic medication, can be used on an as-needed basis for mild-to-moderate abdominal pain associated with IBS. For more persistent and severe pain, low-dose TCAs, such as amitriptyline (answer A), are beneficial. Lubiprostone (answer B) is indicated for patients with IBS-C. SSRIs like fluoxetine (answer D) have shown no improvement in those with abdominal pain and global symptoms related to IBS.

40.3 **B.** Irritable bowel syndrome is a functional disorder with no identifiable organic cause. Colonoscopy in a patient with IBS would show normal colonic mucosa. Colonoscopy is not indicated in a young patient without alarm features or family history of IBD or colon cancer. Focal ulcerations (answer A) adjacent to normal mucosa describe skip lesions and cobblestoning, which are found in Crohn disease. Patients with Crohn disease often present with abdominal pain, weight loss, diarrhea, oral ulcers, malabsorption, and manifestations outside the GI system, including arthritis and eye and skin disorders. Pseudopolyps (answer C) and mucosal inflammation can be found in patients with ulcerative colitis (UC). Patients with UC may present with fever, bloody stool, weight loss, and colicky abdominal pain. Intestinal villous atrophy (answer D) is found in celiac disease. Patients with celiac disease may present with diarrhea, abdominal distention, malabsorption, and nutritional deficiencies.

40.4 **C.** Linaclotide is a recommended pharmacologic therapy in IBS-C. Patients may try this medication after initial treatment with lifestyle modifications. Patients may choose to discontinue treatment due to diarrhea as a common side effect. Loperamide (answer D) can be used in IBS-D, and hyoscyamine (answer A) can be used to treat mild-to-moderate abdominal pain associated with IBS. Evidence regarding the efficacy of fluoxetine (answer B) in treating IBS has shown conflicting results; sertraline has been shown to be moderately effective, especially for IBS-C and when there are comorbid conditions such as depression and/or anxiety.

40.5 **D.** This patient presents with alarm signs of blood in the stool and weight loss. Although a psychiatric diagnosis or IBS is possible, more serious conditions should be evaluated and ruled out. Therefore, neither answer A (cognitive behavioral therapy) for a psychiatric diagnosis nor answer B (loperamide) for the diarrhea is the best treatment at this time. Evaluation should include a colonoscopy, complete blood count, basic metabolic panel, stool cultures, C-reactive protein, and fecal calprotectin to rule out malignancy, infection, or IBD. Recommending fiber supplementation (answer C) or keeping a food diary with later follow-up (answer E) is not appropriate at this time.

CLINICAL PEARLS

▶ The cornerstone of management of IBS is the therapeutic relationship between patient and the clinician, who can collaborate on an individualized plan of care that best manages the patient's symptoms. In the absence of alarm features, laboratory testing may not be required to make an accurate diagnosis.

▶ Alarm features include fever, weight loss, bloody stools, severe abdominal pain, and denial of recent antibiotic use. These may indicate an underlying organic pathology and require additional diagnostic workup such as laboratory, radiographic, and/or endoscopic evaluation.

▶ Treatment should be symptom specific and should include dietary and lifestyle changes, examination of any psychosocial factors that contribute to IBS symptoms, and appropriate pharmacotherapy.

REFERENCES

Böhn L, Störsrud S, Liljebo T, et al. Diet low in FODMAPs reduces symptoms of irritable bowel syndrome as well as traditional dietary advice: a randomized controlled trial. *Gastroenterology*. 2015;149:1399.

Chey WD, Kurlander MD, Eswaran S. Irritable bowel syndrome: a clinical review. *N Engl J Med*. 2015;313(9):949-958.

Heidelbaugh JJ. These 3 tools can help you streamline management of IBS. *J Fam Pract*. 2017;66(6): 346-348, 350-353.

Heidelbaugh JJ, Hungin P, eds. *ROME IV: Functional Gastrointestinal Disorders for Primary Care and Non-GI Clinicians*. Rome Foundation, 2016.

Hungin APS, Becher A, Cayley B, et al. Irritable bowel syndrome: an integrated explanatory model for clinical practice. *Neurogastroenterol Motil*. 2015;27(6):750-753.

Lembo AJ, Lacy BE, Zuckerman MJ, et al. Eluxadoline for irritable bowel syndrome with diarrhea. *N Engl J Med*. 2016;374:242-253.

Weinberg DS, Smalley W, Heidelbaugh JJ, Sultan S. American Gastroenterological Association Institute guideline on the pharmacological management of irritable bowel syndrome. *Gastroenterology*. 2014; 147(5):1146-1148.

A 20-year-old woman who is a college student is brought to the emergency department (ED) complaining of chest pain that started 45 minutes ago. She describes the chest pain as substernal, 10/10 in intensity, radiating to her jaw, and associated with headache, sweating, nausea, and palpitations. She was given oxygen, aspirin, and nitroglycerin by emergency medical services in route to the ED and received morphine on her arrival at the ED. The patient is accompanied by her roommate, who mentions that the patient came back from a concert about an hour ago and complained of feeling nauseated, anxious, and somewhat paranoid. The patient has no history of health problems and has not had similar episodes in the past. She is currently sexually active with one male partner and takes oral contraceptive pills for birth control. She reports drinking alcohol and smoking cigarettes occasionally. On questioning about use of illicit drugs, she hesitates, then says that she drank "a few beers," smoked "a few joints," and "took a capsule" at the concert. She swears that this is the first time she has used any illicit substances.

On examination, she is anxious and restless with heightened alertness. Her temperature is 101 °F (38.3 °C), pulse is 119 beats/min, respiratory rate is 24 breaths/min, blood pressure is 165/90 mm Hg, oxygen saturation is 97% on room air, height is 60 inches, and weight is 100 lb. Eye examination reveals dilated pupils bilaterally with sluggish light reflex, along with occasional twitching of her right eye. Extraocular movements are found to be normal. Her heart examination reveals tachycardia with no murmurs. Respiratory examination reveals tachypnea with shallow breathing, but lung fields are clear to auscultation. Neck is without carotid bruit or jugular venous distention. Distal extremity pulses are brisk and symmetrical. The remainder of her examination is unremarkable.

▶ What is the differential diagnosis for this case?
▶ What is your first diagnostic step?
▶ What is the next step in management of this patient?

ANSWERS TO CASE 41:
Substance Use Disorder

Summary: A 20-year-old woman presents with

- No significant past medical history
- Symptoms of coronary ischemia and other symptoms that signify increased sympathetic activity (substernal chest pain, 10/10 in intensity, radiating to her jaw, and associated with headache, sweating, nausea, and palpitations)
- Report of drinking alcohol, smoking "a few joints," and ingesting unknown substances
- Fever, tachycardia, and hypertension
- Dilated pupils bilaterally with sluggish light reflex, along with occasional twitching of her right eye

Differential diagnosis: Cocaine-induced myocardial ischemia; cocaine- and ecstasy-induced mental status changes (eg, anxiety, paranoia); panic attack; cardiac arrhythmia; and pulmonary embolism.

First diagnostic step: 12-lead electrocardiogram (ECG); markers of myocardial damage, including serum troponin I, creatine kinase, and creating kinase MB isoenzyme (CK-MB) performed stat; urine toxicology screen; blood alcohol level; comprehensive metabolic panel (electrolytes, glucose, kidney and liver function tests); complete blood count (CBC); prothrombin time (PT); partial thromboplastin time (PTT); international normalized ratio (INR); and a chest x-ray.

Next step in management: Telemetry, oxygen, assessment of ABC's, aspirin, sublingual nitroglycerin, and morphine. Beta-blockers should be avoided initially, especially if cocaine intoxication is suspected, rule out acute coronary syndrome with serial ECG and cardiac enzymes.

ANALYSIS

Objectives

1. Be able to state the definition and epidemiology of substance use disorders (SUDs). (EPA 12)

2. Be able to state the most commonly used illicit and prescription drugs, as well as their adverse and toxic effects. (EPA 2)

3. Be able to name the components of a validated ambulatory care screening protocol, history taking, physical examination, and laboratory findings in patients consistent with substance intoxication and SUDs. (EPA 1, 3)

4. Be able to name the medications available to control alcohol use disorder (AUD). (EPA 4)

Considerations

This is a healthy young woman who presents with acute chest pain unrelated to respiration and position but associated with nausea, fever, tachycardia, tachypnea, anxiety, heightened alertness, paranoia, and mydriasis. The events preceding her arrival include ingestion of alcohol and other likely illicit substances that might have caused her to have chest pain. The initial management of this patient will be the same as for any other patient presenting with acute chest pain, as she should be placed on telemetry and oxygen. Airway, breathing, and circulation should be ensured followed by administration of aspirin, sublingual nitroglycerin, and morphine. Beta-blockers should be avoided initially, especially if cocaine intoxication is suspected, due to risk of unopposed alpha constriction, which can induce ischemia. Ruling out acute coronary syndrome with serial ECG and cardiac enzymes should occur every 8 hours over three intervals. She should be monitored closely for mental status changes and withdrawal symptoms of potentially ingested illicit drugs. After ruling out the cardiac causes of chest pain, it is very important to screen for signs and symptoms of acute illicit drug intoxication and drug abuse in this patient. Urine toxicology screening should be performed to detect the most commonly abused illicit substances.

When people consume two or more psychoactive drugs together, such as cocaine, ecstasy, and alcohol, the danger of experiencing adverse effects of each drug is compounded. In this patient, the history and physical examination suggest that she may have used a combination of cocaine and alcohol, which may have led to the formation of a third substance, cocaethylene, which intensifies cocaine's euphoric effects. Cocaethylene is associated with a greater risk of coronary vasospasm than cocaine alone, resulting in myocardial ischemia and sudden death.

APPROACH TO:
Substance Use Disorder

DEFINITIONS

DETOXIFICATION: A process that enables the body to rid itself of a drug.

RELAPSE: Resumption of illicit drug use after an attempt or multiple attempts to quit.

SUBSTANCE USE DISORDER: The *Diagnostic and Statistical Manual of Mental Disorders, Fifth Edition* (*DSM-5*) no longer uses the terms *substance abuse* and *substance dependence*. Instead, the term *substance use disorder* is used, with SUD defined as mild, moderate, or severe to indicate the level of severity. SUDs occur when the recurrent use of alcohol and/or drugs causes clinical and functional impairment, such as health problems, disability, and failure to meet major responsibilities at work, school, or home. A diagnosis of SUD is based on evidence of the craving of a substance, failure to be able to control use, social impairment, risky use, and pharmacological criteria.

CLINICAL APPROACH

Pathophysiology

Primary care providers are well positioned to identify patients at risk for drug abuse early in the course. Since addiction and dependence are equal opportunity afflictions, clinicians should screen all new patients for substance abuse. Abrupt changes in behavior or functioning of the patient should also prompt the provider to screen for substance use. As with many other chronic illnesses, early recognition and management of the substance abuse leads to better outcomes. The most common SUDs in the United States are AUD, tobacco use disorder (see Case 7), cannabis use disorder, stimulant use disorder, hallucinogen use disorder, and opioid use disorder (see Case 59).

Vulnerability and affinity to addiction differs from person to person and is considered multifactorial in origin. Factors include gender, ethnicity, developmental stage, and socioeconomic environment. **Genetic susceptibility accounts for between 40% and 60% of a person's vulnerability to addiction.** Populations at increased risk of drug abuse include adolescents and persons with psychiatric disorders. Table 41–1 includes the most commonly abused substance categories, street names, route of administration, intoxication effects, and potential health complications.

Screening. The **United States Preventive Services Task Force (USPSTF) recommends adults 18 and above be screened both for AUD (Grade B) and for illicit drug use (Grade B).** Screening, brief intervention, and referral to treatment (SBIRT) is broadly recommended by multiple federal agencies, the USPSTF, and all of the primary care physician groups. The National Commission on Prevention Priorities ranked SBIRT among its top five priorities, ahead of 20 other effective services, including colorectal cancer screening, hypertension screening and treatment, and influenza immunization.

Clinician offices can integrate annual tobacco, alcohol, and substance use screening. Tobacco and alcohol screening and brief interventions are measures for the Merit-Based Incentive Payment System (MIPS) used for reimbursement for value-based population health medicine. Annual SBIRT screens are reimbursed by all major insurers. If an individual is identified as having an SUD, the history should be geared to determine what, how, and when the patient is using the drug; the level of counseling and treatment should be based on the pattern and severity of use. Information about co-occurring psychiatric or medical conditions and a personal or family history of substance abuse should be obtained. The clinician should ask open-ended questions and should remain nonjudgmental, respectful, and empathetic at all times. Information should also be elicited about health, family, social, career, financial, and legal impacts of the drug use.

Alcohol Use Disorder. Excessive alcohol use can increase a person's risk of developing serious health problems in addition to those issues associated with intoxication behaviors and alcohol withdrawal symptoms. According to the Centers for Disease Control and Prevention, excessive alcohol use causes 88,000 deaths a year. Data from the National Survey on Drug Use and Health show that in 2017, slightly more than half of Americans ages 12 and up drank alcohol. Most people drink alcohol in moderation, but an estimated 16.7 million are considered heavy drinkers

Table 41–1 • COMMONLY ABUSED ILLICIT AND PRESCRIPTION DRUGS

Category and Name	Commercial and Street Names	Route of Administration	Intoxication Effects and Potential Health Consequences
Cannabinoids			
Hashish	Boom, chronic, gangster, hash, hash oil, hemp	Swallowed, smoked	**Common features:** *euphoria, slowed thinking and reaction time, confusion, impaired balance and coordination* and cough, frequent respiratory infections; impaired memory and learning; tachycardia, anxiety; panic attacks; **tolerance, addiction**
Marijuana	Blunt, dope, ganja, grass, herb, joints, Mary Jane, pot, reefer, sinsemilla, skunk, weed	Swallowed, smoked	
Depressants			
Barbiturates	*Amytal, Nembutal, Seconal, Phenobarbital* and barbs, red, phennies, tooies, yellow jackets	Injected, swallowed	**Common features:** *reduced anxiety; feeling of well-being; lowered inhibitions; slowed pulse and breathing; lowered blood pressure; poor concentration* and fatigue; impaired coordination, memory, judgment; **addiction;** respiratory depression and arrest; death. **Also, for Barbiturates:** *sedation, drowsiness* and depression, excitement, poor judgment, dizziness, life-threatening **withdrawal. Also, for Benzodiazepines:** *sedation, drowsiness* and dizziness. **Also, for GHB:** *drowsiness, nausea* and vomiting, headache, loss of consciousness, loss of reflexes, seizures, coma, death. **Also, for Methaqualone:** *euphoria* and depression, poor reflexes
Benzodiazepines	*Ativan, Halcion, Librium, Valium, Xanax* and candy, downers, sleeping pills, tranks	Swallowed, injected	
GHB	*γ-Hydroxybutyrate* and G, Georgia homeboy, grievous bodily harm, liquid ecstasy	Swallowed	
Methaqualone	*Quaalude, Sopor, Parest* and ludes, mandrex, quad, quay	Injected, swallowed	
Dissociative Anesthetics			
Ketamine	*Ketalar SV* and cat Valiums, K, Special K, vitamin K	Injected, snorted, smoked	**Common features:** *tachycardia, increased blood pressure, impaired motor function,* and memory loss; numbness; vomiting. **Also, for Ketamine:** at high doses, delirium, depression, respiratory depression, and arrest. **Also, for PCP and analogs:** *possible decrease in blood pressure and heart rate, panic, aggression* and loss of appetite, depression, nystagmus
PCP and analogs	*Phencyclidine* and angel dust, boat, hog, love boat, peace pill	Injected, swallowed, smoked	

(Continued)

Table 41–1 • COMMONLY ABUSED ILLICIT AND PRESCRIPTION DRUGS (continued)

Category and Name	*Commercial* and Street Names	Route of Administration	*Intoxication Effects* and Potential Health Consequences
Opioids and Morphine Derivatives			
Codeine	*Codeine with Empirin or Fiorinal, Robitussin A-C, Tylenol with Codeine* and Captain Cody, doors and fours, loads, pancakes and syrup	Injected, swallowed	**Common features:** *pain relief, euphoria, drowsiness, miosis,* and nausea, constipation, confusion, sedation, respiratory depression and arrest, **tolerance, addiction,** unconsciousness, coma, death. **Also, for Codeine:** less analgesia, sedation, and respiratory depression than morphine. **Also, for Heroin:** staggering gait
Heroin	*Diacetyl-morphine* and brown sugar, dope, H, horse, junk, skag, skunk, smack, white horse	Injected, smoked, snorted	
Fentanyl and analogs	*Actiq, Duragesic, Sublimaze* and Apache, China girl, China white, dance fever, friend, goodfella, jackpot, murder 8, TNT, Tango and Cash	Injected, smoked, snorted	
Morphine	*Roxanol, Duramorph, MS-Contin* and M, Miss Emma, monkey, white stuff	Injected, swallowed, smoked	
Opium	*Laudanum, paregoric,* big O, black stuff, block, gum, hop	Swallowed, smoked	
Oxycodone HCl	Oxycontin and Oxy, OC, killer	Swallowed, injected	
Hydrocodone acetaminophen	*Vicodin, Anexsia, Lorcet, Lortab, Norco,* and Vike, Watson-387	Swallowed	
Hallucinogens			
LSD	*Lysergic acid diethylamide* and acid, blotter, boomers, cubes, microdot, yellow sunshines	Swallowed, absorbed through mouth tissues	**Common features:** altered states of perception and feeling; nausea; persisting perception disorder (flashbacks). **Also, for LSD and Mescaline:** increased body temperature, heart rate, blood pressure; loss of appetite, sleeplessness, numbness, weakness, tremors; persistent mental disorders. **Also, for Psilocybin:** nervousness, paranoia
Mescaline	Buttons, cactus, mesc, peyote	Swallowed, smoked	
Psilocybin	Magic mushroom, purple passion, shrooms	Swallowed	

(Continued)

Table 41–1 • COMMONLY ABUSED ILLICIT AND PRESCRIPTION DRUGS (continued)

Category and Name	*Commercial* and Street Names	Route of Administration	*Intoxication Effects* and Potential Health Consequences
Stimulants			
Amphetamines	*Biphetamine, Dexedrine* and bennies, black beauties, crosses, hearts, LA turnaround, speed, truck drivers, uppers	Injected, swallowed, smoked, snorted	**Common features:** *increased heart rate, blood pressure, metabolism; feelings of exhilaration, energy, increased mental alertness* and rapid or irregular heartbeat; reduced appetite, weight loss, heart failure, nervousness, insomnia. **Also, for Amphetamines:** *rapid breathing* and tremor, loss of coordination; irritability, anxiousness, restlessness, delirium, panic, paranoia, impulsive behavior, aggressiveness, **tolerance, addiction. Also, for Cocaine:** *increased temperature* and chest pain, respiratory failure, nausea, abdominal pain, strokes, seizures, headaches, malnutrition, panic attacks, mydriasis. **Also, for MDMA:** *mild hallucinogenic effects, increased tactile sensitivity, empathic feelings* and impaired memory and learning, hyperthermia, cardiac toxicity, renal failure, liver toxicity. **Also, for Methamphetamine:** *aggression, violence, psychotic behavior* and memory loss, cardiac and neurological damage; impaired memory and learning, tolerance, addiction. **Also, for Nicotine:** additional effects attributable to tobacco exposure; adverse pregnancy outcomes; chronic lung disease, cardiovascular disease, stroke, cancer, tolerance, addiction
Cocaine	*Cocaine hydrochloride* and blow, bump, C, candy, Charlie, coke, crack, flake, rock, snow, toot	Injected, smoked, snorted	
MDMA	*Methylenedioxy-methamphetamine* and Adam, clarity, ecstasy, Eve, lover's speed, peace, STP	Swallowed	
Methamphetamine	*Desoxyn* and chalk, crank, crystal, fire, glass, go fast, ice, meth, speed	Injected, swallowed, smoked, snorted	
Methylphenidate	*Ritalin* and JIF, MPH, R-ball, Skippy, the smart drug, vitamin R	Injected, swallowed, snorted	
Nicotine	cigarettes, cigars, smokeless tobacco, snuff, spit tobacco, bidis, chew	Smoked, snorted, taken in snuff and spit tobacco	

(Continued)

Category and Name	Commercial and Street Names	Route of Administration	Intoxication Effects and Potential Health Consequences
Table 41–1 • COMMONLY ABUSED ILLICIT AND PRESCRIPTION DRUGS (continued)			
Other Compounds			
Anabolic steroids	Anadrol, Oxandrin, Durabolin, Depo-Testosterone, Equipoise, roids, juice	Injected, swallowed, applied to skin	**Common features:** no intoxication effects and hypertension, blood clotting and cholesterol changes, liver cysts and cancer, kidney cancer, hostility and aggression, acne; in adolescents, premature stoppage of growth; in males, prostate cancer, reduced sperm production, shrunken testicles, breast enlargement; in females, menstrual irregularities, development of beard and other masculine characteristics, hirsutism, virilization
Dextromethorphan	Found in some cough and cold medications; Robotripping, Robo, Triple C	Swallowed	**Common features:** distorted visual perceptions to complete dissociative effects and at higher doses see "dissociative anesthetics"
Inhalants	Solvents (paint thinners, gasoline, glues); gases (butane, propane, aerosol propellants, nitrous oxide); nitrites (isoamyl, isobutyl, cyclohexyl); laughing gas, poppers, snappers	Inhaled through nose or mouth	**Common features:** stimulation, loss of inhibition; headache; nausea or vomiting; slurred speech, loss of motor coordination; wheezing and unconsciousness, cramps, weight loss, muscle weakness, depression, memory impairment, damage to cardiovascular and nervous systems, sudden death

Data from Commonly Abused Drugs. (Revised March 2020). Retrieved from the National Institute on Drug Abuse (NIDA). https://www.drugabuse.gov/drugs-abuse/commonly-used-drugs-charts. Accessed May 26, 2020.

and are at high risk for AUD. The definitions for the different levels of drinking include the following:

- **Moderate drinking:** Up to one drink per day for women and up to two drinks per day for men.

- **Binge drinking:** Drinking four to five or more alcoholic drinks on the same occasion on at least 1 day in the past 30 days. Binge drinking produces blood alcohol concentrations of greater than 0.08 g/dL. This usually occurs after four drinks for women and five drinks for men over a 2-hour period.

- **Heavy drinking**: Drinking five or more drinks on the same occasion on each of 5 or more days in the past 30 days.

Cannabis Use Disorder. Marijuana is the most-used drug after alcohol and tobacco in the United States. In 2017, there were 26 million people ages 12 and up who reported using marijuana during the previous month. In 2014, based on marijuana use, 4.2 million people ages 12 and up met criteria for an SUD. Cannabis use disorder is defined as continued use despite impairment in psychological, physical, or social functioning. About 10% of users experience addiction. As adult use increases due to state legalization, the use increases in children and adolescents.

Stimulant Use Disorder. Stimulants increase alertness, attention, and energy, as well as elevate blood pressure, heart rate, and respirations. They include a wide range of drugs that have historically been used to treat conditions such as obesity, attention deficit hyperactivity disorder, and depression. Like other prescription medications, stimulants can be diverted for illegal use. The most commonly abused stimulants are amphetamines, methamphetamine, and cocaine. Stimulants can be synthetic (eg, amphetamines) or can be plant derived (eg, cocaine). They are usually taken orally, are snorted, or are delivered intravenously. In 2017, an estimated 1.8 million people ages 12 and older misused stimulants, and 2.2 million were users of cocaine. Withdrawal symptoms that occur after stopping or reducing use include fatigue, vivid and unpleasant dreams, sleep problems, increased appetite, and irregular problems in controlling movement.

Hallucinogen Use Disorder. Hallucinogens can be chemically synthesized (as with lysergic acid diethylamide, also known as LSD) or may occur naturally (as with psilocybin mushrooms, peyote). These drugs can produce visual and auditory hallucinations, feelings of detachment from one's environment and oneself, and distortions in time and perception. In 2017, approximately 1.4 million Americans had recent hallucinogen use.

Clinical Presentation

Some findings on the physical examination may aid in the diagnosis of illicit drug use. Eye examination is crucial, especially in an unconscious patient suspected to be under the influence of drugs. Dilated pupils may indicate stimulant or hallucinogen use or withdrawal from opioids. Constricted pupils are a hallmark of opioid use. Physical examination can also reveal signs such as damage to nasal mucosa, septum perforation due to nasal inhalation, or injection "track marks." Sequelae of cirrhosis, including spider angiomas, caput medusa, hepatomegaly, and/or ascites, due to viral hepatitis or alcohol abuse, may also be found.

Laboratory Values. Several laboratory tests are available for determining the presence of alcohol and other drugs in body fluids and other substances, such as urine, hair, and blood. **Urine drug toxicology tests measure recent substance use rather than chronic use or dependence.** These tests can have false negatives since synthetic substances ingested are often not detected in point-of-care urine drug toxicology tests. These tests can also have false positives and should be interpreted with caution. There is no conclusive test to determine SUDs. Useful laboratory tests may include breath or blood alcohol tests, urine toxicology, liver enzymes, electrolytes, renal function, CBC, PT/INR and PTT, and vitamin-deficiency screening.

Treatment

Substance use disorder is challenging and requires an understanding of the natural history of recovery, including high rates of relapse with the need for multiple long-term interprofessional interventions to achieve optimal outcomes. Although initial symptoms from withdrawal may not be very different from one class of drug to another, there are significant differences in complications and management of withdrawal from different substances. Therefore, it is crucial to identify the abused substance early in the treatment. The treatment is a long-term process, regardless of the substance being abused, and it often requires many behavioral changes and multiple attempts to quit.

Medication and behavioral therapy, especially when combined, are important elements of an overall therapeutic process that often begins with detoxification. This includes management of the withdrawal symptoms, followed by treatment and relapse prevention. A key to preventing relapse is to minimize the withdrawal symptoms, which is often the first step of treatment in a patient who acknowledges addiction. Tapering doses of long-acting agents for the abused drugs is frequently used to treat drug withdrawal. Antidepressants, anxiolytics, mood stabilizers, and antipsychotic medications may be critical for treatment success when patients have co-occurring psychiatric disorders.

Collaboration With Patients. Treatment of drug addiction is provided in various settings with different medication and behavioral therapy options, which should be discussed with the patient at the initiation of the treatment. Considering the wishes and readiness of the patient to acquire treatment, the provider should recommend a comprehensive plan, preferably including both medication and behavioral therapy. General categories for drug treatment programs include detoxification and medically managed withdrawal, long-term residential treatment, short-term residential treatment followed by long-term outpatient treatment, or exclusively outpatient treatment.

Pharmacotherapy. Detoxification is an important first step in substance abuse treatment with three goals: initiating abstinence, reducing withdrawal symptoms and severe complications, and retaining the patient in treatment. Ongoing treatment is needed thereafter to maintain abstinence. The aims are to restore normal cognitive and emotional function, to diminish cravings, and to prevent relapse. Medication helps make patients more receptive to the behavioral treatment and to avoid drug-seeking and related criminal behavior. See Table 41–2 for substance withdrawal symptoms, medications used to treat withdrawal symptoms, long-term treatment, and relapse prevention.

Behavioral Therapies. Behavioral treatment is an important adjunct to addiction treatment. Clinicians help by providing motivational interviewing to encourage behavior change, reduce relapse, modify lifestyles related to drug abuse, and help develop coping mechanisms to handle stressful situations. Additional behavioral therapy models include group therapy, cognitive behavioral therapy, and the 12-step model, which is used by organizations such as Alcoholics Anonymous and Narcotics Anonymous.

Table 41–2 • ADDICTION: WITHDRAWAL SYMPTOMS AND PHARMACOLOGY FOR DRUG WITHDRAWAL AND RELAPSE PREVENTION

Addictions

Withdrawal Symptoms	Generic Name	(Brand Name) Treatment Characteristics
Opioids		
Muscle cramps, arthralgia, anxiety, nausea, vomiting, malaise, drug seeking, mydriasis, piloerection, diaphoresis, rhinorrhea, lacrimation, diarrhea, insomnia, elevated blood pressure and pulse	**Methadone**	(Dolophine, Methadose) Long-acting synthetic opioid; given in dosage sufficient to prevent opioid withdrawal, block the effects of illicit opioid use, decrease opioid craving.
	Buprenorphine	(Subutex, Suboxone) Partial agonist at opioid receptors, lowers the risk of overdose, reduces or eliminates withdrawal symptoms, no euphoria and sedation caused by other opioids (including methadone).
	Naltrexone	(Revie) Long-acting synthetic opioid antagonist; used in outpatient settings; prevents an addicted individual from feeling the effects associated with opioid use, which is the notion behind this treatment; diminished craving and addiction.
Tobacco		
Headaches, irritability, craving, depression, anxiety, cognitive and attention deficits, sleep disturbances, and increased appetite	**Nicotine replacement therapies**	(Gums, patch, spray, lozenges) Used in maintaining low levels of nicotine in the body and reduce the withdrawal symptoms.
	Bupropion	(Wellbutrin, Zyban) Mild stimulant effects, blocks reuptake of norepinephrine and dopamine, marketed initially as antidepressants, showed efficacy in reducing tobacco craving, promoting cessation without concomitant weight gain.
	Vareniciline	(Chantix) Partial agonist/antagonist at nicotinic receptors; minimal stimulation of nicotine receptor but not enough to stimulate dopamine release, which is related to the rewarding effects of nicotine; reduces craving.

(Continued)

Table 41–2 • ADDICTION: WITHDRAWAL SYMPTOMS AND PHARMACOLOGY FOR DRUG WITHDRAWAL AND RELAPSE PREVENTION (continued)

Addictions

Withdrawal Symptoms	Generic Name	(Brand Name) Treatment Characteristics
Alcohol		
<12 hours: insomnia, tremulousness, mild anxiety, gastrointestinal upset, headache, diaphoresis, palpitations, anorexia **12 to 24 hours:** visual, auditory, or tactile hallucinations	Naltrexone	(Revie) Used to reduce relapse in heavy drinkers (defined as 4 or more drinks/day in women and 5 or more drinks/day in men), relapse reduction up to 36% in first 3 months, not very effective in maintaining abstinence.
24 to 48 hours: Generalized tonic-clonic seizures **48 to 72 hours: Delirium Tremens;** hallucinations (predominantly visual), disorientation, tachycardia, hypertension, low-grade fever, agitation, diaphoresis	Acamprosate	(Campral) Reduces withdrawal by acting on GABA and glutamate pathway; very effective in maintaining abstinence in dependent drinkers, even in severe cases, for several weeks to months.
	Disulfiram	(Antabuse) Causes retention of acetaldehyde by interfering with the degradation of alcohol; flushing, nausea, and vomiting experienced on alcohol intake; nonadherence is common.
	Topiramate	(Topamax) Thought to have similar mode of action as acamprosate, not FDA approved for alcohol addictions treatment.
	Chlordiazepoxide, diazepam, lorazepam	(Librium, Valium, Ativan) Benzodiazepines (preferably long acting); decreased severity of withdrawal symptoms; reduced risk of seizures and delirium tremens.
	Carbamazepine, valproate	(Tegretol, Depakote) Anticonvulsants; decreased severity of withdrawal symptoms.
	Atenolol, propranolol	(Tenormin, Inderal) Beta-blockers; used as adjunctive agents, improvement in vital signs; reduction in craving.
	Clonidine	(Catapres) Alpha-agonists; used as adjunctive agents, decreased severity of withdrawal symptoms.

(Continued)

Table 41–2 • ADDICTION: WITHDRAWAL SYMPTOMS AND PHARMACOLOGY FOR DRUG WITHDRAWAL AND RELAPSE PREVENTION (continued)		
Addictions		
Withdrawal Symptoms	**Generic Name**	**(*Brand Name*) Treatment Characteristics**
Stimulants		
Paranoia, depression, somnolence, anxiety, irritability, difficulty to concentrate, psychomotor retardation, increased appetite	**Methylphenidate, amantadine**	(*Ritalin, Symmetrel*) Indirect dopamine agonists; treatment retention was improved in one study of each agent; data are very limited.
	Propranolol	(*Inderal*) Adrenergic antagonists; treatment retention was improved and cocaine use was reduced in patients with severe withdrawal symptoms.
	Desipramine, bupropion	(*Norpramin, Wellbutrin*) Antidepressants; medications are well tolerated but do not appear to be effective during stimulant withdrawal.

CASE CORRELATION

- See Case 7 (Tobacco Use and Cessation) and Case 59 (Opioid Use Disorder and Chronic Pain Management).

COMPREHENSION QUESTIONS

41.1 An 18-year-old young woman who is captain of her high school cheerleading squad presents to the clinic with her mother, who is concerned about her daughter's erratic behavior and emotional outbursts. She states that her daughter rarely sleeps on the weekends but sleeps heavily at the beginning of the week and is frequently late for school. She has no significant medical or psychiatric history. Her mother states that she has tried to discuss these issues, but her daughter gets angry and leaves home. She wants to have her daughter tested for drug use. You speak to the patient alone, and she endorses the symptoms her mother reports. Her vital signs are within normal limits, and the physical examination is unremarkable. She consents to a urine toxicology screen, which is positive for methamphetamine. The patient admits she last used about 1 week ago and has only used twice in her life. What is the most appropriate next step in managing this patient?

A. Confront the patient in the presence of her mother about her addiction problem.

B. Refer the patient for an immediate psychiatry evaluation.

C. Prescribe oral propranolol to prevent withdrawal symptoms.

D. Offer behavioral therapy and drug rehabilitation to the patient alone.

E. Obtain an ECG, comprehensive panel, and CBC.

41.2 A 40-year-old woman presents to the clinic complaining of feeling depressed and jittery. She has been feeling this way on and off for the last year since her husband passed away in a car accident. She reports a recent increase in head-aches, insomnia, loss of appetite, and increased irritability. When asked about substance use, she says she drinks wine at night to help her sleep. Further ques-tioning leads her to disclose that she started drinking more after her husband's death, and she currently drinks, on average, 1.5 bottles of wine each evening. She denies previous history of psychiatric disorder. The patient's physical examination is unremarkable with the exception an elevated blood pressure of 140/90 mm Hg. A comprehensive metabolic panel reveals an alanine amino-transferase (ALT; also known as SGPT) of 30 U/L (normal 10-40) and an aspartate aminotransferase (AST; also known as SGOT) of 84 U/L (normal 10-30). The remaining laboratory studies are negative. There is no family his-tory of liver disease. Which one of the following pharmacologic agents could help reduce this patient's alcohol consumption and increase abstinence?

A. Acamprosate

B. Amitriptyline

C. Paroxetine

D. Promethazine

E. Venlafaxine

41.3 Which one of the following is effective in preventing seizures associated with alcohol withdrawal syndrome?

A. Carbamazepine (Tegretol)

B. Chlordiazepoxide

C. Clonidine (Catapres)

D. Gabapentin (Neurontin)

E. Phenytoin (Dilantin)

ANSWERS

41.1 **D.** This patient should be presented with the results of the urine toxicology screen and options about substance abuse treatment. This should be done with the patient alone and not in the presence of her parent (answer A). She appears reasonable and psychologically stable during the appointment and thus does not require an immediate psychiatry evaluation (answer B). An ECG and serologic evaluation (answer E) will not likely add to the investigation of this patient since she is asymptomatic upon presentation. Similarly, she does not appear acutely intoxicated, and propranolol has no role in the prevention of withdrawal symptoms for methamphetamine intoxication (answer C).

41.2 **A.** Pharmacological treatment is used as an adjunct in treatment of alcohol dependence. Naltrexone, disulfiram, and acamprosate are approved by the Food and Drug Administration (FDA) for this indication. Consistent, good-quality, patient-oriented evidence has found naltrexone or acamprosate to be the most effective treatment of alcohol dependence when used in conjunction with behavioral therapy. Antidepressants (answer C, paroxetine; answer B, amitriptyline; and answer E, venlafaxine) may be beneficial in patients with coexisting depression. The antiemetic ondansetron (not promethazine, answer D) may also help decrease alcohol consumption in patients with AUD. An AST to ALT ratio greater than 2:1 suggests alcoholic liver disease, and a ratio of 3:1 or higher is highly suggestive of alcoholic liver disease. With most hepatocellular disorders, including nonalcoholic fatty liver disease, viral hepatitis, and iron overload disorder, the patient will have an AST to ALT ratio < 1.

41.3 **B.** Benzodiazepines can prevent alcohol withdrawal seizures. Anticonvulsants such as carbamazepine (answer A), gabapentin (answer D), and phenytoin (answer E) have less abuse potential than benzodiazepines but do not prevent seizures. Clonidine (answer C), an alpha-adrenergic agonist, reduces the adrenergic symptoms associated with withdrawal but does not prevent seizures.

CLINICAL PEARLS

▶ No single treatment for SUD is appropriate for all individuals.

▶ Individual and/or group counseling and other behavioral therapies are critical components of effective treatment for SUD.

▶ Medications are an important element of treatment for many patients, especially when combined with counseling and other behavioral therapies.

▶ Individuals with SUD with coexisting mental disorders should have both disorders treated in an integrated way.

▶ Medical detoxification is only the first stage of SUD treatment and by itself does little to change long-term drug use.

▶ Recovery from SUD is often a long-term process and frequently requires interprofessional care management and multiple episodes of treatment.

REFERENCES

Illicit Drug Use, Including Nonmedical Use of Prescription Drugs: Screening. US Preventive Services Task Force draft recommendation statement. https://www.uspreventiveservicestaskforce.org/uspstf/draft-recommendation/drug-use-in-adolescents-and-adults-including-pregnant-women-screening. Accessed May 26, 2020.

Muncie HL, Yasinian Y, Oge L. Outpatient management of alcohol withdrawal syndrome. *Am Fam Physician.* 2013;88(9):589-595.

Phillips KA, Bonci A. Cocaine and other commonly used drugs. In: Jameson J, Fauci AS, Kasper DL, Hauser SL, Longo DL, Loscalzo J, eds. *Harrison's Principles of Internal Medicine.* 20th ed. New York, NY: McGraw Hill; 2018: Chap. 447. http://accessmedicine.mhmedical.com/content.aspx?bookid=2129&sectionid=192534128. Accessed January 21, 2019.

Schuckit MA. Alcohol and alcohol use disorders. In: Jameson J, Fauci AS, Kasper DL, Hauser SL, Longo DL, Loscalzo J, eds. *Harrison's Principles of Internal Medicine.* 20th ed. New York, NY: McGraw Hill; 2018: Chap. 445. http://accessmedicine.mhmedical.com/content.aspx?bookid= 2129&sectionid=192534023. Accessed January 21, 2019.

Substance Abuse and Mental Health Services Administration. (2019). *Key Substance Use and Mental Health Indicators in the United States: Results From the 2018 National Survey on Drug Use and Health* (HHS Publication No. SMA 19-5068, NSDUH Series H-53). Rockville, MD: Center for Behavioral Health Statistics and Quality, Substance Abuse and Mental Health Services Administration. September 2018. https://www.samhsa.gov/data/sites/default/files/cbhsq-reports/NSDUH NationalFindingsReport2018/NSDUHNationalFindingsReport2018.pdf. Accessed May 26, 2020.

Unhealthy Alcohol Use in Adolescents and Adults: Screening and Behavioral Counseling Interventions. US Preventive Services Task Force. November 2018. https://www.uspreventiveservicestaskforce .org/uspstf/recommendation/unhealthy-alcohol-use-in-adolescents-and-adults-screening-and-behavioral-counseling-interventions. Accessed August 20, 2019.

Winslow BT, Onysko M, Hebert M. Medications for alcohol use disorder. *Am Fam Physician.* 2016;93(6):457-465.

Zoorob RJ, Grubb RJ, Gonzalez SJ, Kowalchuk AA. Using alcohol screening and brief intervention to address patients' risky drinking. *Fam Pract Manag.* 2017;24(3):12-16.

CASE 42

A 35-year-old woman presents to your office complaining of skipped or "irregular heartbeats" for the past few weeks. At first, she attributed her symptoms to job-related stress and thought they would disappear. Instead, the skipped beats have increased in frequency to twice a day, lasting up to 2 minutes per episode. Her father, who has coronary heart disease, urged her to see a doctor. She denies chest pain, shortness of breath, or presyncopal symptoms. She drinks two cups of caffeinated coffee per day, does not smoke, and rarely drinks alcohol. She recently tried some over-the-counter diet pills to lose weight but stopped taking them when her symptoms became more frequent. On examination, her temperature is 98.6 °F (37 °C), blood pressure is 130/85 mm Hg, heart rate is 92 beats/min, respiratory rate is 16 breaths/min, and body mass index (BMI) is 27 kg/m². Neck examination is without thyromegaly, nodule, or mass and without jugular venous distention or bruit. Lung examination is bilaterally clear to auscultation. Cardiac examination reveals regular rate and rhythm with normal S_1 and S_2. A midsystolic click followed by a late systolic crescendo murmur is heard at the fifth intercostal space at the midclavicular line. Abdominal examination is unremarkable. Examination of the extremities reveals palpable symmetric distal pulses in all four extremities. Neurologic examination reveals no resting tremor, and reflexes are within normal limits.

▶ What is the most likely diagnosis?
▶ What is the most appropriate initial diagnostic step?
▶ What is the most appropriate initial step in therapy?

ANSWERS TO CASE 42:

Palpitations

Summary: A 35-year-old woman presents with

- Palpitations for weeks that have increased in frequency
- Symptoms that are not associated with chest pain, syncope, dyspnea, or dizziness
- No pertinent past medical history
- Potential triggers of caffeine consumption, diet pill use, and stress
- A midsystolic click followed by a late systolic crescendo murmur
- Family history of coronary heart disease in her father

Most likely diagnosis: Mitral valve prolapse syndrome.

Initial diagnostic step: Obtain 12-lead electrocardiogram (ECG) and echocardiogram.

Initial step in therapy: Restrict caffeine and alcohol; eliminate any amphetamine-based stimulants and/or diuretics; keep a diary of symptoms or possible triggers; follow up with patient to discuss results; monitor for complications; and consider antibiotic prophylaxis for future dental procedures.

ANALYSIS

Objectives

1. Define palpitations. (EPA 1, 12)

2. Identify benign cardiac rhythms and those associated with sudden cardiac death. (EPA 1, 10)

3. Identify the most common structural heart diseases associated with sudden cardiac death. (EPA 10)

4. Develop a rational approach that considers cardiac and noncardiac causes for palpitations. (EPA 2, 3)

Considerations

An otherwise healthy 35-year-old woman gives a history of frequent palpitations without associated dizziness, syncope, or chest pain. We are given clues to noncardiac factors that may contribute to her symptoms, including caffeine consumption, use of diet pills, and job-related stress. Obtaining a clear family history is important because some arrhythmias and structural heart diseases (eg, hypertrophic cardiomyopathy) can run in families. A family history of premature cardiac death or unexplained sudden death may suggest such an inheritance.

A mid-systolic click associated with or without a late systolic murmur suggests the presence of **mitral valve prolapse** (MVP). Usually asymptomatic, it is the **most common valvular heart defect** in the United States, occurring in 3% to 6% of the population. While many are asymptomatic, patients may present with palpitations, fatigue, chest discomfort, and dyspnea. This symptom complex is defined as **mitral** valve prolapse syndrome. These patients may also present with panic attacks. Two percent of patients with MVP will have complications, including mitral regurgitation, atrial fibrillation (AF; if the left atrium becomes enlarged), systolic heart failure, pulmonary hypertension, or infective endocarditis.

Mitral valve prolapse is also associated with Marfan syndrome, as these patients often have aortic root dilations and are at risk for aortic arch aneurysm rupture. Marfan syndrome should be suspected in patients who are tall and thin and have scoliosis; pectus excavatum; long, thin digits (arachnodactyly); a high-arched palate; and an arm wingspan exceeding their height.

APPROACH TO:
Palpitations

DEFINITIONS

ARRHYTHMIA: Primary rhythm disturbances that represent a change from the normal sequence of electrical impulses within the heart.

PALPITATIONS: A common subjective sensation of unduly strong, slow, rapid, or irregular heartbeats that may be related to a cardiac arrhythmia. The sensation may last seconds, minutes, hours, or days and is often intermittent and not clinically concerning.

CLINICAL APPROACH

Pathophysiology

Palpitations are a very common outpatient complaint, comprising as many as 16% of visits to primary care physicians (Table 42–1). Approximately 40% of patients complaining of palpitations have an underlying primary rhythm disturbance. An underlying mental health problem (eg, anxiety, panic disorder) is attributable in 31% of symptomatic patients. Less common etiologies include drugs and alcohol (6%), structural problems within the heart (3%), or noncardiac causes (4%), and 16% are idiopathic. Palpitations associated with syncope, occurring at work or physical activity, affecting sleep, or in the context of known heart disease are more likely due to a cardiac cause. Clinicians are commonly alerted to cardiac palpitations because they may increase the risk of sudden cardiac death.

Cardiac Causes

Benign arrhythmias account for the majority of cases of palpitations. Sinus tachycardia, sinus bradycardia, premature atrial contractions, and premature ventricular contractions (PVCs) represent the most common etiology of benign palpitations, while sinus tachycardia and bradycardia are also common benign dysrhythmias that can manifest as palpitations.

Premature Ventricular Contractions. PVCs occurring at rest and disappearing with exercise are usually benign. They are commonly seen in athletes and require

Table 42–1 • CARDIAC AND NONCARDIAC CAUSES OF PALPITATIONS	
Arrhythmias	Atrial fibrillation/flutter
	AV reentrant tachycardia
	Congenital arrhythmias (ie, Wolff-Parkinson-White, Brugada, long QT syndromes)
	Multifocal atrial tachycardia
	Paroxysmal supraventricular tachycardia
	Premature atrial contractions (PAC) (most common)
	Premature ventricular contractions (PVCs)
	Sinus bradycardia
	Sick sinus syndrome
	Sinus tachycardia
	Ventricular fibrillation
	Ventricular tachycardia (VT)
Medications	Anticholinergics (ie, nasal decongestants)
	Beta-blocker withdrawal
	Inhalers (ie, short acting beta-agonists)
	Sympathomimetics (ie, epinephrine)
	Vasodilators (ie, nitrates)
Metabolic derangement	Electrolyte abnormalities
	Hyper-/hypothyroidism
	Hypoglycemia
	Pheochromocytoma
Other substances	Alcohol
	Amphetamines
	Cocaine
	Marijuana
	Nicotine
Other noncardiac	Anemia
	Exercise
	Fever
	Hypovolemia
	Stress
	Vasovagal syncope
	Paget disease of bone
	Pregnancy
	Pulmonary disease
Psychiatric disorders	Generalized anxiety disorder
	Other anxiety disorders
	Panic disorder
	Somatization disorder
Structural heart disease	Cardiomyopathy (ie, hypertrophic)
	Tumor (ie, atrial myxoma)
	Valvular disease (ie, MVP)

no investigation. PVCs in the presence of known cardiac disease, metabolic disease, or worrisome symptoms (eg, syncope) require appropriate investigation due to increased risk of fatal arrhythmias, including ventricular tachycardia (VT) or ventricular fibrillation.

Supraventricular Tachycardia. Supraventricular tachycardia (SVT) refers to any tachycardia that is not of ventricular origin. This definition includes sinus tachycardia, which can be a physiologic reaction to conditions like stress, fever, infection, or hyperthyroidism. Most SVTs are paroxysmal and have a sudden, almost immediate onset and regular rhythm. A person experiencing paroxysmal SVTs (PSVT) may feel their heart rate go from 60 to 200 beats/min instantaneously. PSVTs are most commonly atrioventricular (AV) nodal reentry tachycardias or part of Wolff-Parkinson-White (WPW) syndrome. WPW syndrome is caused by an accessory track that bypasses the AV node and conducts electrical impulses between the atria and ventricles. The classic ECG finding is a slurred upstroke of the QRS complex known as a "delta wave." WPW increases susceptibility to dangerous arrhythmias and can lead to sudden cardiac death. It can be treated by catheter ablation of the accessory track.

Prolonged QT Interval. Prolongation of the QT interval is another common finding that predisposes to cardiac events. Prolonged QT interval has been linked to a wide variety of medications, including macrolide antibiotics, antiemetics, antiarrhythmics, antipsychotics, and antidepressants. Prolonged QT interval is defined as QT_c^1 greater than 470 **milliseconds** in men or 480 **milliseconds** in women. **Any patient with a QT interval greater than 500 milliseconds is at increased risk for dangerous arrhythmias.**

QT_c is defined as measured QT interval corrected for heart rate:

$$QT_c = \frac{QT \text{ (in msec)}}{\sqrt{RR \text{ interval (in msec)}}}$$

A variety of less common genetic arrhythmias may present in young adults or even children. While most cases of long QT interval are acquired, **long QT interval syndrome** is a rare genetic cause, most often inherited in an **autosomal dominant pattern.** Patients may present with either palpitations or syncope and typically have a family history of syncope or sudden cardiac death.

Noncardiac Causes

Psychiatric Causes. Psychiatric causes should be considered in the differential diagnosis for palpitations and may be overlooked if not screened for in the initial history. Panic disorder is more common in women of childbearing age. Patients with panic attacks commonly present with complaints of palpitations, chest pain, and shortness of breath. They will report brief episodes of overwhelming panic or a sense of impending doom associated with tachycardia, dyspnea, or dizziness. Still, these complaints merit a formal cardiac workup and risk stratification. Criteria for panic disorder are often comorbid with SVT, and women are more likely to be misdiagnosed with an anxiety disorder when presenting with a cardiac event.

Medications and Substances. Numerous medications and substances may contribute to palpitations, including alcohol, nicotine, caffeine (especially energy drinks), and illicit drugs (eg, cocaine). A careful medication review and inquiry about any over-the-counter medications, herbs, or supplements are important to an evaluation of palpitations.

Structural Causes. Structural causes of palpitations include cardiomyopathy, atrial or ventricular septal defects, congenital heart disease, pericarditis, valvular disease (eg, MVP, aortic stenosis, aortic insufficiency), and heart failure. The presence of restrictive, hypertrophic, or dilated cardiomyopathies may lead to sudden cardiac death. **Hypertrophic obstructive cardiomyopathy (HCM) is the most common cause of sudden cardiac death in adolescents** in the United States but is often not detected on routine physical examination (Case 29). Echocardiography demonstrating a thickened intraventricular septum with outlet obstruction remains the gold standard for diagnosis; however, current evidence does not support routine echocardiography screening in athletes.

Clinical Presentation

History and Physical Examination. The patient's age at onset of palpitations is important to note, as an **age older than 50 years is associated with greater risk of coronary artery disease.** Palpitations associated with syncope are usually pathologic, so hospitalization with cardiac monitoring and cardiology evaluation should be considered. The clinical examination should focus on vital signs (blood pressure and heart rate), including orthostatic readings. The neck should be examined for abnormalities, including thyroid enlargement or nodule or carotid bruit. The presence of resting tremor or brisk reflexes may suggest hyperthyroidism. The cardiac examination should evaluate potential murmurs and point of maximum impulse since displacement may suggest cardiomegaly. Heart rate, rhythm, and extra sounds should be documented.

Laboratory Values. Laboratory screening of all patients with new palpitations should include a **complete blood count, comprehensive metabolic panel, and thyroid-stimulating hormone level.** If a pheochromocytoma is suspected, plasma and/or 24-hour urine metanephrines evaluation is indicated.

Electrocardiogram. **A 12-lead ECG is appropriate in all patients with palpitations, even if they are symptom free during the provider encounter.** The presence of left ventricular hypertrophy, atrial enlargement, AV block, prior myocardial infarction, and delta waves should trigger additional testing. Prolonged QT interval should trigger a thorough review of medications, as well as consultation with a cardiologist. Other cardiac testing may be appropriate based on the history, examination, and results of the initial evaluation. Ambulatory electrocardiographic rhythm monitoring can be accomplished for periods of 24 to 72 hours using a **Holter monitor.** A **cardiac event monitor** can be worn by a patient for up to 30 days and might be useful when the palpitations do not occur daily. The monitor is worn continuously and is activated by the patient when palpitations are felt.

Imaging and Stress Testing. An **echocardiogram** can be useful in identifying patients with suspected structural abnormalities of heart chambers or valves, which could trigger heart rhythm disturbances. Cardiac examination findings consistent with structural or valvular disease merit an echocardiogram; however, a normal examination does not rule out these pathologies. Exercise **stress testing** in age- and risk-appropriate patients may be important for identifying arrhythmias triggered by exercise. This test may be of particular importance in patients with suspected coronary artery disease. Anyone with suspected structural problems should be evaluated by a surface echocardiogram prior to undergoing stress testing. Patients with suspected HCM or severe aortic stenosis should avoid exercise stress testing.

Electrophysiology Testing. Finally, **electrophysiology studies** may be needed to re-create rhythm disturbances and identify hyperactive foci and accessory tracts such seen in WPW syndrome. These areas can subsequently be electrically ablated.

Treatment

The treatment of palpitations is dependent on the etiology. Reduction in exposure to triggers (eg, medications, excessive caffeine) may provide significant relief in those with benign causes. Anxiety or panic disorder may be treated by a combination of pharmacologic and behavioral interventions. If structural cardiac disease is suspected, referral to a cardiologist is indicated.

Symptomatic PSVT can often be terminated with vagal stimulation techniques. Carotid sinus massage, Valsalva maneuver, and cold applications to the face (diver's reflex) can trigger vagus nerve stimulation, which may break an episode of SVT. Intravenous adenosine is the treatment of choice to break SVT, while beta-blockers or calcium channel blockers are used as first-line therapy for hemodynamically stable SVT. Synchronized cardioversion is recommended in cases of acute SVT or wide-complex tachycardia when the patient is hemodynamically unstable or when medical therapy is either ineffective or contraindicated.

Ventricular Arrhythmias. Ventricular arrhythmias can be life threatening and require immediate treatment. The most common cause of ventricular arrhythmias is ischemia. VT may be reversed with antiarrhythmic therapy in hemodynamically stable patients. Amiodarone can be used to convert VT to sinus rhythm or for maintenance of sinus rhythm after electrical cardioversion. Patients with VT who are unstable require immediate cardioversion. Ventricular fibrillation is imminently fatal and requires defibrillation. An automatic implantable cardioverter-defibrillator may be implanted in patients with a history of VT or with conditions that commonly result in ventricular arrhythmias, including advanced dilated cardiomyopathy, long QT syndrome, and HCM.

Atrial Fibrillation. Chronic AF should be treated with medication (commonly beta-blockers or calcium channel blockers) to optimize a ventricular rate below 100 beats/min. Rhythm control (ie, conversion to sinus rhythm) has failed to show superiority to rate control in a number of trials and may be associated with an increased risk of hospitalization. In select patients, rhythm control may be attempted by electrical cardioversion or antiarrhythmic drugs, including amiodarone. A transesophageal echocardiogram should be done prior to cardioversion in order to rule out the presence of an atrial thrombus. **Most patients with AF will require anticoagulation** because they are at an increased risk of embolic stroke from blood clots that form in the cardiac atrium, in accordance with the CHADS2-VASC risk calculation (www.chadsvasc.org).

> **CASE CORRELATION**
> • See Case 29 (Adolescent Health Maintenance).

COMPREHENSION QUESTIONS

42.1 A 35-year-old man presents to establish health care with a new family provider. He has no pertinent past medical or family history, and he does not smoke or drink alcohol. When prompted, he states that he has noticed an intermittent "fluttering" in his chest for the past 3 months that spontaneously resolves. He has had increased stress at work and has been drinking six cups of caffeinated coffee a day to complete his workload. He has not had time to exercise, and his diet consists of what he can find in the office cafeteria. He denies any history of anxiety. Which of the following is the most likely underlying etiology of his palpitations?

    A. Excessive caffeine

    B. Structural heart disease

    C. Coronary artery disease

    D. Primary rhythm disturbance

    E. Work stress

42.2 A 42-year-old asymptomatic woman is being seen in the office for an annual health maintenance examination. She is noted to have an abnormal finding on ECG. Which of the following is an indication for referral to a cardiologist or cardiac electrophysiologist?

    A. PVCs on a resting ECG that resolve with exercise

    B. Delta waves on an ECG

    C. Isolated unifocal PVCs on exercise ECG

    D. Sinus tachycardia

42.3 Which of the following patients should undergo an exercise stress test for evaluation of palpitations?

    A. A 60-year-old man with symptomatic PVCs but without syncope

    B. A 35-year-old woman with hypertrophic cardiomyopathy seen on an echocardiogram

    C. A 32-year-old man who is tall and slender with pectus excavatum and a midsystolic click on examination

    D. A 68-year-old man with suspected aortic stenosis

42.4 A 16-year-old young man comes to your office for a sports physical. He plans to try out for his high school football team but requires medical clearance. He has no cardiovascular complaints, and his history is unremarkable except for a family history of an uncle dying suddenly while jogging at age 25. His physical examination is remarkable for a harsh systolic murmur loudest over his left lower sternal border, which increases with the Valsalva maneuver. You obtain an ECG, which shows left ventricular hypertrophy. Which of the following is the most appropriate next step in diagnostic evaluation?

A. An exercise stress test

B. An echocardiogram

C. A chest radiograph

D. A left-heart catheterization

E. Reassurance that he is cleared to play football

42.5 You are called to the bedside of a 55-year-old man who is hospitalized for the evaluation of chest pain. When you arrive, you find the patient confused and not answering questions. The nurse informs you that the patient was speaking coherently a few minutes ago. The patient's pulse is 180 beats/min, his systolic blood pressure is 60 mm Hg, and his diastolic blood pressure cannot be measured. Telemetry reveals wide-complex tachycardia. Which of the following is the most appropriate next step in the management of this patient?

A. Adenosine

B. Cardiology consultation

C. Emergent cardioversion

D. Negative chronotropic agent

E. 12-lead ECG

ANSWERS

42.1 **D.** Primary rhythm disturbances are the most common cause of palpitations, making up approximately 40% of cases. Other common causes include psychiatric etiologies (eg, anxiety, panic disorder); medications; metabolic causes (eg, electrolytes, thyroid hormone imbalance); and structural heart disease (answer B). Many cases of palpitations remain undiagnosed despite appropriate evaluation. The other causes (answer A, excessive caffeine; answer C, coronary artery disease; and answer E, work stress) are less common.

42.2 **B.** The presence of delta waves indicates WPW syndrome and the presence of an accessory track that can be ablated by an electrophysiologist. Although the patient is currently asymptomatic, the presence of this finding indicates a high potential for a tachyarrhythmia. Answer A (PVCs on resting ECG) and answer C (unifocal PVCs on exercise) are fairly common findings and not indications for referral. A patient with answer D (sinus tachycardia) needs to be further investigated regarding etiology but does not need a referral to a cardiologist; for example, the patient may have anemia or hyperthyroidism.

42.3 **A.** A 60-year-old with PVCs, especially if they are of new onset, may be showing the initial presentation of coronary artery disease and should undergo stress testing. All the other conditions listed (answer A, hypertrophic cardiomyopathy; answer B, likely Marfan syndrome; and answer D, suspected aortic stenosis) are contraindications to stress testing.

42.4 **B.** This young man has signs suggestive of hypertrophic cardiomyopathy. A systolic murmur is not uncommon, but the intensity should *decrease* with Valsalva; when the murmur increases with Valsalva, this is concerning since HCM is one of the leading causes of sudden death of young athletes. The confirmatory test for it is an echocardiogram. Coronary catheterization (answer D) and stress testing (answer A) are tests for coronary artery disease and are not recommended for this patient. A beta-blocker or calcium channel blocker would worsen the patient's hemodynamic status. Chest x-ray (answer C) is often normal with HCM. Reassurance (answer E) is inappropriate since this patient is at risk for sudden death.

42.5 **C.** This patient likely has VT (wide-complex tachycardia) with clinical deterioration and hemodynamic instability. He needs immediate electrical cardioversion. If the patient were in a stable VT, then medical cardioversion could be conducted using intravenous amiodarone. Answer B (cardiology consultation) may be considered after the patient is stabilized, but immediate correction of the rhythm is critical due to the patient's instability. Answer E (12-lead ECG) is also indicated, but the rhythm strip is sufficient to make a diagnosis, and delay for the 12-lead study may cause patient compromise. Answer A (adenosine) is contraindicated with ventricular tachycardia and can lead to asystole. Answer D (negative chronotropic agent) is typically used for supraventricular tachycardia and would have no effect on VT, and it could possibly cause hypotension.

CLINICAL PEARLS

▶ Patients with palpitations require a detailed evaluation into potential cardiac etiologies, as psychosocial stress cannot be assumed as the sole etiology.

▶ Workup for palpitations includes laboratory testing for common metabolic etiologies and a 12-lead ECG.

▶ A 24- to 72-hour Holter monitor is appropriate in a patient with frequent (eg, daily) palpitations; a 30-day event monitor is a better test in someone with infrequent episodes.

▶ Hypertrophic cardiomyopathy is the most common cause of sudden cardiac death in adolescents. An adolescent with a systolic heart murmur that increases in intensity with Valsalva maneuver should have their activity restricted until a diagnostic echocardiogram can be performed.

REFERENCES

Al-Khatib SM, Stevenson WG, Ackerman MJ, et al. 2017 AHA/ACC/HRS guideline for management of patients with ventricular arrhythmias and the prevention of sudden cardiac death. *J Am Coll Cardiol.* 2018;72(14):e91-e220.

Bouknight DP, O'Rourke RA. Current management of mitral valve prolapse. *Am Fam Physician.* 2000;61(11):3343-3350, 3353-3354.

Field JM, Hazinski MF, Sayre MR, et al. Part 1: executive summary: 2010 AHA guidelines for CPR and ECC. *Circulation.* 2010;122(18 suppl 3):S640-S656.

January CT, Wann LS, Alpert JS, et al. 2014 AHA/ACC/HRS guideline for the management of patients with atrial fibrillation. *J Am Coll Cardiol.* 2014;64(21):e1-e76.

Lip GY, Halperin JL. Improving stroke risk stratification in atrial fibrillation. *Am J Med.* 2010;123(6):484-488.

Michaud GF, Stevenson WG. Approach to supraventricular tachyarrhythmias. In: Jameson J, Fauci AS, Kasper DL, Hauser SL, Longo DL, Loscalzo J, eds. *Harrison's Principles of Internal Medicine.* 20th ed. New York, NY: McGraw Hill; 2018: Chap. 241. http://accessmedicine.mhmedical.com/content.aspx?bookid=2129&sectionid=188731341. Accessed May 19, 2019.

Miller JM, Zipes DP. Diagnosis of cardiac arrhythmias. In: Libby P, Bonow RO, Mann DL, et al, eds. *Braunwald's Heart Disease.* 8th ed. Philadelphia, PA: Saunders Elsevier; 2008:763-831.

Page RL, Joglar JA, Caldwell MA, et al. 2015 ACC/AHA/HRS guideline for the management of adult patients with supraventricular tachycardia. *J Am Coll Cardiol.* 2016;67(13):e27-e115.

Wexler RK, Pleister A, Raman SV. Palpitations: evaluation in the primary care setting. *Am Fam Physician.* 2017;96(12):784-789.

The mother of a 16-year-old girl calls the practice answering service on a Saturday afternoon. She states that her daughter was stung by a wasp on her left forearm several hours ago. The patient has no significant medical history or history of previous allergic reactions to insect stings or bites. She is having no difficulty breathing or swallowing and has not been dizzy or light-headed. Her mother's primary concern is that the area around the sting or bite is now red, itchy, and becoming increasingly swollen, extending in a circular pattern several centimeters in diameter. The red area is moderately warm to the touch, so her mother is concerned that it is infected. She gave her daughter some ibuprofen for the pain and would like you to phone a prescription for an antibiotic and something to prevent the redness from spreading.

▶ Is an antibiotic indicated for this patient, and if so, which one?
▶ What are the next steps in therapy?
▶ What guidance should be given regarding immunizations for this patient?

ANSWERS TO CASE 43:
Sting and Bite Injuries

Summary: A 16-year-old girl presents with

- A report over the phone of being stung by a wasp
- Painful and itchy localized reaction without symptoms of anaphylaxis
- No history of previous allergic reactions
- A request from the patient's mother for you to manage the situation over the phone by prescribing antibiotics

Is an antibiotic indicated: No antibiotic treatment is indicated, as this is a localized reaction to a wasp sting, with a high likelihood for a histamine-mediated reaction and a low likelihood of a bacterial infection, given the mechanism of injury and time course.

Next steps in therapy: Local application of ice, administration of oral and/or topical antihistamines for itching and swelling, and nonsteroidal anti-inflammatory drugs (NSAIDs) or acetaminophen for pain.

Immunization guidance: Tetanus-diphtheria-pertussis (Tdap) booster is not required because insect stings are considered minor and clean injuries that do not warrant prophylaxis. However, if the patient is not up to date on routine vaccination, Tdap vaccination should be considered.

ANALYSIS

Objectives

1. Be able to list the insects, arachnids, and arthropods that commonly cause sting and bite injuries. (EPA 12)
2. Be able to differentiate local from systemic reactions to stings and bites. (EPA 1, 10)
3. Know the management of common insect bites and stings, as well as animal bite injuries. (EPA 4)

Considerations

This adolescent without a history of allergies has sustained a wasp sting, and no therapy is required other than symptomatic treatment. The differential diagnosis for this case includes various beestings (different people will have different reactions), nonvenomous insect bites (eg, mosquito), and spider bites. Insects of the order *Hymenoptera* cause the majority of cases of sting- or bite-induced anaphylaxis and cause more mortality than all other types of insect bites and stings. Localized reactions occur as a result of the toxic properties of the venom, whereas more severe reactions tend to be caused by an allergic reaction to venom allergens.

Several types of beestings result in the retention of the stinger in the victim, which can result in continued injection of the bee venom. If the patient presents within seconds to a few minutes of the sting, stingers should be promptly removed with caution, as grasping the base of the stinger may result in compression of a venom-containing sac and increased venom release. Thus, it is suggested that scraping or brushing the stinger off of the skin is preferable to grasping the stinger. **Rapidly removing the stinger is preferable to taking the time to locate a scraping implement** if one (eg, a credit card or driver's license) is not immediately at hand. If the patient presents more than 3 to 5 minutes after the sting, extraction is not urgent because venom injection is complete.

Spider bites may present in the same fashion as many insect stings. Typically, the development of pruritus and histamine-mediated swelling within the first few hours of the bite are absent. Cellulitis within days is common, as is the development of an eschar at the site of the bite. Most spider bites, especially those associated with the brown recluse spider, are associated with methicillin-resistant *Staphylococcus aureus* (MRSA) infection.

APPROACH TO:
Stings and Bites

DEFINITIONS

HYMENOPTERA: Order of insects that includes wasps, yellow jackets, hornets, honeybees, bumblebees, and fire ants and comprises the majority of insects responsible for stings.

LARGE LOCALIZED ALLERGIC REACTIONS: Erythema and warmth of the skin at the site of an insect sting, mediated by immunoglobulin (Ig) E reaction to the *Hymenoptera* or other venom.

CLINICAL APPROACH TO STINGS AND BUG BITES

Localized Reactions

Almost all *Hymenoptera* stings will result in a **localized reaction,** which includes erythema, swelling, pain, and itching at the site of the injury. These reactions **tend to occur almost immediately and can last from hours to days.** The localized tissue response is a consequence of a histamine-mediated reaction caused by the venom that is released by the sting. Local reactions can be treated with ice and oral or topical antihistamines for itching. Tetanus prophylaxis was previously recommended, but due to the superficial nature of the stings and absence of confirmed cases of tetanus following beestings, insect stings are no longer an indication for tetanus prophylaxis.

Delayed Reactions

Large localized allergic reactions are mediated by IgE reactive to the *Hymenoptera* venom. These reactions may be confused with cellulitis, as large areas (≥ 10 cm in diameter) of redness and warmth (angioedema) can develop over 24 to 48 hours.

These reactions are not infectious and will not respond to antibiotics. They are **best treated with oral antihistamines and in some cases a short course of oral corticosteroids** initiated early after the sting, as these reactions may last up to 5 to 10 days. A person with a history of a large localized reaction to a beesting is likely to have similar or more severe reactions to subsequent stings. However, the history of this type of reaction does not result in an increased risk of anaphylaxis to subsequent stings. The risk of systemic nonanaphylactic reactions with future stings is 4% to 10%, while the risk of anaphylaxis is 1% to 3%; however, the risk of anaphylaxis with prior systemic reaction is high.

Anaphylaxis

Up to 4% of the population may experience a systemic reaction to a *Hymenoptera* sting. Those who have had a previous systemic reaction have a 50% or greater risk of having an anaphylactic reaction to future stings. Systemic reactions can vary from mild symptoms, including nausea, generalized urticaria, or angioedema, to severe and life-threatening hypotension, shock, airway edema, and death. Severe immediate hypersensitivity reactions usually occur within minutes of the sting.

Treatment. Treatment of anaphylaxis should include assessment and management of the ABCs (airway, breathing, and circulation), with intubation if necessary, intravenous access, and fluid resuscitation as soon as possible. **Intramuscular epinephrine should be administered as quickly as possible (0.3-0.5 mL of 1:1000 solution for adults; 0.01 mg/kg for children with 0.3 mg maximum dose)** and repeated in 5 to10 minutes if needed. Antihistamines, corticosteroids (if severe), and bronchodilators may also be required. Anyone with an anaphylactic reaction should be observed in a hospital setting for 12 to 24 hours, as the symptoms can recur after treatment.

Prevention. Persons with known anaphylactic reactions should be prescribed epinephrine injector kits to carry with them for immediate access at all times. They should be instructed to avoid wearing perfumes and bright clothing and to avoid walking barefoot when in areas prevalent with bees. Any person with a history of systemic reaction should be referred to an immunologist or allergist for evaluation for venom immunotherapy, which can reduce the risk of future severe reactions by up to 50%.

Arthropod Bites

Most arthropod bites do not cause significant injury or illness. When suspected, the area should be cleansed with warm water and soap, and a cool compress should be applied. Use of NSAIDs or acetaminophen is also recommended. When angioedema and pain develop around the site of injection, MRSA cellulitis should be considered, and the patient should be treated with oral trimethoprim-sulfamethoxazole, doxycycline, or clindamycin. If oral antibiotics do not adequately treat the cellulitis, abscess should be considered, and if present, incision and drainage should be performed. In these cases, as well as for those cases resistant to oral antibiotics, intravenous vancomycin should be started.

Mites

Patients may also present with bites from parasitic insects; these bites may be barely visible or invisible to the naked eye. Two common sources of pruritic rash in the primary care setting are mites (especially *Sarcoptes scabiei*) and fleas. *Sarcoptes scabiei* (scabies) infestation commonly manifests as an intensely pruritic papular rash with predilection for volar wrists, finger webs, axilla, and gluteal cleft. Patients may report that the pruritis, typically worse at night, is often severe enough to disturb sleep. Afflicted patients may report close contacts with similar rashes, and prolonged bodily contact (as in sexual contact or parent holding child) is considered high risk for transmission.

Certain populations are at especially high risk for scabies infection, including the homeless, although infestation affects patients across all socioeconomic and age groups. Close quarters in institutional settings (eg, prisons, extended care facilities, subacute rehabilitation facilities, day cares) provide an ideal setting for local outbreak. The diagnosis of scabies is often made clinically, although insect identification and skin-scraping techniques exist to visualize mites, eggs, or mite fecal matter under the microscope. **Topical permethrin is the treatment of choice for uncomplicated scabies** infection for the patient and high risk contacts.

Fleas

Fleabites typically present as papular urticaria in a patient with a pet dog or cat or recent contact with animals. Symptomatic treatment of the rash with topical or oral antihistamines is advised, and if a house pet is the suspected source, consultation with a veterinarian is recommended for eradication. In addition, patients should be instructed to thoroughly clean and vacuum the home and use commercially available insecticides.

Bedbugs

Consideration should also be given to a diagnosis of bedbug bites in the patient who presents with a papular pruritic rash. These rashes can be differentiated from fleabites by the appearance of a small hemorrhagic punctum at the center of the lesion. As in the treatment of flea infestation, treatment is symptomatic (including topical antihistamines or corticosteroids) and often resolves spontaneously within weeks. Consultation with a pest control professional for eradication is recommended.

CLINICAL APPROACH TO ANIMAL BITES

Pathophysiology

Nearly five million animal bites occur in the United States each year. The most common animals involved are dogs and cats, while human bites are also common. Cat and rodent bites are notorious for being "injection"-type bites, while those from dogs and humans are commonly "crush"-type bites, based upon the teeth involved in the bite. The risk of infection from an animal or human is dependent on numerous factors. Larger and deeper wounds are more likely to become infected than smaller, superficial wounds. Bite wounds on the hand tend to have an increased risk of infection due to thin skin and close proximity to small joint spaces. Host factors,

CASE FILES: FAMILY MEDICINE

such as the presence of chronic illnesses or immune suppression, also play a role in susceptibility to infection.

Many different bacteria can be involved in bite wound infections. Cat and human bites have a higher risk of infection and should always be treated empirically with antibiotics, whereas only approximately 20% of dog bite wounds become infected. All cat bite wounds should be suspected to be contaminated with *Pasteurella multocida*. Both cats and dogs carry multiple species of staphylococci and streptococci, as well as anaerobic bacteria. Humans carry staphylococci, streptococci, *Haemophilus* species, *Eikenella* species, and anaerobic bacteria.

Treatment

The initial management of the patient who has been bitten should focus on the ABCs and on protection of the current injury (eg, splinting of fractures, protection of cervical spine, etc), as well as local wound care, including control of bleeding and assessment of the injuries incurred. History should be gathered on the type of animal that caused the bite, the situation regarding the bite (whether provoked or unprovoked), and the vaccination status of the animal, particularly to document rabies vaccination status (if known). Almost all cases of human rabies in the United States since 1960 have been caused by bats, skunks, dogs, foxes, and raccoons.

Local cleaning of the wound(s) with soap and water, irrigation with sterile saline solution, and debridement of devitalized tissue should occur as soon as possible. For minor and superficial to shallow wounds, these treatments are often sufficient. Primary closure of bite wounds is controversial and should be limited to lacerations less than 12 hours old. Deep puncture wounds and those with signs of infection should be well irrigated with sterile solution and not primarily closed. Tetanus vaccination should be updated in all patients as needed. Hepatitis B and HIV postexposure prophylaxis should be considered for patients who sustained a human bite from a high-risk person. Animal control authorities should be contacted for guidance regarding rabies vaccination.

All patients who sustain cat bites should be treated for 10 to 14 days with oral amoxicillin-clavulanate. Although clear evidence of efficacy is lacking for the treatment of dog and human bites, current recommendations are for antibiotic prophylaxis with amoxicillin-clavulanate for 5 to 7 days for patients with moderate-to-severe wounds. When cellulitis is present, longer courses of antibiotic therapy, usually 10 to 14 days, are required. Hospitalization, intravenous antibiotics, and surgical intervention may be required for more severe infections, including widespread cellulitis, osteomyelitis, or septic joint infections, and in patients with complicating medical conditions, including immunosuppression.

CASE CORRELATION

- See Case 13 (Skin Lesions) and Case 48 (Fever and Rash).

COMPREHENSION QUESTIONS

43.1 A 31-year-old homeless woman presents with an intensely pruritic rash and is diagnosed with a scabies infestation. She is currently sexually active with one male partner and inquires whether he should be treated as well. What advice should you give her?

A. Treat him only if he manifests symptoms.

B. Treat him presumptively, as sexual contact carries a high risk for transmission.

C. Do not treat him, as resistance to permethrin is increasing.

D. Do not treat him, given potential risks of adverse medication reaction.

43.2 A 22-year-old woman develops a progressively enlarging red, hot area on her right leg following a sting from a yellow jacket. She states that the sting was of brief duration, and she was able to fully remove the stinger with tweezers. She has no previously known allergic reaction to beestings and is not suffering from any symptoms of systemic anaphylaxis. She sees you in the office the day after the sting and states that the area of the sting is still enlarging despite using over-the-counter corticosteroid cream and an oral antihistamine. Which of the following is the most appropriate next treatment for this patient?

A. Oral prednisone

B. Topical antihistamine

C. Antibiotic directed against gram-positive cocci

D. Portable epinephrine kit for future stings

E. Reassurance

43.3 A 7-year-old boy is brought to the office by his father the day after the child was bitten on the left forearm by his pet dog. The dog has had all of its vaccinations, including rabies. The child has had no fever, has full movement of the injured limb, and has no sign of neurologic or vascular injury. The wound is not deep and is not bleeding, but it has developed 2 cm of erythema surrounding the site. Which of the following is the most appropriate treatment?

A. Intravenous vancomycin for 10 to 14 days

B. Oral trimethoprim-sulfamethoxazole for 10 to 14 days

C. Oral amoxicillin-clavulanate for 10 to 14 days

D. Local wound care without antibiotics

43.4 A 43-year-old man comes to the office; he was involved in an altercation 2 days ago and sustained a deep laceration wound around his right knuckles from where he struck the face of another man. He was intoxicated at the time, and upon return home he did not clean the wound and went straight to sleep. The injury site has now developed purulent drainage, pain, and erythema, and the man has a low-grade fever. There is no surrounding rash, and he has not noted any spreading of the erythema. A plain film radiograph of the hand shows a hairline fracture of the fifth metacarpal head with swelling and bruising noted over the affected area. Which of the following is the most likely organism causing infection?

A. Methicillin-resistant *Staphylococcus aureus*

B. *Streptococcus* species

C. *Eikenella corrodens*

D. *Escherichia coli*

E. *Peptostreptococcus*

43.5 A mother brings in her 6-year-old child; the child was bitten on the hand yesterday while playing with a rabbit that was recently obtained from a neighbor. The child's wound is on the volar surface of the right second finger just distal to the proximal interphalangeal joint. Which of the following steps in the management of bite wounds is most effective in preventing wound infection?

A. Tetanus prophylaxis

B. Rabies prophylaxis

C. Saline irrigation and wound care

D. Prophylactic antibiotics

E. Irrigation and primary closure

ANSWERS

43.1 **B.** This patient has an uncomplicated reaction to a scabies infestation. Empiric treatment of close contacts of those with confirmed scabies infestation is recommended; this includes sexual partners and family members with prolonged physical contact (ie, a baby held by the patient). Treatment of household members is also recommended given significant latency in the development of clinical symptoms (some patients with active infestation do not manifest symptoms for 4-6 weeks) (answer A). Though permethrin resistance has increased over time (answer C), treatment of close contacts is still recommended to avoid the cycle of eradication and reinfestation. Topical permethrin administration carries few risks to the patient (answer D).

43.2 **A.** This patient is having a large, local reaction to her sting. This is an IgE-mediated reaction that should respond to a course of oral corticosteroids. There is at least a 50% chance that a similar reaction will occur if she is stung again, but she is unlikely to develop anaphylactic reactions in the future and does not need anaphylaxis prophylaxis (answer D). The patient should be informed that the localized reaction may take 5 to 10 days to completely resolve. Her history of a sting makes cellulitis less likely, and thus antibiotics (answer C) are not needed. The patient should have therapy rather than simply be observed (answer E). Topical antihistamine (answer B) is unlikely to be effective since the reaction is already fairly significant despite an oral antihistamine and topical steroid cream.

43.3 **C.** This child is developing cellulitis from the bite wound. Based on his presentation with lack of fever or systemic illness, he does not appear to require hospitalization and intravenous antibiotics (answer A). He can be treated with oral antibiotics for 1 to 2 weeks, with the drug of choice being amoxicillin/clauvulanic acid for some of the common bacteria encountered, including staphylococcal and streptococcal species and *Pasteurella* species.

43.4 **C.** While each of these bacteria (answer A, MRSA; answer B, *Streptococcus* spp; answer D, *E. coli*; and answer E, *Peptostreptococcus*) can be isolated in injuries from human bites, *Eikenella* species appear to be most common in closed fist injuries. For patients presenting after a "fistfight" with bite injuries, prophylaxis with amoxicillin-clavulanate is indicated due to inoculation with oral flora into the skin and subcutaneous tissues.

43.5 **C.** Rodents and lagomorphs (rabbits) neither are reservoirs of the rabies virus nor have been shown to transmit the rabies virus to humans (answer B). The most important step in preventing the infectious complications of bite wounds is proper wound care with inspection, irrigation, and debridement. Tetanus prophylaxis (answer A) should be considered in all bite wounds but is not the most important step. Likewise, antibiotic prophylaxis (answer D) may also be indicated, especially in high-risk bites (those located on the hand, late presentation, cat bites), and should be directed against staphylococci, streptococci, anaerobes, and *Pasteurella* species as appropriate. Primary closure of a contaminated wound (answer E) should not occur unless performed within 6 hours of injury and only when the wound is appropriate cleaned.

CLINICAL PEARLS

▶ Anyone with a history of anaphylactic reactions should be given a prescription for an epinephrine injector kit and instructed in the importance of keeping it at hand. These prescriptions need to be updated often, as the medication expires within 6 to 12 months.

▶ Local cleaning of the wound(s) with soap and water, irrigation with saline, and debridement of devitalized tissue should occur as soon as possible.

▶ Human "bite" wounds are not always the result of a bite. A punch to the mouth can cause inoculation and infection to the knuckles of the puncher.

▶ All cat and human bites should be empirically treated with amoxicillin-clavulanate due to high rates of infection, whereas approximately 20% of dog-bite wounds will become infected.

▶ Cellulitis following spider bites with the suspicion of MRSA should be treated with oral trimethoprim-sulfamethoxazole, doxycycline, or clindamycin.

REFERENCES

Brook I. Management of human and animal bite wounds: an overview. *Adv Skin Wound Care.* 2005;18(4):197-203.

Goddard, J. Bed bugs (*Cimex lectularius*) and clinical consequences of their bites. *JAMA.* 2009; 301(13):1358.

Golden DBK. Stinging insect allergy. *Am Fam Physician.* 2003;67:2541-2546.

James Q. Puncture wounds and bites. In: Tintinalli JE, Stapczynski J, Ma O, Yealy DM, Meckler GD, Cline DM, eds. *Tintinalli's Emergency Medicine: A Comprehensive Study Guide.* 8th ed. New York, NY: McGraw Hill; 2016: Chap. 46. http://accessmedicine.mhmedical.com/content.aspx?bookid= 1658&sectionid=109449392. Accessed May 20, 2019.

Juckett G. Arthropod bites. *Am Fam Physician.* 2013;88(12):841-847.

Liang JL, Tiwari T, Moro P, et al. Prevention of pertussis, tetanus, and diphtheria with vaccines in the United States: recommendations of the Advisory Committee on Immunization Practices (ACIP). *MMWR Recomm Rep.* 2018;67:1.

Manning SE, Rupprecht CE, Fishbein D, et al. Human rabies Prevention—United States 2008: recommendation of the Advisory Committee on Immunization Practices; CDC. *MMWR Recomm Rep.* 2008;57:1-28.

Schneir A, Clark RF. Bites and stings. In: Tintinalli JE, Stapczynski J, Ma O, Yealy DM, Meckler GD, Cline DM, eds. *Tintinalli's Emergency Medicine: A Comprehensive Study Guide.* 8th ed. New York, NY: McGraw Hill; 2016: Chap. 211. http://accessmedicine.mhmedical.com/content.aspx?bookid= 1658&sectionid=109385845. Accessed May 20, 2019.

Suchard JR. "Spider bite" lesions are usually diagnosed as skin and soft-tissue infections. *J Emerg Med.* 2011;41(5):473-481.

A 60-year-old man is brought to the emergency department (ED) by ambulance because of slurred speech and left-side weakness that began approximately 6 hours ago. His wife states her husband went to bed the night before and was well. When they awoke, she noticed that he had some difficulties talking and moving his left arm and leg. He has a past medical history of poorly controlled hypertension, a myocardial infarction 10 years ago, hyperlipidemia, and moderate obesity. His daily medications include a baby aspirin, an angiotensin-converting enzyme inhibitor, and a statin. He consumed alcohol heavily in the past but stopped drinking completely after his heart attack. He has smoked a pack of cigarettes daily since his teenage years. His wife remembers that 3 months ago he complained of bilateral leg pain during their morning walk and had to stop after 15 minutes, and that 1 month ago he had a "slight right eye blackout" for 5 minutes.

On presentation to the ED, his temperature is 99.8 °F (37.6 °C), blood pressure is 195/118 mm Hg, pulse is 106 beats/min, respiratory rate is 18 breaths/min, and oxygen saturation is 97% on room air. Although his pupils are equally round and reactive and extraocular movements are intact, he is unable to turn his eyes voluntarily toward the left side. His neck is supple, there is no jugular venous distention, and there are no bruits. His lungs are clear, heart sounds are regular without murmurs, and abdomen is nontender. His extremities are warm, but distal pulses in his feet are difficult to palpate. The neurologic examination reveals that he is awake, alert, and oriented, although he does not recognize that he is ill. He is right-handed and shows loss of awareness and attention with respect to objects or stimuli on his left side. He has mild dysarthria, but his speech is fluent, and he understands and follows commands appropriately. There is mild weakness on the left side of the face and left-sided homonymous hemianopsia, no nystagmus or ptosis, and no tongue or uvula deviation. He is not able to move his left arm and leg and has left-sided hyperreflexia. His left great toe is upgoing on Babinski test.

▶ What is the most likely diagnosis?
▶ What is your initial diagnostic step?
▶ What is your initial step in therapy?

ANSWERS TO CASE 44:

Cerebrovascular Accident/Transient Ischemic Attack

Summary: This 60-year-old man presents with

- A history of coronary artery disease, myocardial infarction, hypertension, and hyperlipidemia
- Presentation to the ED with a 6-hour history of slurred speech and an inability to move his left arm and leg
- An episode of amaurosis fugax (fleeting, painless, transient monocular vision loss) in his right eye 1 month prior to presentation of these symptoms
- Being right-handed and alert and oriented, but with no awareness of his disability (anosognosia) and left-sided neglect
- Significant hypertension, dysarthria, and left hemiparesis
- Left-sided homonymous hemianopsia, conjugate rightward gaze deviation, left hemifacial weakness, and left hyperreflexia

Most likely diagnosis: Cerebrovascular accident (CVA).

Initial diagnostic step: Obtain a stat computed tomography (CT) scan of the brain without contrast.

Initial step in therapy: Determine advisability for acute treatment with thrombolytic agents.

ANALYSIS

Objectives

1. Recognize the significance of a correct diagnosis and evaluation of transient ischemic attacks (TIAs) and CVAs based upon risk factors. (EPA 1, 2, 3)
2. Recognize the conditions that can mimic TIAs and CVAs. (EPA 1, 2)
3. Understand that the clinical evaluation gives the most important clues about diagnosis of TIA or stroke. (EPA 1, 10)
4. Be familiar with the accepted approach for the early management of patients with ischemic stroke. (EPA 4)
5. Be familiar with the current strategies for prevention of CVA and TIA. (EPA 4, 12)

Considerations

This 60-year-old patient has developed focal neurologic deficits, which represents the most common presentation of a patient with a stroke. Considering that he has a history of uncontrolled hypertension, hypercholesterolemia, and vascular manifestations of atherosclerosis, such as coronary artery disease and peripheral vascular disease (lower extremity claudication), ischemic stroke is the most probable diagnosis. Furthermore, he had a TIA (amaurosis fugax) 1 month prior to presentation, which places him at an even greater risk for an ischemic stroke. His neurologic deficits are compatible with an ischemic stroke in the territory of the right middle cerebral artery, which is his nondominant hemisphere and the reason he is not aphasic.

Of immediate importance, after securing the ABCs (airway, breathing circulation), the clinician should confirm that the neurologic impairments are secondary to an ischemic stroke and not another condition, specifically an intracranial hemorrhage. A brain CT without contrast should be obtained as soon as possible to exclude hemorrhage, tumor, abscess, and mass effect, which would preclude administration of thrombolytic therapy. Serum glucose, urine toxicology screen, coagulation studies, serum electrolytes, renal function tests, lipid profile, and a complete blood count are also indicated. A 12-lead electrocardiogram (ECG) should be obtained to exclude acute myocardial infarction or arrhythmia such as atrial fibrillation, and the patient should be placed on telemetry.

Since it has been more than 4.5 hours from the onset of symptoms, this patient is not a candidate for thrombolytic therapy. Although this patient's blood pressure is markedly elevated, in the setting of an acute ischemic CVA, blood pressure management should be cautious, as compensatory hypertension can be permitted to avoid increasing risk of ischemic injury from hypoperfusion.

This patient should be admitted to the hospital for further evaluation and management, preferably to a dedicated stroke unit. Aspirin should be given within 48 hours of the onset of stroke, and deep venous thrombosis (DVT) prophylaxis should started with subcutaneous low-molecular-weight heparin. An evaluation of the patient's speech and swallowing function and an early physical therapy consultation should be obtained. Further imaging with brain magnetic resonance imaging (MRI), magnetic resonance angiography (MRA), or CT angiography can help to clarify the etiology of the stroke and guide treatment. In this patient, carotid duplex ultrasonography is indicated since he had an episode of amaurosis fugax, caused by a blockage of the ophthalmic artery, which branches from the internal carotid artery.

Management of this patient's chronic medical conditions is critical to reduce his risk of subsequent strokes. In this patient, these measures include tight control of his hypertension and hypercholesterolemia, along with immediate smoking cessation. Since this patient had a stroke while taking daily aspirin, an alternative antiplatelet agent should be considered.

APPROACH TO:
Cerebrovascular Accident/Transient Ischemic Attack

DEFINITIONS

HEMORRHAGIC STROKE: Central nervous system (CNS) damage secondary to intracerebral or subarachnoid hemorrhage.

ISCHEMIC STROKE: An infarction of the CNS with resultant neurological deficit that persists beyond 24 hours or is interrupted by death within 24 hours.

TRANSIENT ISCHEMIC ATTACK: A transient episode of neurologic dysfunction caused by focal brain, spinal cord, or retinal ischemia, **without** acute infarction. There is no time cutoff that reliably distinguishes whether a symptomatic ischemic event will result in ischemic infarction.

TRANSIENT SYMPTOMS WITH INFARCTION (TSI): A transient episode of neurologic dysfunction associated with irreversible ischemic brain injury as evident by imaging changes even after resolution of symptoms.

CLINICAL APPROACH

Epidemiology

Strokes are the fifth leading cause of death in the United Sates and are a major cause of disability. A stroke is presumed to have occurred if the symptoms persist for more than 24 hours, while most TIAs last for less than an hour. However, there is an unreliable correlation between symptom duration and actual infarction. **Patients with a TIA are at increased risk of a subsequent stroke.** Patients with a TIA often require hospital admission, further evaluation, and the same long-term management as stroke patients. **An assessment called the ABCD^2 (age, blood pressure, clinical features, duration of symptoms, and diabetes) score** can be used to identify patients at high risk of ischemic stroke in the first 7 days after TIA. The ABCD^2 score is as follows:

- Age ($\geq$ 60 years = 1 point)
- Blood pressure elevation when first assessed after TIA (systolic $\geq$ 140 mm Hg or diastolic $\geq$ 90 mm Hg = 1 point)
- Clinical features (unilateral weakness = 2 points; isolated speech disturbance = 1 point; other = 0 points)
- Duration of neurologic symptoms ($\geq$ 60 minutes = 2 points; 10 to 59 minutes = 1 point; < 10 minutes = 0 points)
- Diabetes (present = 1 point)

Estimation of 2-day stroke risk is determined by the ABCD^2 score as follows:

- Score 0 to 3: Low stroke risk (1%)
- Score 4 to 5: Moderate risk (4%)
- Score 6 to 7: High risk (8%)

Risk Factors. **Hypertension is the single most important risk factor for stroke,** and the incidence of stroke in the United States has decreased as a result of improved strategies to control hypertension (Table 44–1). Other risk factors include diabetes mellitus, older age, male gender, family history, hyperlipidemia, tobacco abuse, alcohol abuse, cocaine abuse, and prothrombotic disorders. Many cardiovascular conditions also predispose people to stroke, usually through formation of an embolic clot. These conditions include atrial fibrillation, myocardial infarction, endocarditis, carotid stenosis, rheumatic heart disease, presence of a mechanical

Table 44–1 • RISK FACTORS FOR STROKE AND TRANSIENT ISCHEMIC ATTACK	
Modifiable Risk Factors	Nonmodifiable Risk Factors
Atherosclerotic cardiovascular disease (coronary, carotid, or peripheral)	Age
	Ethnicity
Atrial fibrillation	Family history
Cigarette smoking	Gender
Heart failure	History of prior stroke, TIA, or myocardial infarction
Diabetes mellitus	
Hyperlipidemia	
Obesity	
Physical inactivity	
Poor diet	
Sickle cell disease	

valve, advanced dilated cardiomyopathy, and a patent foramen ovale or atrial septal defect, which can expose the systemic arterial system to a paradoxical embolus from a venous source. Sickle cell disease is also a risk factor for stroke, as patients with this condition commonly experience strokes as children.

Pathophysiology

Ischemic Strokes. Ischemic strokes are classified as **thrombotic or embolic origin.** Strokes that affect the small branches of the main arteries of the brain are termed lacunar infarcts or small-vessel strokes. These strokes often forewarn a larger, more debilitating stroke. The causes of the emboli are usually of cardiovascular origin and include the previously mentioned conditions as well as dissection of various vessels. While most emboli result from blood clots, emboli can also occur from vegetations from infective endocarditis, sterile vegetations from Libman-Sacks endocarditis (which occurs in systemic lupus erythematosus), and marantic endocarditis (which occurs with cancer).

Hemorrhagic Strokes. Intracerebral hemorrhage means bleeding into the brain parenchyma, which most commonly is caused by weakened arterial vessels associated with hypertension. Arterial aneurysms most commonly occur at junctions of arterial branching (circle of Willis). Less common causes of hemorrhagic strokes include bleeding from arteriovenous malformations. Intracerebral bleeding often occurs in the thalamus, putamen, cerebellum, and brain stem.

Differential Diagnosis. The differential diagnosis of acute neurologic signs and symptoms is broad. Along with CVAs, such symptoms can be caused by seizures, acute confusional states, delirium, syncope, metabolic and toxic encephalopathy (eg, hypoglycemia, poisoning), brain tumors, CNS infections, migraines, multiple sclerosis, and subdural hematoma. Migraines with neurologic symptoms can be especially difficult to differentiate from stroke since migraines do not have to be accompanied by a headache. However, the symptoms of stroke are usually of a much more rapid onset than those of a migraine. Stroke victims are also usually alert and aware of what is happening to them, unlike people suffering from delirium or various types of encephalopathies. When it is determined that a stroke is the cause of the presentation, **it is crucial to differentiate between ischemic and hemorrhagic stroke because of the implications for further treatment.**

The initial assessment should establish if the patient is eligible for thrombolytic treatment; establishing the time of symptom onset is the most important factor. The onset of symptoms is assumed to be the time that the patient was last known to be free of symptoms, such as when they went to bed.

Clinical Presentation

Signs and Symptoms. Sudden onset of focal neurologic deficits is the usual presentation of stroke patients, although some patients can have a gradual worsening of symptoms. Unless there is a hemispheric infarction, basilar artery occlusion, or cerebellar stroke with edema, nearly all of the patients are alert. If the middle cerebral artery territory is affected, the patient will generally experience aphasia (when the dominant hemisphere is involved), contralateral hemiparesis, sensory loss, spatial neglect, and contralateral impaired conjugate gaze. When the territory of the anterior cerebral artery is affected, lower extremity deficits are more frequent than upper extremity deficits. These patients often have associated cognitive and personality changes. Vertebrobasilar stroke symptoms and signs include motor or sensory loss in all four extremities, crossed signs, disconjugate gaze, nystagmus, dysarthria, and dysphagia. If the cerebellum is affected by ischemic stroke, then ipsilateral limb and gait ataxia are commonly present.

Assessment of vital signs is important in the initial examination. Severe high blood pressure can be suggestive of hypertensive encephalopathy or intracranial hemorrhage. A fever may lead to consideration of an infectious cause. A rapid or irregularly irregular pulse may suggest atrial fibrillation as a potential cause of the stroke. A timely general physical examination and comprehensive neurologic examination should follow, as well as subsequent interval evaluations.

CT Scans. **A CT scan of the brain without contrast is the initial imaging test of choice in the evaluation of acute stroke.** A CT scan of the brain may not show evidence of an ischemic stroke for up to 72 hours but can immediately exclude most cases of intracranial hemorrhage, tumors, or abscesses. CT is more cost effective, takes less time than MRI, and can be used to detect a hemorrhagic transformation of an infarct in a patient with an ischemic stroke whose symptoms deteriorate. If neurologic symptoms have resolved, MRI evaluation within 24 hours is the preferred imaging study due to its increased sensitivity for differentiating between a TIA and a TSI stroke.

Other Imaging. Further imaging studies may be indicated to clarify the etiology of the stroke and to detect intracranial or extracranial arterial occlusions, which may affect treatment decisions. Evaluation of the cerebrovascular system can be accomplished with MRA, CT angiography, catheter angiography, or transcranial Doppler ultrasonography. Echocardiography may also be necessary to assess the structure of the heart. Transesophageal echocardiography is particularly useful in detecting cardiac sources of embolism, such as thrombus caused by myocardial infarction, endocarditis, rheumatic heart disease, valvular prostheses, and atrial septal defects. A carotid duplex ultrasonography evaluation is also recommended to evaluate for carotid plaques or stenosis.

Other Tests. A 12-lead ECG should be performed in all stroke patients to detect or rule out acute myocardial infarctions, which can either cause a stroke or result from a stroke. An ECG will also aid in the diagnosis of atrial fibrillation or other arrhythmias that may cause a stroke. A comprehensive metabolic panel (including electrolytes, liver and kidney evaluation, and serum glucose value) and a urine toxicology screening are important to exclude hypoglycemia and metabolic or toxic encephalopathy. If the patient is on anticoagulant therapy, the prothrombin time, partial thromboplastin time, and complete blood count with platelets should be obtained before considering thrombolytic therapy. A lipid panel, erythrocyte sedimentation rate, antinuclear antibodies, and serologic tests for syphilis may also be indicated. In young patients without an identifiable cause for a stroke, a workup for coagulation disorders or antiphospholipid syndrome may be indicated. A lumbar puncture is contraindicated if subarachnoid or intracranial hemorrhage is suspected.

Treatment

Addressing the ABCs. As in every critically ill patient, **the initial survey should assess the ABCs.** If hypoxia is detected, supplemental oxygen should be administered to maintain oxygen saturation above 94% and the cause of the hypoxia investigated (eg, partial airway obstruction, aspiration pneumonia, atelectasis). An endotracheal tube should be placed if the airway is threatened. **The patient should be placed on telemetry to detect atrial fibrillation or any other arrhythmias.**

Treating Hypertension. Unless hypertensive encephalopathy, aortic dissection, acute renal failure, or pulmonary edema is present, the **treatment of arterial hypertension should be cautious.** Prior to intravenous thrombolytic treatment, blood pressure should be lowered if systolic blood pressure is > 185 mm Hg or diastolic blood pressure is > 110 mm Hg. After thrombolytic treatment, systolic blood pressure should be kept less than 180 mm Hg and diastolic blood pressure less than 105 mm Hg. Pharmacologic options for treatment of hypertension in patients with acute ischemic stroke include intravenous labetalol, nicardipine, and sodium nitroprusside. Hypotension or hypovolemia should be corrected with parenteral fluids.

Treating Fever and Hyperglycemia. Fever and elevated serum glucose after a stroke are often associated with less favorable outcomes and should be controlled during the poststroke period. An infectious source for the fever should be investigated. Serum glucose should be treated to a target of 140-180 mg/dL, with careful avoidance of hypoglycemia.

Pharmacologic Treatment of Ischemic Stroke. **Judiciously selected patients can benefit from intravenous administration of recombinant tissue-type plasminogen activator (rtPA)** if they can be treated within 3 to 4.5 hours of the onset of ischemic stroke. Time from onset of symptoms to administration of rtPA has a powerful impact on outcomes; treatment should only be delayed to obtain a noncontrast head CT and a blood glucose level. Contraindications to the use of thrombolytic therapy include recent surgery, trauma, gastrointestinal bleeding, prior ischemic stroke in the past 3 months, use of anticoagulants, and uncontrolled hypertension. Direct intra-arterial thrombolysis or mechanical thrombectomy may be considered when available.

Most patients with a nonhemorrhagic stroke should receive aspirin within the first 48 hours. Generally, patients who receive rtPA should receive aspirin 24 hours later. Poststroke cerebral edema can lead to herniation of the brain stem, resulting in death. Cerebral edema should be treated with mannitol or decompression neurosurgery.

Poststroke Management. Acute treatment in a dedicated stroke unit results in better outcomes and decreased mortality. Early poststroke treatment care includes mobilization once the patient is stable and evaluation of the patient's ability to speak and swallow. After a stroke, the patient is often immobile and needs intensive medical care in order to avoid malnutrition, skin breakdown, and infection. A patient's neurologic deficits commonly improve after a stroke and may continue to improve for up to 6 months to a year. Prior strokes also predispose patients to seizures, and some patients may initially present with a seizure as the first symptom of stroke. When thrombolytic therapy is not used, DVT prophylaxis should be provided. Family support and treatment of depression should also be initiated when appropriate.

Prevention

A history of a previous TIA or CVA confers a high risk for future events. Aggressive risk factor control should be undertaken in these patients. All patients should be counseled to quit smoking and to reduce alcohol intake. Hypertensive patients should be treated per guidelines (see Case 30). All patients with a TIA or ischemic stroke of atherosclerotic origin should be treated with a high-intensity statin regardless of baseline low-density lipoprotein (LDL) cholesterol level. Strict diabetic control should aim for a hemoglobin A_{1c} level less than 7.0%. Antiplatelet agents such as aspirin (81-325 mg/day), the combination of aspirin and extended-release dipyridamole (Aggrenox), or clopidogrel (Plavix) should be started in patients with a history of noncardioembolic ischemic stroke or TIA.

Carotid endarterectomy (CEA) can reduce the risk of stroke in a patient with a history of previous TIA or CVA and symptomatic carotid artery stenosis greater than 60% to 70%. A noninvasive carotid balloon angioplasty and stenting procedure is an alternative to CEA in select patients.

Anticoagulation with warfarin reduces the risk of stroke and stroke recurrence in patients with appropriate risk factors, including patients with advanced congestive heart failure, ischemic stroke caused by a myocardial infarction with existence of a left ventricular thrombus, and rheumatic heart disease or a mechanical heart valve. Atrial fibrillation is the most common cause of cardioembolic stroke, and anticoagulation in these patients can be achieved with warfarin or one of the non–vitamin K antagonist, direct-acting oral anticoagulants.

CASE CORRELATION
- See Case 20 (Chest Pain) and Case 30 (Hypertension).

COMPREHENSION QUESTIONS

44.1 A 72-year-old man is brought to the ED because of weakness and numbness of the right arm. He had no other symptoms or signs of neurological compromise. The emergency physician states that the patient has either a stroke or TIA. Which of the following would be most commonly expected in a patient with a TIA?

   A. Resolution of symptoms within 1 hour

   B. Stroke within 90 days in less than 1% of patients

   C. Computed tomographic evidence of infarction

   D. Computed tomographic evidence of ischemia

   E. MRI evidence of infarction

44.2 An 84-year-old woman is brought into the emergency center for confusion. Her daughter-in-law found the patient walking down the street a few blocks from her house. The daughter-in-law noticed that the patient did not appear to know where she was and did not recognize her. Upon prompting by you, she seems confused and does not speak. The patient experienced a CVA 1 year previously and had mild residual weakness on her left arm and leg. She takes medications for hypertension, hyperlipidemia, constipation, and gout. The patient has a blood pressure of 195/106 mm Hg, pulse of 86 beats/min, respiratory rate of 18 breaths/min, and temperature of 97.9 °F (36.6 °C). She does not follow commands and is oriented only to person. She complains of headache, yet a CT of the brain does not show evidence of an acute hemorrhage. Which of the following is the most appropriate next step in management?

   A. Lumbar puncture

   B. Chest radiograph

   C. Intravenous labetalol

   D. MRI of the brain

   E. Intravenous mannitol

44.3 An 82-year-old man with a suspected stroke is transferred from a small rural hospital to a major medical center. Three hours have elapsed since initial presentation. His blood pressure is 144/92 mm Hg, and he is awake, alert, oriented, and moving all four extremities. He has slurred speech and right arm weakness. A CT scan of the brain is negative. Which of the following is the most important next step in the management of this patient?

   A. Avoidance of acetaminophen

   B. Aggressive blood pressure management

   C. Thrombolysis

   D. A speech and swallowing evaluation

44.4 A 65-year-old man was hospitalized due to sudden weakness of the right arm and was diagnosed with an ischemic stroke. Carotid duplex ultrasonography revealed 40% to 59% bilateral stenosis. Which of the following is the best strategy regarding prevention of future strokes in this patient?

A. Warfarin

B. Carotid endarterectomy

C. Clopidogrel

D. Long-acting nitrates

44.5 A man is brought to the ED by ambulance. Coworkers at his office stated that he was acting normally until approximately 1 hour ago, when he became confused and had trouble walking. One coworker thought that his right leg seemed weak. His temperature is 97.4 °F (36.3 °C), pulse is 118 beats/min, and blood pressure is 90/65 mm Hg. The patient is arousable, but he does not follow commands and is not oriented. He has a medical alert bracelet on his arm indicating that he is a diabetic and allergic to penicillin. A serum glucose level obtained at the bedside is 50 mg/dL. Which of the following should be your immediate first step in management?

A. Immediately give the patient intravenous D50 or glucagon.

B. Immediately obtain a CT scan to assess possibility for giving rtPA.

C. Immediately perform a lumbar puncture to assess for subarachnoid hemorrhage.

D. Immediately give the patient mannitol.

E. Immediately start cardiopulmonary resuscitation (CPR) with chest compressions.

ANSWERS

44.1 **A.** Although by definition a TIA is defined as a temporary neurological deficit with resolution within 24 hours, TIAs typically are less than 1 hour in duration. These events do not cause infarction. The occurrence of stroke after TIA is as high as 5.3% within 2 days and 10.5% within 90 days (not less than 1%, as in answer B). Warfarin is indicated in specific circumstances, such as the presence of atrial fibrillation, but it is not routinely used following a TIA. There will not be evidence of infarction (answers C and D [CT scan] and answer E [MRI scan]). The majority of CT imaging of the brain will be normal in TIA. The main purpose of the CT scan is to rule out a tumor or hemorrhagic stroke.

44.2 **C.** Intravenous labetalol should be started to achieve appropriate blood pressure control since this patient has signs of hypertensive encephalopathy. Caution should be exercised not to lower the blood pressure too much, but out of the danger zone. Routine chest x-rays (answer B) are not recommended as routine initial workup of a suspected CVA. CT of the brain *without* contrast can exclude most cases of intracranial hemorrhage, tumors, or abscesses; it is the initial test of choice in the workup of suspected stroke, but it can miss up to 15% of subarachnoid hemorrhages. When a subarachnoid hemorrhage is suspected but not seen on CT, a lumbar puncture (answer A) is indicated for diagnosis. Answer D (MRI of the brain) may be helpful, but initially the blood pressure control is most important. Answer E (intravenous mannitol) helps to decrease intracerebral pressure, but currently the patient does not have evidence of this condition.

44.3 **C.** This patient is a candidate for thrombolysis since the symptoms have been present for less than 3 to 4.5 hours. Use of thrombolytics < 3 hours since the onset of symptoms has the best efficacy. Early mobilization of stroke patients should be started when they are considered medically stable after the patient has been adequately evaluated and treated. In the setting of an acute stroke, management of high blood pressure should be cautious and not required in this instance since the blood pressure is not in the severe range (answer B). At this point, 4 hours after symptoms, when the patient is speaking without difficulty, a swallowing evaluation (answer D) is not immediately warranted. Avoidance of acetaminophen (answer A) is the intervention for analgesic-associated headache, which is not this patient's problem.

44.4 **C.** Patients with stroke but no detected sources of embolism benefit from antiplatelet agents and not anticoagulants such as warfarin (answer A). Aspirin, clopidogrel, or a combination of aspirin and dipyridamole are acceptable regimens. For patients with recent TIA or ischemic stroke and ipsilateral severe (> 70%) carotid artery stenosis, CEA (answer B) is recommended. When the degree of stenosis is less than 50%, there is no indication for CEA. Patients with a history of symptomatic cerebrovascular disease should be treated with a statin to achieve an LDL goal of less than 100 mg/dL.

44.5 **A.** The patient has severe hypoglycemia and needs to be treated immediately with intravenous glucose or glucagon. If the patient does not recover with glucose or glucagon infusion, then other tests, such as a CT scan (answer B), may be warranted. Be aware that hypoglycemia can mimic many of the symptoms of a stroke, including focal weakness. Mannitol (answer D) is used in cases of cerebral edema and not for raising blood sugar. The patient is tachycardic, likely from hypoglycemia, and does not require CPR (answer E).

CLINICAL PEARLS

▶ Hypertension is the single most important modifiable risk factor for stroke.

▶ Although most strokes are cerebral infarctions, it is crucial to differentiate between ischemic and hemorrhagic stroke because of the implications for further treatment.

▶ Judiciously selected patients can benefit from intravenous administration of rtPA.

▶ Computed tomography of the brain without contrast is the initial imaging test of choice in most suspected strokes, followed by lumbar puncture for analysis of cerebrospinal fluid.

▶ Unless hypertensive encephalopathy, aortic dissection, acute renal failure, or pulmonary edema is present, the treatment of arterial hypertension should be cautious.

REFERENCES

Adam SS, McDuffie JR, Ortel TL, Williams JW Jr. Comparative effectiveness of warfarin and new oral anticoagulants for the management of atrial fibrillation and venous thromboembolism: a systematic review. *Ann Intern Med.* 2012;157(11):796-807.

Donnan G, Fisher M, Macleod M, Davis S. Stroke. *Lancet.* 2008;371(9624):1612-1623.

Johnston SC, Rothwell PM, Nguyen-Huynh MN, et al. Validation and refinement of scores to predict very early stroke risk after transient ischaemic attack. *Lancet.* 2007;369(9558):283.

Powers WJ, Rabinstein AA, Ackerson T, et al. 2018 guidelines for the early management of patients with acute ischemic stroke: a guideline for healthcare professionals from the American Heart Association/American Stroke Association. *Stroke.* 2018;49(3):e46-e110.

Simmons BB, Cirignano B, Gadegbeku AB. Transient ischemic attack: Part I. Diagnosis and evaluation. *Am Fam Physician.* 2012;86(6):521-526.

Simmons BB, Gadegbeku AB, Cirignano B. Transient ischemic attack: Part II. Risk factor modification and treatment. *Am Fam Physician.* 2012;86(6):527-532.

Smith WS, Johnston S, Hemphill J III. Cerebrovascular diseases. In: Jameson J, Fauci AS, Kasper DL, et al, eds. *Harrison's Principles of Internal Medicine.* 20th ed. New York, NY: McGraw Hill; 2018: Chap. 419.

Stone NJ, Robinson JG, Lichtenstein AH, et al. 2013 ACC/AHA guideline on the treatment of blood cholesterol to reduce atherosclerotic cardiovascular risk in adults. A report of the American College of Cardiology/American Heart Association Task Force on Practice Guidelines. *Circulation.* 2013;129:S1-S45.

Whelton PK, Carey RM, Aronow WS, et al. 2017 ACC/AHA/AAPA/ABC/ACPM/AGS/APhA/ASH/ASPC/NMA/PCNA guideline of the prevention, detection, and management of high blood pressure in adults. A report of the American College of Cardiology/American Heart Association Task Force on Clinical Practice Guidelines. *JACC.* 2018;71(19):e127-e248.

A 39-year-old man presents to the emergency department (ED) with a nonproductive cough and subjective fever. He states that he is homeless, and his illness has been worsening over the past 2 weeks. Originally, he had dyspnea on exertion, and now he is short of breath at rest. On questioning, he tells you that he lives in a homeless shelter when he can, but he frequently sleeps on the streets. He has used intravenous drugs (primarily heroin) "on and off" for many years and has had unprotected anal receptive intercourse with multiple partners. He denies any significant medical history and only gets medical care when he comes to the ED for an illness or injury. On review of systems, he endorses chronic fatigue, weight loss, and diarrhea. On examination, he is a thin, disheveled man appearing much older than his stated age. His temperature is 100.4 °F (38.0 °C), blood pressure is 100/50 mm Hg, pulse is 105 beats/min, and respiratory rate is 24 breaths/min. His initial oxygen saturation is 89% on room air, which improves to 94% on 4 L of oxygen by nasal cannula. Significant findings on examination include dry mucous membranes, a tachycardic but regular cardiac rhythm, a soft and nontender abdomen, and cachectic-appearing extremities. His pulmonary examination is significant for tachypnea and fine crackles bilaterally, but there are no visible signs of cyanosis on extremities. His chest radiograph reveals diffuse, bilateral, interstitial infiltrates that look like "ground glass."

▶ What is the most probable cause of this patient's current pulmonary complaints?
▶ What underlying illness does this patient most likely have?
▶ What diagnostic testing and treatment should be started?

ANSWERS TO CASE 45:
HIV, AIDS, and Other Sexually Transmitted Infections

Summary: A 39-year-old man presents with

- Fever, cough, dyspnea, and fatigue
- Tachypnea and hypoxemia
- A history of homelessness and intravenous drug use
- Chest radiograph that reveals bilateral interstitial infiltrates that look like ground glass

Most probable cause of pulmonary complaints: *Pneumocystis jirovecii* pneumonia.

Most likely underlying illness: Acquired immunodeficiency syndrome (AIDS).

Diagnostic testing and treatment: Complete blood count (CBC) and platelets, comprehensive metabolic panel, arterial blood gas; human immunodeficiency virus (HIV) enzyme-linked immunosorbent assay (ELISA) with confirmatory Western blot; CD4/CD8 cell count; HIV RNA assay; induced sputum culture for *P. jirovecii* and acid-fast bacilli; urine testing for *Chlamydia trachomatis*, *Neisseria gonorrheae*, and *Trichomonas*; serum rapid plasma reagin (RPR); start treatment with oral trimethoprim-sulfamethoxazole (TMP-SMX) and consider starting highly active antiretroviral therapy (HAART) with appropriate case management, including intensive treatment for substance use disorder, counseling, and social work.

ANALYSIS

Objectives

1. List the common risk factors for and modes of transmission of HIV/AIDS. (EPA 12)

2. Recognize common presentations of persons infected with HIV. (EPA 1, 2)

3. List the most common sexually transmitted infections (STIs). (EPA 12)

4. Describe common treatment regimens for sexually transmitted infections. (EPA 4)

Considerations

The case described is that of a 39-year-old homeless man with substance use disorder who has had unprotected intercourse with multiple partners, including anal receptive intercourse. He has had chronic fatigue and weight loss, and he now presents with fever, tachypnea, and hypoxemia. It is likely that he is infected with HIV and has an opportunistic infection, namely *P. jirovecii* pneumonia.

   Pneumocystis jirovecii (formerly *Pneumocystis carinii*) pneumonia is an AIDS-defining illness in persons infected with HIV. *Pneumocystis jirovecii* is a fungus that may colonize many people, but it typically causes disease only in those with profound immune deficiencies, such as AIDS or cancers treated with chemotherapy. *Pneumocystis jirovecii* pneumonia usually presents with nonproductive cough, fever, and dyspnea that worsens over a few days to a few weeks. Patients usually are found to be febrile, tachypneic, and hypoxic, but their lung examination may be unremarkable (other than tachypnea). The presence of **bilateral interstitial infiltrates on chest radiograph, often described as having a "ground-glass" appearance,** is pathognomonic for *P. jirovecii* pneumonia. The identification of the organism in sputum is diagnostic, but treatment is usually started prior to definitive diagnosis in those with a classic clinical picture and high suspicion.

As *P. jirovecii* pneumonia occurs after the CD4 and CD8 counts have markedly reduced, patients often will have signs and symptoms of other AIDS-related complications as well. In patients with AIDS, it is common to see additional comorbid conditions, including oral or esophageal candidiasis, chronic infectious diarrhea, Kaposi sarcoma, wasting syndrome, and weight loss. Although typically occurring in the setting of advanced disease, *P. jirovecii* pneumonia remains a common presenting illness in patients who did not know that they were infected with HIV and is a frequent initial opportunistic infection in those with known HIV disease. The incidence of *P. jirovecii* pneumonia is decreasing in the United States with more widespread awareness of HIV disease, broader usage of antiretroviral therapy, and prophylactic use of TMP-SMX in patients with CD4 counts of less than 200 cells/μL.

APPROACH TO:

HIV, AIDS, and Other Sexually Transmitted Infections

DEFINITIONS

ACQUIRED IMMUNODEFICIENCY SYNDROME: The advanced stage of the HIV infection, in which opportunistic infections occur with specific criteria for its designation.

HUMAN IMMUNODEFICIENCY VIRUS: A retrovirus that infects the helper T cells of the immune system, which are defined by the presence of the cell-signaling protein CD4, and causes a decline in both their number and their effectiveness.

CLINICAL APPROACH TO HIV/AIDS

Epidemiology

As of 2017, over 36 million people in the world were living with HIV infection and/or AIDS. Mortality from AIDS-related illnesses has declined in the past decade, with an estimated 940,000 deaths occurring in 2017 (down from 1.5 million in 2013), but a disproportionate amount of deaths due to HIV occurs in sub-Saharan Africa. HIV-1 is more common worldwide, whereas HIV-2 has been reported in western Africa, Europe, South America, and Canada. As of 2017, in the United States 1.5 million people were living with HIV. Approximately **15% do not know their status**, compared to an estimated 25% in 2011. Populations at

Table 45–1 • CDC HIV SCREENING RECOMMENDATIONS
For Patients in All Health Care Settings
• HIV screening is recommended for patients in all health care settings after the patient is notified that testing will be performed unless the patient declines (opt-out screening).
• Persons at high risk for HIV infection should be screened for HIV at least annually.
• Separate written consent for HIV testing should not be required; general consent for medical care should be considered sufficient to encompass consent for HIV testing.
• Prevention counseling should not be required with HIV diagnostic testing or as part of HIV screening programs in health care settings.
For Pregnant Women
• HIV screening should be included in the routine panel of prenatal screening tests for all pregnant women.
• HIV screening is recommended after the patient is notified that testing will be performed unless the patient declines (opt-out screening).
• Separate written consent for HIV testing should not be required; general consent for medical care should be considered sufficient to encompass consent for HIV testing.
• Repeat screening in the third trimester is recommended in certain jurisdictions with elevated rates of HIV infection among pregnant women.

Reproduced from Branson BM, Handsfield HH, Lampe MA, et al. Revised recommendations for HIV testing of adults, adolescents and pregnant women in health-care settings. MMWR Recomm Rep. 2006;55(RR-14):1-17.

elevated risk of contracting HIV include men who have sex with men, intravenous drugs users, female sex workers, and transgender women. In sub-Saharan Africa, most infections among adolescents aged 15 to 19 are in girls, and young women aged 15 to 24 are twice as likely to be living with HIV than men.

Due to the large number of undiagnosed HIV infections, the Centers for Disease Control and Prevention (CDC) expanded screening recommendations, summarized in Table 45–1. The United States Preventive Services Task Force (USPSTF) recommended screening all persons aged 15 to 65, and those of other ages who are at risk, for HIV (Grade A), although the frequency of screening was not defined.

Pathophysiology

HIV infects the helper and cytotoxic T cells of the immune system, which are defined by the presence of the cell-signaling proteins CD4 and CD8, respectively, and causes a decline in both their number and their function in supporting the immune system. This decline in functional helper and cytotoxic T cells disables the cell-mediated arm of the immune system and leaves the body vulnerable to infection from multiple opportunistic organisms. This advanced stage of HIV infection, in which such opportunistic infections occur, is known as AIDS.

Transmission. **HIV is transmitted from person to person through contact with infected blood and body fluids.** Sexual transmission varies by practice, with the highest estimated rate of transmission for receptive anal intercourse, followed by insertive anal intercourse, receptive vaginal-penile intercourse, and insertive vaginal-penile intercourse. Transmission is possible with receptive or insertive penile-oral intercourse but is very rare. The risk of HIV transmission is increased by the presence of genital or anal lesions caused by other STIs.

The risk of transmission can be reduced by the proper and consistent use of latex condoms. Male circumcision has been shown to decrease the rate of HIV transmission.

Sharing needles by intravenous drug users is the third most common source of transmission of HIV behind penile-anal and penile-vaginal transmission. Vertical transmission from an infected woman to her baby can occur during delivery and rarely from breastfeeding. Blood and blood-product transfusions have been linked to infection, although the routine screening of donor blood for HIV now makes this an extremely rare event.

Health care workers have been infected with HIV through accidental punctures with needles or by infected blood entering through open skin wounds or mucous membranes. The risk of transmission to health care workers is low and is related to the viral load of the patient, the amount of blood to which the worker is exposed, and the depth of the inoculum. Postexposure risk of developing HIV infection can be reduced by immediate and careful cleaning of the exposure/puncture site along with postexposure prophylactic (PEP) treatment, with antiretroviral therapy started within 72 hours after exposure. Regimens for PEP include two to three antiretroviral medications taken for 28 days.

Clinical Categorization of HIV/AIDS Infections. **The CDC defines four clinical stages for adults aged > 13. For classification purposes, a patient's HIV is defined by the highest clinical stage in which the patient has ever qualified.**

Stage 1: No AIDS-defining illness and either CD4 cell count $\geq$ 500 cells/μL or percentage of total lymphocytes > 29

Stage 2: No AIDS-defining illness and either CD4 cell count of 200 to 499 cells/μL or percentage between 14 and 28 (see Table 45–2 for some HIV conditions)

Stage 3 (AIDS): CD4 cell count < 200 cells/μL or percentage < 14 and documentation of AIDS-defining condition (Table 45–3)

Stage 4: Unknown laboratory parameters with an AIDS-defining condition

Table 45–2 • SOME EXAMPLES OF HIV-RELATED CONDITIONS THAT ARE NOT AIDS DEFINING
Bacillary angiomatosis
Oropharyngeal candidiasis
Persistent, recurrent, or difficult-to-treat vaginal candidiasis
Cervical dysplasia or carcinoma in situ
Oral hairy leukoplakia
Idiopathic thrombocytopenic purpura
Listeriosis
Pelvic inflammatory disease (especially if complicated by tubo-ovarian abscess)
Peripheral neuropathy
Herpes zoster, two or more episodes involving more than one dermatome

Data from Centers for Disease Control and Prevention. 1993 revised classification system for HIV infection and expanded surveillance case definition for AIDS among adolescents and adults. MMWR Recomm Rep. 1992;41(RR-17):1-19.

Table 45–3 • EXAMPLES OF AIDS-DEFINING CONDITIONS
Candidiasis of bronchi, trachea, or lungs
Coccidioidomycosis (disseminated or extrapulmonary)
Cytomegalovirus disease
Disseminated or extrapulmonary histoplasmosis
Burkitt lymphoma
Mycobacterium avium complex (disseminated or extrapulmonary)
Pneumonia, recurrent
Toxoplasmosis of brain
Esophageal candidiasis
Extrapulmonary *Cryptococcus*
HIV-related encephalopathy
Intestinal isosporiasis (> 1-mo duration)
Immunoblastic lymphoma
Mycobacterium tuberculosis (any site)
Progressive multifocal leukoencephalopathy
Wasting syndrome caused by HIV
Invasive cervical cancer
Intestinal cryptosporidiosis (> 1-mo duration)
Herpes simplex: chronic ulcer, bronchitis, pneumonitis, or esophagitis
Kaposi sarcoma
Primary brain lymphoma
Pneumocystis jiroveci pneumonia
Recurrent *Salmonella* septicemia

Data from Centers for Disease Control and Prevention. Guidelines for the prevention and treatment of opportunistic infections among HIV-exposed and HIV-infected children: recommendations from the National Institutes of Health, the HIV Medicine Association of the Infectious Diseases Society of America, the Pediatric Infectious Diseases Society, and the American Academy of Pediatrics, 2009. MMWR Recomm Rep. 2009;58(RR-11):1-166.

Clinical Presentation

Following initial exposure to HIV, some patients will complain of nonspecific influenza-like symptoms, such as low-grade fever, fatigue, sore throat, or myalgias. This illness typically occurs 6 to 8 weeks following the infection and is commonly self-limited. The primary infection is also known as acute seroconversion syndrome, as the symptoms are thought to be related to the development of antibodies to the virus.

Following the resolution of the primary infection symptoms, there is a period of clinical latency that can last from 6 months to up to 10 years following the transmission of the virus. During this time, most infected persons are asymptomatic, although some may develop lymphadenopathy. While the patient is asymptomatic, a decline in helper and suppressor T-cell number and immune function usually occurs in the untreated patient, as many patients initially present with profound immunodeficiency and opportunistic infections.

Late Disease. HIV and its comorbid opportunistic infections can affect every organ system in the body. Some infections, such as tuberculosis and pneumococcal pneumonia, also affect healthy people but are greatly increased in incidence and severity in the presence of HIV disease. Many mildly pathogenic organisms such as *Candida* species cause unusual, severe infections in parts of the body, including the esophagus and lungs. Kaposi sarcoma, cytomegalovirus retinitis, primary brain lymphoma, and cryptococcal meningitis are unique to extreme immunodeficiency and very low T-cell counts. Cancers in healthy subjects, including cervical cancer, are common in HIV-positive people, while others, such as primary central nervous system (CNS) lymphoma, are extremely rare outside of persons infected with HIV. Although the natural history of AIDS is universal fatality, with the advent of HAART most treated patients with HIV are able to achieve normal life expectancies.

Diagnostic Evaluation. The standard screening test for HIV infection is the detection of HIV antibodies using the ELISA; **positive samples must be confirmed by Western blot testing.** When HIV is diagnosed, a complete history and physical examination should be performed. Emphasis should be placed on identifying possible mechanisms of exposure, comorbid conditions, presence of STIs, determining the presence of AIDS-defining conditions, encouraging safe sexual practices, treating any addiction, and assisting with coping strategies. **HIV infection is reportable to local health authorities, while partner notification laws vary by state.**

Laboratory Values. **Before instituting therapy, laboratory testing should include HIV genotype testing to identify strains that may be resistant to therapy.** A quantitative assay of HIV RNA levels (viral load) can help to assess disease activity. CD4 and CD8 lymphocyte counts and viral load should be measured at baseline and every 3 to 6 months thereafter to monitor for disease staging, progression, and the risk of complications and opportunistic infections. A CBC, comprehensive metabolic panel, and urinalysis should be performed at baseline and periodically thereafter to monitor for complications of HIV and efficacy as well as side effects of treatment. Serology for toxoplasmosis and cytomegalovirus should also be obtained to identify organisms at risk for reactivation following immunosuppression.

STI Screening. Screening for **other STIs** (*C. trachomatis*, *N. gonorrhea*, syphilis, herpes simplex, hepatitis B and C) should be performed initially and repeated based upon any ongoing risks. Hepatitis A and B vaccinations should be offered to those who lack immunity. A purified protein derivative (PPD) test should be performed and, if initially negative, repeated annually. However, a PPD may be falsely negative if the patient is very immunosuppressed or very ill. If positive, a chest radiograph and an interferon gamma release assay test should be performed for confirmation of potential active tuberculosis disease.

Treatment

Preexposure Prophylaxis. Patients at high risk of contracting HIV can be prescribed preexposure prophylaxis (PrEP), which reduces risk of infection in the event of exposure by 90%. PrEP includes a combination of antiretroviral agents (tenofovir and emtricitabine) that inhibit RNA-dependent DNA polymerase, resulting in prevention of HIV DNA replication. Patients should be screened for high-risk sexual behaviors (condomless penile-anal or penile-vaginal sex with partners other than their main partner, sex during drug use) and inquired about total number of sex partners to determine their candidacy for PrEP treatment. PrEP should not be prescribed to patients with an existing HIV infection or those with renal impairment (glomerular filtration rate < 60 mL/min).

HAART. Due to the complexity of treatment regimens and frequently changing treatment guidelines, **patients with HIV/AIDS should be referred to an infectious disease specialist or managed by a provider with experience and expertise in treating this condition.** In general, HAART, the combination of several antiretroviral drugs aimed at controlling the viral load of HIV and preventing HIV from multiplying, is used in patients who have AIDS, who have symptoms of disease, or who are pregnant to reduce the risk of vertical transmission. Updated guidelines on HIV/AIDS treatment and monitoring can be obtained online (http://www.aidsinfo.nih.gov).

Prophylaxis for Complications. Prophylactic treatments to reduce the risk of infection are also important in immunosuppressed patients. HIV patients should receive annual attenuated influenza vaccination and pneumococcal vaccination (before the CD4 count falls to less than 200 cells/µL). **Live virus vaccines are contraindicated in both HIV patients with CD4 counts less than 200 and their close (household) contacts.** Prophylaxis against *P. jirovecii* pneumonia should be instituted using TMP-SMX when the CD4 count falls to less than 200 cells/µL or if there is a history of oropharyngeal candidiasis. *Mycobacterium avium*–intracellulare complex prophylaxis, using azithromycin or clarithromycin, is recommended if the CD4 count falls to less than 50 cells/µL.

CLINICAL APPROACH TO OTHER SEXUALLY TRANSMITTED INFECTIONS

Chlamydia

Infection with *C. trachomatis* is the most frequently reported STI in the United States. Chlamydia can be passed from person to person by vaginal, anal, or oral intercourse and is frequently asymptomatic. The USPSTF recommends screening for chlamydia in all sexually active women ages 16 to 24 and in those at increased risk for infection; there is insufficient evidence to support routine screening in asymptomatic men. Risk factors for infection include multiple sexual partners, young age, history of another STI, and non-Hispanic black race. The risk of transmission can be reduced by the proper use of latex condoms with every sexual encounter. Untreated chlamydia infections in women can lead to ascending infections (eg, pelvic inflammatory disease [PID]), with an increased risk of ectopic pregnancy or infertility. Chlamydia can also cause cervicitis in women, epididymitis in men, and urethritis and pharyngitis in both men and women.

Testing for chlamydia is performed via samples from the cervix, vagina, or pharynx, or by *C. trachomatis* nucleic acid amplification testing of properly collected urine samples; urethral samples are no longer required. Patients diagnosed with chlamydia and their sexual partner(s) should be treated to reduce the risk of complications and to prevent further spread of the disease. The standard treatment for chlamydia is either oral azithromycin 1 g single dose or oral doxycycline 100 mg twice daily for a week. Doxycycline should not be used in pregnant women.

Gonorrhea

Gonorrhea is caused by N. gonorrhoeae. This infection may pass from person to person by vaginal, oral, or anal intercourse. In men, gonorrhea may cause dysuria and penile discharge. In women, the infection may be asymptomatic until complications such as PID occur. The USPSTF recommends routinely screening sexually active women age 24 and under and older women at risk; there is insufficient evidence to support routine screening in asymptomatic men. Testing for gonorrhea is performed similarly to, and usually in tandem with, testing for chlamydia. The recommended treatment for gonorrhea is single-dose ceftriaxone 250 mg intramuscularly along with treatment for chlamydia as described previously due to a high risk of coinfection.

Syphilis

Syphilis is the manifestation of infection by the spirochete *Treponema pallidum*, and infections may be symptomatic or asymptomatic (latent). Symptomatic syphilis is often divided into three stages based on the symptom and length of time from exposure.

- Primary: Characterized by a painless ulcer, or chancre, at the site of infection (usually on the genitalia)

- Secondary: Characterized by skin rash notably on the palms and soles, or condyloma lata on mucus membranes

- Tertiary: Characterized by cardiac or granulomatous lesions (gummas)

Commonly, syphilis is diagnosed on serologic testing of an asymptomatic person; this is called latent syphilis. If latent syphilis can be diagnosed within a year of infection, it is known as "early latent"; all other latent syphilis is either "late latent" or "latent syphilis of unknown duration." Notably, neurosyphilis can occur at any stage; thus, any patient with syphilis with neurological symptoms or signs should have investigation for CNS involvement.

Syphilis can be diagnosed by either direct identification of the *Treponema* spirochete or serologic testing. Spirochetes can be identified by dark-field microscopy of tissue or exudate from a chancre. Initial screening is performed via RPR or the Venereal Disease Research Laboratory (VDRL) test with confirmation of positive results via fluorescent treponemal antibody absorption (FTA-ABS) test. Screening for syphilis is recommended for all pregnant women in order to lower the risk of congenital syphilis. Screening should be performed for anyone who has another STI or is otherwise at high risk for infection.

Single-dose intramuscular penicillin G is the recommended treatment for early stage syphilis, with longer courses required for late latent, latent disease of unknown duration, and tertiary stage. For penicillin-allergic patients, doxycycline, tetracycline, or ceftriaxone may be used as alternatives for patients with early disease or late latent disease.

Herpes

Genital herpes is a viral infection caused most commonly by herpes simplex virus (HSV) type 2. The diagnosis is often made clinically as HSV causes painful vesicles or ulcers. Most persons infected with HSV-2 have not been clinically diagnosed due to presence of mild or unrecognized infection. These persons may shed virus and therefore may transmit the infection to others while being asymptomatic.

Serologic antibody testing to HSV-2 can yield both false-positive and false-negative results, allowing for challenging clinical interpretation. HSV infections may be diagnosed by culture or polymerase chain reaction testing of samples from clinically evident lesions.

Antiviral therapy be used for both acute management of symptomatic outbreaks and suppression to reduce the frequency of outbreak or reduce the risk of viral transmission to an uninfected partner. Pregnant women with a history of HSV should be placed on suppressive therapy late in pregnancy to decrease the risk of symptomatic outbreak or viral shedding at the time of delivery to reduce the risk of neonatal herpes in the newborn. Women with clinically evident genital herpes at the time of delivery should be offered cesarean delivery.

Trichomonas

Trichomoniasis, or "trich," is a very common, curable STI caused by the protozoan *Trichomonas vaginalis*. This infection is asymptomatic in approximately 70% of those infected. Symptomatic women may have vaginal itching, burning, or discharge. On examination, the clinician may see a "frothy" discharge and the characteristic erythematous "strawberry" cervix. Symptomatic men may have urethral itching, burning, or discharge.

A saline wet mount of vaginal discharge allows for the direct visualization of the motile, flagellated trichomonads. Treatment is with 2 g of metronidazole in a single oral dose (preferred) or 500 mg twice a day for 7 days. Tinidazole is an alternative treatment.

Human Papilloma Virus

Human papilloma virus (HPV) infection is the most common STI. It can be passed during anal, vaginal, or oral intercourse. **Most infections with HPV are asymptomatic and cleared by the body's immune system.** HPV infections can lead to genital warts, cervical cancer in women, penile cancer in men, and anal or oropharyngeal cancers in both. See Case 1 for guidelines on HPV vaccination.

CASE CORRELATION

- See Case 1 (Adult Male Health Maintenance) and Case 22 (Vaginitis and Other Vaginal Infections).

COMPREHENSION QUESTIONS

45.1 A 42-year-old HIV-infected woman has a CD4 count of 125 cells/mm^3 and is taking HAART. She has not experienced any AIDS-defining illness. She continues to struggle with heroin and alcohol dependence. She does not regularly take her HAART and has been nonadherent with follow-up appointments. Which of the following treatments is most appropriate at this time?

A. Initiate fluconazole for candidiasis prophylaxis

B. Initiate antiviral treatment for herpes zoster prophylaxis

C. Initiate TMP-SMX for *P. jirovecii* pneumonia prophylaxis

D. Initiate clarithromycin for *M. avium*–intracellulare complex prophylaxis

45.2 A 25-year-old previously healthy man presents to the emergency department after experiencing a generalized tonic-clonic seizure that lasted 30 seconds. He has been experiencing headaches over the past 6 months but no other associated symptoms. His mother states that she witnessed him having two previous seizures. The patient has a history of being sexually promiscuous and using intravenous drugs. The result of his last HIV test is unknown. On neurologic examination, he is noted to have increased tone on the right and decreased right arm swing when walking. The remainder of his neurologic examination is unremarkable. A computed tomography scan with contrast of the brain reveals a ring-enhancing lesion measuring 15 mm over the left motor strip region and a 12-mm ring-enhancing lesion in the left basal ganglia. Which of the following would be an AIDS-defining condition in this patient?

A. Glioblastoma multiforme

B. Subarachnoid hemorrhage

C. Herpes zoster encephalitis

D. Listeriosis with brain abscess

E. Primary brain lymphoma

45.3 During a routine screening, a 22-year-old asymptomatic woman tests positive for gonococcal cervicitis. The chlamydia assay is negative. She has no known drug allergies. Which of the following treatments should be prescribed?

A. Penicillin G 1.2 million units IM for 1 dose

B. Ceftriaxone 250 mg IM for 1 dose

C. Ciprofloxacin 250 mg orally for 1 dose

D. Ceftriaxone 250 mg IM for 1 dose and azithromycin 1 g orally for 1 dose

45.4 A 45-year-old asymptomatic man has an STI screening performed at a local free clinic because of having sex with a new partner 2 months ago. He has never been tested for STIs previously. He tests negative for HIV, gonorrhea, and chlamydia but is notified that he has a positive RPR test. What is the next appropriate step for him?

A. Treatment with intramuscular penicillin G

B. FTA-ABS testing

C. Notification of his STI to the local health department

D. Repeat his STI panel because this is likely a false-positive test

ANSWERS

45.1 **C.** This patient has a CD4 cell count of 125 cells/mm^3. With this level of cell count (below 200 cells/mm^3), the patient should continue antiretroviral therapy and start *P. jirovecii* pneumonia prophylaxis with TMP-SMX. The CD4 level is not yet low enough, which most experts identify as below 50 cells/mm^3, to recommend *M. avium*–intracellulare complex prophylaxis (answer D). Fluconazole for candidiasis prophylaxis (answer A) is not indicated unless there is severe or recurrent disease, since resistance may occur. Antiviral prophylaxis for herpes zoster (answer B) is not indicated, but rather prophylaxis for herpes simplex virus for recurrent infections.

45.2 **E.** Primary brain lymphoma is an AIDS-defining condition. Glioblastoma multiforme (answer A) and subarachnoid hemorrhage (answer B) may present with these symptoms but are not AIDS-defining conditions. Listeriosis (answer D) and herpes zoster encephalitis (answer C) can be associated with HIV, but they are not AIDS-defining conditions.

45.3 **D.** Patients who test positive for gonorrhea should be treated for both gonorrhea and chlamydia. Ceftriaxone 250 mg IM with azithromycin is the appropriate treatment for gonorrhea, with or without evidence of chlamydia. Some countries are reporting increasing resistance and recommend ceftriaxone 500 mg IM alone, but this is not considered standard management at present. Her sexual partner(s) should also be offered treatment. Penicillin (answer A) is the treatment for syphilis and is ineffective for gonorrhea. Ceftriaxone 250 mg IM alone (answer B) is prone to gonorrhea resistance and treatment failure. Ciprofloxacin orally (answer C) had been used previously, but it is no longer recommended due to resistance.

45.4 **B.** This patient has tested positive on his initial screening test for syphilis with a nontreponemal test. Most of these initial screening tests are assessing for antibodies against phospholipids and can have false positives; this can be due to a recent viral infection or autoimmune conditions such as systemic lupus erythematosus. A confirmatory test with a specific treponemal test (FTA-ABS) should be performed prior to making the diagnosis or implementing treatment. If positive, he should then be treated with penicillin (answer A) and the health department should be notified (answer C).

Repeating the STI panel (answer D) would not help confirm syphilis since another non-treponemal test would be performed.

CLINICAL PEARLS

▶ Due to the complexity of the drug regimens and the ever-changing guidelines, persons with HIV should be comanaged with an infectious disease specialist or a clinician with experience and expertise in the field.

▶ The best treatment for uncomplicated gonococcal cervicitis or proctitis is intramuscular ceftriaxone and oral azithromycin due to the emerging resistance of gonorrhea.

▶ Patients who test positive for a nontreponemal syphilis screening test should have a confirmatory test (treponemal test) prior to treatment.

▶ Live virus vaccines are contraindicated in both HIV patients with CD4 counts less than 200 cells/mm^3 and their close (household) contacts.

▶ The risk of transmission of HIV to health care workers by accidental needlesticks from HIV-infected patients is very low. It is important to report these injuries promptly, as early prophylactic treatment can significantly lower the risk of developing HIV disease.

▶ Someone who tests positive for gonorrhea should be treated for both gonorrhea and chlamydia because of the high risk of coinfection.

REFERENCES

AIDS Education and Training Centers. Peer education trainer's manual. 2015 ed. http://www.aidsetc .org/resource/peer-education-trainers-manual. Accessed December 28, 2018.

Armstrong C. CDC updates guidelines on diagnosis and treatment of sexually transmitted diseases. *Am Fam Physician*. 2011;84(1):123-125.

Centers for Disease Control and Prevention. Sexually transmitted diseases. https://www.cdc.gov/std/. Accessed December 28, 2018.

Cohen MS, Shaw GM, McMichael AJ, Haynes BF. Acute HIV-1 infection. *N Engl J Med*. 2011;364:1943-1954.

Fauci AS, Folkers GK, Lane H. Human immunodeficiency virus disease: AIDS and related disorders. In: Jameson J, Fauci A, Kasper D, Hauser S, Longo D, Loscalzo J, eds. *Harrison's Principles of Internal Medicine*. 20th ed. New York, NY: McGraw Hill; 2018: Chap. 226. http://accessmedicine.mhmedical .com/content.aspx?bookid=1130&Sectionid=79738808. Accessed December 29, 2018.

Mattei PL, Beachkofsky TM, Gilson RT, Wisco OJ. Syphilis: a reemerging infection. *Am Fam Physician*. 2012;86(5):433-440.

Roett MA, Mayor MT, Uduhiri KA. Diagnosis and management of genital ulcers. *Am Fam Physician*. 2012;85(3):254-262.

United States Preventive Services Task Force. Human Immunodeficiency Virus (HIV): Screening. Available at: https://www.uspreventiveservicestaskforce.org/uspstf/recommendation/human-immunodeficiency-virus-hiv-infection-screening. Accessed May 26, 2020.

United States Preventive Services Task Force. Chlamydia and Gonorrhea: Screening. Available at: https://www.uspreventiveservicestaskforce.org/uspstf/recommendation/chlamydia-and-gonorrhea-screening. Accessed May 26, 2020.

World Health Organization. Global health observatory data. http://www.who.int/gho/hiv/en/. Accessed December 28, 2018.

World Health Organization. Guidelines on post-exposure prophylaxis for HIV and the use of co-trimoxazole prophylaxis for HIV-related infections among adults, adolescents, and children. http://www.who.int/hiv/pub/guidelines/arv2013/arvs2013upplement_dec2014/en/. Accessed December 28, 2018.

CASE 46

A 33-year-old man presents to the office for an acute visit with reports of nausea and diarrhea for the past week. In addition, he has had a low-grade fever and some right upper quadrant abdominal pain, and he has noticed that the whites of his eyes appear yellow. He has no significant medical history and takes no medications daily but takes acetaminophen occasionally for headaches. He drinks 1 to 2 beers a week but denies tobacco or intravenous drug use. He is a pastor and went on a mission in rural Central America about 4 weeks ago. Although he primarily ate cooked foods of local cuisine and occasionally raw fruit, he reports several days of nausea and "traveler's diarrhea" while on the trip. On examination, he is a well-developed and tan-pigmented man in no apparent distress. His temperature is 99.8 °F (37.6 °C), blood pressure is 110/80 mm Hg, pulse is 90 beats/min, and respiratory rate is 14 breaths/min. He has a prominent yellow color to his sclera and under his tongue. Lung and cardiac examinations are unremarkable. His abdominal examination reveals moderate tenderness in the right upper quadrant, normal bowel sounds, and a palpable liver edge just below the costal margin. There are no abdominal masses palpated, and there is no rebound tenderness or guarding. On rectal examination, he has soft stool that is guaiac negative.

▶ What is the most likely diagnosis?
▶ When and how did he most likely contract this illness?
▶ How can you confirm the diagnosis?
▶ What are the options for treatment?

ANSWERS TO CASE 46:

Jaundice

Summary: A 33-year-old man presents with

- Diarrhea, abdominal pain, and jaundice a month after traveling to Central America
- Scleral icterus and tender hepatomegaly
- Abdominal examination that reveals moderate tenderness in the right upper quadrant
- Normal bowel sounds and a palpable liver edge just below the costal margin
- No significant medical history
- Report that he drinks 1 to 2 beers a week but denial of tobacco or intravenous drug use

Most likely diagnosis: Acute hepatitis A infection.

Most likely timing and source of infection: Ingestion of contaminated food or water while on his mission to Central America 4 weeks earlier.

Confirming the diagnosis: Anti–hepatitis A immunoglobulin (Ig) M.

Treatment options: Supportive care and symptomatic treatment for the patient; report infection to local health department; consider giving hepatitis A vaccine or Ig prophylaxis to close household or sexual contacts or persons sharing illicit drugs with an infected patient. Hepatitis A immunization will not be required for the patient.

ANALYSIS

Objectives

1. Develop a differential diagnosis for adults with jaundice, with and without pain. (EPA 1, 2)

2. List the symptoms, management, complications, and modes of transmission of hepatitis A, B, and C. (EPA 1, 4, 10)

3. Be able to interpret the results of hepatitis viral serology tests. (EPA 3)

Considerations

This presentation of nonbloody diarrhea along with nonspecific, crampy abdominal pain is most often caused by viral gastroenteritis and is self-limited. However, this patient has several signs and symptoms that prompt consideration of other diagnoses. The finding of scleral icterus should prompt an evaluation for causes of jaundice. The differential diagnosis for jaundice with abdominal pain and diarrhea includes viral, bacterial, or parasitic infections, illicit drug or alcohol abuse, adverse drug reactions, toxins, and autoimmune disease.

Diagnosis of this patient's condition requires laboratory evaluation since it cannot be made on clinical grounds alone. A systematic approach to jaundice begins with a serum fractionated bilirubin. When evaluating a patient with jaundice, fractionated bilirubin can help classify the etiology by indicating whether there is excess unconjugated or conjugated bilirubin.

APPROACH TO:
Jaundice

DEFINITIONS

CAPUT MEDUSAE: Dilated superficial paraumbilical veins that usually result from shunting associated with severe portal hypertension and liver failure.

JAUNDICE: A yellowish-brown staining of the skin, sclera, and mucous membranes from excess bilirubin pigment when serum bilirubin is elevated.

SPIDER ANGIOMA/TELANGIECTASIAS: Dilated, small, superficial veins with the distribution of the superior vena cava that appear as red, blue, or purple web-like formations on the face, neck, upper trunk and abdomen, and lower extremities. They are a result of increased serum estrogen levels, which remain elevated due to the inability of the impaired liver to metabolize conjugated estrogens. This is often seen in cirrhotic patients.

CLINICAL APPROACH TO JAUNDICE

Pathophysiology

To understand jaundice, it is imperative to understand bilirubin, which is a breakdown product of red blood cells. Heme is further broken down into bilverdin, then to unconjugated bilirubin. Unconjugated bilirubin is highly water insoluble and is noncovalently bound to albumin in the plasma and never enters the urine. Albumin carries unconjugated bilirubin to the liver, where bilirubin gets conjugated with glucuronic acid into a water-soluble form. Conjugated bilirubin is excreted by hepatocytes into bile and then largely excreted into the stool.

The degree of jaundice generally correlates with the total serum bilirubin level. Fractionated bilirubin provides direct (conjugated) and indirect concentrations. Conjugated bilirubin is excreted in the urine as urobilinogen, whereas unconjugated bilirubin is bound to albumin and does not enter glomerular filtration. An elevated urobilinogen level in a jaundiced patient suggests a conjugated hyperbilirubinemia; the absence of urobilinogen suggests an unconjugated hyperbilirubinemia.

Jaundice is characterized by prehepatic, intrahepatic, or posthepatic causes. Prehepatic jaundice most often results from hemolysis of red blood cells, which overwhelms the liver's ability to conjugate and clear the bilirubin through its normal pathways. This results in a state of hyperbilirubinemia that is primarily unconjugated.

Hepatic causes of jaundice represent over one-half of acute jaundice in adults and can lead to either unconjugated or conjugated hyperbilirubinemia. Congenital defects in enzymes involved in glucoronidation can lead to unconjugated hyperbilirubinemia. Alcoholic liver disease, drug-induced liver injury, and viruses, including hepatitis, reduce the liver's ability to transport bilirubin after it has been conjugated, resulting in a conjugated hyperbilirubinemia.

Posthepatic jaundice is usually caused by obstruction to the flow of bile through the bile ducts. This can be caused by bile duct stones, strictures, or tumors that narrow or block the ducts. Posthepatic jaundice is therefore a conjugated hyperbilirubinemia.

Clinical Presentation

History. The history and physical examination provide the most important information in the diagnostic evaluation of jaundice. **Any medications, whether prescription, nonprescription, or herbal supplements, should be reviewed.** Acetaminophen and aspirin are widely used over-the-counter agents that, in toxic amounts, can cause hepatocellular damage. Numerous herbal agents (eg, Jamaican bush tea, kava, and ma huang) have also been associated with liver damage.

Social history is of critical importance in a patient with jaundice. Alcohol abuse and hepatitis C are the most common causes of cirrhosis in the United States. Intravenous drug use, transfusions of blood or blood products, and unsafe sexual practices can lead to infection with hepatitis B or C. Viral hepatitis has also been linked to tattooing when unsterilized or shared equipment is used. Travel history, especially the location and timing of any international travel, and recent exposure to persons with jaundice or contaminated foods (eg, raw produce) can lead to the consideration of hepatitis A. Occupational exposures to aflatoxin or vinyl chloride are risk factors for hepatocellular carcinoma.

Signs and Symptoms. It is necessary to clarify the onset of jaundice as acute or gradual, noting gastrointestinal symptoms, including abdominal pain, nausea, vomiting, diarrhea, or changes in stool or urine color. Skin pruritus is common in patients with jaundice and may precede its onset. Fever and prodromal viral symptoms such as anorexia, fatigue, and myalgias can suggest viral hepatitis. Fever and chills in the setting of right upper quadrant abdominal pain may point to gallbladder-related pathology, including acute cholangitis, cholecystitis, or choledocolithiasis. Fever can be a sign of underlying sepsis. Unintentional weight loss and lymphadenopathy may suggest underlying malignancy. Bruising or bleeding disorders may suggest severe hepatic dysfunction interfering with the production of clotting factors. Increasing abdominal girth may be caused by ascites, and peripheral edema may be caused by obstruction of venous return from the lower extremities and hypoalbuminemia. These findings may suggest portal hypertension and are indicative of more severe pathology.

Jaundice. Jaundice is often noticeable on examination at serum levels greater than double the normal range. Yellow discoloration can be noticed in the sclera, especially in persons of darker complexion, and can also been seen in oral mucus membranes, including under the tongue and in the hard palate. Skin examination may reveal tanning or bronzing, as well as needle track marks, ruptured veins, or cellulitis, which can suggest intravenous drug use. Signs that suggest chronic liver disease on skin examination include caput medusae, spider angioma, palmar erythema, and easy bruising or bleeding.

Physical Examination. Abdominal examination should include the evaluation of the general contour of the abdomen, the presence of ascites or hepatosplenomegaly, and any rebound, guarding, or localized tenderness. Hepatomegaly may suggest cirrhosis, acute hepatitis, malignancy, or hepatic congestion due to right-sided heart failure. Splenomegaly may suggest portal hypertension from cirrhosis, malignancy, or splenic sequestration of damaged red blood cells. On chest examination, gynecomastia may also suggest cirrhosis due to increased estrogen. Neurologic examination should evaluate for asterixis and encephalopathy.

Laboratory Testing. **The most important initial laboratory test in the evaluation of jaundice is a serum bilirubin level.** Other important components of laboratory evaluation in the jaundiced patient include a complete blood count (CBC) and platelet count, alanine transaminase (ALT), aspartate transaminase (AST), alkaline phosphatase, gamma-glutamyltransferase (GGT), prothrombin time (PT) with international normalized ratio (INR), albumin, and protein. Elevated ALT and/or AST can suggest hepatocellular damage but may be normal in chronic liver disease. Elevated alkaline phosphatase can indicate biliary obstruction, and GGT is used to determine if an elevated alkaline phosphatase is due to a biliary process. PT/INR, albumin, and protein are indicators of synthetic function of the liver, which, if abnormal, can suggest hepatic decompensation.

CLINICAL APPROACH TO UNCONJUGATED HYPERBILIRUBINEMIA

Gilbert Syndrome

Unconjugated hyperbilirubinemia is caused by impaired conjugation in a state of normal red blood cell turnover and normal hepatic function. Gilbert syndrome is a congenital reduction of conjugation of bilirubin in the liver due to an autosomal recessive mutation in a gene for an enzyme involved in **glucuronidation.** It is a benign condition occurring in approximately 5% of the population, often discovered incidentally, as it has no clinical significance. Patients with Gilbert syndrome may develop moderate hyperbilirubinemia (less than 5 mg/dL) and clinical jaundice during times of stress, illness, or fasting that self-resolves with the removal of the stressor or illness. In these patients, other parts of the physical examination and laboratory evaluation are normal. In an asymptomatic patient with mildly elevated unconjugated bilirubinemia, an unremarkable physical examination, and normal ALT, AST, thyroid-stimulating hormone (TSH), and CBC, no further workup is indicated.

Hemolysis

Hemolysis can cause an unconjugated hyperbilirubinemia in proportion to the amount of hemolysis that occurs. It is most often diagnosed by the identification of anemia along with the presence of red cell fragments on peripheral smear and elevated serum lactate dehydrogenase and decreased haptoglobin. The serum bilirubin level typically remains below 5 mg/dL in hemolytic conditions, such as spherocytosis, thalassemias, sickle cell disease, glucose-6-phosphate dehydrogenase deficiency, malaria, thrombotic thrombocytopenic purpura, and hemolytic uremic syndrome. The treatment is to address the underlying cause of the hemolysis.

CLINICAL APPROACH TO CONJUGATED HYPERBILIRUBINEMIA

Conjugated hyperbilirubinemia can be categorized into causes of intrahepatic origin and extrahepatic origin. Viral hepatitis is one of the most prevalent causes of intrahepatic damage. Other intrahepatic causes of cholestasis and conjugated hyperbilirubinemia include drug-induced liver injury, Wilson disease (decreased copper metabolism), autoimmune hepatitis, and primary biliary cirrhosis.

Hepatitis A

Epidemiology. Hepatitis A is an acute viral infection of the liver primarily transmitted via fecal-oral contamination and accounts for nearly one-half of viral hepatitis cases in the United States, although rates have been declining since introduction of the vaccine. Since the virus is shed in stool, contaminated food and water are the primary sources of infection. Hepatitis A can also be transmitted through personal contact (within the household or in day care settings), sexual contact with another infected individual (especially in men who have sex with men), and intravenous drug use. Hepatitis A virus (HAV) is also more widespread in low socioeconomic areas, likely due to inadequate sanitation and hygiene practices. It is common in travelers to Africa, Asia, Greenland, Middle East, Mexico, and Central and South America. Travelers to these areas are at risk for infection and should be immunized prior to travel with two doses of vaccine given 6 months apart.

Clinical Presentation. Hepatitis A causes a **self-limited illness** characterized by jaundice, fever, fatigue, malaise, nausea, vomiting, diarrhea, anorexia, weight loss, right upper quadrant abdominal discomfort, and dark urine. On physical examination, jaundice is found in 70% of patients. Hepatomegaly and splenomegaly may also be present. The average incubation period for hepatitis A is 28 days, and transmission is possible 2 weeks prior to the development of symptoms and for 1 week after jaundice appears. Acute illness is generally limited to less than 2 months. There is no chronic stage of hepatitis A, although 10% to 15% of patients may experience a relapse within the following 6 months after the acute infection has resolved. Although very uncommon, HAV infection can lead to fulminant hepatic failure; however, this is more likely in patients who have chronic hepatitis B or C infection. Fatality due to hepatitis A is rare for all ages.

Hepatitis A is diagnosed based on clinical features and the detection of anti–HAV IgM. Other laboratory findings that support the diagnosis include the presence of a conjugated hyperbilirubinemia and elevated serum transaminases in the range of 500 to 5000 U/L. An elevated anti–HAV IgG but negative IgM indicates a prior hepatitis A infection or vaccination, but not an acute illness.

Treatment. While there is no specific treatment for hepatitis A, supportive care and symptomatic treatments are indicated. Patients who develop fulminant hepatitis should be hospitalized in a facility with liver transplant capability. Effective measures in preventing HAV transmission include adequate handwashing, avoidance of contaminated foods and water, and proper food handling and preparation. Hepatitis A vaccination recommendations are discussed in Cases 1, 11, and 29.

Hepatitis B

Epidemiology. Hepatitis B is a viral infection **transmitted via percutaneous or mucosal contact with contaminated blood or body fluids.** Hepatitis B is a prominent condition, with 350 million chronic carriers worldwide and an estimated 1 million chronic carriers in the United States. Areas of the world with intermediate to high rates of infections are Eastern Europe, Asia, sub-Saharan Africa, Middle East, and the Pacific islands. Sexual contact (eg, men having sex with men, multiple partners, and sexual contact with an infected person) and needle sharing are common mechanisms of infection in the United States. Hepatitis B may also be vertically transmitted from mother to baby. The incubation period from exposure to clinical symptoms is about 90 days, and only 30% to 50% of infections are symptomatic. Along with acute-phase symptoms similar to hepatitis A, hepatitis B can cause a chronic infection. The risk of developing **chronic hepatitis B is inversely related to the age at infection**: 90% of infected infants, 30% of children younger than age 5 years, and less than 5% of infected adults develop chronic hepatitis B. Worldwide, there are about 600,000 deaths each year in chronic carriers due to cirrhosis, liver failure, and hepatocellular carcinoma.

Clinical Presentation. On serologic evaluation, hepatitis B surface antigen (HBsAg) is present in both acute and chronic infections, and viral load is associated with risk of transmission to others. HBsAg typically becomes detectable in 1 to 9 weeks following hepatitis B virus (HBV) exposure (average of 4 weeks) and disappears in 4 months after onset of symptoms in those who spontaneously recover. Persistent detection of HBsAg more than 6 months postexposure generally indicates chronic HBV infection. Hepatitis B e antigen (HBeAg) is a marker for HBV replication and degree of infectivity. Antibody to the hepatitis B core antigen (HBcAg IgM) is diagnostic of an acute HBV infection and is the only serological marker detectable during the window period of seroconversion. A measurable level of HBsAg with a negative HBcAg IgM is diagnostic of chronic hepatitis B. **Antibody to the surface antigen (anti–HBsAb) in the absence of HBsAg indicates a resolved HBV infection or successful immunity from HBV vaccination.** Figures 46–1 and 46–2 highlight the serologic studies associated with both acute and chronic hepatitis B infection.

Treatment. Acute hepatitis B infection is treated supportively. Persons with chronic hepatitis B may be candidates for antiviral therapy and should be referred to a hepatologist. Hepatitis B vaccination is universally recommended for children (Case 5) and adults at high risk. Postexposure prophylaxis with hepatitis B immunoglobulin and/or vaccination is recommended for all unvaccinated persons who are exposed to infected bodily fluids.

Hepatitis C

Epidemiology. Hepatitis C virus (HCV) infection is most prevalent in persons born between 1945 and 1965, the majority of whom were likely infected during the 1970s and 1980s. Approximately 71 million people worldwide have chronic HCV infection, and nearly 400,000 individuals die annually from HCV due to cirrhosis or hepatocellular carcinoma. Transmission occurs via exposure to infected blood or body fluids via sexual contact and use of illicit drugs (60% of acute cases

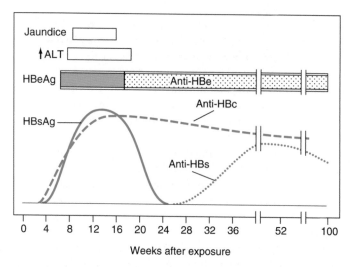

Figure 46–1. Serologic markers in acute hepatitis B infection. (Reproduced with permission, from Braunwald E, Fauci AS, Kasper DL, et al, eds. *Harrison's Principles of Internal Medicine*, 16th ed. 2005. Copyright © McGraw Hill LLC. All rights reserved.)

in the United States), sharing of needles and other drug paraphernalia, tattooing, accidental exposure of health care workers, unprotected sex in HCV-positive men who have sex with men, or vertical transmission from mother to baby. Blood or blood product transfusion and organ transplantation from infected donors were common sources of exposure prior to 1992, before universal screening of blood donors became routine.

Clinical Presentation. HCV can be detected in the blood through HCV antibody testing or RNA polymerase chain reaction within 2 to 3 weeks of exposure. Clinical onset is generally 2 to 12 weeks postexposure. Most infections are asymptomatic,

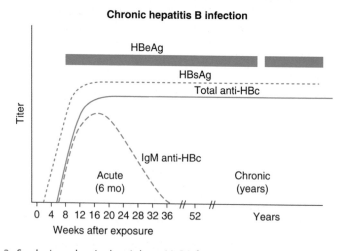

Figure 46–2. Serologic markers in chronic hepatitis B infection.

yet hepatitis C can also cause an acute illness in 20% to 30% of patients with jaundice, abdominal pain, fatigue, malaise, and anorexia. **Of those infected with hepatitis C, 80% will develop a chronic infection,** with measurable levels of HCV RNA for more than 6 months.

Of patients with chronic hepatitis C, 20% will develop cirrhosis, hepatic decompensation, and hepatocellular carcinoma during a 20- to 30-year time frame, making hepatitis C the current leading cause for liver transplantation in the United States. Fortunately, rates are declining due to the advent of effective antiviral pharmacotherapy. Patients with HCV infection should avoid alcohol consumption and should receive hepatitis A and B vaccinations. The progression of chronic HCV infection can be assessed by the amount of inflammation and cirrhosis seen on liver biopsy, commonly performed to evaluate the extent of fibrosis and to determine candidacy for antiviral treatment.

Treatment. Treatment and cure results are highly variable depending upon virus genotype, extent of fibrosis, patient risk factors, and chronic health conditions. Treatment goals are to reduce all-cause mortality and long-term complications of chronic infection by inducing a sustained remission of HCV. There is currently no vaccination available for hepatitis C. The United States Preventive Services Task Force recommends screening of adults aged 18 to 79 with an anti-HCV antibody test (Grade B recommendation).

Hepatitis D

Epidemiology. Hepatitis D virus (HDV) is an uncommon cause of viral hepatitis in the United States; it uses the viral envelope of hepatitis B to infect its host and thus requires coinfection with hepatitis B. It is transmitted through percutaneous or mucosal contact with blood or body fluid from an infected individual. Approximately 5% of HBV carriers worldwide may be coinfected with HDV.

Clinical Presentation. The clinical manifestations of HBV and HDV coinfection typically resemble that of an HBV infection. In coinfection, 5% or less will become chronically infected with HDV. Superinfection of HDV in a patient with chronic HBV may progress to severe liver disease and cirrhosis more rapidly than in patients with chronic HBV alone. There is currently no vaccination available for hepatitis D.

Hepatitis E

Hepatitis E virus (HEV) is transmitted via the fecal-oral route, and while it is rare in the United States, it has a high prevalence in Asia, Africa, Middle East, and Central America, where it is associated with contaminated water supply in areas of poor sanitation. The clinical signs and symptoms of HEV infection are similar to those seen in HAV. Diagnosis of acute HEV infection can be confirmed by detection of HEV in serum or stool or IgM anti-HEV. Prevention relies primarily on good sanitation, and treatment is generally supportive.

Alcohol Use Disorder

Alcohol use disorder is a pattern of alcohol use that involves controlling one's alcohol use and is associated with persistent or unsuccessful attempts to cut down or control alcohol use. It can cause an acute hepatitis, chronic fatty liver disease, cirrhosis, and fibrosis. Alcohol leads to a conjugated hyperbilirubinemia by impairing bile acid secretion and uptake as well as by causing hepatocellular damage. Common physical findings include ascites, jaundice, cutaneous telangiectasias, palmar erythema, testicular atrophy, gynecomastia, a contracted nodular liver, splenomegaly, and malnutrition. **Transaminase levels from alcohol abuse typically show an AST out of proportion to ALT, commonly with a ratio of 2 or greater.** In viral hepatitis, there is usually a greater elevation of the ALT (see Case 41).

Nonalcoholic Fatty Liver Disease

Epidemiology. Nonalcoholic fatty liver disease (NAFLD) results from deposition of fat within the hepatocytes and can cause intrahepatic cholestasis, resulting in conjugated hyperbilirubinemia. It is commonly associated with obesity, physical inactivity, and metabolic syndrome, including diabetes mellitus, hyperlipidemia, and hypertriglyceridemia. NAFLD is the most common liver disease in Western countries. Thirty to forty percent will progress to nonalcoholic steatohepatitis, and approximately 40% will progress to advanced fibrosis and cirrhosis.

Clinical Presentation. While most cases are asymptomatic and detectable only via elevated serum transaminases, symptoms may include right upper quadrant pain, jaundice, and pruritus. NAFLD is diagnosed via ultrasound and confirmed with liver biopsy. First-line treatments for NAFLD include appropriate nutrition, weight management, and exercise. Patients are also encouraged to limit alcohol, acetaminophen, and nonsteroidal anti-inflammatory drug use and to receive immunizations for HAV and HBV.

Extrahepatic Obstruction

Physical obstructions of bile drainage can cause conjugated hyperbilirubinemia through extrahepatic obstruction. On laboratory evaluation, patients commonly have an elevated alkaline phosphatase, suggesting a cholestatic pattern. Common etiologies of obstruction include gallstones that become impacted in the bile ducts, postoperative biliary strictures, or extrinsic compression of the bile ducts by neoplasms, such as pancreatic cancer. Pancreatic cancer is the most common cause of painless jaundice in a patient with biliary obstruction; cancer in the head of the pancreas compresses on the biliary ducts. Imaging of the biliary tree with ultrasound, computed tomographic scan, magnetic resonance imaging, or magnetic resonance cholangiopancreatography is usually diagnostic. Endoscopic retrograde cholangiopancreatography (ERCP) can be diagnostic and, in some cases, therapeutic.

CASE CORRELATION

- See Cases 1 (Adult Male Health Maintenance), Case 5 (Well-Child Care), Case 11 (Adult Female Health Maintenance), Case 29 (Adolescent Health Maintenance), and Case 41 (Substance Use Disorder).

COMPREHENSION QUESTIONS

46.1 A 32-year-old man with asthma and hypertension presents for evaluation of an elevated bilirubin level detected on blood work required for a preemployment physical. Total bilirubin level was 2.5 mg/dL (normal up to 1 mg/dL). Fractionated bilirubin results revealed an elevated unconjugated component. He is currently asymptomatic but reports that he recently "had the flu." He generally drinks one beer per night, is monogamous with his wife, has no history of intravenous drug abuse, and has one tattoo. His sclerae are anicteric, and there are no signs of jaundice. His transaminases, electrolytes, TSH, and CBC are normal. Which of the following is the initial step in the evaluation of this patient?

    A. Reassurance

    B. Recommend alcohol abstinence

    C. Abdominal ultrasound

    D. Hepatitis serologies

    E. Referral to a hepatologist

46.2 A 45-year-old woman was diagnosed 6 months ago with acute hepatitis B infection. She is unaware of how she contracted the virus. She takes no medications and since the diagnosis has started taking a multivitamin and exercising. She now has the following serologies: HBsAg negative; anti-HB surface antibody positive; HBeAg negative; and anti-HB core antibody positive. Which of the following is the correct diagnosis?

    A. Chronic active infection with low infectivity

    B. Chronic active infection with high infectivity

    C. Resolved acute infection with low infectivity

    D. Resolved acute infection with high infectivity

    E. Resolved infection but at risk for reinfection in the future

46.3 A 35-year-old woman presents to her primary care provider with a several-day history of dark colored urine, vomiting, and right upper quadrant pain. She has a history of hypothyroidism, and her current medications include levothyroxine and birth control pills. She does not drink alcohol; she has a smoking history of 10 pack-years, though she quit smoking 5 years ago; and she admits to intravenous drug use in her teens. Her temperature is 98.4 °F, blood pressure is 123/82 mm Hg, pulse is 70 beats/min, and body mass index is 31 kg/m². Her sclerae and skin are icteric. Laboratory evaluation indicates an elevated total bilirubin of 10 mg/dL (normal 1 mg/dL) with direct bilirubin of 7 mg/dL (normal 0-0.3 mg/dL), elevated alkaline phosphatase seven times the upper limit of normal, and normal albumin, AST, ALT, and PT. Which is the best next step in establishing the diagnosis?

A. Viral hepatitis panel

B. Abdominal ultrasound

C. Liver biopsy

D. Evaluation of peripheral smear

E. Endoscopic retrograde cholangiopancreatogram

46.4 A 21-year-old college student plans to take a trip to Thailand with his friends; the trip is scheduled for 2 months from now. He confesses that he has experimented with drugs, including smoking marijuana as well as intranasal and intravenous cocaine and heroin. He is excited about the upcoming trip and wants to find out which immunizations he will need prior to his departure. Based on his history and upcoming plans, which of the following vaccinations and serologic tests will you recommend to him at this time?

A. Hepatitis A vaccination, hepatitis A and B serologies

B. Hepatitis A and B vaccination, hepatitis A and B serologies

C. Hepatitis B vaccination, hepatitis B and C serologies

D. Hepatitis A and B vaccination, hepatitis B and C serologies

ANSWERS

46.1 **A.** This patient has a classic presentation of Gilbert disease, which is a benign disease for processing bilirubin (decreased activity of bilirubin uridine diphosphate glucuronosyltransferase enzyme). Typically, the patient has a benign mild elevation of **unconjugated** bilirubin, triggered by stress such as exercise or not eating. In the face of otherwise normal history, examination, and liver enzymes, no further workup is indicated. People with Gilbert syndrome can have icteric sclerae and jaundice that worsens with stress or illness. Answer B (alcohol abstinence) is not required for this condition. Answer C (abdominal ultrasound) can be useful for identifying gallstones but is not useful for this condition. Answer D (hepatitis serologies) would be indicated for a patient with icterus with a conjugated (direct) bilirubin and high liver transaminase levels. Answer E (referral to a hepatologist) is not indicated in this case due to the very likely diagnosis of Gilbert disease.

46.2 **C.** These serologies are consistent with resolved hepatitis B infection and ongoing immunity; the anti–HBsAg antibodies indicate immunity. The anti–HBV core antibody indicates antibodies against the core antigen. The HBV vaccine only contains surface antigen and not core antigen, so patients who are vaccinated only and are without history of HBV infection would not have a positive HBV core antibody. This patient has both negative surface and e antigens, so she does not have chronic active infection (answers A and B) and is not at risk of spreading the disease to others (answer D). Because of the presence of anti-HBs antibody, the patient is immune to future reinfection (answer E).

46.3 **B.** This patient has an elevated conjugated (direct) hyperbilirubinemia with an elevated alkaline phosphatase with otherwise normal liver function. This particular pattern suggests cholestasis, and these patients should be evaluated with a right upper quadrant abdominal ultrasound to determine whether obstruction is intrahepatic or extrahepatic. Patients with viral hepatitis (answer A) usually have elevated transaminases. Liver biopsy (answer C) should be considered when liver function abnormalities remain unexplained despite noninvasive evaluation. A peripheral smear (answer D) is useful in the setting of unconjugated hyperbilirubinemia and hemolytic anemia. ERCP (answer E) is useful in patients who have an obstruction due to cholelithiasis or malignancy established by initial imaging.

46.4 **D.** Both hepatitis A and B vaccinations are recommended with travel to Asia. This patient has a high likelihood of hepatitis B and C infection given his history of intranasal and intravenous drug use. Vaccination recommendations can change, and it is best to review travel recommendations online (https://wwwnc.cdc.gov/travel). An appointment with a primary care provider or travel clinic should be made 4 to 6 weeks prior to taking any international trips to determine the appropriate vaccinations needed and general health information. However, if a patient has not been immunized against hepatitis A, two separate vaccines 6 months apart are required to confer immunity. The other answer choices only provide partial vaccination or serology recommendations.

CLINICAL PEARLS

▶ Unconjugated hyperbilirubinemia found on routine blood work in an asymptomatic individual may suggest the benign diagnosis of Gilbert syndrome. Management involves reassurance and supportive care.

▶ Patients with chronic hepatitis B or C should be referred to a hepatologist for evaluation of appropriate antiviral therapy and monitoring for hepatocellular carcinoma.

▶ The acute onset of painless jaundice in a patient older than age 50 years should prompt an examination for pancreatic cancer (malignancy in the head of the pancreas causing compression of the bile ducts).

▶ All pregnant women should be screened for the presence of HBsAg. If positive, treating the newborns with hepatitis B immunoglobulin and vaccination can reduce the risk of vertical transmission.

▶ The greatest risks for developing cirrhosis include alcohol abuse, hepatitis C, and NAFLD.

▶ Anyone with chronic hepatitis C should be counseled to avoid all alcohol intake.

▶ All adults between ages 18 and 79 should be screened for hepatitis C.

REFERENCES

Centers for Disease Control and Prevention. Traveler's health. https://wwwnc.cdc.gov/travel. Accessed May 2, 2019.

Dienstag JL. Acute viral hepatitis. In: Jameson JL, Fauci A, Kasper D, Hauser S, Longo D, Loscalzo J, eds. *Harrison's Principles of Internal Medicine.* 20th ed. New York, NY: McGraw Hill; 2018: Chap. 332. https://accessmedicine.mhmedical.com/content.aspx?sectionid=159214492&bookid= 2129&Resultclick=2. Accessed May 2, 2019.

Fargo MV, Grogan SP, Saguil A. Evaluation of jaundice in adults. *Am Fam Physician.* 2017;95(3):164-168.

United States Preventive Services Task Force. Hepatitis C: draft recommendation statement. https:// www.uspreventiveservicestaskforce.org/Page/Document/draft-recommendation-statement/hepatitis-c-screening1. Accessed September 5, 2019.

Wilkins T, Akhtar M, Gititu E. Diagnosis and management of hepatitis C. *Am Fam Physician.* 2015; 91(12):835-842.

Wilkins T, Tadkod A, Hepburn I, Schade RR. Nonalcoholic fatty liver disease: diagnosis and management. *Am Fam Physician.* 2013;88(1):35-42.

Wilkins T, Zimmerman D, Schade RR. Hepatitis B: diagnosis and treatment. *Am Fam Physician.* 2010;81(8):965-972.

A 52-year-old man presents to the office with approximately 2 weeks of upper abdominal pain. His symptoms include some "discomfort" in the epigastric region that comes and goes. He has had some "heartburn" and nausea, but no vomiting or diarrhea. He has noticed that his stools appear darker than they used to, but he has not had bloody stools or rectal bleeding. He has recently noticed early satiety. He takes an over-the-counter nonsteroidal anti-inflammatory drug (NSAID) several times daily because of arthritis in his knees. He smokes a pack of cigarettes a day and drinks three to four beers per night. On examination, he is pale appearing but in no acute discomfort and not presyncopal. He is afebrile, blood pressure is 120/80 mm Hg, pulse is 95 beats/min, and respiratory rate is 14 breaths/min. Head, ears, eyes, nose, and throat examination is notable only for pale conjunctivae. Cardiac and pulmonary examinations are unremarkable. His abdomen has normal bowel sounds and moderate tenderness in the epigastrium with slight guarding but no rebound. Rectal examination reveals normal sphincter tone, no masses, and dark black stool that is guaiac positive.

▶ What is the most likely diagnosis?
▶ What evaluation and treatment are indicated at this point?
▶ What can be suggested to reduce the risk of recurrence of this problem?

ANSWERS TO CASE 47:
Dyspepsia and Peptic Ulcer Disease

Summary: A 52-year-old man presents with

- Vague upper abdominal discomfort, nausea, and early satiety
- Daily NSAID use and regular cigarette smoking and alcohol consumption
- Pale appearance, which suggests that he may be anemic
- Mild abdominal tenderness and melanotic stool on examination, which should raise suspicion for an upper gastrointestinal (GI) bleed
- Rectal examination with normal sphincter tone, no masses, and dark black stool that is guaiac positive

Most likely diagnosis: Bleeding peptic ulcer, upper GI bleed.

Evaluation and treatment: Since this patient has a high likelihood of having an upper GI bleed, hemodynamic stability should be ensured immediately. This patient's vitals suggest he is currently hemodynamically stable, but if he develops hypotension and/or tachycardia he may require intravenous fluid resuscitation. Initial testing should include a stat complete blood count (CBC), blood type and screen, consultation for an esophagogastroduodenoscopy (EGD), discontinuation of his NSAID, and testing for *Helicobacter pylori*. He should be treated with a proton pump inhibitor (PPI) and antibiotics for *H. pylori* if tests confirm its presence. He may require a blood transfusion if found to be significantly anemic.

Suggestions to reduce risk of recurrence: Discontinuation and avoidance of NSAIDs and aspirin or, if unable to completely discontinue, use of a PPI along with the NSAID; cessation of smoking and drinking alcohol; and eradication of *H. pylori* if positive.

ANALYSIS

Objectives

1. Learn the common presenting signs and symptoms of peptic ulcer disease (PUD), functional dyspepsia, and gastroesophageal reflux disease (GERD). (EPA 1, 2)

2. Learn the risk factors for the development of PUD. (EPA 12)

3. Learn how to diagnose and treat PUD and GERD, as well as know the risks of pharmacotherapy. (EPA 3)

4. Understand the role of *H. pylori* in PUD, including methods for testing for and treatment of PUD. (EPA 4)

5. Know the alarm symptoms and extraesophageal symptoms for GERD and PUD. (EPA 10)

Table 47–1 • "ALARM" SYMPTOMS FOR WHICH EARLY UPPER GASTROIN-TESTINAL ENDOSCOPY IS RECOMMENDED

Unintentional weight loss

Progressive dysphagia

Recurrent/persistent vomiting

Odynophagia

Unexplained anemia

Gastrointestinal bleeding/hematemesis

Family history of cancer, specifically upper gastrointestinal cancer

History of gastric surgery

Jaundice

Considerations

Approximately 40% of dyspepsia is caused by PUD, while 60% is attributable to functional (nonulcer) dyspepsia. Reflux esophagitis accounts for 5% to 15% of cases of dyspepsia, while gastric or esophageal cancer is found in less than 2% of cases. PUD is characterized by mucosal damage (eg, from NSAIDs or aspirin) with chronic exposure of the damaged mucosa to pepsin and gastric acid secretion. It usually occurs in the stomach or proximal duodenum. Less commonly, it occurs in the lower esophagus, the distal duodenum in unopposed hypersecretory states such as Zollinger-Ellison syndrome, or ectopic gastric mucosa (eg, Meckel diverticula). Symptoms of functional dyspepsia are essentially the same as those of PUD, but with no evidence of organic or structural disease to explain the symptoms.

Upper endoscopy should be considered for patients with new-onset GERD or dyspepsia who are older than age 50 years or who have symptoms that may be associated with upper GI malignancy (Table 47–1). The cutoff age may be more appropriate at 40 or 45 years for Asian or African American patients. For persons younger than age 50 years and without alarm symptoms, testing for *H. pylori* via immunoglobulin (Ig) G serology is the initial step, followed by stool antigen or ^{13}C urea breath test if inconclusive. For those who test positive, treating the *H. pylori* infection via combination antibiotic and acid-suppression therapy is indicated. For persons who test negative, empiric therapy with a PPI for 8 weeks is a cost-effective intervention. Endoscopy or reconsideration of the diagnosis should be considered for those who continue to be symptomatic following these interventions.

APPROACH TO:
Peptic Ulcer Disease and GERD

DEFINITIONS

DYSPEPSIA: One or more of the following symptoms: postprandial fullness, early satiety, and epigastric pain or burning.

GASTROESOPHAGEAL REFLUX DISEASE (GERD): Stomach acid that has regurgitated into the esophagus that leads to heartburn, esophagitis, and an increased risk for esophageal adenocarcinoma.

H$_2$ RECEPTOR ANTAGONIST: Competitive antagonists of histamine binding to gastric parietal cell H$_2$ receptors, which prevent activation of the pathway that mediates release of acid into the gastric lumen.

PEPTIC ULCER DISEASE (PUD): Mucosal erosion of the stomach or duodenum that is 0.5 cm or greater in diameter and often due to increased acidity, but also may be due to decreased mucosal defenses. Often related to infection from *H. pylori*.

PROTON PUMP INHIBITOR (PPI): Suppresses gastric acid production by irreversibly inhibiting the H$^+$/K$^+$ adenosine triphosphatase (ATPase) proton pump in gastric parietal cells.

CLINICAL APPROACH TO PUD

Pathophysiology

Peptic ulcer disease is a term generally used to describe both duodenal and gastric ulcers. **Duodenal ulcers are more prevalent overall, whereas gastric ulcers are more common in frequent NSAID users.** Risk factors for the development of PUD include *H. pylori* infection, the use of NSAIDs and aspirin, cigarette smoking, alcohol consumption, and personal or family history of PUD. Black and Hispanic populations have a higher likelihood of developing PUD as well. The lifetime risk of developing PUD in the United States is approximately 12% for men and 10% for women. Table 47–2 summarizes other causes of PUD.

Helicobacter pylori is a corkscrew-shaped gram-negative bacillus that is the causative agent of most non–NSAID-related ulcers and is associated with the development of gastric cancer. **The presence of the organism is associated with a five to seven times increased risk of the development of PUD.** *H. pylori* infection is commonly acquired during childhood and is more common in developing countries.

Clinical Presentation

Signs and Symptoms. Dyspepsia symptoms are common, and there is significant overlap between the symptoms of PUD, GERD, and functional dyspepsia. Patients with symptoms primarily of heartburn or acid regurgitation are more likely to have GERD. **Classic symptoms associated with PUD include epigastric abdominal pain that is improved with the ingestion of food or pain that develops a few hours after eating.** Patients with PUD classically describe the pain as burning or gnawing. Nocturnal symptoms are also common with PUD, when the circadian stimulation of acid secretion is maximal prior to awakening. The symptoms of PUD are often gradual in onset and may be present for weeks or months. Patients often self-medicate with over-the-counter acid suppression medications, which usually provide some relief, prior to presenting to the clinician.

Physical Examination. The examination of the patient with dyspepsia should confirm the suspicion of PUD and rule out other diagnoses that may present with

Table 47–2 • CAUSES OF PEPTIC ULCERS

Causes	Etiology	Comments
Common causes	*Helicobacter pylori* infection	Gram-negative, motile spiral rod found in >70% of patients with peptic ulcer disease
	NSAIDs	5% to 20% of patients who use NSAIDs over long periods develop peptic ulcer disease NSAID-induced ulcers and complications more common in the elderly, those with concomitant *H. pylori* infection, or those on steroids or anticoagulants
Other/rare causes	Other medications	Steroids, bisphosphonates, potassium chloride, chemotherapeutic agents (eg, intravenous fluorouracil)
	Acid-hypersecretory states/gastrinomas (eg, Zollinger-Ellison syndrome)	Multiple gastroduodenal, jejunal, or esophageal ulcers that are difficult to heal
	Malignancy	Gastric cancer, lymphomas, lung cancers
	Stress	After acute illness, multiorgan failure, ventilator support, extensive burns (Curling ulcer), or head injury (Cushing ulcer)

Data from Kurata JH, Nogawa AN. Meta-analysis of risk factors for peptic ulcer. Nonsteroidal anti-inflammatory drugs, Helicobacter pylori, and smoking. J Clin Gastroenterol. 1997;24:2-17.

abdominal pain. Most patients with dyspepsia and GERD will have unremarkable abdominal examinations, and those with PUD may only have the examination finding of mild-to-moderate epigastric tenderness. A severely tender and rigid abdomen suggests perforation. The presence of upper GI bleeding may be documented by guaiac-based fecal occult blood testing (FOBT); however, the bleeding from PUD may be episodic, and a single negative FOBT does not completely rule out an upper GI bleed. Signs of anemia (eg, pale conjunctiva and skin, tachycardia, orthostatic hypotension) should be evaluated and treated according to severity and underlying risk factors. If a patient with known coronary artery disease becomes symptomatic and has a hemoglobin level less than 7 g/dL, then blood transfusion should be considered.

Laboratory Testing. **Serologic testing for anti–*H. pylori* IgG antibodies** is inexpensive, noninvasive, and readily available, and it should be the first test performed in a previously uninvestigated patient. It is a highly sensitive and specific test, yet it **cannot distinguish an active infection from a treated infection.** Once the test is positive, it will almost always stay positive and should not be repeated. **Stool antigen testing** has an excellent positive predictive value and is most often used 8 to 14 weeks posttreatment in cases suspected to be refractory to treatment. For this test to be most accurate, patients must not have been treated with PPIs for at least 2 weeks prior to stool collection. Active *H. pylori* infection can be confirmed by ^{13}C **urea breath testing.** This test is highly sensitive and specific but is the most expensive option, so it should be reserved for patients who have already been treated and have inconclusive stool antigen testing.

Endoscopy. The gold standard for diagnosis of *H. pylori* is endoscopy with gastric mucosal biopsy; however, this is often not required unless in the setting of an upper GI bleed. Endoscopy also allows for direct visualization of ulcers and evaluation for the presence of malignancy or other pathology in the esophagus, stomach, or duodenum. It should be considered when a patient has high suspicion for esophageal or gastric complications of PUD or GERD, rather than purely for diagnosis of *H. pylori*.

Treatment

Management in the Hospital. A CBC should be obtained to determine a baseline hemoglobin value and should be repeated every 6 to 8 hours in a hospitalized patient to monitor for anemia and GI blood loss, even in the setting of negative fecal occult blood. Liver transaminases, serum amylase, and lipase levels should be obtained when biliary or pancreatic disease is suspected. **Alternative etiologies of epigastric pain, such as myocardial infarction or cholecystitis, should be considered** and ruled out with appropriate testing. A chest radiograph can be obtained to rule out abdominal visceral perforation, characterized by free air under the diaphragm. Patients with significant anemia, hemodynamic instability (eg, hypotension, tachycardia, orthostasis), or a suspected acute abdomen should be immediately hospitalized. Urgent surgical evaluation should be obtained if an acute abdomen is present.

Pharmacologic Management. Dyspepsia in patients younger than age 60 years with no alarm symptoms can be managed with a noninvasive *H. pylori* "test-and-treat" protocol with serologic testing followed by acid suppression using a PPI if symptoms remain. Generally, PPIs have greater efficacy in suppressing acid production and promoting ulcer healing than H$_2$ blockers. If symptoms resolve, no further testing is indicated. Along with treatment, NSAIDs, tobacco, and alcohol should be discontinued.

Treatment. If testing for *H. pylori* is positive, appropriate treatment to eradicate the infection, along with a PPI to suppress acid production, should be prescribed (Table 47–3 lists *H. pylori* treatment regimens). Patients should be asked about previous antibiotic exposure when deciding which antibiotic regimen to begin.

Long-Term Treatment. Most patients with *H. pylori* infection who have been treated successfully will require chronic acid suppressive therapy to combat symptoms of dyspepsia. Chronic acid suppressive therapy with PPIs has been associated with increased risk of hypomagnesemia and vitamin B$_{12}$ and iron deficiency. Studies have suggested a link to community-acquired pneumonia, *Clostridium difficile*–associated diarrhea, osteoporosis, and renal impairment, yet prospective studies have not shown a causal relationship or consistent results.

Complications

Approximately 25% of patients with PUD have a serious complication, such as hemorrhage, perforation, or gastric outlet obstruction. Silent ulcers and complications are more common in older patients and in patients taking chronic NSAIDs and aspirin. Surgical treatment for PUD is rarely indicated yet may be warranted in cases of severe hemorrhage that cannot be controlled via endoscopy or in cases of perforation or obstruction. Clinically relevant upper GI bleeding occurs in

Table 47–3 • RECOMMENDED FIRST-LINE THERAPIES FOR *HELICOBACTER PYLORI* INFECTION

Regimen	Drugs (Doses)	Dosing Frequency	Duration (Days)	FDA Approval
Clarithromycin triple	PPI (standard or double dose)	BID	14	Yes[a]
	Clarithromycin (500 mg)			
	Amoxicillin (1 g) or metronidazole (500 mg TID)			
Bismuth quadruple	PPI (standard dose)	BID	10-14	No[b]
	Bismuth subcitrate (120-300 mg) or subsalicylate (300 mg)	QID		
	Tetracycline (500 mg)	QID		
	Metronidazole (250-500 mg)	QID (250) TID to QID (500)		
Concomitant	PPI (standard dose)	BID	10-14	No
	Clarithromycin (500 mg)			
	Amoxicillin (1 g)			
	Nitroimidazole (500 mg)[c]			
Sequential	PPI (standard dose)	BID	5-7	No
	PPI, clarithromycin (500 mg) + nitroimidazole (500 mg)[c]	BID	5-7	
Hybrid	PPI (standard dose) + amoxicillin (1 g)	BID	7	No
	PPI, amoxicillin, clarithromycin (500 mg), nitroimidazole (500 mg)[c]	BID	7	
Levofloxacin triple	PPI (standard or double dose) + amoxicillin (1 g)	BID	5-7	No
	Levofloxacin (500 mg)	QD		
	Amoxicillin (1 g)	BID		
Levofloxacin sequential	PPI (standard or double dose) + amoxicillin (1 g)	BID	5-7	No
	PPI, amoxicillin, levofloxacin (500 mg QD), nitroimidazole (500 mg)[c]	BID	5-7	
LOAD	Levofloxacin (250 mg)	QD	7-10	No
	PPI (double dose)	QD		
	Nitazoxanide (500 mg)	BID		
	Doxycycline (100 mg)	QD		

Abbreviations: BID, twice daily; FDA, Food and Drug Administration; LOAD, levofloxacin, omeprazole, Alinia, doxycycline; PPI, proton pump inhibitor; QD, once daily; QID, four times daily; TID, three times daily.
[a]*Several PPI, clarithromycin, and amoxicillin combinations have achieved FDA approval. The PPI, clarithromycin, and metronidazole combination is not an FDA-approved treatment regimen.*
[b]*PPI, bismuth, tetracycline, and metronidazole combined treatment with a PPI for 10 days is an FDA-approved treatment regimen.*
[c]*Metronidazole or tinidazole.*
Source: Chey WD, Leontiadis GI, Howden CW, Moss SF. ACG clinical guideline: treatment of Helicobacter pylori infection. Am J Gastroenterol. 2017;112:212.

15% to 20% of patients with PUD and is the most common indication for surgical intervention; it is also the most common cause of death. The risk of rebleeding in PUD is the greatest within 48 hours of the initial bleed, and the risk of death increases proportionally with advanced age, medical comorbidities, and compromised hemodynamic status.

CLINICAL APPROACH TO GERD

Pathophysiology

Gastroesophageal reflux disease, the most common GI condition, is a chronic digestive condition in which gastric acid and stomach contents regurgitate from the stomach into the esophagus. A presumptive diagnosis can be accurately made in the setting of the classic symptoms of heartburn and regurgitation.

Treatment

Pharmacologic Management. Patients with typical symptoms of GERD who do not have a history of PUD should not be tested for *H. pylori*. Patients with GERD often begin self-directed acid-suppressive therapy with either an over-the-counter H_2 antagonist or a PPI before seeking advice from a health care provider. The test-and-treat strategy for GERD posits starting with the lowest possible dose of an H_2 antagonist once daily to control symptoms with increasing frequency and potency, followed by transition to a PPI if symptoms are not adequately controlled (step-up therapy). If a patient is on chronic PPI therapy, they should be "stepped down" to a H_2 antagonist if possible. Of note, patients should be informed that a PPI is most effective if taken 30 to 60 minutes before a meal.

Endoscopy and Lifestyle Modifications. When a patient requires acid-suppressive therapy for 8 weeks to control symptoms and cannot undergo step-down therapy or stop medication, then they should undergo upper endoscopy to rule out potential complications. Patients with heartburn or regurgitation should be advised to avoid smoking, alcohol, spicy foods, citrus foods, fatty foods, large meals, chocolate, and peppermint, and they should avoid eating or drinking 3 to 4 hours prior to lying down. Elevation of the head of the bed 6 to 8 inches and avoiding tight clothing around the waist may also help to improve symptoms.

Complications

Up to 40% of patients with chronic GERD will experience heartburn and regurgitation on a monthly basis. Most patients with GERD will have nonerosive reflux disease, while others will progress to erosive esophagitis. Caucasian males age 45 years or older who have chronic GERD, smoke cigarettes, and drink alcohol are at the greatest risk of development of Barrett esophagus, which is a precursor for esophageal adenocarcinoma. Patients with Barrett esophagus should be placed on lifelong PPI therapy and undergo surveillance with upper endoscopy to monitor for the development of esophageal adenocarcinoma.

Patients older than age 50 years or those with alarm symptoms for either PUD or GERD should be referred for upper GI endoscopy to exclude complications of esophageal stricture, erosive disease, or malignancy. Endoscopy is preferred over radiographic procedures due to direct visualization and the ability to perform a biopsy.

Gastric ulcers tend to present later in life than duodenal ulcers and have a higher chance of being a sign of malignancy. Endoscopy also can be therapeutic, as a stricture can be dilated or a visible source of bleeding can be identified and cauterized. **Any patient 50 years of age or older who has hematemesis, hematochezia, or melena should undergo a colonoscopy, regardless of the upper endoscopic findings,** to evaluate for a lower GI cause of bleeding, including diverticulosis, vascular malformation, or malignancy.

CASE CORRELATION

- See Case 23 (Lower Gastrointestinal Bleeding) and Case 40 (Irritable Bowel Syndrome).

COMPREHENSION QUESTIONS

47.1 A 30-year-old healthy woman recently attended a health fair, where she tested positive for *H. pylori* on a blood test. She denies any recent abdominal discomfort, nausea, vomiting, diarrhea, or melena. Occasionally, she uses over-the-counter acid suppressive therapy after eating spicy foods or drinking alcohol when she develops mild heartburn, and her symptoms typically resolve within a week. Which of the following is the most appropriate advice to give this patient regarding *H. pylori*?

    A. Based on this test result, it is not possible to tell if she has an active infection.

    B. She should undergo stool antigen testing to prove infection.

    C. She should undergo upper endoscopy to prove infection.

    D. She should be prescribed a PPI for 8 weeks.

    E. She should be prescribed triple therapy to treat infection.

47.2 A 62-year-old man presents with increasing shortness of breath and fatigue over the last several days. Cardiac examination reveals regular rate and rhythm, and lungs are clear to auscultation bilaterally. No jaundice, jugular venous distention, or peripheral edema is noted. Mucous membranes are pink with no evidence of cyanosis, and capillary refill is brisk. CBC reveals a microcytic anemia, and a gastric ulcer is diagnosed on upper GI endoscopy. Gastric mucosa biopsy confirms an *H. pylori* infection. This patient's last colonoscopy was 10 years ago and was unremarkable. Which of the following is the next most appropriate step in the workup of this patient?

    A. Barium esophagram

    B. Abdominal ultrasound

    C. Colonoscopy

    D. Urea breath test

    E. Stool antigen test

47.3 A 41-year-old man presents to your office for upper GI discomfort that has been present for the last 2 months. He says that he has a "full" sensation in the epigastric region. He recently began smoking again due to increased stress at work. He denies blood in his stool, denies vomiting, and has not had dysphagia. He has unintentionally lost 10 lb in the last few weeks, which he attributes to not eating. There is no family history of GI disorders. He has never had an upper endoscopy or colonoscopy. Which of the following is the most appropriate next step in workup of this patient?

A. *H. pylori* test and treat

B. Proton pump inhibitor therapy for 8 weeks

C. Fecal occult blood test

D. Upper endoscopy

E. Urea breath test

47.4 A 25-year-old woman arrives at the emergency center with a 15-hour history of nausea, vomiting, and severe epigastric abdominal pain that awoke her from sleep. She admits to heavy alcohol consumption the prior evening, which is common for her on the weekends. She takes no medications, including NSAIDs. Her temperature is 39 °C (102.2 °F), blood pressure is 100/60 mm Hg, pulse rate is 130 beats/min, and respirations are 14 breaths/min. An acute abdominal series radiograph upon admission displayed a substantial amount of free air under the right hemidiaphragm. Which of the following is the most likely diagnosis?

A. Perforated peptic ulcer

B. Alcohol-related gastritis

C. Appendicitis

D. Gastroenteritis

E. Kidney stones

ANSWERS

47.1 **A.** *H. pylori* serologic testing cannot distinguish active infections from old infections or diagnose the presence of ulcers. Treating a positive serum test in an asymptomatic person is not indicated, but rather education of the patient regarding the need for further testing to confirm the diagnosis. Stool antigen testing (answer B), upper endoscopy (answer C), daily PPI therapy (answer D), and triple therapy (answer E) are not indicated in a patient without symptoms of dyspepsia.

47.2 **C.** The presence of blood in the stool or anemia in a patient older than age 50 years, even when an ulcer is found, is an indication for colonoscopy, as this may also represent a presentation of a concomitant colon cancer. A urea breath test (answer D) may be beneficial after completion of treatment to confirm eradication of the infection. Answer A (barium esophagram) is often useful to diagnose GERD or a hiatal hernia, but it is not useful in this patient with proven PUD. Answer B (abdominal ultrasound) is useful in the assessment of gallstones or biliary tract disease but not in evaluating PUD. Answer E (stool antigen test) is helpful 8 to 14 weeks posttreatment in cases suspected to be refractory to treatment; it is also useful for diagnosing *C. difficile* infection.

47.3 **D.** This patient has abdominal pain and alarm symptoms of unintended weight loss and early satiety. He should be referred for upper endoscopy and possible colonoscopy. Test-and-treat strategies for *H. pylori* and/or GERD (answer A) or a urea breath test (answer E) are not indicated in the setting of alarm symptoms, which require prompt workup. A FOBT (answer C) is not indicated, as endoscopy is warranted. Likewise, PPI therapy for 8 weeks (answer B) would potentially delay the diagnosis of a potentially dangerous condition.

47.4 **A.** The acute abdominal symptoms and free air under the diaphragm indicate a perforated viscus. This patient has a perforated ulcer with hemodynamic instability. Additional workup includes a chemistry panel, CBC, and urgent laparotomy. Answer B (alcohol-related gastritis) would present as epigastric pain, possibly melena or coffee ground emesis, but not with air under the diaphragm. Answer C (appendicitis) presents as periumbilical pain that radiates or moves to the right lower quadrant; it may lead to perforation but often is localized in the right lower quadrant area and does not often present with free air. Answer D (gastroenteritis) presents with diarrhea and sometimes with vomiting. Answer E (kidney stones) presents as costovertebral angle tenderness with radiation to the groin area and often with hematuria; there is no free air in this disease.

CLINICAL PEARLS

▶ Persons who require long-term NSAID therapy and/or aspirin should be monitored for signs and symptoms of dyspepsia and PUD.

▶ Persons with chronic symptoms of dyspepsia who have not been taking NSAIDs or aspirin or those who are from Mexico, Central America, Africa, or other endemic areas should be tested for *H. pylori* infection via IgG serologic testing and treated if positive.

▶ Commonly held beliefs, such as ulcers being caused by a stressful lifestyle or spicy foods, are incorrect. Certain foods may contribute to functional dyspepsia, but the vast majority of ulcers are caused by *H. pylori* and NSAIDs.

▶ Patients who experience heartburn and regurgitation should be treated with acid-suppressive therapy in a step-up fashion, with attempts at step-down therapy when symptoms are controlled.

▶ Acid-suppression therapy may carry long-term risks of community-acquired pneumonia; *C. difficile*–associated diarrhea; demineralization of bone; decreased absorption of calcium, magnesium, and iron; and interaction with the metabolism of clopidogrel. Risks and benefits of therapy should be discussed with patients.

REFERENCES

American Gastroenterological Association medical position statement on the management of Barrett's esophagus. *Gastroenterology.* 2011;140:1084-1091.

Anderson WD, Strayer SM, Mull SR. Common questions about the management of gastroesophageal reflux disease. *Am Fam Physician.* 2015;91(10):692-697.

Aziz I, Palsson O, Sperber A, Whitehead WE, Simren M. Epidemiology, clinical characteristics, and associations for symptom-based Rome IV functional dyspepsia in adults in the USA, Canada, and the UK: a cross-sectional population-based study. *Lancet Gastroenterol Hepatol.* 2018;3(4):252-262.

Chey WD, Leontiadis GI, Howden CW, Moss SF. ACG clinical guideline: treatment of *Helicobacter pylori* infection. *Am J Gastroenterol.* 2017;112(2):212-239.

Fashner J, Gitu AC. Diagnosis and treatment of peptic ulcer disease and *H. pylori* infection. *Am Fam Physician.* 2015;91(4):236-242.

Heidelbaugh JJ, Kim AH, Chang R, Walker PC. Overutilization of proton pump inhibitors: what the clinician needs to know. *Ther Adv Gastroenterol.* 2012;5(4):219-232.

Katz PO, Gerson LB, Vela MF. Guidelines for the diagnosis and management of gastroesophageal reflux disease. *Am J Gastroenterol.* 2013;108(3):308-328.

Loyd RA, McClellan DA. Update on the evaluation and management of functional dyspepsia. *Am Fam Physician.* 2011;83(5):547-552.

Sandhu DS, Fass R. Current trends in the management of gastroesophageal reflux disease. *Gut Liver.* 2018;12(1):7-16.

Valle J. Peptic ulcer disease and related disorders. In: Jameson J, Fauci AS, Kasper DL, Hauser SL, Longo DL, Loscalzo J, eds. *Harrison's Principles of Internal Medicine.* 20 ed. New York, NY: McGraw Hill; 2018: Chap. 317. http://accessmedicine.mhmedical.com/content.aspx?bookid=2129& sectionid=192282176. Accessed May 25, 2019.

An 18-month-old girl is brought to the office by her mother because of a rash. The patient has had a subjective high fever for the past 3 days, along with some mild respiratory symptoms of cough and rhinorrhea. She was given acetaminophen for the fever but no other medications. The fever has gone down in the past day, but today she developed an erythematous rash that developed suddenly, starting on the trunk and spreading to the extremities. The child has no significant medical history and no known sick contacts, although she attends day care 3 days a week. On examination, she is mildly fussy but is easily consolable in her mother's lap. Upon inspection, the rash consists of small macules and papules that blanch on palpation. The remainder of her examination is unremarkable.

▶ What is the most likely diagnosis?
▶ What is the most likely cause of this illness?
▶ What is the appropriate treatment?

ANSWERS TO CASE 48:
Fever and Rash

Summary: An 18-month-old girl presents with

- A rapidly spreading rash that started after 3 days of fever
- Diffuse, blanching, erythematous macules and papules
- Mild respiratory symptoms of cough and rhinorrhea
- No significant medical history and no known sick contacts
- History of attending day care 3 days a week

Most likely diagnosis: Roseola.

Most likely cause of the illness: Human herpesvirus 6 (HHV-6).

Treatment: Supportive care only, as the rash is likely to completely resolve in 24 to 48 hours.

ANALYSIS

Objectives

1. Be able to identify common rashes associated with viral infections in children. (EPA 1, 2)

2. Know the appropriate management of febrile illness associated with rashes in children. (EPA 4)

Considerations

This toddler has a history of fever and a diffuse, erythematous, maculopapular rash. The rash is most likely due to roseola, caused by HHV-6, which is a ubiquitous virus that infects most children between 6 months and 3 years (although most infections are asymptomatic). The virus has an incubation period of 1 to 2 weeks and causes a prodromal illness associated with mild respiratory symptoms and a sudden high fever (39 °C to 40 °C), which, in rare cases, can cause febrile seizures. A few days after inoculation, the fever typically resolves, and the erythematous rash appears.

APPROACH TO:
Fever and Rash

DEFINITIONS

ENANTHEM: An eruption on a mucus membrane as a symptom of a disease.

EXANTHEM: An eruption on the skin as a symptom of a disease.

CLINICAL APPROACH TO PEDIATRIC FEVER AND RASH

Pathophysiology

Febrile illnesses and rashes are extremely common presentations in family medicine and pediatric practices. In most cases, these presentations represent mild, self-limited illnesses that require no specific therapy. However, some cases will represent serious infections that require urgent intervention. Rashes associated with fever may be caused by viruses, bacteria, spirochetes, drug reaction, or autoimmune disease. The patient history should attempt to identify any exposures that may cause these syndromes, focusing on duration of the illness, other associated constitutional symptoms, sick contacts, history of recent travel, use of medications, or exposure to animals and insects (eg, ticks).

Clinical Presentation

History. A review of immunization status is critical, as many diseases preventable by vaccines can cause fever and rash. **Immunization does not always guarantee complete lifelong immunity,** but it should confer a less severe presentation of the disease. Education on the importance of immunizations is paramount, given some increasing reluctance to vaccinate children coupled with outbreaks of chicken pox, mumps, and measles in recent years.

   Physical Examination. A thorough physical examination with a complete skin examination should be performed. Examination findings can both lead to a specific diagnosis and identify complications of the causative agent. For example, the presence of exudative pharyngitis along with fever and rash may suggest scarlet fever caused by a group A streptococcus infection, while wheezes or rhonchi on lung examination in a patient with crops of vesicles at different stages may lead to a diagnosis of varicella (chicken pox) complicated by pneumonitis. Understanding the definitions of macules, papules, pustules, and vesicles allows for increased accuracy in diagnosis and ability to cogently discuss challenging cases with colleagues. Case 13 highlights definitions of many common skin lesions.

CLINICAL APPROACH TO COMMON VIRAL INFECTIONS

Roseola

Human herpesvirus 6 is a ubiquitous virus that infects most children before the age of 3 years, although most infections are asymptomatic. The virus has an incubation period of 1 to 2 weeks and causes a prodromal illness associated with mild respiratory symptoms and a high fever. This prodromal illness typically does not last longer than 5 days. **Following defervescence, a characteristic erythematous maculopapular rash appears suddenly** on the trunk and spreads rapidly to the extremities, sparing the face. The rash commonly disappears in 1 to 2 days. The diagnosis is primarily clinical, based on the history and examination. Due to the short-lived nature of the disease, no treatment is usually required other than acetaminophen and reassurance.

Varicella Zoster

Pathophysiology. The varicella zoster virus is a highly contagious virus that causes two clinical syndromes, chicken pox (varicella) and shingles (zoster). **Chicken pox** occurs more commonly in children. The diagnosis of varicella is usually clinical but may be confirmed with Tzanck smear or identification of the virus by DNA polymerase chain reaction.

Clinical Presentation. Varicella begins with the development of clusters of **vesicles on an erythematous base,** described as "dewdrops on a rose petal." The initial exanthem is rapidly followed by malaise, fever (38 °C to 42 °C), and anorexia. The vesicles progress to shallow, crusted erosions and ulcerations. The contagious period continues 4 to 5 days after the appearance of the rash and lasts until all lesions have crusted over. It takes an average of 10 to 21 days after contact with an infected person for someone to develop chicken pox. Patients with varicella may also develop enanthems, with lesions on the oral, nasal, or gastrointestinal mucosa.

Treatment. Antiviral therapy using acyclovir, valacyclovir, or famciclovir may shorten the course of the illness in patients older than 2 years of age if started within 24 hours of onset of the exanthem. Varicella vaccination is now universally recommended at age 12 to 15 months with a booster dose at age 4 years. While the vaccine has significantly reduced the incidence of childhood chicken pox, breakthrough infections can occur in vaccinated individuals. These infections are usually much less severe, with fewer vesicles and little to no fever. The varicella vaccine is a live, attenuated virus and should not be given to immunocompromised or pregnant patients.

Complications. In rare cases, serious complications may develop, which include encephalitis, meningitis, and pneumonitis. Superinfection of the vesicles with bacteria, most commonly group A streptococcus and *Staphylococcus aureus,* is a particularly common and potentially dangerous complication. Varicella, while less common in adolescents and adults, can cause severe disease and complications in older patients.

Herpes Zoster

Herpes zoster, or shingles, is a reactivation of the varicella virus, which remains dormant in the dorsal root ganglia following the initial infection. The reactivated virus causes a vesicular eruption, usually along a single dermatome that does not cross the midline. The reaction can occur at any age but is more common in the elderly or immunosuppressed. The rash can be extremely painful and can result in a chronic postherpetic neuralgia that can last long after resolution of the rash. Antiviral therapy started within 72 hours of onset of the rash may reduce the incidence of the postherpetic neuralgia. Gabapentin is an effective treatment for postherpetic neuralgia. The herpes zoster vaccine is recommended for people over 50 years old.

Erythema Infectiosum

Parvovirus B19 causes a characteristic syndrome known as erythema infectiosum or **fifth disease,** typically among children younger than 10 years of age. It is spread by respiratory droplets, with peak incidence in winter and spring. A mild prodromal fever and upper respiratory symptoms precede a rash. The rash usually starts as confluent erythematous macules on the face, often sparing the nose and periorbital regions, resulting in a classic **"slapped cheek"** appearance. Two to four days after the facial rash, a lacy, pruritic exanthem spreads to the trunk and extremities. This usually lasts for 1 to 2 weeks but can have a relapsing course for several months. Parvovirus B19 in adults and older adolescents tends to cause a more severe illness, with rheumatic complaints, including arthralgias. In patients with sickle cell disease, parvovirus B19 infection can lead to an aplastic crisis with anemia and leukopenia. The virus can also be transmitted from mother to fetus during pregnancy, resulting in fetal hydrops and pregnancy loss. Unfortunately, there is no treatment other than supportive measures. If there is significant fetal anemia, consideration can be given to intrauterine transfusion if indicated.

CLINICAL APPROACH TO COMMON BACTERIAL INFECTIONS

Group A Beta-Hemolytic Streptococcus

Group A beta-hemolytic streptococcus (GABS) is associated with numerous diseases, particularly in children. It is the causative agent of streptococcal pharyngitis, impetigo, erysipelas, and cellulitis. Invasion and multiplication within the fascia can lead to necrotizing fasciitis. Feared complications of GABS infection include rheumatic fever and postinfectious glomerulonephritis. GABS infections can be confirmed by rapid antigen testing or culture via a pharyngeal swab. Laboratory evaluation is rarely necessary yet may reveal leukocytosis with neutrophilia and possibly eosinophilia, as well as elevated erythrocyte sedimentation rate, C-reactive protein, and antistreptolysin O titer.

Scarlet Fever. GABS is the causative agent of scarlet fever. The rash of **scarlet fever** usually starts approximately 2 days after the onset of sore throat and fever. The rash consists of punctate, raised, erythematous eruptions that can become confluent and feel like sandpaper. The rash tends to start on the upper trunk and spreads to the rest of the trunk and the extremities. The exanthem can also be associated with an enanthem: oral mucositis resulting in a "strawberry tongue." Several weeks later, the rash fades before widespread desquamation of the skin begins, sometimes lasting 1 to 2 months.

Treatment. The first-line treatment for GABS infections is penicillin, with cephalosporins or macrolides as alternatives in penicillin-allergic patients. Patients may be counseled to return to school or work 24 hours after initiation of antibiotics if they are afebrile. Exposed individuals should be monitored for fever and other symptoms for at least a week and should receive treatment if they have a positive throat culture. Household and close contacts with similar symptoms should be empirically treated.

Impetigo. Impetigo is a skin infection caused by streptococcus or staphylococcus, with characteristic "honey-crusted" lesions. Contact precautions should be employed to minimize spread. Treatment options include oral penicillins or cephalosporins or topical mupirocin.

Neisseria meningitidis

Blood infection with *Neisseria meningitidis* (meningococcemia) can cause an **acute, life-threatening illness,** with high fevers, hypotension, and altered mental status.

Most people with meningococcemia develop frank bacterial meningitis, with associated signs of meningeal irritation (eg, headache, stiff neck). The **rash of meningococcemia often starts as an erythematous maculopapular eruption that does not blanch with compression and that progresses to form petechiae.** Meningococcemia can lead to disseminated intravascular coagulation, resulting in complications, including gangrene and autoamputation of limbs (purpura fulminans), adrenal hemorrhage (Waterhouse-Friedrichsen syndrome), deafness, stroke, and renal infarctions.

Persons with suspected meningococcemia should be immediately hospitalized and quarantined, usually in the intensive care unit. The ABCs (airway, breathing, and circulation) should be urgently evaluated, blood and cerebrospinal fluid cultures collected, and empiric antibiotic therapy instituted until an organism is isolated via culture and drug sensitivities are obtained. **Treatment should not be delayed by performing a lumbar puncture, as early and appropriate antibiotic treatment markedly improves the outcome of meningococcal infections.** A common empiric regimen for presumed meningitis in infants less than 30 days old is ampicillin plus gentamicin. Vancomycin plus ceftriaxone should be used in older children and adults. Antibiotic coverage can be later tailored based on culture results. The first choice for culture-proven meningococcal meningitis is penicillin G. A meningococcal vaccine is recommended for routine childhood immunization and also should be offered to patients at risk for the disease (eg, asplenia, those living in dormitories or military barracks). Close contacts of someone with meningococcal infection should be offered prophylaxis with ciprofloxacin or rifampin.

CLINICAL APPROACH TO TICK-BORNE DISEASES

Rocky Mountain Spotted Fever

Rocky Mountain spotted fever (RMSF) is an acute, life-threatening infection caused by the organism *Rickettsia rickettsii*, commonly transmitted by the *Dermacentor* tick. The infection occurs more often in the summer months, when people are more likely to be outdoors. Despite its name, RMSF is most common in the southeastern United States but is found throughout the Western Hemisphere.

The initial illness consists of nonspecific signs and symptoms, such as fever, headache, myalgias, arthralgias, and fatigue. Some patients, especially children, may complain of abdominal pain. **This prodrome is followed by a macular, papular, or petechial eruption that starts on the wrists and ankles then spreads to the trunk, palms, and soles.** The rash usually develops between the third and fifth day of the illness. Laboratory evaluation often reveals leukopenia, thrombocytopenia, hyponatremia, and elevated liver transaminases. The diagnosis is confirmed with serology; however, the clinical utility of this test is limited by cost and delayed results. As risk of mortality sharply increases around day 5 of illness, likely cases should be treated empirically with doxycycline. Therapy should be continued for at least 3 days after the patient becomes afebrile.

Lyme Disease

Lyme disease is endemic in many areas of the United States, including New England and the mid-Atlantic region. The causative spirochete, *Borrelia burgdorferi*, is transmitted via the bite of deer ticks of the *Ixodes* species. Because the ticks are very small, infected persons are often unaware of a history of a tick bite. The characteristic rash, **erythema migrans,** develops 3 to 30 days following infection. The exanthem is typically an expanding erythematous macule with central clearing, often described as appearing like a "bull's-eye." Following this, dissemination of the spirochete can occur, resulting in multiple symptoms and signs, including diffuse arthralgias and myalgias, Bell palsy, aseptic meningitis, carditis, and even complete heart block in the weeks following initial infection. Late disease is most characteristically marked by polyarthritis months to years after inoculation. Diagnosis is confirmed by serologic testing. The treatment of choice for Lyme disease is doxycycline, amoxicillin, or cefuroxime. Patients treated with appropriate antibiotic therapy in the early stages of Lyme disease commonly recover completely and without lasting sequelae. Approximately 10% to 20% of patients who present late in the disease, despite appropriate antibiotic therapy, may have persistent or recurrent symptoms known as posttreatment Lyme disease syndrome. Table 48–1 provides a summary of some of the most common causes of rash and fever in children.

Table 48–1 • INFECTIOUS CAUSES OF FEVER AND RASH			
Disease	Causative Organism	Rash	Distinguishing Features
Roseola	Human herpesvirus 6 (HHV-6)	Erythematous, maculopapular rash, starting on the trunk and sparing the face	High fever followed by rash
Chicken pox	Varicella zoster virus	Papules or vesicles on an erythematous base: "dewdrops on a rose petal"	Varicella: vesicles in multiple stages
Shingles	Varicella zoster virus	Vesicular rash in a dermatomal pattern	Zoster: dermatomal vesicles in single stage Postherpetic neuralgia
Erythema infectiosum	Parvovirus B19	Erythematous macular rash on cheeks ("slapped cheek"), followed by a lacy, reticulated rash over trunk and extremities	Congenital: hydrops fetalis Child: mild upper respiratory symptoms Adult: mild arthralgias
Measles	Measles virus	Erythematous maculopapular rash starting at the forehead and moving down the body	Koplik spots, fever, and malaise
Rubella	Rubella virus	Erythematous macular rash starting at the face and neck and moving to the trunk and extremities	"3-day/German measles" Congenital: patent ductus arteriosus, sensorineural deafness, hematopoietic "blueberry muffin" rash

(Continued)

Table 48–1 • INFECTIOUS CAUSES OF FEVER AND RASH (continued)			
Disease	Causative Organism	Rash	Distinguishing Features
Smallpox	Variola virus	Macules, papules, or pustules at the same stage of development	Eradicated in 1980
Hand-foot-and-mouth disease	Coxsackie A virus	Vesicular enanthem on tongue, on lips, and in mouth; maculovesicular rash on hands, feet, buttocks, and groin	Rash on palms and soles
Scarlet fever	Group A streptococcus	Erythematous papular rash starting on neck and moving to trunk and extremities	"Strawberry tongue" enanthem "Sandpaper" rash
Rheumatic fever	Group A streptococcus	Erythema marginatum: erythematous, serpiginous macules with pale centers	Carditis, polyarthritis, subcutaneous nodules, and Sydenham chorea
Meningococcemia	*Neisseria meningitidis*	Erythematous maculopapular rash progressing to form petechiae	Meningitis, disseminated intravascular coagulation, and adrenal crisis
Toxic shock syndrome	*Staphylococcus aureus*	Diffuse erythematous macular rash with peeling palms and soles	Vomiting, diarrhea, and hypotension
Typhoid fever	*Salmonella enterica*	Maculopapular rash on lower chest and abdomen: "rose spots"	Diarrhea, abdominal pain, and hepatosplenomegaly Carrier state in gallbladder
Rocky Mountain spotted fever	*Rickettsia rickettsii*	Maculopapular rash starting on the wrists and ankles with centrifugal spread	Rash on palms and soles
Lyme disease	*Borrelia burgdorferi*	Erythema migrans-erythematous macule with central clearing: "bull's-eye"	Bell's palsy, meningitis, arthritis, carditis, and heart block

CASE CORRELATION

- See Case 13 (Skin Lesions).

COMPREHENSION QUESTIONS

48.1 A 4-year-old boy is brought to your office by his mother for evaluation of a rash on his face that his mother first noticed one day previously. His mother comments that it looks like somebody "slapped him." The mother reports that he has had a cold for the last couple of days. The child's physical examination is unremarkable except for an erythematous macular rash over both cheeks and a temperature of 102 °F (38.9 °C). The mother admits that the child is behind on his immunization schedule. Which of the following is the most likely cause?

A. Varicella zoster virus

B. Parvovirus B19

C. Human herpesvirus 6

D. Rubella virus

E. Child abuse warranting immediate contact with social services

48.2 A 6-year-old girl is brought to your office by her mother because of a rash first noticed a week ago. Her mother reports that several children in her child's school have chicken pox, but that her child has received all of her immunizations, including two doses of the varicella vaccine. You observe the child actively playing with the toys in the waiting room before both the mother and child are brought back to the examination room. The child has a temperature of 100.4 °F (38 °C), a pulse of 90 beats/min, a blood pressure of 100/70 mm Hg, and a respiratory rate of 20 breaths/min. The physical examination is unremarkable except for about 20 vesicles on erythematous bases sparsely scattered on the child's trunk and limbs. Which of the following is the most appropriate treatment?

A. Supportive care

B. Antiviral therapy

C. Antibiotic therapy

D. Immune globulin

48.3 An 18-year-old adolescent young man is brought to the emergency department from his college dorm by his roommate. The patient is confused and cannot give a history. He has a temperature of 104 °F (40 °C), pulse of 110 beats/min, blood pressure of 90/60 mm Hg, and respiratory rate of 24 breaths/min. His head cannot be moved because of severe nuchal rigidity. Multiple petechiae are observed on his buttocks and legs. After initiation of treatment for the patient, what is the most appropriate advice to give to this patient's roommate?

A. Provide reassurance that he does not require prophylaxis.

B. The patient should take acyclovir for prophylaxis.

C. The patient should take penicillin for prophylaxis.

D. The patient should take rifampin for prophylaxis.

E. The patient should take cefuroxime for prophylaxis.

48.4 A 7-year-old boy is brought to a hospital in Charlotte, North Carolina, with a fever of 104 °F (40 °C). A maculopapular rash is seen on his wrists and ankles, but the palms and soles are spared. His laboratory results show leukopenia, hyponatremia, and elevated liver transaminases. His parents say that he was on a camping trip 1 week ago, but they vigorously used insect repellants and filtered all of their water. His father came in contact with poison oak, but the boy denies any pruritus. Which of the following is the best treatment for this patient's rash?

A. Penicillin

B. Acyclovir

C. Ceftriaxone

D. Vancomycin

E. Doxycycline

ANSWERS

48.1 **B.** This question describes erythema infectiosum, or fifth disease, which is caused by parvovirus B19. It often has a prodrome of fever and upper respiratory symptoms, mistaken by the mother in this question as a "cold." While the child does need to be caught up on his immunizations, there are currently no vaccinations for parvovirus B19. Answer A (varicella zoster) usually presents with upper respiratory symptoms, fatigue, and a vesicular rash with different stages of healing. Answer C (HHV-6 infection) is the etiologic agent of roseola infantum and presents as a maculopapular rash and fever in children under the age of 2 years. Answer D (rubella infection) presents in children as a low-grade fever, sore throat, rhinorrhea, and a maculopapular rash that begins in the face and spreads to the rest of the body. There is no evidence of child abuse (answer E) in this case.

48.2 **A.** The child has chicken pox caused by the varicella zoster virus. While the varicella vaccine is effective, sporadic breakthrough cases do occur. However, these cases are usually much less severe and have fewer complications than in unimmunized patients. Supportive care is advised, as this illness is self-limited. Antivirals (answer B) have been shown to reduce duration and severity only if initiated early. Antibiotics (answer C) and immune globulin (answer D) have no role in the treatment of this patient.

48.3 **D.** Based on this patient's history of living in a dorm and the clinical presentation of high fever, nuchal rigidity, and petechial/purpural rash, the most likely diagnosis is meningitis and meningococcemia caused by *N. meningitidis*. The patient is severely affected and is in septic shock. All people in close contact with the patient should receive ciprofloxacin or rifampin prophylaxis (not penicillin [answer C], cefuroxine [answer E], or no prophylaxis [answer A]). Acyclovir would be a prophylactic medication for herpes simplex virus (answer B).

48.4 **E.** This patient has RMSF and should be treated with doxycycline. The disease is commonly found in North Carolina and is carried by ticks that the boy could have picked up during the camping trip. RMSF has a characteristic rash that starts on the wrists and ankles and can eventually involve the palms and soles. Typically, the rash of RMSF spreads centripetally from the wrists and ankles to involve the trunk and extremities. Penicillin (answer A) is used to treat syphilis or group A streptococcal disease. Acyclovir (answer B) is used to treat herpes simplex virus infections. Answer C (ceftriaxone) is used to treat gonorrhea. Answer D (vancomycin) is used to treat methicillin resistant *S. aureus*.

CLINICAL PEARLS

▶ Shingles that approaches the eye (herpes zoster ophthalmicus) should be evaluated by an ophthalmologist because of the risk of a reactivation involving the trigeminal nerve. A clue that the eye may become involved is seeing characteristic lesions approaching the tip of the nose.

▶ Parvovirus B19 infection often presents in a child as a high fever and a slapped cheek appearance.

▶ Many vaccine-preventable illnesses, including measles, rubella, and varicella, have characteristic rashes associated with them. Always obtain a vaccination history on children presenting with fever and rash and strive to keep vaccinations up to date in children and adults.

▶ Roseola typically has a red maculopapular rash that appears suddenly after defervescence, starting on the trunk and moving to the extremities, avoiding the face.

▶ Varicella develops as clusters of vesicles on an erythematous base, progressing to crusted erosions, and lesions are in different stages of healing.

▶ Herpes zoster affects a single dermatome and does not cross the midline. Antiviral therapy begun within 72 hours can reduce the complications.

▶ Meningococcemia can cause meningitis and a disseminated rash leading to DIC and petechiae.

▶ Lyme disease begins from a tick bite and the characteristic rash is erythema migrans (bull's eye).

REFERENCES

Allmon A, Deane K, Martin KI. Common skin rashes in children. *Am Fam Physician*. 2015;92(3):211-216.

Biesbroeck L, Sidbury R. Viral exanthems: an update. *Dermat Ther*. 2013;26:433-438.

Chen LF, Sexton DJ. What's new in Rocky Mountain spotted fever. *Infect Dis Clin North Am*. 2008;22(3):415-432.

Cohen JI. Herpes zoster. *N Engl J Med.* 2013;369:255-263.

Dandache P, Nadelman RB. Erythema migrans. *Infect Dis Clin North Am.* 2008;22(2):235-260.

Ely JW, Stone MS. The generalized rash: part I. Differential diagnosis. *Am Fam Physician.* 2010;81(6):726-734.

Ely JW, Stone MS. The generalized rash: part II. Diagnostic approach. *Am Fam Physician.* 2010;81(6):735-739.

Folster-Holst R, Kreth HW. Viral exanthems in childhood—infectious (direct) exanthems. Part 1: classic exanthems. *J Dtsch Dermal Ges.* 2009;7(4):309-316.

Folster-Holst R, Kreth HW. Viral exanthems in childhood—infectious (direct) exanthems. Part 2: other viral exanthems. *J Dtsch Dermal Ges.* 2009;7(5):414-419.

Mann K, Jackson MA. Meningitis. *Pediatr Rev.* 2008;29(12):417-429.

McKinnon HD, Howard T. Evaluating the febrile patient with a rash. *Am Fam Physician.* 2000; 62:804-816.

Shapiro ED. Lyme disease. *N Engl J Med.* 2014;370:1724-1731.

Survey JT, Reamy BV, Hodge J. Clinical presentation of parvovirus B19 infection. *Am Fam Physician.* 2007;75(3):373-376.

Zerr DM, Meier AS, Selke SS, et al. A population-based study of primary human herpesvirus 6 infection. *N Engl J Med.* 2005;352(8):768-776.

A 32-year-old woman presents for evaluation of a right breast lump that she noticed on self-examination. While she does not often perform breast self-examination (BSE), she thinks that this lump is new. She denies nipple discharge or breast pain and states the lump is mildly tender on palpation. She has never noticed any breast masses previously and has never had a mammogram. She has no personal or family history of breast disease. She takes oral contraceptive pills regularly but no other medications. She does not smoke cigarettes or drink alcohol. She has never been pregnant. On examination, she is a well-appearing, somewhat anxious, thin woman. Her vital signs are within normal limits. On breast examination, in the lower outer quadrant of the right breast there is a 2-cm, firm, well-circumscribed, freely mobile mass without overlying erythema that is mildly tender to palpation. There is no skin dimpling, retraction, or nipple discharge. While no other discrete breast masses are palpable, the bilateral breast tissue is noted to be firm and glandular throughout. There is no evidence of axillary, supraclavicular, or cervical lymphadenopathy. The remainder of her physical examination is unremarkable.

▶ What is the most likely diagnosis of this breast lesion?
▶ What is the first step in evaluation?
▶ What is the recommended follow-up for this patient?

ANSWERS TO CASE 49:
Breast Diseases

Summary: A 32-year-old woman presents with

- A right breast lump detected on breast self-examination that is estimated to be 2 cm in size, firm, and freely mobile
- No lymphadenopathy noted on physical examination
- No personal or family history of breast disease
- Regular medication of oral contraceptive pills but no other medications

Most likely diagnosis: Simple breast cyst.

First step in evaluation: Triple-test evaluation, including clinical breast examination (CBE), ultrasound imaging, and tissue sampling via fine-needle aspiration (FNA) of the cyst.

Recommended follow-up: If aspiration of the cyst results in complete resolution of the mass, and if the fluid is clear or yellow, then follow-up clinical examination in 1 to 2 months is recommended to ensure no recurrence; if the mass persists despite aspiration, if the fluid is bloody, or if the lesion recurs, then further evaluation with additional imaging and biopsy is indicated.

ANALYSIS

Objectives

1. Describe how to evaluate a breast mass. (EPA 1, 3)

2. Know the risk factors for breast cancer. (EPA 12)

3. Know the physical examination findings suggestive of benign and malignant breast masses. (EPA 1)

4. Know how to manage benign breast diseases. (EPA 4)

Considerations

The majority of breast concerns seen by family health care providers—most frequently, palpable masses, nipple discharge, and mastalgia—commonly represent benign conditions. However, a palpable mass is the most common presenting symptom of breast cancer and can be alarming for patients. Breast cancer is the most common nonskin cancer and the second leading cause of cancer death in US women behind lung cancer. An estimated **one in eight women will develop breast cancer in their lifetime,** with a median age of diagnosis of 62 years. In 2018, an estimated 266,000 new cases were diagnosed. The rate of new diagnosis, 126 in 100,000, has been fairly stable over the past 30 years. The estimated number of breast cancer deaths in 2018 was 41,000, but the death rate has declined over the past 30 years due to effective screening guidelines that have led to earlier detection and treatment. The 5-year survival of breast cancer is 90%.

The most common benign breast diseases are fibrocystic changes and fibroadenomas; other lesions include intraductal papilloma, duct ectasia, and galactocele. Breast tissue may also develop simple cysts, abscesses, lipomas, and trauma-induced fat necrosis. Malignant lesions may be in situ, including ductal or lobular carcinoma in situ; or invasive, including invasive ductal carcinoma or invasive lobular carcinoma. Inflammatory carcinoma, which causes inflammatory skin changes, can be confused with cellulitis or mastitis.

In the case presented, several clues suggest the likelihood of a benign process, including younger age—especially in the context of no personal or family breast cancer history—and benign characteristics on physical examination that are most consistent with a cystic lesion. Regardless of these reassuring findings, a thorough evaluation of the lesion is imperative.

APPROACH TO:
Breast Diseases

DEFINITIONS

DUCT ECTASIA: Inflammation of a subareolar mammary duct, which can lead to duct obstruction, a tender mass, duct discharge, and fever; a residual nodule may persist after resolution.

FIBROADENOMA: The most common benign breast tumor, typically affecting premenopausal women. Composed of fibrous and glandular tissue, it is classically rubbery and well encapsulated and may grow in pregnancy due to estrogen sensitivity.

FIBROCYSTIC CHANGE: Irregularity of breast tissue, described as feeling "lumpy."

GALACTOCELE: A milk-containing cyst caused by lactiferous duct obstruction, typically occurring during lactation or upon cessation of breastfeeding.

GALACTORRHEA: The spontaneous release of breast milk that is unassociated with lactation.

INTRADUCTAL PAPILLOMA: A benign growth of papillary cells into a mammary duct, classically presenting as a small palpable mass with unilateral bloody nipple discharge in premenopausal women.

MASTITIS: Inflammation of breast tissue that presents as a painful, swollen, erythematous breast. This may progress to infection and fever. Most common in lactating women, who can develop obstruction to milk drainage secondary to trauma associated with breastfeeding.

CLINICAL APPROACH

Palpable Breast Masses

Monthly BSEs are no longer recommended, as they have been shown to increase discovery of palpable lesions, raise anxiety, and increase the number of biopsies without decreasing mortality. The American Cancer Society (ACS) guidelines recommend that women practice "breast self-awareness," which refers to being familiar with how their breasts normally appear and feel and report any changes to their provider. Selected women may still opt to perform BSEs or be advised to do so (eg, those with breast implants); these women should perform BSEs when their breasts are not tender or swollen (eg, avoid the first week of the menstrual cycle). Women of average breast cancer risk should follow mammography screening guidelines per the US Preventive Services Task Force or ACS (Case 11). Women with increased breast cancer risk (see Table 49–1) may be subject to earlier or more frequent screening or risk-reducing medications such as tamoxifen, raloxifene, or aromatase inhibitors.

A new solid breast mass should be evaluated by **triple-test assessment, which includes (1) CBE, (2) imaging via ultrasound or mammography, and (3) tissue sampling for pathologic assessment.** Each of these components of the triple test is scored on a three-point scale (benign = 1 point, suspicious = 2 points, malignant = 3 points). Thus, a total triple test score of three to four is consistent with a benign lesion, but

Table 49–1 • RISK FACTORS FOR BREAST CANCER	
Demographic factors	Increasing age
	Female gender (1% of breast cancers occur in males)
	Race (greatest in non-Hispanic whites, followed by African Americans, and lowest among Asian/Pacific Islanders)
Personal medical history	Prior breast disease, including malignancy, carcinoma in situ, or atypical hyperplasia
	History of chest radiation
	Known genetic mutation associated with increased breast cancer (eg, *BRCA1* or *BRCA2*)
	Dense breast tissue visualized on mammogram
Intrinsic estrogen exposure	Early menarche (prior to age 12)
	Late menopause (after age 55)
	Nulliparity
	Increased age at time of first live birth (after age 30)
	Note: breastfeeding associated with *decreased* risk
Extrinsic estrogen exposure	Use of pharmacologic estrogen therapy, although recent studies question whether oral contraceptives pose significant risk
Family history	Breast cancer in a first-degree relative (eg, mother, sister, or daughter), especially if the cancer occurred prior to age 55
Lifestyle factors	Obesity
	Tobacco use
	Alcohol use (3 or more drinks per week)
	Note: physical activity associated with *decreased* risk

Table 49–2 • TYPICAL CHARACTERISTICS OF BREAST LUMPS ON PHYSICAL EXAMINATION		
Characteristic	More Likely Benign	Suspicious for Malignancy
Consistency	Soft	Firm/hard
Surface	Smooth, regular	Irregular
Mobility	Mobile	Fixed or tethered
Symptoms	Tender	Painless
Age	< 30 y	> 50 y

Data from Fauci AS, Braunwald E, Kasper DL, et al., eds. Harrison's Principles of Internal Medicine. *17th ed. 2008.*
Copyright © McGraw Hill LLC. All rights reserved.

a score greater than five likely warrants surgical intervention due to high suspicion of malignancy.

Clinical Breast Examination. Evaluation starts with a complete history, emphasizing factors that may confer an increased risk of breast cancer as well as changes in size over time, relation to menstrual cycle, and associated skin changes (eg, peau d'orange), nipple discharge, or constitutional symptoms. Specific characteristics of any palpable lumps, including size, location, tenderness, mobility, firmness, and distinction of the mass from the surrounding tissue should be noted, as well as any axillary or supraclavicular lymphadenopathy. These observations assist both in developing a diagnosis and in comparing serial examinations. The characteristics of the mass and the age of the woman will provide initial clues toward the likely diagnosis (Table 49–2). Additional associated findings suggestive of malignancy include overlying skin changes (dimpling, retraction, or erythema); bloody nipple discharge; and axillary or supraclavicular lymphadenopathy.

Imaging. The next component of the triple test is imaging. Generally, women under age 30 and pregnant women should be imaged with ultrasonography, whereas nonpregnant women over 30 should undergo mammography. Ultrasound is useful for distinguishing between cystic and solid lesions. Mammography enables identification of radiologic features of lesions that are suggestive of malignancy.

Tissue Sampling. **Fine-needle aspiration** provides the least invasive and simplest breast tissue evaluation. It is warranted for masses that are cystic and symptomatic. FNA that (1) returns clear, yellow, or green-tinged fluid and (2) results in complete resolution of the mass is diagnostic of a benign cyst. In this setting, the fluid can be discarded, and no further workup is necessary unless it recurs. Appropriate follow-up includes repeat CBE within 4 to 6 weeks to ensure no recurrence of the lesion.

Further evaluation via **stereotactic core-needle or excisional biopsy** is warranted if the mass does not completely resolve, the aspirated fluid is bloody, no fluid is aspirated, the lesion is complex (containing both cystic and solid components), or the lesion recurs on follow-up CBE. While more invasive and costlier than FNA, this procedure is more likely to provide a diagnostic sample. **Surgical excision** is the most invasive and expensive diagnostic method and is indicated when stereotactic biopsies detect **atypical ductal hyperplasia.** Surgical excision can be therapeutic by offering complete removal of the lesion.

Breast Pain

Breast pain (mastalgia) is the most frequent breast-related complaint for which women seek evaluation. As with breast lumps, the patient's primary fear is that the pain is a manifestation of breast cancer. However, **breast pain is not a common presentation of breast cancer,** particularly if bilateral. Regardless, the evaluation of mastalgia should include a careful history with attention to breast cancer risk factors, CBE, and screening mammography per guidelines to rule out malignancy.

Breast pain is categorized as cyclic, noncyclic, or extramammary. **Cyclic mastalgia,** pain that fluctuates with the woman's menstrual cycle, is usually diffuse and bilateral. Pain typically occurs during the late luteal phase when hormonal changes stimulate physiologic proliferation of glandular breast tissue and resolves with the onset of menses. It may also be attributable to hormonal contraceptives. **Noncyclic mastalgia** may be either continuous or intermittent but does not vary with the menstrual cycle. Common causes include stretching of Cooper ligaments by large breasts; various benign breast diseases (eg, cyst, abscess, fat necrosis, duct ectasia, or mastitis, as described previously); pregnancy; or hormone replacement therapy. **Extramammary pain** is defined as breast pain secondary to nonbreast pathology, such as musculoskeletal chest wall pain or radicular nerve pain. The etiology of most cases of chronic mastalgia is unknown and likely multifactorial.

Laboratory evaluation is generally limited to pregnancy testing in reproductive-age women. Many women require no further treatment beyond reassurance, but some experience significant pain that interferes with sexual activity, physical activity, social life, or professional life. First-line therapy is conservative and includes wearing a well-fitting supportive brassiere, reducing or discontinuing pharmacologic hormone therapy, stress reduction, and oral or topical analgesics. For refractory cases, second-line therapies include danazol (the only medication approved by the Food and Drug Administration for treatment of mastalgia) or tamoxifen; however, these are associated with significant side effects. Neither evening primrose oil nor caffeine reduction has been shown to provide significant relief.

Nipple Discharge and Galactorrhea

Benign Nipple Discharge. Nipple discharge is **usually caused by a benign process.** Up to 25% of women will have this symptom during their life. Nipple discharge that occurs only with nipple stimulation; that is clear, yellow, or green; and that appears from multiple ducts is usually physiologic and does not require further investigation. This discharge often resolves with efforts to reduce nipple stimulation, including refraining from checking to see if the discharge will continue to occur.

Pathologic Nipple Discharge. Nipple discharge that is spontaneous, persistent, bloody, from a single duct, associated with a mass, or present in women over age 40 is more likely to represent a pathologic process and requires prompt evaluation. The most common causes of pathologic discharge include intraductal papilloma, duct ectasia, cancer, and infection. If the discharge is not obviously bloody, then testing for occult blood via a guaiac-based assay should be performed.

Following the initial history and physical examination, mammography should be performed to evaluate for malignancy in all women with suspected pathologic nipple discharge. **The treatment of most cases of unilateral, spontaneous, or bloody**

nipple discharge is surgical excision of the involved terminal duct, allowing for both resolution and diagnosis.

Galactorrhea. Galactorrhea specifically refers to milky nipple discharge that occurs longer than 1 year postpartum, after breastfeeding cessation, or in the absence of parturition. The condition is most common in women aged 20 to 35 years old and in parous women. Galactorrhea is associated with various medical conditions, including hypothyroidism, hypothalamic-pituitary disorders, hormone-secreting neoplasms (eg, pituitary adenoma), and chronic renal failure; however, galactorrhea **is not associated with breast cancer.** Numerous pharmacologic agents can cause galactorrhea via pituitary dopamine inhibition. Common complicit medications include antidepressants such as selective serotonin reuptake inhibitors or tricyclic antidepressants; antipsychotics such as risperidone; H_2 receptor antagonists such as cimetidine; gastrointestinal motility agents such as metoclopramide; antiandrogenic medications such as spironolactone; and opiates. Additionally, hormonal contraceptives may cause galactorrhea by directly stimulating the pituitary lactotrophs and suppressing hypothalamic secretion of prolactin inhibitory factor.

The first step in the workup of galactorrhea is to rule out pregnancy. Next, the clinician must evaluate for endocrinopathies, such as hypothyroidism and prolactinoma, through history, examination, and laboratory testing of thyroid-stimulating hormone (TSH) and prolactin levels. Potentially offending pharmacologic agents should be discontinued if possible. Treatment of galactorrhea should be aimed at the underlying etiology: levothyroxine for hypothyroidism, dopamine agonists for hyperprolactinemia, and rarely, surgical resection of prolactinoma.

CASE CORRELATION

- See Case 11 (Adult Female Health Maintenance) and Case 28 (Family Planning—Contraceptives).

COMPREHENSION QUESTIONS

49.1 A 34-year-old nulliparous woman presents with 1 month of bilateral milky nipple discharge. Review of systems is negative for breast, endocrine, or neurologic symptoms. She was prescribed risperidone 2 months ago for newly diagnosed schizophrenia. CBE reveals expressible milky discharge. The thyroid gland is not palpable. Urine pregnancy test is negative. Serum TSH and free T_4 levels are within normal limits. Which of the following is the most accurate advice to give to this woman?

A. The nipple discharge likely contains occult blood due to a benign breast disease.

B. Her clinical presentation is highly suspicious for breast malignancy.

C. This condition is likely attributable to her antipsychotic medication.

D. Her normal examination and serologic testing are indicative of a physiologic process.

49.2 A 52-year-old woman presents to her family health care provider with a palpable breast mass. Menarche occurred at age 10, and she had her first child at age 24. She takes low-dose oral contraceptive pills and calcium supplements daily. Her mother was diagnosed with breast cancer at age 45. She has never smoked tobacco and drinks alcohol socially. An attempt at FNA does not result in aspiration of fluid. Her mammogram is normal. Which of the following is the appropriate next step in evaluation of this patient?

A. Repeat clinical examination in 4 to 6 weeks

B. Repeat mammogram routinely in 1 year

C. Refer for core-needle biopsy

D. Discontinue her hormonal contraceptive medication

49.3 A 29-year-old woman presents with unilateral breast pain. Which of the following histories, if true, is most concerning for a malignant process?

A. Associated symptoms include fever, chills, malaise, and erythema of the skin of the affected breast. The pain is severe enough that it prohibits her from breastfeeding her 3-month-old infant on that breast.

B. She initially attributed the pain to bruising over the left breast secondary to trauma sustained in a recent motor vehicle accident in which she was the restrained driver, but she became concerned when she incidentally noted a new irregular mass in the breast tissue underlying the healing bruises.

C. The pain is associated with erythema, swelling, warmth, and dimpling of the skin over the affected breast. She recently noted a nontender lump in the ipsilateral axilla.

D. The pain is localized to a spot in the upper outer quadrant of the right breast. She recently also noted a well-circumscribed, mobile lump there that has grown in size over the past few weeks. She is especially concerned about her health because she is 6 months pregnant.

49.4 A 22-year-old woman presents with the complaint of a palpable, firm, mobile, 2-cm mass in the 12 o'clock position on her right breast. She states that it has been present for almost 6 months, does not change with her menstrual cycle, and is not painful. She smokes approximately 8 to 10 cigarettes daily, drinks three or four cups of caffeinated coffee daily, and rarely drinks alcohol. She has no personal or family history of breast cancer. Which of the following is the most appropriate initial evaluation of this mass?

A. Surgical excision

B. Mammogram

C. Ultrasound

D. Fine-needle aspiration

ANSWERS

49.1 **C.** This woman's galactorrhea likely represents a side effect of her antipsychotic medication. Discharge that is spontaneous, unilateral, persistent, bloody, or associated with a mass is more likely due to pathologic processes—either benign (eg, intraductal papilloma, duct ectasia) or malignant—and requires full evaluation. In this case, the discharge is unlikely to be physiologic (answer D) in the absence of pregnancy or breastfeeding history. Initial workup has appropriately ruled out pregnancy and hypothyroidism; the prolactin level should also be tested. A milky discharge is not indicative of cancer (answer B). Milky breast discharge is almost always benign and non-bloody (answer A).

49.2 **C.** Biopsy is the next most appropriate step. Tissue diagnosis is a required element of the triple-test evaluation for breast malignancy, especially given her history of early menarche and known first-degree relative with breast cancer diagnosed at a young age. A negative mammogram (answer B) is not diagnostic of a benign process and does not rule out breast cancer. Monitoring for changes through serial clinical examinations (answer A) will inappropriately delay workup. The lump is not attributable to her hormonal medications (answer D).

49.3 **C.** Inflammatory carcinoma presents with erythematous, warm, tender, thickened, and dimpling breast skin that resembles an orange peel (described as a "peau d'orange" appearance). The axillary lump is concerning for lymphadenopathy. Mastitis classically causes fever, malaise, and breast pain in lactating women (answer A). A new lump following breast trauma (answer B) likely represents fat necrosis, but it should be fully evaluated in case the trauma just brought attention to a preexisting lesion. Fibroadenomas are well-circumscribed, mobile, sometimes tender masses that are estrogen responsive and thus may grow during pregnancy (answer D).

49.4 **C.** Ultrasound is the most appropriate first step in the evaluation of this lesion. In a 22-year-old woman with the characteristics of a 1- to 2-cm non-tender mobile breast mass, the most likely diagnosis is a fibroadenoma, which is a benign smooth muscle tumor. Breast sonography can characterize whether the lesion is cystic or solid. If it is cystic, then FNA (answer D) may be considered. If it is solid, then mammography (answer B) may be considered, but for a 22-year-old patient, the fibrous tissue may make mammography less reliable. Hence, if the ultrasound findings are very diagnostic for a fibroadenoma, then observation with careful monitoring is often employed. Answer A (surgical excision) may eventually be the treatment, but initially, characterizing the lesion is the first step.

CLINICAL PEARLS

▶ Breast health maintenance should be discussed with all female patients, including the need for breast self-awareness, age-appropriate mammography screening, understanding of personal breast cancer risk, and the lack of evidence to support regular BSEs.

▶ It may be natural for women to worry that their breast-related complaint represents cancer. Clinicians must not only properly work up and manage the presenting condition, but they should also provide appropriate reassurance.

▶ All breast masses require evaluation and should never simply be dismissed. Triple-test workup, including CBE, imaging, and tissue sampling, provides complete evaluation of breast lesions and informs treatment decisions.

▶ Approximately 1% of breast cancer occurs in men. A new palpable mass in a man's breast should prompt a diagnostic evaluation.

REFERENCES

ACS releases guideline on breast cancer screening. *Am Fam Physician*. 2016;93(8):712.

American Cancer Society. Breast cancer facts and figures 2017–2018. http://www.cancer.org/content/cancer/en/research/cancer-facts-statistics.html. Accessed February 9, 2019.

Bleyer A, Welch HG. Effect of three decades of screening mammography on breast-cancer incidence. *N Engl J Med*. 2012;367:1998-2005.

Cancer stat facts: female breast cancer. National Cancer Institute. https://seer.cancer.gov/statfacts/html/breast.html. Published 2018. Accessed February 9, 2019.

Reid CM, Grigorian A, de Virgilio C, Hari DM. New palpable mass in right breast. In: deVirgilio C, Frank PN, Grigorian A, eds. *Surgery: A Case Based Clinical Review*. New York, NY: Springer; 2015: 25-36.

Salzman B, Collins, Hersh L. Common breast problems. *Am Fam Physician*. 2019;99(8):505-514.

US Preventive Services Task Force. Final Recommendation Statement: Breast Cancer: Medication Use to Reduce Risk. https://www.uspreventiveservicestaskforce.org/uspstf/recommendation/breast-cancer-medications-for-risk-reduction. Accessed June 30, 2020

A 28-year-old nulliparous woman presents for evaluation of irregular menstrual cycles for the past year. They occur on average only once every 2 or 3 months, and she has gone as long as 4 months without a cycle. Currently, she states her last cycle occurred 11 weeks ago. Her cycles have been "mostly" regular, usually occurring every 30 days. Her menarche occurred at age 13, and she has never been on hormonal contraception. She does not smoke, does not drink alcohol, and does not exercise. She is sexually active in a monogamous relationship with a male partner who uses condoms for contraception. On review of systems, she reports a 30-lb weight gain in the past 18 months but denies other constitutional symptoms. On examination, she is noted to be obese, with a body mass index of 36 kg/m^2, and her other vital signs are within normal limits. She has fine hair growth on her face and a velvety thickening of the skin on her neck. Her general physical examination is unremarkable. A pelvic examination reveals normal external genitalia, no vaginal or cervical discharge, no cervical motion tenderness, and no uterine or adnexal masses.

▶ What is the most likely diagnosis?
▶ What is the initial step in evaluation of this condition?
▶ What therapy can best regulate her menstrual cycle?

ANSWERS TO CASE 50:
Menstrual Cycle Irregularity

Summary: A 28-year-old woman presents with

- Irregular menstrual cycles over the past year
- Obesity, with a 30-lb weight gain in the past 18 months
- Hirsutism
- Acanthosis nigricans, a skin condition characterized by dark, velvety discoloration in body creases whereby the skin becomes thickened
- A monogamous relationship with a male partner who uses condoms for contraception
- An unremarkable pelvic examination

Most likely diagnosis: Anovulatory menstrual cycles secondary to polycystic ovary syndrome (PCOS).

Initial step in evaluation: Pregnancy test.

Therapy to regulate menstrual cycle: Oral contraceptive pills.

ANALYSIS

Objectives

1. Learn the common causes of irregular menstrual cycles. (EPA 1, 2)

2. Develop an understanding of a rational workup of menstrual cycle abnormalities. (EPA 3)

3. Learn the management of common menstrual cycle disorders. (EPA 5)

Considerations

Menstrual cycles are considered normal if they occur at regular intervals of 21 to 35 days in length. During their reproductive years, most women will at some point experience early, late, or missed menstrual cycles, and this is considered normal. When this occurs on a rare occasion and pregnancy is ruled out, watchful waiting is usually indicated, with resumption of normal menstrual cycles almost always occurring.

The differential diagnosis of persistent menstrual cycle irregularities is broad. Pregnancy must be ruled out in a woman with a significant menstrual pattern change. After pregnancy is excluded, numerous neuroendocrine and genitourinary conditions must be considered.

In our case of an obese, hirsute woman with ongoing weight gain and irregular menses, PCOS should be the initial consideration after pregnancy has been excluded. PCOS is defined as a syndrome of insulin resistance and androgen excess and has substantial metabolic impact. It is associated with infertility, hirsutism, acne, obesity, and metabolic syndrome. PCOS is diagnosed via the Rotterdam criteria, requiring two of the following three manifestations:

- Hyperandrogenism, evidenced by hirsutism or elevated serum androgen levels (eg, testosterone, androstenedione, or dehydroepiandrostenedione)

- Oligomenorrhea with cycle length greater than or equal to 35 days

- Multifollicular ovaries on pelvic ultrasound, defined as 12 or greater small follicles in an ovary

Anovulation is the menstrual cycle irregularity associated with PCOS. Without ovulation, there is a failure of luteal production of progesterone, resulting in an absence of normal menstruation. Women with PCOS can have induced menstrual bleeding by providing periodic supplemental progesterone or by using combination oral contraceptive pills (estrogen and progesterone). Weight loss is very important in women with PCOS to increase fertility, as a loss of even 2% to 5% of body weight can greatly increase rates of pregnancy. Insulin resistance in PCOS is treated with metformin. Infertility secondary to PCOS is treated with clomiphene or letrozole.

APPROACH TO:
Menstrual Cycle Irregularity

DEFINITIONS

ABNORMAL UTERINE BLEEDING (AUB): Heavy and irregular vaginal bleeding, defined as greater than 80 mL of blood, that leads to anemia without iron supplementation.

AMENORRHEA: Absence of menstrual bleeding for 6 or more months, or the length of three or more cycles, when a woman is not pregnant.

HEAVY MENSTRUAL BLEEDING (HMB) PREVIOUSLY CALLED MENORRHAGIA: Heavy menstrual flow occurring at regular intervals or prolonged duration of flow (> 7 days), occurring at regular intervals.

METRORRHAGIA: Bleeding occurring at irregular intervals.

OLIGOMENORRHEA: Menses that have an interval of greater than 35 days.

PALM COEIN: A mnemonic to list the various causes of AUB, with the PALM representing anatomical causes (polyps, adenomyosis, leiomyomata, malignancy) and COEIN indicating other causes (coagulopathy, ovulatory, endometrial, iatrogenic, not otherwise specified).

CLINICAL APPROACH

Normal Menstrual Cycles

In a normal (highly simplified) menstrual cycle, the hypothalamus secretes gonadotropin-releasing hormone, which stimulates the anterior pituitary to secrete follicle-stimulating hormone (FSH) and luteinizing hormone (LH). As the FSH level rises, it causes an ovarian follicle to mature and release estrogen, which induces endometrial proliferation. A midcycle LH surge causes ovulation, and the follicle is transformed into the corpus luteum, which secretes progesterone, which compacts and matures the endometrium. If pregnancy does not occur, the production of progesterone abruptly decreases, resulting in sloughing of the endometrium and a menstrual bleed. Abnormal bleeding can occur with regular menstrual cycles or irregular menstrual cycles; causes are discussed in the material that follows.

History and Physical Examination

History. A thorough history is the initial component of the evaluation of menstrual irregularities. The history of the presenting complaint should examine both the specific abnormality that is occurring and when it was first noted. Encouraging the woman with menstrual irregularities to use a menstrual calendar can be very valuable in this setting. Associated symptoms, including weight gain or loss, galactorrhea, and heat or cold intolerance, should be documented. A complete past medical history should be obtained, including a complete reproductive health history detailing age at menarche; history of any previous menstrual cycle abnormalities; medications (especially anticoagulants, phenytoin, antipsychotics, tricyclic antidepressants, and corticosteroids); contraception; infections; surgeries; and sexual practices, along with pregnancies and their outcomes. A social history focusing on psychosocial stressors, substance use, exercise, eating habits, and sexual activity should be documented.

General Physical Examination. The general physical examination should attempt to identify medical conditions that can cause menstrual abnormalities. Extremes of body mass index—both obese and underweight conditions—can directly affect menstruation. Hirsutism and/or acne should prompt the clinician to consider a workup for androgen excess. The thyroid gland should be examined for size, consistency, and the presence of nodules. Skin and hair changes may also occur with thyroid and other endocrine conditions. Breasts should be examined for galactorrhea. Unexplained bruising or easy bleeding may occur with concomitant coagulopathies.

Pelvic Examination. The pelvic examination is a critical component in the evaluation of the woman with menstrual irregularities. Initial efforts should be made to determine whether the blood is coming from the uterus or another anatomic site, as urethral, rectal, vaginal wall, or cervical bleeding can easily be mistaken for menstrual abnormality. Signs of pelvic infection should be noted and cultures collected, as cervicitis may predispose to cervical bleeding. A Papanicolaou (Pap) smear should be performed according to current cervical cancer screening guidelines. A bimanual examination should note the size and consistency of the uterus and the presence of any uterine or adnexal masses or tenderness. In women who have never been sexually active, the pelvic examination should be conducted carefully. Unless the bleeding is severe, in which case examination under anesthesia may be warranted, the examination may be deferred until after a trial of medical therapy. A pelvic ultrasound may also be considered to evaluate for potential anatomic abnormalities, including uterine fibroids or masses, adnexal masses, or tumors.

PALM COEIN. This mnemonic is a useful way of characterizing the various causes and helping clinicians to be more systematic in classifying the etiology and grading the severity. For example, part of the PALM COEIN nomenclature for

AUB caused by leiomyomata (fibroids) is designated AUB-L, and further sub-divided from numbers 0 (submucosal < 50% intramural within the body of the uterus) up to 7 (subserosal and pedunculated).

Abnormal Bleeding Associated With Regular Menstrual Cycles

Causes of Heavy Menstrual Bleeding. HMB with regular intervals between bleeding suggests that regular ovulation is occurring. This implies that the endocrine pathways are functioning normally and that the problem may be anatomic within the genital or hematologic system. **Leiomyomata** (uterine fibroids), especially those that are submucosal in the uterus, are a common cause of heavy uterine bleeding. They create an increased endometrial surface area with a resultant increase in menstrual bleeding. **Endometrial polyps** may cause HMB by a similar mechanism. **Coagulopathy that is inherited (most commonly von Willebrand disease) or due to medications (eg, warfarin) is also a common cause of abnormal menstrual bleeding.** Liver disease, thrombocytopenia, and hematologic disorders predisposing to bleeding may also contribute to HMB.

Causes of Oligomenorrhea. Reduced volume of menstrual bleeding associated with regular ovulation is a less common occurrence. **Asherman syndrome** occurs with scarring within the uterine cavity caused by trauma from uterine curettage. It can result in the reduction in the size of the uterus as the walls become scarred and adherent to each other. This may result in minimal or even absent menstruation in the setting of normal hormonal function. A scarred and obstructed cervical os can cause a similar clinical picture.

Abnormal Bleeding Associated With Irregular Menstrual Cycles

Pathophysiology. Bleeding that is unpredictable in terms of timing and flow is known as dysfunctional uterine bleeding (DUB) and generally implies an abnormality within the hypothalamic-pituitary-ovarian axis. This pattern commonly occurs shortly after menarche and as a woman approaches menopause. At other times, it signals anovulation. In this setting, the endometrium is continuously stimulated by estrogen and sloughs off irregularly. Chronic anovulation should be evaluated with serum prolactin and LH levels.

Continuous estrogen stimulation can also lead to endometrial hyperplasia and endometrial carcinoma. **Risk factors for endometrial carcinoma include an age older than 50 years, hypertension, thyroid disease, diabetes, Lynch syndrome, or any history of unopposed exogenous estrogen, such as tamoxifen therapy, early menarche, late menopause, nulliparity, or anovulatory menstrual cycles.**

Evaluation. The **evaluation of a woman with DUB is dependent on age and risk factors.** In the period after menarche, watchful waiting is usually indicated, with correction of the problem usually occurring within 1 to 2 years. In women younger than 35 years who are not at increased risk of endometrial cancer, treatment including hormonal cycling may be offered without workup beyond the history and physical examination.

Further evaluation is indicated for women with risk factors for endometrial cancer, women younger than age 35 years with continued symptoms despite treatment, and postmenopausal women with uterine bleeding. The standard workup includes a pelvic ultrasound and an endometrial biopsy. **Transvaginal pelvic ultrasound** provides information on uterine size and the presence of masses and can assess the thickness of the endometrium, which correlates with the risk of hyperplasia. An **endometrial biopsy** can be performed quickly and easily in the office setting, using a thin, disposable sampling device. The combination of sonographic measurement of endometrial thickness and endometrial biopsy is highly sensitive and specific for the diagnosis of endometrial cancer. **Hysteroscopy** (endoscopic evaluation of the uterine cavity) can directly visualize endometrial masses, polyps, or other abnormalities and allows for directed biopsy. It is often performed with **dilation and curettage**, which sharply removes almost the entire endometrial lining for diagnostic and therapeutic purposes.

Treatment. When the workup does not reveal malignancy, **anovulatory bleeding is usually responsive to treatment with either combined estrogen and progestin oral contraceptives or progestin alone.** A progestin can be given for 7 to 10 days with a subsequent withdrawal bleed expected to occur within a week following the completion of the course. Both of these regimens have been shown to reduce the risk of developing endometrial hyperplasia and carcinoma. When medical treatments fail, or when symptoms are severe, surgical options may be required. Hysterectomy provides definitive treatment and is necessary in the case of a malignancy. Endometrial ablative procedures are also available and widely used.

CASE CORRELATION

- See Case 11 (Adult Female Health Maintenance), Case 28 (Family Planning—Contraceptives) and Case 29 (Adolescent Health Maintenance).

COMPREHENSION QUESTIONS

50.1 A 42-year-old obese gravida 2, para 2 (G2P2) woman presents for evaluation of irregular menstrual bleeding for a year. She has had painless vaginal bleeding in various amounts at various times of the month. She has a history of smoking a half a pack of cigarettes per day for 10 years. She has two children, is on no medications, and has no significant medical history. She took an oral contraceptive agent for 5 years during her teen years. Her examination reveals her uterus to be slightly enlarged, but without masses or tenderness. The remainder of her examination is unremarkable. A pregnancy test is negative. Which of the following is the most significant risk factor for the patient developing endometrial cancer?

    A. Smoking

    B. Parity

    C. Body habitus

    D. History of oral contraceptive use

50.2 A 35-year-old nulliparous woman has had irregular menstrual cycles since high school. She frequently misses cycles and has never been pregnant. When she has cycles, they are very light and last for only a few days. She has had mild-to-moderate comedonal and pustular acne since late adolescence and in recent years has developed some hair growing under her chin. She denies taking any medications or history of other gynecologic or medical problems. Which of the following is the most appropriate evaluation for the initial workup of her problem?

A. Serum thyroid-stimulating hormone (TSH)

B. Serum karyotype

C. Serum estradiol

D. Urine cortisol

E. Serum FSH

50.3 A 28-year-old woman complains of irregular spotting between cycles for the past 2 months. She has been previously healthy and has never been pregnant. She has been sexually active for the past 6 months with the same male partner. On examination, her only positive findings are a mildly enlarged and moderately tender uterus. Her pregnancy test is negative. Which of the following is the most probable diagnosis?

A. Uterine leiomyoma

B. Cervical carcinoma

C. Endometritis

D. Endometrial cancer

E. Urinary tract infection

ANSWERS

50.1 **C.** This patient's obesity is the most significant risk factor for endometrial cancer due to chronically elevated unopposed estrogen levels stored in adipose tissue. Parity (answer B) is protective for endometrial cancer. Risk factors for endometrial cancer include anovulatory menstrual cycles, obesity, nulliparity, age greater than 35 years, and use of tamoxifen or unopposed exogenous estrogen. Interestingly, smoking (answer A) is a negative risk factor for endometrial cancer. Answer D (history of oral contraceptive use) decreases the risk of endometrial cancer since the progestin exposure decreases endometrial mitosis, hyperplasia, and cancer.

50.2 **A.** Thyroid-stimulating hormone is indicated in AUB workup. Both total serum testosterone levels and prolactin are useful. In general, a pregnancy test, TSH, and prolactin level are the initial tests for the evaluation of menstrual irregularities. Estrogen (answer C) does not have a role in the initial workup for anovulation. Serum karyotype (answer B) is useful for premature ovarian insufficiency but not for anovulation. Answer E (serum FSH) is useful if there is a possibility of premature ovarian insufficiency, which usually presents with a history of hot flushes and oligomenorrhea. Urine cortisol (answer D) may help in the diagnosis of Cushing disease but is not generally indicated unless the patient has other stigmata of corticosteroid excess, such as abdominal striae, easy bruisability, and buffalo hump.

50.3 **C.** Endometritis is a common cause of vaginal spotting. It is generally a poly-microbial infection caused by an ascending infection of normal vaginal flora. Commonly isolated organisms include *Neisseria gonorrhoeae, Chlamydia tra-chomatis, Ureaplasma urealyticum, Peptostreptococcus, Gardnerella vaginalis,* and group B streptococcus. The patient's history makes cervical cancer (answer B) less likely. Leiomyoma (answer A) or polyps are possible, but these are less likely with her history of recent spotting and sexual activity. Endometrial cancer (answer D) would also be unlikely in a patient with previously regular menses. While a urinary tract infection (answer E) may cause hematuria in cases of severe cystitis, it would not cause uterine enlargement or tenderness. The diagnosis of endometritis can be confirmed with an endometrial biopsy showing inflammatory cells, particularly plasma cells.

CLINICAL PEARLS

▶ The first test performed on a woman with menstrual cycle irregularities should be a pregnancy test.

▶ The newer terminology for abnormal menses that is heavy, prolonged, and associated with anemia is AUB.

▶ The mnemonic PALM COEIN is a useful model in categorizing AUB and determining severity.

▶ Heavy menstrual bleeding is the newer terminology for menorrhagia and refers to heavy vaginal bleeding at regular intervals.

▶ A history of anovulatory cycles does not confer absolute protection against pregnancy. Ovulation may occur intermittently and irregularly. If a woman does not want to become pregnant, she should be counseled on contraceptive options.

▶ In general, the most common cause of AUB that is irregular is PCOS.

▶ Women with PCOS should be treated and monitored appropriately due to an elevated risk of metabolic syndrome and cardiovascular disease.

REFERENCES

Braun MM, Overbeek-Wager EA, Grumbo RJ. Diagnosis and management of endometrial cancer. *Am Fam Physician.* 2016;93(6):468-474.

Ely JW, Kennedy CM, Clark EC, Bowdler NC. Abnormal uterine bleeding: a management algorithm. *J Am Board Fam Med.* 2006;19:590-602.

Hall JE. Disorders of the female reproductive system. In: Jameson J, Fauci AS, Kasper DL, Hauser SL, Longo DL, Loscalzo J, eds, *Harrison's Principles of Internal Medicine*. 20th ed. New York, NY: McGraw Hill; 2018: Chap. 385. http://accessmedicine.mhmedical.com/content.aspx?bookid=2129&sectionid=192287740. Accessed December 13, 2018.

Hall JE. Menstrual disorders and pelvic pain. In: Jameson J, Fauci AS, Kasper DL, Hauser SL, Longo DL, Loscalzo J, eds. *Harrison's Principles of Internal Medicine*. 20th ed. New York, NY: McGraw Hill; 2018: Chap. 386. http://accessmedicine.mhmedical.com/content.aspx?bookid=2129&sectionid=192287811. Accessed December 13, 2018.

Hickey M, Higham JM, Fraser I. Progestogens with or without estrogen for irregular uterine bleeding associated with anovulation. *Cochrane Database Syst Rev*. 2012;(9):CD001895.

Klein DA, Poth MA. Amenorrhea: an approach to diagnosis and management. *Am Fam Physician*. 2013;87(11):781-788.

Norman RJ, Dewailly D, Legro RS, Hickey TE. Polycystic ovary syndrome. *Lancet*. 2007;370:685-697.

Osayande AS, Mehulic S. Diagnosis and initial management of dysmenorrhea. *Am Fam Physician*. 2014;89(5):341-346.

Sweet MG, Schmidt-Dalton TA, Weiss PM. Evaluation and management of abnormal uterine bleeding in premenopausal women. *Am Fam Physician*. 2012;85(1):35-43.

Teede H, Deeks A, Moran L. Polycystic ovary syndrome: a complex condition with psychological, reproductive, and metabolic manifestations that impacts on health across the lifespan. *BMC Med*. 2010;8:41.

Williams T, Mortada R, Porter S. Diagnosis and treatment of polycystic ovary syndrome. *Am Fam Physician*. 2016;94(2):106-113.

Wong CL, Farquhar C, Roberts H, Proctor M. Oral contraceptive pill as treatment for primary dysmenorrhea. *Cochrane Database Syst Rev*. 2009;(4):CD002120.

A 34-year-old obese woman presents to your office with a chief complaint of recurrent yeast infections and increased thirst. She also has noticed increased urinary frequency, but she believes this is related to her yeast infection. Over the last several years, she has gained more than 40 lb despite having tried numerous diets, most recently a low-carbohydrate, high-protein and fat diet. The patient's only other pertinent history is that she was told to "watch her diet" during pregnancy because of excessive weight gain. Her baby had to be delivered at 38 weeks via cesarean section 2 years ago because he weighed more than 10 lb (> 4500 g). Her family history is unknown, as she is adopted. On physical examination, her blood pressure is 155/94 mm Hg, her pulse is 72 beats/min, and her respiratory rate is 16 breaths/min. Her height is 65 inches, and her weight is 223 lb (body mass index [BMI] = 37.1 kg/m²). On examination, she has darkened skin that appears to be thickened on the back of her neck and moist, reddened skin beneath her breasts. Her pelvic examination reveals a thick, white vaginal discharge. A wet preparation from the vaginal discharge shows branching hyphae consistent with *Candida* species. A urinalysis is negative for leukocyte esterase, nitrites, protein, and glucose.

▶ What is the most likely primary diagnosis for this patient?
▶ What physical findings are suggestive of the diagnosis and have implications for management?
▶ What diagnostic studies should be ordered at this time?

ANSWERS TO CASE 51:

Diabetes Mellitus

Summary: A 34-year-old woman presents with

- Recurrent yeast infections, polydipsia, and polyuria
- A 40-lb weight gain despite efforts to lose weight
- Obesity—BMI of 37.1—and a report that she was told to watch her diet during pregnancy 2 years ago
- Acanthosis nigricans, *Candida* vaginitis, and a negative urinalysis
- Blood pressure of 155/94 mm Hg and other vital signs within normal limits

Most likely primary diagnosis: Type 2 diabetes mellitus.

Physical findings: Obesity, acanthosis nigricans, blood pressure that is elevated for a diabetic, *Candida* vaginitis, and likely *Candida* skin infection under her breasts.

Diagnostic studies: Fasting serum glucose measurement and glycosylated hemoglobin level (HbA_{1c}); comprehensive metabolic panel, including electrolytes and renal function; fasting lipid panel; and urine microalbumin/creatinine ratio.

ANALYSIS

Objectives

1. List the diagnostic criteria for diabetes mellitus, including classic signs and symptoms, physical findings, and diagnostic studies. (EPA 1, 3)

2. Compare and contrast the pathophysiologic and epidemiologic differences between type 1 and type 2 diabetes mellitus. (EPA 12)

3. List the treatment options for diabetic patients. (EPA 4, 12)

4. Describe the acute emergencies that can occur in diabetic patients and how to manage them. (EPA 1, 4, 10)

Considerations

Diabetes mellitus is one of the most common diseases encountered in medical practice. It was the seventh leading cause of death in the United States in 2015. There are an estimated 30.3 million diabetics in the United States, of which 23.1 million were diagnosed and 7.2 million were undiagnosed. Nearly one in four adults in the United States also qualifies as "prediabetic"; therefore, over 35% of the US population can be classified as either diabetic or prediabetic. Diabetes affects all ethnic groups, but there is a disproportionate burden of disease in African Americans, Native Americans, and Hispanics. While some diabetics exhibit the classic symptoms of polyuria, polydipsia, polyphagia, and weight loss, many patients are diagnosed when asymptomatic.

The complications of diabetes are myriad. Diabetics are 6 to 10 times more likely than nondiabetics to be hospitalized for cardiovascular disease and 15 times more likely to be hospitalized for peripheral vascular disease. **It is the leading cause of blindness in working-age adults in the United States,** most of which is preventable. It is also the leading cause of end-stage renal disease requiring dialysis and of nontraumatic amputations. It is estimated that patients with diabetes have an average of 2.3 times higher medical expenditures than they would in the absence of diabetes.

Other common complications of diabetes include neuropathic, gastrointestinal, and immunologic disease. **Peripheral neuropathy**, leading to reduced sensation or pain, can result in the development of injuries, ulcerations, infections, or amputations of the extremities. Gastroparesis is a chronic problem that commonly causes nausea and vomiting and impairs the patient's ability to maintain an adequate nutritional status. Poorly controlled diabetics suffer relative immunosuppression that makes them more prone to opportunistic infections, including bacterial and fungal skin and genitourinary infections.

Impaired glucose tolerance, or elevated serum glucose levels, may be present for years prior to a formal diagnosis of type 2 diabetes mellitus. In the case presented, the history of excessive weight gain during pregnancy with a fetal macrosomia (> 4500 g or 9 lb, 4 oz) and advice to watch her diet should prompt the clinician to suspect a history of gestational diabetes. Women who have gestational diabetes are at a three-fold increased risk of developing diabetes later in life.

The symptoms of polydipsia and polyuria should lead the clinician to an increased suspicion for the evaluation of diabetes. High serum glucose levels function as an osmotic diuretic, resulting in frequent urination. Patients with diabetes also may present with polyphagia, as their insulin deficiency prevents food intake from being properly metabolized, resulting in a state of hunger for which they will frequently eat but not feel satiated.

APPROACH TO:
Diabetes Mellitus

DEFINITIONS

GESTATIONAL DIABETES: New-onset glucose intolerance during pregnancy that often resolves after delivery but is associated with a significantly increased risk for developing postpartum diabetes.

TYPE 1 DIABETES: Often referred to as "juvenile diabetes" but can occur in adults; the exact pathophysiologic mechanism is unknown, but it is thought to be autoimmune. Current theories support the notion that an infection or an environmental or genetic trigger causes the body to mistakenly attack pancreatic beta cells that make insulin.

TYPE 2 DIABETES: Often referred to as "adult onset;" primarily due to insulin resistance and a resulting relative deficiency of insulin. It is strongly associated with obesity and has an even more significant genetic component than type 1 diabetes.

CLINICAL APPROACH

Diagnosis

Diabetes mellitus is a general term for several different variations of disease along a spectrum; these variations result in high blood glucose levels that, if uncontrolled over a period of time, eventually lead to microvascular and macrovascular complications. The major classifications of diabetes mellitus are type 1 diabetes, type 2 diabetes, and gestational diabetes.

The American College of Endocrinology diagnostic criteria for diabetes are any of the following:

1. A fasting plasma glucose ≥ 126 mg/dL (no caloric intake for at least 8 hours)

2. A 2-hour plasma glucose ≥ 200 mg/dL after a 75-g glucose load (ie, glucose tolerance test [GTT])

3. Random plasma glucose ≥ 200 mg/dL plus symptoms (eg, polydipsia, polyuria)

4. Glycosylated hemoglobin (HbA$_{1c}$) ≥ 6.5%

Glycosylated hemoglobin A$_{1c}$ is used to estimate the average glucose levels over the past 3 months for appropriate monitoring and goal setting in those who are diagnosed with diabetes. A hemoglobin A$_{1c}$ < 6% is considered a normal value, while values between 6% and 6.5% are considered "prediabetes." In patients with hemoglobinopathies (eg, sickle cell anemia), recent blood loss, or a recent drastic change in diet (eg, no or extremely low-carbohydrate diet), serum fructosamine levels should be obtained; these levels indicate average glucose levels over a 2- to 3-week period.

Measurement of C-peptide and insulin levels can be used to distinguish type 2 from type 1 diabetes when the history, physical examination, and other tests, such as serum ketones and osmolality, are not enough. Extremely low insulin and C-peptide levels support a diagnosis of type 1 rather than type 2 diabetes mellitus. The American Diabetes Association recommends lipid profiles (at the time of diagnosis and at least annually thereafter); serum creatinine; urinalysis; urine microalbumin/creatinine ratios (at time of diagnosis in type 2 diabetics and annually thereafter; in type 1 diabetics who have had disease for 5 years and annually thereafter); annual dilated eye examinations; monofilament foot examinations; electrocardiogram (in adults); and thyroid disease screening with a thyroid-stimulating hormone level in type 1 diabetics.

Glucosuria occurs when the blood glucose level is greater than the renal threshold of excretion, often estimated at a serum level of 180 mg/dL, the level that approximates a glycosylated hemoglobin level of 8%. Overt signs of insulin resistance (eg, acanthosis nigricans, elevated blood pressure, obesity) also make the diagnosis of type 2 diabetes more likely.

The general approach to managing diabetes mellitus is aimed at secondary prevention of macrovascular (eg, accelerated coronary artery disease, accelerated cerebral and peripheral vascular disease) and microvascular (eg, retinopathy, nephropathy, and neuropathy) complications.

Type 1 Diabetes

Type 1 diabetes, or insulin-dependent diabetes mellitus (IDDM), is a chronic disease of carbohydrate, fat, and protein metabolism due to a lack of insulin resulting from autoimmune destruction of insulin-producing pancreatic beta cells. Due to the lack of insulin, which is required for glucose and carbohydrate metabolism, type 1 diabetics are prone to metabolizing fats, with the resultant production of ketones. This process may lead to **diabetic ketoacidosis (DKA),** a syndrome characterized by hyperglycemia usually greater than 250 mg/mL, high levels of serum acetone and beta-hydroxybutyrate, and an anion gap metabolic acidosis. Patients often present with vomiting, abdominal pain, extreme thirst, and, in severe cases, labored deep breathing (Kussmaul breathing). DKA often occurs during times of physical stress, such as an infection or myocardial infarction, or when the patient does not properly take insulin. DKA is a medical emergency requiring hospitalization, vigorous intravenous hydration with normal saline, correction of the acidosis and electrolyte disturbances, aggressive insulin management, and evaluation for the underlying cause of the condition.

Type 2 Diabetes

Type 2 diabetes was previously called adult-onset diabetes mellitus (AODM) and is still commonly called non–insulin-dependent diabetes mellitus (NIDDM). These patients, in contrast to type 1 diabetics in whom there is a lack of insulin, exhibit **insulin resistance in peripheral tissues, often related to visceral adiposity and obesity.** Type 2 diabetics often manifest signs of insulin resistance for many years prior to the diagnosis of overt diabetes. This type of diabetes accounts for at least 90% of the diagnosed cases and virtually all cases of undiagnosed diabetes in the United States.

Type 2 diabetes has a stronger familial predisposition than type 1. It is strongly associated with obesity and its complications, including cardiometabolic syndrome: hyperinsulinemia, hypertension, dyslipidemia, hyperglycemia, and central obesity/visceral adiposity.

Hyperosmolar Hyperglycemic Nonketotic Syndrome. Uncontrolled type 2 diabetics can achieve extremely high blood sugars without developing ketosis and acidosis; as a result, DKA does not usually occur in type 2 diabetes. **Hyperosmolar hyperglycemic nonketotic syndrome (HHNS)** occurs when blood glucose levels become substantially elevated, frequently approaching 1000 mg/dL (glucose levels are often much higher than those expected in DKA). HHNS may be the presenting symptom of some cases of type 2 diabetes, or it may result from either a concurrent illness or failure to take medications. Patients with HHNS typically present with severe dehydration, altered mental status, and visual disturbances. Serum osmolality is elevated, and the patient has a large fluid deficit. In severe cases, coma or death can occur due to electrolyte abnormalities, dehydration, and the toxic effects of metabolic acidosis. HHNS must be managed with hospitalization, aggressive rehydration with normal saline, correction of electrolyte abnormalities, treatment of any underlying illnesses, and the judicious use of insulin.

Gestational Diabetes

Gestational diabetes mellitus (GDM) occurs in approximately 7% of all pregnancies, resulting in over 200,000 cases annually in the United States. Elevated levels of human placental lactogen, estrogen, and progesterone produced by the placenta during pregnancy act as insulin antagonists, leading to increased insulin resistance and carbohydrate intolerance. Maternal and fetal complications related to GDM are numerous. Maternal complications include hyperglycemia, DKA, increased urinary tract infection (UTI) risk, increased pregnancy-induced hypertension/preeclampsia, and retinopathy. Fetal effects include congenital malformations (if hyperglycemia during conception/embryogenesis), macrosomia, respiratory distress syndrome, neonatal hypoglycemia, hyperbilirubinemia, hypocalcemia, polycythemia, and polyhydramnios. Women with GDM are more prone to develop non–pregnancy-related type 2 diabetes. They should be screened with a GTT postpartum and should undergo annual diabetic screening.

Risk factors for GDM include advanced maternal age, member of a high-incidence ethnic group (eg, Native American, African American, Hispanic American, South or East Asian, Pacific Islander), BMI of 25 kg/m^2 or greater, history of glucose intolerance, previous history of GDM, prior birth of a macrosomic infant, and history of diabetes mellitus in a first-degree family member. Patients with polycystic ovary syndrome, metabolic syndrome, hypertension, or acanthosis nigricans are also at increased risk.

The American College of Obstetricians and Gynecologists recommends screening all women for gestational diabetes between 24 and 28 weeks' gestation with an oral 50-g, 1-hour GTT. If the 1-hour glucose challenge is greater than 140 mg/dL, then an oral 100-g, 3-hour GTT should be performed. The 3-hour GTT requires serum glucose levels be obtained at fasting, 1-, 2-, and 3-hour intervals. The diagnosis of GDM is made based on two or greater abnormal results in the 3-hour GTT, defined as glucose levels of > 95 mg/dL while fasting, > 180 mg/dL at 1 hour, > 155 mg/dL at 2 hours, and > 140 mg/dL at 3 hours. GDM is treated with strict dietary management and aerobic exercise for at least 30 minutes 5 days a week. When necessary, oral agents (metformin, glyburide) or insulin may be used. Increased surveillance for fetal demise in pregnant women with GDM is mandatory, particularly at > 32 weeks' gestation and when fasting glucose levels exceed 105 mg/dL.

Treatment

The overall goals for the diabetic patient are to achieve a "controlled" status:

- Strict glycemic control with a goal of HbA$_{1c}$ of ≤ 7.0%

- Low-density lipoprotein cholesterol (LDL-C) level ≤ 100 mg/dL

- Blood pressure < 130/80 mm Hg (per American College of Cardiology/American Heart Association [ACC/AHA] guidelines) or < 140/90 mm Hg (per American Diabetic Association [ADA] guidelines)

- Lifestyle modifications, including a calorie-restricted diet consisting of low carbohydrates and low saturated fats and physical activity counseling (at least 150 min/wk of moderate-intensity aerobic physical activity [50% to 70% maximum heart rate] and resistance training [three times/week])

Table 51–1 • INSULIN PREPARATIONS

Type of Insulin	Onset of Action	Peak of Action	Duration of Action
Rapid acting (lispro or aspart insulin)	15 min	30-90 min	3-5 h
Short acting (regular insulin)	30-60 min	60-120 min	5-8 h
Intermediate acting (neutral protamine Hagedorn [NPH] insulin)	13 h	7-15 h	18-24 h
Long acting (glargine insulin; insulin detemir)	1 h	None	24 h

Data from the National Institutes of Health. https://www.diabetes.org/diabetes/medication-management/insulin-other-injectables/insulin-basics. Accessed June 10, 2020.

Treatment for Type 1 Diabetes. The treatment for **type 1 diabetes requires insulin administration.** In most cases, combination therapy using short-acting insulin prior to meals and long-acting basal insulin confers the greatest outcomes in minimizing complications. Insulin pump therapy, which provides a continuous subcutaneous infusion of short-acting insulin, is also an alternative for patients with labile glucose control. Insulin management requires careful and frequent self-monitoring of glucose, often with adjustment of insulin dosage based on the glucose levels, amount of physical activity, and caloric/carbohydrate intake (Table 51–1). Patients must monitor glucose levels regularly in order to ensure proper glycemic control and to prevent unnecessary (and dangerous) insulin administration in the setting of normoglycemia or hypoglycemia.

Treatment for Type 2 Diabetes. Patients with type 2 diabetes mellitus and those at risk of developing diabetes should be educated on the importance of an appropriate calorie-restricted and low-carbohydrate diet and exercise as key components of their management. In some cases, this strategy may be all that is required to achieve appropriate glycemic control. When lifestyle changes alone do not result in adequate glycemic control, oral agents should be considered as first-line treatment in patients with HbA_{1c} level of less than or equal to 9.0%. For HbA_{1c} levels greater than 9%, dual therapy with insulin and oral agents should be considered.

Medications for the prevention of diabetes mellitus are currently not recommended but can be considered when lifestyle modifications prove unsuccessful. Many medications are available for treating type 2 diabetes (Table 51–2). **Metformin is the initial treatment** unless contraindications (eg, renal disease) are present.

Biguanides. Biguanides (eg, metformin) act on the liver to **decrease glucose output during gluconeogenesis.** Secondary actions include improved insulin sensitivity in the liver and muscle and a hypothesized decrease in intestinal absorption of glucose. Other advantages to metformin include no potential risk of hypoglycemia, reduced serum insulin levels, potential modest weight loss, and a reduction in triglycerides and LDL-C. The most common side effects of metformin are gastrointestinal, including nausea and diarrhea. These side effects may be reduced by starting at low doses and taking the medication with meals. The most dangerous side effect attributable to metformin is the development of lactic acidosis. Metformin should be withheld 48 hours prior to any imaging that requires iodinated contrast.

Table 51-2 • AGENTS USED FOR TREATMENT OF TYPE 1 OR TYPE 2 DIABETES

	Mechanism of Action	Examples[a]	HbA$_{1c}$ Reduction (%)[b]	Agent-Specific Advantages	Agent-Specific Disadvantages	Contraindications
Oral						
Biguanides[c*]	↓ Hepatic glucose production	Metformin	1-2	Weight neutral, do not cause hypoglycemia, inexpensive, extensive experience, ↓ CV events	Diarrhea, nausea, lactic acidosis, vitamin B$_{12}$ deficiency	Renal insufficiency (see text for GFR < 45 mL/min), HF, radiographic contrast studies, hospitalized patients, acidosis
Alpha-glucosidase inhibitors[c**]	↓ GI glucose absorption	Acarbose, miglitol, voglibose	0.5-0.8	Reduce postprandial glycemia	GI flatulence, rarely associated with liver enzyme elevation, needs monitoring of liver function tests for at least first year	Renal/liver disease
Dipeptidyl peptidase IV inhibitors[c***]	Prolong endogenous GLP-1 action; ↑ Insulin, ↓ glucagon	Alogliptin, linagliptin, saxagliptin, sitagliptin, vildagliptin	0.5-0.8	Well tolerated, do not cause hypoglycemia	Angioedema/urticarial and immune-mediated dermatologic effects	Reduced dose with renal disease
Insulin secretagogues: Sulfonylureas[e]	↑ Insulin secretion	Glibornuride, gliclazide, glimepiride, glipizide, gliquidone, glyburide, glyclopyramide	1-2	Short onset of action, lower postprandial glucose, inexpensive	Hypoglycemia, weight gain	Renal/liver disease
Insulin secretagogues: Nonsulfonylureas[c***]	↑ Insulin secretion	Mitiglinide, nateglinide, repaglinide	0.5-1.0	Short onset of action, lower postprandial glucose	Hypoglycemia	Renal/liver disease

	Mechanism	Examples	HbA$_{1c}$ reduction (%)[b]	Other health benefits	Disadvantages/adverse effects	Contraindications
Sodium-glucose cotransporter 2 inhibitors***	↑ Renal glucose excretion	Canagliflozin, dapagliflozin, empagliflozin, ertugliflozin	0.5–1.0	Do not cause hypoglycemia, ↓ weight and BP; acute kidney injury, UTI's, bone fractures	Urinary and genital infections, polyuria, dehydration, exacerbate tendency to hyperkalemia and DKA; see text	Moderate renal insufficiency, insulin-deficient DM
Thiazolidinediones***	↓ Insulin resistance, ↑ glucose utilization	Pioglitazone, rosiglitazone	0.5–1.4	Lower insulin requirements	Peripheral edema, HF, weight gain, fractures, macular edema	HF, liver disease
Parenteral						
Amylin agonists[c,d]****	Slow gastric emptying, ↓ glucagon	Pramlintide	0.25–0.5	Reduce postprandial glycemia, weight loss	Injection, nausea, ↑ risk of hypoglycemia with insulin	Agents that also slow GI motility
GLP-1 receptor agonists[c]****	↑ Insulin, ↓ glucagon, slow gastric emptying, satiety	Albiglutide, dulaglutide, exenatide, liraglutide, lixisenatide, semaglutide	0.5–1.0	Weight loss, do not cause hypoglycemia; rarely pancreatitis, thyroid cancers	Injection, nausea, ↑ risk of hypoglycemia with insulin secretagogues	Renal disease, agents that also slow GI motility; medullary carcinoma of thyroid, pancreatic disease
Insulin[c,d]****	↑ Glucose utilization, ↓ hepatic glucose production and other anabolic actions	See text and Table 51–1	Not limited	Known safety profile	Injection, weight gain, hypoglycemia	
Medical nutrition therapy and physical activity[a]	↓ Insulin resistance, ↑ insulin secretion	Low-calorie, low-fat diet, exercise	1–3	Other health benefits	Compliance difficult, long-term success low	

Reproduced with permission, from Jameson J, Fauci AS, Kasper DL, et al. Harrison's Principles of Internal Medicine, 20th ed. 2018. Copyright © McGraw Hill LLC. All rights reserved.

Abbreviations: ACE, angiotensin-converting enzyme; BP, blood pressure; HF, heart failure; CV, cardiovascular; CVD, cardiovascular disease; DKA, diabetic ketoacidosis; GFR, glomerular filtration rate; GI, gastrointestinal; HbA$_{1c}$, hemoglobin A$_{1c}$.

Note: Some agents used to treat type 2 DM are not included in table (see text).

[a]*Examples are approved for use in the United States; others are available in other countries. Examples may not include all agents in the class.*

[b]*HbA$_{1c}$ reduction (absolute) depends partly on starting HbA$_{1c}$.*

[c]*Used for treatment of type 2 diabetes.*

[d]*Used in conjunction with insulin for treatment of type 1 diabetes. Cost of agent in the United States: *low, **moderate, ***high, ****variable.*

Metformin is classified as category B in pregnancy and is thought to be safe in nursing mothers. It is the oral agent of choice in type 2 diabetes in children older than age 10 years.

Sulfonylureas. Sulfonylureas were the first oral agents available for the treatment of type 2 diabetes. Their principal action is to function as **insulin secretagogues** that stimulate pancreatic beta cells to secrete insulin. Disadvantages include a significant risk of hypoglycemia, weight gain, poor response in 20% of patients, and a tendency for the medications to lose effectiveness over time.

Glucagon-like Peptide-1 Agonists. Glucagon-like peptide-1 (GLP-1) agonists, or GLP-1 incretin mimetics, are synthetic peptides that **stimulate insulin release.** This class can be used as adjunctive therapy for type 2 diabetics with inadequate glycemic control while also taking metformin, a sulfonylurea, and/or a thiazolidinedione (TZD). A distinct benefit of this class is early satiety and subsequent weight loss, which can improve dietary management. This class should be avoided in patients with diabetic gastroparesis. Side effects include hypoglycemia when added to a sulfonylurea (but not when added to metformin), nausea, vomiting, diarrhea, and acute pancreatitis.

Dipeptidyl Peptidase-4 Inhibitors. The dipeptidyl peptidase-4 (DPP-4) inhibitors work via an enzyme that **inactivates incretin hormones GLP-1 and glucose-dependent insulinotropic polypeptide (GIP).** GIP and GLP-1 stimulate insulin synthesis and release from pancreatic beta cells in a glucose-dependent manner. GLP-1 also decreases glucagon secretion from pancreatic alpha cells in a glucose-dependent manner, leading to reduced hepatic glucose production. This class can be used as monotherapy or in combination with metformin, a sulfonylurea, or a TZD as **second-line** therapy. Adverse effects include upper respiratory tract symptoms and severe hypersensitivity (eg, requires titration to balance hypoglycemia and preprandial glycemic control, anaphylaxis, and/or angioedema).

Thiazolidinediones. TZD, or glitazones, **activate PPARs (peroxisome proliferator-activated receptors), leading to improved insulin sensitivity in muscle and adipose tissue.** Secondary actions include decreased hepatic gluconeogenesis and increased peripheral glucose utilization. Since their release, several members of this class of medication have been withdrawn from the market due to increased risk of cardiovascular events.

Other Medications. **Meglitinides** are **short-acting secretagogues that increase insulin secretion from the pancreas** and work in a similar fashion to sulfonylureas. **Alpha-glucosidase inhibitors** (eg, acarbose) **delay carbohydrate absorption** by inhibiting alpha-glucosidase in the small intestine, which decreases postprandial hyperglycemia. **Pramlintide** is an amylinomimetic agent that has physiologic actions equivalent to those of human amylin, a glucoregulatory hormone synthesized by pancreatic beta cells and released with insulin in response to a meal. It **inhibits inappropriately high glucagon secretion during episodes of hyperglycemia** (eg, after a meal) in patients with type 1 or type 2 diabetes mellitus and does not impair normal glucagon response to hypoglycemia.

Comorbidity Treatment and Prevention. Other treatments are as important as tight glucose control in the effort to reduce adverse events, including heart attacks and strokes. **Strict blood pressure control is important.** Diabetics with elevated blood pressure should be treated, usually with **angiotensin-converting enzyme inhibitors or angiotensin receptor blockers** as the first-line medication. Diabetes is considered a coronary heart disease risk equivalent for decisions regarding **lipid management.** The LDL-C goal is less than 100 mg/dL, and all diabetics, with few exceptions, should be on a high-intensity statin medication. All diabetics should be advised to be immunized with the 23-valent **pneumococcal vaccine** (PPSV23) and get an annual **influenza** vaccination. Diabetics should be screened annually for diabetic neuropathy with a monofilament examination of the feet, should have annual microalbumin screening for diabetic nephropathy, and should have an annual dilated ophthalmologic evaluation to screen for diabetic retinopathy. Diabetic patients should be encouraged to quit smoking, monitor their weight on weekly basis, and perform regular foot inspections.

Treatment of Hypoglycemia

Hypoglycemic symptoms are related to the central and sympathetic nervous systems. Decreased levels of glucose lead to deficient cerebral glucose availability, which can manifest as confusion, difficulty with concentration, irritability, hallucinations, focal impairments (eg, hemiplegia), and eventually coma and death. Stimulation of the sympathoadrenal nervous system leads to sweating, palpitations, tremulousness, anxiety, and hunger. Causes of hypoglycemia include fasting, exogenous insulin, elevated C-peptide levels, autoimmunity, sulfonylurea abuse, and hormonal deficiency (eg, hypoadrenalism, hypopituitarism, glucagon deficiency).

When hypoglycemia is suspected and the patient is conscious and cooperative, sugar-containing products (eg, juice, soda, or candy) can rapidly alleviate the symptoms on a temporary basis and should be followed by a regular meal. If the person is not able to take something by mouth, rapid administration of **intramuscular glucagon** can be effective. Glucagon should be prescribed to patients at significant risk for clinical hypoglycemia. It can be easily administered by caregivers or family members in the case of an emergency. In the hospital setting or when intravenous access is available, a rapid injection of 50% dextrose (D_{50}) quickly restores normal serum and brain glucose levels. Following any of these therapies, the patient should be closely monitored, as the hypoglycemia may recur (especially if the patient uses a long-acting insulin or oral hypoglycemic agent) unless additional glucose and/or carbohydrates are administered.

CASE CORRELATION

- See Case 30 (Hypertenstion), Case 33 (Obesity), and Case 35 (Hyperlipidemia).

COMPREHENSION QUESTIONS

51.1 A 16-year-old girl has had an increased craving for sweets. She often consumes two to three ice cream sundaes and four large regular sodas a day but has still managed to maintain her weight. Friends often notice her using the bathroom more frequently to urinate, but she denies any episodes of purging and states that she just has to urinate after drinking so much cola. On physical examination, she is 5 ft 8 in and 110 lb, and her thyroid is not palpable. Which of the following test results would confirm your suspicion of diabetes mellitus?

A. A single fasting glucose reading of 115 mg/dL

B. A 2-hour oral GTT greater than 200 mg/dL with a 100-g glucose load

C. A random glucose greater than 200 mg/dL with symptoms such as polydipsia or polyuria

D. A HbA$_{1c}$ of 6% or greater

51.2 A 7-year-old boy is brought to the office with symptoms of polydipsia, polyphagia, polyuria, and weight loss of 8 lb. For the past 24 hours, he has had abdominal pain and vomiting. A urinalysis performed in the office shows the presence of glucose and ketones. A finger-stick blood glucose is 530 mg/dL. Which of the following is the most appropriate initial management in this patient?

A. Discharge home with oral metformin and a prompt referral to a dietician

B. Hospitalization with administration of intravenous 5% dextrose and subcutaneous regular insulin

C. Discharge home with a prescription for insulin, advice to hydrate aggressively, and office follow-up in 24 hours

D. Hospitalization with determination of electrolytes and potential anion gap acidosis and administration of intravenous normal saline and regular insulin

E. Hospitalization with immediate endocrinology consult for insulin dosing

51.3 An 83-year-old man was diagnosed with type 2 diabetes mellitus 3 months ago. He has modified his diet and tries to walk at least half a mile every evening. He drinks a glass of wine with lunch and dinner daily. For the past week, he has felt dizzy upon standing and has fallen on two occasions but never lost consciousness. After the last episode of falling, he presented to the local emergency department, where his blood pressure was 155/76 mm Hg, heart rate was 74 beats/min, and respiratory rate was 16 breaths/min. A finger stick showed a random glucose level of 54 mg/dL. Which of the following classes of medications has the lowest incidence of causing hypoglycemia when used as single-agent therapy?

A. Biguanide

B. Insulin

C. Sulfonylurea

D. Meglitinide

51.4 A 39-year-old gravida 1, para 0 (G1P0) woman who is a new patient presents to the office at 10 weeks' gestation. She is known to have type 2 diabetes mellitus and currently takes metformin. Her last HbA_{1c} was 10.4% one month ago. Her urinalysis is negative for ketones and leukocytes and reveals only trace protein. She has no other medical problems and does not drink or smoke. On physical examination, she is 5 ft 4 in and weighs 202 lb with a BMI of 34.7 kg/m². She asks you about the risk of diabetes to her fetus. Compared to GDM, this patient is at an increased risk for developing which of the following?

A. Fetal malformations

B. Fetal macrosomia

C. Polyhydramnios

D. Shoulder dystocia

E. Preterm labor

51.5 A 56-year-old man with type 2 diabetes presents to discuss his management. His last HbA_{1c} was 8.8%, and he currently takes metformin twice daily. He adamantly does not want to take insulin. He has seen a lot of commercials for diabetic agents and wants to try one that will help to curb his appetite. Which of the following agents will likely cause early satiety?

A. Acarbose

B. Rosiglitazone

C. Nateglinide

D. Sitagliptin

E. Exenatide

ANSWERS

51.1 **C.** Diabetes mellitus can be defined by the measurement of an 8-hour fasting glucose greater than 125 mg/dL (not 115 mg/dL, as in answer A); a random glucose of 200 mg/dL or more with classic symptoms; or a 2-hour GTT of 200 mg/dL or more after a 75-g glucose load (not 100-g glucose load, as in answer B); or a HbA$_{1c}$ of ≥ 6.5% (not > 6%, as in answer D).

51.2 **D.** This is a classic presentation of DKA, a common initial presentation of type 1 diabetes mellitus, and is a medical emergency. This child requires immediate hospitalization, determination of electrolytes and potential anion gap metabolic acidosis, intravenous normal saline, and insulin. Intravenous dextrose (answer B) should not be administered until the fluid deficit is corrected with normal saline and the anion gap has been reversed. Metformin (answer A) will not clinically improve this patient. An endocrinologist (answer E) is not required for dosing of insulin. Discharging the patient home (answer C) would not be appropriate management in this emergent situation.

51.3 **A.** Biguanides (eg, metformin) are effective medications for the treatment of type 2 diabetes, and they do not cause hypoglycemia when given as monotherapy. Insulin (answer B), insulin secretagogues such as meglitinide (answer D), and sulfonylureas (answer C) carry a risk of hypoglycemia as a complication of therapy.

51.4 **A.** This patient has pregestational diabetes mellitus and is presenting in the first trimester of pregnancy. Pregestational diabetes is associated with increased fetal malformations due to the higher serum glucose levels during organogenesis (5- to 10-week gestational age). In contrast, gestational diabetes tends to be associated with hyperglycemia after 24-weeks' gestation, when the fetal organs have already formed. Gestational diabetes is more likely to lead to fetal macrosomia (answer B) and polyhydramnios (answer C). Both gestational and pregestational diabetes are associated with shoulder dystocia (answer D). Preterm labor (answer E) occurs at the same frequency in diabetics as nondiabetics.

51.5 **E.** Exenatide, a GLP-1 agonist, has been shown to cause early satiety and weight loss; it would therefore be beneficial in this patient. However, GLP-1 agonists should be avoided in patients with diabetic gastroparesis. The other medications (answer A, acarbose; answer B, rosiglitazone; answer C, nateglinide; answer D, sitagliptin) may cause nausea, diarrhea, or other gastrointestinal side effects, but they do not cause early satiety. Rosiglitazone, a TZD, has been associated with significant weight gain.

CLINICAL PEARLS

▶ Diabetes is one of the most common diseases encountered in clinical practice and is often diagnosed in asymptomatic patients. The threshold criteria for diagnosis have been lowered to decrease microvascular and macrovascular complications, including death.

▶ Type 1 diabetes is a problem of insulin deficiency, most commonly due to autoimmune destruction of the beta islet cells of the pancreas.

▶ Type 2 diabetes is characterized by insulin resistance and accounts for more than 90% of all cases of diabetes in the United States. The increasing prevalence of obesity greatly contributes to more patients who will develop diabetes over the course of their lives.

▶ Gestational diabetes mellitus can lead to fetal macrosomia and polyhydramnios, while pregestational diabetes is more frequently associated with fetal malformations.

▶ Biguanides are the mainstay of oral diabetic agents in patients with type 2 diabetes due to tolerability, low cost, efficacy, and demonstrated reduction in morbidity and mortality. However, they are contraindicated in patients with renal insufficiency.

▶ Newer oral diabetic agents can play an important role in adjunctive therapy when modest reductions in HbA$_{1c}$ are the goal; they are often selected based on cost and side-effect profile.

▶ Long-acting insulin should be considered in patients with type 2 diabetes who have very poor glycemic control, significant insulin resistance, and metabolic syndrome.

REFERENCES

ACC/AHA/AAPA/ABC/ACPM/AGS/APhA/ASH/ASPC/NMA/PCNA guideline for the prevention, detection, evaluation, and management of high blood pressure in adults: a report of the American College of Cardiology/American Heart Association Task Force on Clinical Practice Guidelines. *J Am Coll Cardiol.* 2018;71:e127-e248.

American College of Obstetrics and Gynecology. ACOG guidelines at a glance: gestational diabetes mellitus. *Obstet Gynecol.* 2013;122:406-416.

American Diabetes Association (ADA). Diagnosis and classification of diabetes mellitus. *Diabetes Care.* 2018;41(suppl 1):S13-S27.

American Diabetes Association (ADA). 8. Pharmacologic approaches to glycemic treatment: standards of medical care in diabetes. *Diabetes Care.* 2018;41(suppl 1):S73-S85.

American Diabetes Association (ADA). 5. Prevention or delay of type 2 diabetes: standards of medical care in diabetes 2018. *Diabetes Care.* 2018;41(suppl 1):S51-S54.

American Diabetes Association (ADA). Standards of medical care in diabetes—2018. *Diabetes Care.* 2018;37(suppl 1):S1-S156.

Garber AJ, Abrahamson MJ, Barzilay JI, et al.. Consensus statement by the American Association of Clinical Endocrinologists and American College of Endocrinology on the comprehensive type 2 diabetes management algorithm—2016 executive summary. *Endocr Pract.* 2016;22(1):84-113.

Handelsman Y, Bloomgarden ZT, Grunberger G, et al. American Association of Clinical Endocrinologists and American College of Endocrinology—clinical practice guidelines for developing a diabetes mellitus comprehensive care plan—2015. *Endocr Pract.* 2015;21(suppl 1):1-87.

Powers AC, Niswender KD, Rickels MR. Diabetes mellitus: management and therapies. In: Jameson JL, Fauci A, Kasper D, Hauser S, Longo D, Loscalzo J, eds. *Harrison's Principles of Internal Medicine.* 20th ed. New York, NY: McGraw Hill; 2018: Chap. 397. https://accessmedicine.mhmedical.com/content.aspx?sectionid=192288412&bookid=2129&Resultclick=2. Accessed March 5, 2019.

Steinberg J, Carlson L. Type 2 diabetes therapies: a STEPS approach. *Am Fam Physician.* 2019; 99(4):237-243.

Yang W, Dall TM, Beronjia K, et al. Economic costs of diabetes in the US in 2017. *Diabetes Care.* 2018;41(5):917-928.

Zoungas S, Chalmers J, Neal B, et al. Follow-up of blood-pressure lowering and glucose control in type 2 diabetes. *N Engl J Med.* 2014;371:1392-1406.

A 74-year-old woman presents with the complaint that she has been developing nontraumatic bruises all over her extremities for the last several days. She has also noticed that her stools seem to be a lot darker, "almost like coffee grounds." She recently relocated to your area to live with her daughter. While this is her initial visit to your office, she has had refills available for all of her current medications and previously been at her baseline state of health. Her past medical history is significant for hypertension, postmenopausal state, an irregular heartbeat that she does not remember the name of, arthritis, and "a touch of diabetes." Her prescribed medications include hydrochlorothiazide and warfarin. Her over-the-counter medications include aspirin, which she started taking since moving to your city, a multivitamin, acetaminophen for her arthritis, and ibuprofen for when her knees really bother her. She also reports that she regularly drinks herbal teas.

▶ What is the differential diagnosis for this patient's presentation?
▶ What diagnostic studies are indicated?
▶ Why are the elderly at an increased risk for the development of adverse drug reactions?

ANSWERS TO CASE 52:

Adverse Drug Reactions and Interactions

Summary: A 74-year-old woman presents with

- Easy bruising and dark coffee-ground stools for several days
- Medications including an antihypertensive medication, an anticoagulant, and multiple over-the-counter medications (likely unaware of any potential drug interactions)
- Past medical history significant for hypertension, postmenopausal state, an irregular heartbeat, arthritis, and "a touch of diabetes"

Differential diagnosis: An adverse drug interaction involving warfarin and aspirin, nonsteroidal anti-inflammatory drugs (NSAIDs), and acetaminophen. Other (much less likely) possibilities include upper gastrointestinal bleeding from a peptic/duodenal ulcer or gastrointestinal malignancy, liver disease, or hematologic abnormality (eg, acute leukemia or severe thrombocytopenia).

Diagnostic studies: This patient should have orthostatic blood pressures measured, a guaiac-based test for occult blood in the stool, a stat complete blood count (CBC) and platelet count, a prothrombin time (PT) with international normalized ratio (INR), a comprehensive metabolic panel, and an electrocardiogram (ECG). Depending upon results of these tests, it may be appropriate to observe this patient in the hospital if she is orthostatic or if other signs suggest blood or volume loss that could predispose her to syncope.

Reasons for increased risk of drug reactions in the elderly: Polypharmacy, decline in renal and hepatic function, and pharmacodynamic considerations, including changes in body composition and volume of distribution that develop with normal aging.

ANALYSIS

Objectives

1. Understand the scope and risk of the problem of drug interactions and adverse effects. (EPA 12)

2. Describe strategies to reduce the risks of adverse drug interactions. (EPA 4, 12)

3. Explain why the elderly are particularly vulnerable to potential adverse drug reactions. (EPA 12)

Considerations

This elderly woman presents with many symptoms suspicious for a bleeding disorder: easy bruising and coffee ground stool. She has numerous risks for the development of adverse events related to her various medications. In addition to her age, the use of warfarin is another risk, and its use should be closely monitored via serial PT/INR measurements. Warfarin also has numerous drug-drug interactions, including an increased risk of bleeding and bruising with the concomitant use of aspirin, NSAIDs, and/or acetaminophen.

The extensive use of multiple medications, or polypharmacy (including prescribed, over-the-counter, herbal, and homeopathic products), makes adverse drug reactions and interactions a significant public health concern. Approximately 40% of people age 60 years and older take at least five medications daily and will experience an average of one unintended adverse drug event each year. Two-thirds of these patients will require medical attention because of it. **Approximately 10% of hospitalized patients experience a documented adverse event secondary to medications.** Physiologic changes and the use of multiple medications simultaneously for multiple medical conditions place aging individuals and the elderly at increased risk of adverse events and drug-drug interactions. **An estimated 3% to 11% of hospital admissions in the elderly are related to adverse drug reactions.**

The presence of bruising (suggesting an increased PT/INR) and the possibility of melena or hematochezia necessitates further evaluation: a rectal examination, a guaiac-based fecal occult blood test (FOBT), and screening for anemia and/or thrombocytopenia. A negative FOBT test does not rule out lower gastrointestinal malignancy. If suspicion becomes high, she should undergo additional testing, including colonoscopy. Due to her age and comorbid conditions, she should have a comprehensive metabolic panel to evaluate her glucose, electrolytes, and renal and liver functions, and she should have an ECG to evaluate for signs of ischemia. With the possibility of significant abnormalities on these tests that may require urgent management, it would be reasonable to place her on observation status in the hospital for monitoring and treatment.

If she is found to have a prolonged PT/INR, several therapeutic options are available, depending on the clinical situation and the magnitude of the abnormality. For over-anticoagulated patients with mildly elevated INR values (eg, 3-4) without evidence of bleeding, temporary discontinuation of warfarin or dose reduction is sufficient. For more elevated INR values in the setting of acute bleeding or spontaneous bruising (> 5), low-dose oral vitamin K and temporarily stopping warfarin will correct most abnormalities within a few days. When the INR value is very high (eg, > 10) or if there is evidence of acute bleeding and hemodynamic compromise, then intravenous vitamin K and replacement of coagulation factors with a transfusion of fresh-frozen plasma will rapidly reverse the coagulopathy.

APPROACH TO:
Adverse Drug Reactions and Interactions

DEFINITIONS

BEERS CRITERIA: The Beers Criteria for Potentially Inappropriate Medication Use in Older Adults (commonly referred to as the *Beers list*) is a guideline for health care providers to improve the safety in medication prescribing for older adults, to minimize unnecessary medications, and to minimize polypharmacy and drug interactions.

CYTOCHROME P450: An enzyme system found mostly in the liver (but also in the small intestine, lungs, and kidneys) that is composed of more than 50 isoenzymes and is responsible for the metabolism of numerous medications. The cytochrome (**CYP**) **isoenzymes can be induced,** resulting in increased drug metabolism and reduced therapeutic benefit of a medication, **or blocked,** resulting in decreased drug metabolism and potential for drug toxicity.

STOPP AND START TOOLS: The Screening Tool of Older People's Prescriptions (STOPP) and Screening Tool to Alert to Right Treatment (START) are lists of potentially inappropriate and interactive medications with therapeutic alternatives.

CLINICAL APPROACH

Etiologies of Adverse Drug Effects

Adverse drug effects (ADEs) are defined as any effects experienced beyond the intended therapeutic scope of the drug that have a negative impact on the patient. ADEs can range from minor symptoms such as nausea or diarrhea to severe or life-threatening symptoms, including cardiac arrhythmias precipitated by antiarrhythmic or stimulant medications.

Benefits. Other side effects from medications have been found to be beneficial. For example, peripheral alpha-adrenergic blockers, initially used as antihypertensives, have been found to minimize lower urinary tract obstructive symptoms from benign prostatic hyperplasia. Minoxidil, an antihypertensive agent, is used in the treatment of hair loss. Fluoxetine, an antidepressant, can be used in the treatment of premature ejaculation.

Drug Interactions. **Drug interactions account for 5% to 10% of adverse reactions.** They may be caused by pharmacokinetic effects, resulting in a change in either the drug's concentration or the drug's effect. Some of these interactions may be predictable, as a consequence of chemical effects secondary to enzymatic effects, protein binding, renal or hepatic interactions, and pharmacodynamic interactions. For example, warfarin may interact with several other medications and dietary factors to increase the active form of this drug to toxic levels, resulting in over-anticoagulation with resultant bruising and hemorrhage.

Synergistic Effects. **Drugs also may have additive or synergistic effects** caused by using two or more agents designed to produce a desired effect (eg, lowering blood pressure), but with an effect greater than anticipated. An example of this is using a beta-adrenergic blocking agent with certain calcium channel blockers (eg, diltiazem, verapamil). Both medications can decrease heart rate, but via different mechanisms of action. Combining the two agents may result in profound bradycardia and hypotension.

Chemical Interactions. Other **interactions may be more directly related to the chemical properties** of the medications or the solutions in which they are delivered. For example, mixing glargine insulin with other insulin types in the same syringe may result in precipitation of the insulin product, rendering them ineffective. Similarly, some intravenous medications must be administered individually to avoid precipitation (eg, calcium and ceftriaxone) or potentiation (eg, potassium and digoxin).

Drug Metabolism

Medications with a high first-pass hepatic clearance may be particularly susceptible to adverse events caused by alterations in hepatic metabolism. Diseases that change the effective circulatory volume (eg, heart failure) may also alter the rate of drug or metabolite elimination due to the effects on hepatic and renal blood flow.

The **CYP system** plays a significant role in many real or potential adverse drug events. Although more than 50 CYP isoenzymes have been identified, 6 of these isoenzymes metabolize 90% of drugs. Alcohol use can produce a hepatotoxic metabolite of acetaminophen. Grapefruit has a substantial impact on the cytochrome P450 3A4 system and should be avoided in patients taking statins, antiarrhythmic agents, immunosuppressants, and calcium channel blockers.

Many drugs are bound to serum albumin. When multiple agents are competing for the same albumin-binding sites, there is a potential to have greater amounts of unbound medication, resulting in higher circulating free drug levels. This causes particular concern for drugs that have a smaller volume of distribution, rapid onset of action, or narrow therapeutic index.

Renal Considerations. Renal considerations are related to the interaction of drugs at renal sites and **decreased renal function.** Renal interactions are often a result of alterations in the elimination of water-soluble drugs because of competition for the renal tubular system. These effects may be either positive or negative. An example of a beneficial effect is the concomitant administration of probenecid with penicillin. Probenecid decreases renal excretion of penicillin, resulting in an increased level and therapeutic effect of the antibiotic.

Other renal considerations include decreased kidney function, secondary to either disease processes or the natural decline in renal function that occurs with aging. Many medications have recommendations for alteration in dosing amount and/or interval based upon the patient's creatinine clearance. Creatinine is a by-product of muscle metabolism, and older patients may have falsely elevated calculated creatinine clearance rates because they have decreased muscle mass. Creatinine clearance is calculated using the following equation:

$$\text{Creatinine clearance} = \frac{[(140 - \text{age}) \times (\text{ideal body weight in kg})] \times (0.85 \text{ for women})}{72 \times \text{serum creatinine in mg/dL}}$$

Interventions to Reduce the Risk of Adverse Drug Events

To minimize risk of adverse medication reactions in the elderly and to identify high-risk medications, an expert consensus panel developed a widely used list of medications that should be avoided, called the **Beers criteria.** Many of these medications are sedating or have anticholinergic effects that increase the risk of falls. Others have narrow therapeutic indices, increasing the risk of developing toxic serum levels. **The STOPP/START criteria** have been used to detect ADEs that are either causal or contributory to acute hospitalization in older people at a rate 2.8 times more frequently than Beers criteria. It is imperative that clinicians are aware of equally effective therapeutic alternatives. If a patient is already on these medications, lowering the dose to the minimum effective dose is another way of minimizing risk. The following are prudent considerations to reduce adverse drug events or interactions, especially in the elderly:

- Use the Beers Criteria and/or STOPP/START criteria as well as pharmacists and additional pharmacy references (eg, Micromedex) to minimize risk.

- Only prescribe medications that are clearly indicated for an appropriate duration of time, yet do not avoid a necessary medication.

- When a patient presents with a new complaint, consider the potential for ADEs in the differential.

- Obtain a history of adverse drug events related to previous and current medications on all patients and routinely perform drug interaction surveys on patients taking multiple medications while documenting and reporting any adverse events.

- Maintain a current list of all medications that a patient is taking, including prescribed, over-the-counter, herbal, and homeopathic medications. **Perform a medication reconciliation at every visit.**

- **Instruct your patients to bring in all of their medications regularly to make sure your medication list is accurate.**

- Consider rational reductions and discontinuation of medications in elderly patients after consultation with the patient, family, and pharmacists.

- Have knowledge of renal, hepatic, and circulatory issues that affect your patients.

- Consider issues related to individual patients, such as unique genetic or ethnic factors.

CASE CORRELATION
- See Case 18 (Geriatric Health Maintenance and End-Of-Life Issues).

COMPREHENSION QUESTIONS

52.1 A 62-year-old man with hypertension, hypercholesterolemia, and benign prostatic hyperplasia (BPH) presents to his provider with increasing muscle aches in his thighs and shoulders and complaints of dark, tea-colored urine. These symptoms started about 10 days ago. He has been drinking plenty of fluids as part of a new diet, specifically grapefruit juice. On routine laboratory evaluation, his serum transaminases are elevated to nearly three times the normal limit, serum creatinine is 1.6 mg/dL (baseline 1.1 mg/dL), and urinalysis reveals 1+ proteinuria. His only medications are lisinopril, simvastatin, and a baby aspirin. Which of the following is the most likely diagnosis in this patient?

A. Drug-induced hepatitis from long-term simvastatin

B. Postrenal azotemia and proteinuria due to BPH

C. Acute kidney injury secondary to aspirin and lisinopril

D. Hepatic enzyme inhibition leading to elevated circulating drug levels

52.2 A 73-year-old man has type 2 diabetes mellitus, coronary heart disease, stage 3 chronic kidney disease, and chronic obstructive pulmonary disease. He has newly diagnosed atrial fibrillation and meets criteria for anticoagulation with warfarin. His current medications include metformin, glipizide, losartan, metoprolol, and ipratropium. Which of the following is the most important consideration in avoiding adverse drug reactions in the elderly?

A. Glomerular filtration rate (GFR)

B. Polypharmacy

C. Cardiac stroke volume

D. Hepatic blood flow

52.3 A 36-year-old woman presents to your office appearing very distressed after having a positive pregnancy test. She says that she has taken her oral contraceptive pills (OCPs) consistently at the same time every day for the past year. She has no significant past medical history except for mild depression. The only medication she takes is a prescribed OCP, but she admits that she also takes vitamins and herbal supplements. Which of the following additional information would be most helpful in discovering why her OCP may have failed?

A. Which OCP she is taking

B. Which herbal supplements she is taking

C. Her number of sexual partners

D. If she has ever been pregnant before

E. What time of day she takes her OCP

ANSWERS

52.1 **D.** Grapefruit juice inhibits the cytochrome P450 3A4 system that metabolizes simvastatin. This patient has rhabdomyolysis from increased circulating levels of simvastatin. Simvastatin may increase transaminases, but associated cases of hepatitis and liver failure are very rare (answer A). The combination of aspirin and lisinopril has not been shown to cause acute kidney injury (answer C); a creatinine level of 0.2 mg/dL above baseline levels does not confer acute kidney injury. Moderate proteinuria and a mild elevation in serum creatinine do not constitute postrenal azotemia and proteinuria due to BPH in this patient (answer B).

52.2 **B.** A multitude of factors result in the elderly being particularly vulnerable to adverse drug events. Included among these are polypharmacy, decreased renal and hepatic function, decreased cardiac output, and pharmacokinetic and pharmacodynamic considerations. Answer A (GFR) is reduced in elderly patients and is an issue with medications that are cleared via the kidney, but these effects are not as dangerous and common as polypharmacy. Answer C (cardiac stroke volume) is decreased in older patients, and answer D (hepatic blood flow) is reduced; nevertheless, these effects, though important, are not as common as polypharmacy in causing adverse events.

52.3 **B.** Asking which herbal supplements patients take is imperative. St. John's wort, a common herbal antidepressant, can induce the hepatic enzymes CYP3A4 and CYP3A5 and cause increased metabolism of estradiol, which then lowers the efficacy of OCPs. The most common reasons for OCP failure are user nonadherence or medications that interfere with their efficacy. Answer A (type of OCP) may be helpful, but the adherence to the schedule is much more important. Answer C (number of sexual partners) is not relevant to the failure of the oral contraceptive. Answer D (pregnancy history) is important in the care of her obstetrical issue but does not impact the contraceptive failure. Answer E (time of day of taking the OCP) is not relevant to the mechanism of the failure.

CLINICAL PEARLS

▶ Factors to consider when prescribing to elderly patients: (1) physiological changes, (2) arthritis (opening child-proof caps), (3) visual acuity, and (4) cognitive deficits.

▶ In elderly patients with new symptoms, consider adverse drug events highly in your differential.

▶ Renal interactions are often a result of alterations in the elimination of water-soluble drugs because of competition for the renal tubular system. These effects may be either positive or negative.

▶ Many practices have pharmacists as a component of the patient-centered medical home model of health care. Pharmacists can be invaluable members of the patient care team in reviewing medications, herbal supplements, vitamins, and potential interactions.

▶ The Beers Criteria and/or STOPP/START criteria are useful in preventing ADEs in patients.

REFERENCES

2019 American Geriatrics Society Beers Criteria® Update Expert Panel. American Geriatrics Society 2019 updated AGS Beers Criteria® for potentially inappropriate medication use in older adults. *J Am Geriatr Soc.* 2019;67(4):674-694.

Hamilton H, Gallagher P, Ryan C, et al. Potentially inappropriate medications defined by STOPP criteria and the risk of adverse drug events in older hospitalized patients. *Arch Intern Med.* 2011;171(11):1013-1019.

Hill-Taylor B, Sketris I, Hayden J, et al. Application of the STOPP/START criteria: a systematic review of the prevalence of potentially inappropriate prescribing in older adults, and evidence of clinical, humanistic and economic impact. *J Clin Pharm Ther.* 2013;38(5):360-372.

Lavan AH, Gallagher P. Predicting risk of adverse drug reactions in older adults. *Ther Adv Drug Saf.* 2016;7(1):11-22.

Lynch T, Price M. The effect of cytochrome P450 metabolism on drug response, interactions, and adverse effects. *Am Fam Physician.* 2007;76:391-396.

Khodyakov D, Ochoa A, Olivieri-Mui BL, et al. STOPP/START medication criteria modified for US nursing home setting. *J Am Geriatr Soc.* 2017;65(3):586-591.

Pretorius RW, Gataric G, Swedlund SK, Miller JR. Reducing the risk of adverse drug events in older adults. *Am Fam Physician.* 2013;87(5):331-336.

Steinman MA, Hanlon JT. Managing medications in clinically complex elders: "There's got to be a happy medium." *JAMA.* 2010;304(14):1592.

Stump AL, Mayo T, Blum A. Management of grapefruit-drug interactions. *Am Fam Physician.* 2006; 74(4):605-608.

A previously healthy 48-year-old man presents to his primary care office with severe low back pain that began the previous day after he helped his daughter move into her college dorm. He denies any trauma or previous back injury. He describes the pain as generally "achy" and sometimes characterized as being "sharp" when he moves suddenly. The pain is located in his lower back and radiates down the back of both legs to the middle of his posterior thighs. He denies any bladder or bowel incontinence or weakness in his legs. He denies fever, chills, weight loss, or malaise. He finds it very difficult to stand for prolonged periods of time because he cannot find a comfortable position. He states that this is the worst back pain he has ever experienced. It has not been relieved with acetaminophen or ibuprofen. His past medical history is significant for hypertension, and his only medication is lisinopril daily. He does not smoke or use illicit drugs and only drinks alcohol on occasion. On physical examination, he is well developed, overweight, and in moderate discomfort. His vitals are within normal limits. On neuromuscular examination, he has moderate tenderness bilaterally in his lumbar paraspinous muscles, and his lumbar flexion and extension are limited by pain. Strength and sensation are within normal limits and are symmetrical bilaterally. He has normal and symmetric knee and ankle deep tendon reflexes. Straight leg raise testing is negative bilaterally, and gait is within normal limits.

- ▶ What is the most likely diagnosis?
- ▶ What is the most appropriate workup?
- ▶ What is the best treatment plan?

ANSWERS TO CASE 53:

Acute Low Back Pain

Summary: A 48-year-old man presents with

- Acute onset of low back pain after strenuous activity
- Previously healthy status
- Appears overweight, unremarkable neurologic examination
- Denial of any systemic complaints
- Past medical history significant for hypertension, with his only medication being lisinopril daily

Most likely diagnosis: Acute low back pain, lumbar sacral strain.

Most appropriate workup: No formal workup is required unless symptoms persist after conservative treatment for at least 1 month.

Best treatment plan: Relative rest (but not bed rest), nonsteroidal anti-inflammatory drugs (NSAIDs) or acetaminophen, and muscle relaxants.

ANALYSIS

Objectives

1. Develop a differential diagnosis for acute low back pain. (EPA 2)

2. List the "red flag" symptoms of low back pain and how to investigate them. (EPA 3, 10)

3. Describe effective treatments for musculoskeletal back pain. (EPA 4)

Considerations

Acute low back pain is the one of the most common diagnoses in primary care practices. Approximately 90% of patients with acute low back pain will fully recover within 4 to 6 weeks of symptom onset. Since the differential diagnosis of low back pain is broad, the role of the clinician is to determine if the pain is caused by a self-limited condition, an acute neurological compromise, or a systemic disease and to consider psychosocial factors that may lead to chronic back pain and complicate the recovery or efficacy of treatment.

This patient's history includes pertinent positive findings of a recent history of repetitive lifting and twisting associated with lumbar sacral strain. His signs, symptoms, and physical examination are all consistent with a localized musculoskeletal condition. His lack of acute neurologic or systemic symptoms is a pertinent negative finding. He denies a history of depression and substance abuse. This clinical scenario is best managed by symptomatic therapies for 4 to 6 weeks without imaging and with close follow-up if symptoms do not resolve. In the majority of patients with acute back pain in the absence of red flag symptoms, laboratory tests and imaging studies are not required. Education in proper lifting techniques and exercise therapy to improve core and lumbar sacral strength and flexibility may help to prevent future strain and injury.

APPROACH TO:
Low Back Pain

DEFINITIONS

CAUDA EQUINA SYNDROME: Damage to nerve bundles below the spinal cord resulting in acute low back pain, perineal anesthesia, bowel and/or bladder incontinence, and bilateral radicular pain.

HERNIATED DISK: Rupture of the fibrocartilage between the vertebrae leading to leakage of the nucleus pulposus, which may impinge on the nerve roots and cause pain.

SCIATICA: A sharp or burning pain that radiates along the path of the sciatic nerve (L4–S2) to the buttocks and to the posterior thigh, usually caused by piriformis compression or a herniated disk of the lumbar region of the spine.

CLINICAL APPROACH

Pathophysiology

Acute low back pain should be evaluated in a systematic manner to avoid missing important red flag symptoms (Table 53–1) and unnecessary imaging, treatments,

Table 53–1 • RED FLAG SYMPTOMS IN LOW BACK PAIN
Unrelenting night pain
Unrelenting pain at rest
Neuromotor deficit
Unexplained fever
Greater than 6 weeks' duration
Age > 70
Loss of bowel or bladder control
Progressive focal neurologic deficits
Suspicion of ankylosing spondylitis
Trauma
History or suspicion of cancer
Osteoporosis
Chronic corticosteroid use
Immunosuppression
Alcohol abuse
Intravenous drug use
Perineal (saddle) anesthesia

Table 53–2 • DIFFERENTIAL DIAGNOSIS OF LOW BACK PAIN
Condition (Prevalence)
Mechanical low back pain (~97%) • Lumbar strain, sprain (70%) • Degenerative facets or disks (10%) • Herniated disk (4%) • Compression fracture (4%) • Spinal stenosis (3%) • Spondylolisthesis (2%) • Spondylolysis (<1%)
Nonmechanical spinal conditions (1%) • Cancer (primary or metastatic) (0.7%) • Inflammatory arthritis (0.3%) • Infection (0.01%)
Visceral disease (2%) • Pelvic organs: prostatitis, PID, endometriosis • Renal disease: nephrolithiasis, pyelonephritis, perinephric abscess • Aortic aneurysm • Gastrointestinal disease: pancreatitis, cholecystitis, peptic ulcer

Abbreviation: PID, pelvic inflammatory disease.
Data from Kinkade S. Evaluation and treatment of acute low back pain. Am Fam Physician. 2008;75:1181-1188, 1190-1192; Deyo RA, Weinstein JN. Low back pain. N Engl J Med. 2001;344(5):363-370.

or referrals. The first step is to generate a differential diagnosis (Table 53–2) and to understand the common signs and symptoms of its components. The history in the patient presenting with acute low back pain should differentiate minor back conditions from those requiring urgent evaluation via a methodological approach.

Cauda Equina Syndrome. Patients presenting with cauda equina syndrome have increasing neurologic deficits and leg weakness, bowel and/or urinary incontinence, anesthesia or paresthesia in a saddle distribution, and bilateral sciatica. Physical findings include pain elicited by the straight leg raise test, reduction in anal sphincter tone, and decreased bilateral ankle reflexes. These patients require immediate evaluation with lumbosacral magnetic resonance imaging (MRI), corticosteroids to decrease pain and inflammation, neurosurgical evaluation, and commonly immediate surgical decompression of the entrapped cauda equina to prevent further neurologic deterioration.

Infection. Fevers, point tenderness directly over the vertebrae, recent infections, and a history of intravenous drug use can point toward an **infectious** process like osteomyelitis, septic diskitis, paraspinous abscess, or epidural abscess. These infections should be promptly considered and evaluated with a complete blood count (CBC), erythrocyte sedimentation rate (ESR), C-reactive protein (CRP), and cultures from blood, abscess contents, and cerebral spinal fluid. Imaging with MRI or computed tomographic (CT) scan will be needed. Treatment usually requires long courses of intravenous antibiotics and sometimes surgical drainage.

Cancer. An underlying **cancer** is much more likely if the patient has a history of cancer with a likelihood of metastasis to bone (eg, prostate, hematologic, breast, lung); unexplained weight loss; worsening pain at night; failure to improve after

1 month of conservative therapy; or an age greater than 50 years. To further evaluate patients with these risk factors, a CBC, ESR, CRP, and plain film radiographs of the lumbosacral spine should be obtained initially. Abnormalities in these tests should be further evaluated by MRI and/or a nuclear medicine bone scan.

Sciatica. **Sciatic pain** is the classic sign of a **herniated disk or piriformis compression.** It is typically characterized by a sharp or burning pain that radiates from the lumbar spine down the back and side of the leg and distal to the knee. Additional symptoms of radiculopathy may include anesthesia, dysesthesia, hyperesthesia, and paresthesia that are confined to a specific lumbosacral dermatome. Sciatica can be examined by performing both a straight leg raise test and a contralateral leg raise test along with sensory, strength, and reflex testing of the lower extremities (L4, knee strength and reflex; L5, great toe and foot dorsiflexion; and S1, plantar flexion and ankle reflexes). Greater than 90% of lumbar disk compression of nerve roots occurs at L4-L5 and L5-S1. MRI is not recommended for patients with sciatica unless the symptoms last for greater than 1 month, if alarm symptoms are present, or if the patient is not a candidate for an epidural corticosteroid injection or surgical intervention.

Spinal Stenosis. **Spinal stenosis** is a congenital or acquired condition of spinal canal narrowing with or without concomitant facet hypertrophy that exerts pressure on the spinal cord and nerve roots. **Degenerative arthritis and spondylolisthesis are the most common acquired causes of lumbar spinal stenosis.** Congenital causes include dwarfism, spina bifida, and myelomeningocele. Spinal stenosis presents as lower back and leg pain, leg weakness, and pseudoclaudication that occurs after walking various distances, while the vascularity of the legs remains uncompromised. The majority of patients with spinal stenosis are symptomatic only when engaged in activities. Pain is often relieved by sitting, performing lumbar flexion (bending over), squatting, or lying down. Patients classically describe increased pain with spine extension (eg, standing straight or walking downhill) with improvement upon spinal flexion (eg, leaning forward, walking uphill, or bending over a shopping cart). It is more common in patients over 60, and its rules of evaluation are the same as for a herniated disk. Spinal stenosis is initially treated with NSAIDs and muscle relaxants, physical therapy, and epidural corticosteroid injections. Surgical therapy is reserved for patients who have failed conservative treatment or those with progressive neurologic deficits.

Conservative treatment for sciatica involves anti-inflammatories including NSAIDs or acetaminophen, muscle relaxants, short-course oral corticosteroids, and activity modifications. Given the lack of proven efficacy, potential adverse drug reactions, and risk of dependence, opioid use is generally reserved for patients who have severe pain and who have exhausted nonnarcotic treatment options. Physical therapy may be appropriate for individuals with persistent moderate symptoms of 3 weeks or more since the majority of the patients are likely to experience spontaneous improvement in the first 2 weeks. Surgical options may be considered in those who suffer from disabling radicular pain of 6 weeks or more or with progressive neuropathic deficits.

Vertebral Compression Fractures. **Vertebral compression fractures** are more common in older adults, especially those with chronic corticosteroid use or osteoporosis (Case 58). These commonly occur after low-impact trauma but may also occur with no trauma history at all. Patients typically present with acute onset of back pain after certain sudden movements such as lifting, bending, or coughing. The pain often follows the distribution of the contiguous nerve and radiates bilaterally into the anterior abdomen or pelvis, also known as the "girdle of pain." The fractures are generally localized to the thoracolumbar segment (T12-L2) of the spine. Vertebral compression fractures are best initially evaluated by plain film radiographs of the thoracolumbar spine. They can be treated medically with pain control, physical therapy, and calcitonin and bisphosphonates, as well as treatment of the underlying osteoporosis. Spinal bracing and surgical management with balloon kyphoplasty can be considered and may have better outcomes than medical management in those with severe pain.

Psychosocial Causes. **Psychosocial factors** and emotional distress should also be evaluated in the patient with low back pain. Depression, fear avoidance (fear that activity will cause permanent damage), job dissatisfaction, current involvement in litigation, reliance on passive treatments, or somatization are predictors of slow recovery and increase the risk for developing chronic low back pain. Acknowledgment and treatment of such factors as applicable may be effective adjuvant therapy.

Lumbar Sacral Strain. The vast majority of patients seeking medical evaluation with back pain will be diagnosed with **lumbar sacral strain.** The exact anatomical cause of the pain is often unknown, but it is often hypothesized that there may be an incomplete tear in the annulus fibrosus that may leak fluids, creating local inflammation, or it may bulge posteriorly and irritate certain lumbar roots. Irritation and spasm of the surrounding muscles, tendons, ligaments, or joint capsule may be concomitantly involved in this painful process.

Treatment

The treatment of acute mechanical low back pain (less than 4 weeks) centers on the use of NSAIDs, acetaminophen, muscle relaxants, heat, and early mobility. Bed rest for any length of time has not been shown to improve pain and may lengthen the duration of pain and prolong recovery. For patients with moderate-to-severe pain, combination therapy of a muscle relaxant and an NSAID may be more effective than monotherapy. Due to their sedative effects, muscle relaxants are typically recommended for nighttime dosing.

In general, patients should be encouraged to resume normal daily activities as tolerated with reasonable restrictions on bending and lifting until the pain resolves. Specific exercises have not been proven to be beneficial in speeding recovery. Massage therapy and spinal manipulation may be of some benefit for acute pain; physical therapy has some benefit for short-term pain relief, but most studies do not show long-term benefit. Although acupuncture and yoga may be reasonable options for chronic back pain, their effectiveness in acute back pain remains unproven. Lumbar support braces have not been shown to prevent low back pain. For prevention of mechanical back pain, exercise has been proven to help prevent first episodes of back pain and recurrences in certain subgroups of workers.

CASE CORRELATION

- See Case 12 (Musculoskeletal Injuries) and Case 58 (Osteoporosis).

COMPREHENSION QUESTIONS

53.1 A 45-year-old man with no significant past medical history presents with severe back pain after lifting heavy boxes at work 2 days ago. Other than his back pain, his review of symptoms is negative. His pain is exacerbated by coughing and sneezing. The pain radiates from his lower back down his right posterior thigh to his great toe when you perform both a straight leg raise and the contralateral leg raise tests. His strength, sensation, and reflexes are intact and symmetrical. Which of the following is the recommended first step in the evaluation of this patient?

A. Plain film radiographs

B. MRI

C. CT scan

D. Nuclear bone scan

E. No imaging indicated

53.2 A 58-year-old Caucasian woman presents complaining of low back pain 4 weeks after a fall. She has no history of fever, unexplained weight loss, diabetes, or cancer. Her past medical history is significant for moderate persistent asthma and nicotine dependence. She had a hysterectomy for uterine fibroids at age 40. Which of the following aspects of the patient's history should prompt further evaluation of her pain?

A. History of corticosteroid use

B. Caucasian ethnicity

C. Time course of back pain

D. History of cocaine use

E. Premenopausal age

53.3 A 67-year-old man with coronary artery disease, dyslipidemia, and eczema comes to you complaining of lower back pain and left leg pain. The pain is worse when he stands for long periods of time but improves when he bends forward to push his shopping cart around the grocery store. He indicates that his feet "burn" and "ache" after walking different distances every day. His lower extremity neuromuscular examination is unremarkable. Which of the following is the most appropriate treatment for this patient?

A. Emergent spinal cord decompression

B. Epidural corticosteroid injection

C. Kyphoplasty

D. Bed rest for 4 days

E. Tramadol

ANSWERS

53.1 **E.** The patient has signs and symptoms of a herniated disk. There is no evidence that imaging within the first month has any morbidity benefit. If symptoms persist after 1 month, then MRI (answer B) would be the correct choice. X-rays (answer A) do not show disks or nerve roots, and CT (answer C) has poorer visualization of soft tissue than MRI. A bone scan (answer D) would not yield any significant information in this case.

53.2 **A.** The patient's history is suspicious for a vertebral compression fracture that could be secondary to osteoporosis caused in part by corticosteroid use in a postmenopausal woman. A patient with moderate persistent asthma may have undergone prolonged treatment with corticosteroids for prior exacerbations and would therefore be at increased risk for osteoporosis. The time course of her pain is 4 weeks; pain for 6 weeks and greater is a red flag symptom for further evaluation with radiographic imaging (answer C). While osteoporosis is more common in Caucasian women, it is not considered a red flag (answer B). Postmenopausal women are at greater risk for osteoporosis than premenopausal women (answer E). Smoking and alcohol dependence are risk factors for osteoporosis; there is no evidence that cocaine use contributes to the development of osteoporosis (answer D).

53.3 **B.** The patient's history is classic for spinal stenosis. Patients often find relief by sitting or stooping, as these positions tend to lead to spinal flexion rather than extension (as in walking straight or downhill). NSAIDs, physical therapy, and epidural corticosteroid injections are used to relieve pain. Surgical decompression (answer A) is used in cauda equina syndrome, and kyphoplasty (answer C) is useful in vertebral fractures. Bed rest (answer D) is not used in the conservative treatment of back pain for any cause and has been shown to increase the duration of pain. Answer E (tramadol) is an opioid-like medication and not indicated in this patient since there is some danger in habituation.

CLINICAL PEARLS

▶ Red flag symptoms in low back pain should prompt an immediate diagnostic workup.

▶ Cauda equina syndrome is a surgical emergency that should be evaluated immediately by MRI and treated with the prompt administration of corticosteroids.

▶ Sciatica due to a suspected herniated disk can be managed conservatively for 4 weeks before radiographic imaging has any proven benefit.

▶ Lumbar sacral strain is the most common cause of back pain, generally resolves within a few weeks, and is treated with NSAIDs, acetaminophen, and/or muscle relaxants.

▶ Bed rest provides no significant benefit for any type of acute back pain and may prolong pain and slow recovery.

REFERENCES

Delitto A, George SZ, Van Dillen LR, et al. Low back pain: clinical practice guidelines linked to the International Classification of Functioning, Disability, and Health from the Orthopaedic Section of the American Physical Therapy Association. *J Orthop Sports Phys Ther*. 2012;42(4):A1-A57.

Kamper SJ, Apeldoorn AT, Chiarotto A, et al. Multidisciplinary biopsychosocial rehabilitation for chronic low back pain: Cochrane systematic review and meta-analysis. *BMJ*. 2015;350h444.

Lemeunier N, Leboeuf-Yde C, Gagey O. The natural course of low back pain: a systematic critical literature review. *Chiropr Man Therap*. 2012;20:33.

Maher C, Underwood M, Buchbinder R. Non-specific low back pain. *Lancet*. 2017:389(10070):736-747.

McCarthy J, Davis A. Diagnosis and management of vertebral compression fractures. *Am Fam Physician*. 2016;94(1):44-50.

Rubinstein SM, de Zoete A, van Middlekoop M, et al. Benefits and harms of spinal manipulative therapy for the treatment of chronic low back pain: systematic review and meta-analysis of randomised controlled trials. *BMJ*. 2019;364:l689.

Traeger A, Buchbinder R, Harris I, Maher C. Diagnosis and management of low-back pain in primary care. *CMAJ*. 2017;189(45):E1386-E1395.

Will JS, Bury DC, Miller JA. Mechanical low back pain. *Am Fam Physician*. 2018;98(7):421-428.

An 18-month-old boy is brought to your office by his mother for a routine well-child examination. This is his first visit to your office, as he has been seen for regular well-child examinations at another clinic since his birth. The child is the product of a spontaneous vaginal delivery at term without complications. His personal and family medical histories are unremarkable, and his immunizations are up to date. He has one older sister, age 6 years, who is in the first grade, with normal growth and development. The child lives at home with both biological parents and his sister. There are no pets in the home, and no one smokes. Overall, he eats a well-balanced diet, although mom reports he is sometimes a picky eater.

The child's mother notes that she is concerned about his development because he still does not speak single words and only babbles, and her other child was using many words by this age. On further history, you discover that he often disregards the calling of his name but does startle at loud noises. The child's mother has read about autism on the Internet and is concerned that her son may have this diagnosis. She also states that because of her concern, if he needs any immunizations today, she does not want them to be given for fear that this might worsen her son's condition.

On physical examination, the patient is in the 50th percentile for height and 75th percentile for weight and head circumference. His entire physical examination is unremarkable. On developmental screening, you observe that he walks and runs well, and the mother reports that he can walk up steps and kick a ball forward. During the examination, he only babbles and does not utter discrete words. When given a toy car, he puts it in his mouth, but never demonstrates rolling the car along the floor or table. When you call the child's name, tap him on the shoulder, say "Look!" and point to a toy in the corner, you are unable to get his attention.

► By what age should an infant use single words?
► What is your next step in the evaluation of this patient?
► Should immunizations be delayed in this patient?

ANSWERS TO CASE 54:

Autism Spectrum Disorder

Summary: An 18-month-old child presents with

- His mother's request for a routine well-child examination
- A delay in language and social skill development
- History of spontaneous vaginal delivery at term without complications
- Unremarkable personal and family medical histories and up-to-date immunizations
- Measurements in the 50th percentile for height and 75th percentile for weight and head circumference
- Often disregarding the calling of his name but startling at loud noises
- His mother's request to delay any immunizations that are due

Age by which a child should use single words: Most children will say "mama/dada" indiscriminately by 9 months of age and use two words other than "mama/dada" by 12 months of age. Speech of no single identifiable words by 16 months of age is a red flag for the presence of an autism spectrum disorder (ASD).

Next step in evaluation: This patient has developmental delays concerning for an ASD. Screening should be completed with a level 1 standardized autism-specific screening tool, such as the Screening Tool for Autism in Toddlers and Young Children (STAT). Due to the concerns noted on examination, the patient should be referred for a comprehensive ASD evaluation, early intervention/early childhood education services, and an audiology evaluation.

Should immunizations be delayed: Despite current controversy, there is no evidence that immunizations are implicated as a cause of autism; thus, the parents should be counseled that the routine immunizations are recommended. Many concerns have been raised that the measles-mumps-rubella (MMR) vaccine may precipitate autism, based on reports of parents who first detected autism in their children following MMR vaccination and a study of 12 autistic patients in which their physicians reported similar suspicions, which has since been retracted for falsification of methods. Subsequent studies have failed to show any evidence of a link between MMR vaccination and the development of autism. To date, there is no evidence to support that the use of thimerosal, a mercury-containing preservative that is no longer used in childhood vaccines (but may still be present in some multidose vials influenza vaccine), causes autism.

ANALYSIS

Objectives

1. State the diagnostic criteria for ASDs and the differential diagnosis of pervasive developmental disorder (PDD). (EPA 2, 3)

2. List the key clinical signs of ASDs. (EPA 1)

3. Forumulate a strategy for the assessment and management of ASDs. (EPA 4)

Considerations

This 18-month-old child presents with significant language and social skills delay. These two findings are highly suspicious for ASD; therefore, he should promptly undergo a comprehensive autism assessment. There is no description of stereotyped movement or findings, yet these are not necessary for the diagnosis of ASD. However, this child should also undergo a formalized audiology evaluation. Since he startles to loud noises, a significant hearing deficit is not likely.

APPROACH TO:
Autism Spectrum Disorder

DEFINITIONS

JOINT ATTENTION: An infant demonstrates enjoyment in sharing with another individual an object/event by looking back and forth between the individual and the object/event.

SOCIAL RELATEDNESS: Internal drive to connect with others and share similar feelings.

CLINICAL APPROACH

Epidemiology

In April 2018, the Centers for Disease Control and Prevention (CDC) released data on **the prevalence of ASD** in the United States, estimating **1 in 59 children (1 in 38 boys and 1 in 152 girls)** has ASD. Recurrence risk is as high as 19% when there is an older sibling with ASD. As evidenced by prevalence statistics, most providers will care for several children with ASD during the course of their career. Furthermore, as a result of increased media attention intended to raise awareness about these disorders and the early signs, more and more parents will begin to raise concerns to their child's clinician. Primary care providers must be able to recognize the key clinical features of these disorders, to formulate a systematic plan to assess them, and to know how to assist families with the ongoing treatment and care of a child with ASD.

Pathophysiology

ASD is a neurodevelopmental disorder that is the result of a combination of environmental and genetic factors. Evidence supports multiple-gene involvement, with environmental factors influencing the wide variation in phenotypic expression. Environmental factors implicated include exposures to teratogens in utero and maternal illnesses during pregnancy, but no studies have verified a causal role.

Under the *Diagnostic and Statistical Manual of Mental Disorders, Fifth Edition* (*DSM-5*), ASD no longer includes the subdiagnoses of autistic disorder (AD), Asperger syndrome (AS), and pervasive developmental disorder not otherwise specified (PDD-NOS). Diagnosis of ASD requires persistent deficits and impairments in social skills and limited, repetitive, and stereotyped behavior patterns.

Clinicians should also specify if there is an accompanying intellectual impairment, language impairment, or catatonia; an association with a known medical or genetic condition or environmental factor; or an association with another neurodevelopmental, mental, or behavioral disorder.

Clinical Presentation

Although there is no pathognomonic feature, ASD is universally characterized by deficits in social relatedness, and the early social deficits, such as delayed or absent joint attention, appear to be reliable red flag symptoms. However, these characteristics frequently go unnoticed by parents, and it is commonly a delay in speech that prompts them to raise a concern with their child's health care provider.

In order to diagnose ASD, a child must demonstrate abnormal behavior in the early developmental period, delays in social communication and interaction, and restricted, repetitive behavior. Diagnosis requires three behavioral criteria under category A and at least two in category B.

A. **Impaired social communication and interaction:**
   1. Lack of social-emotional reciprocity.
   2. Deficient use of nonverbal communicative behaviors such as facial expressions, eye contact, and gestures used in social interaction.
   3. Deficits in establishing, cultivating, and understanding relationships.

B. **Restricted, repetitive patterns of behavior:**
   1. Stereotyped or repetitive use of objects, speech, or motor movements.
   2. Inflexible adherence to monotony, routines, or ritualized patterns of behavior.
   3. Restricted patterns of interests that is atypical in either intensity or focus.
   4. Over- or underreaction to certain sensation stimuli or abnormal interests to certain environmental sensations, such as obsession with lights or negative response to different textures.

C. Symptoms must be observed in the early developmental period but may not be fully expressed until later due to exceeding social demands or compensation by learned strategies.

D. Symptoms result in clinically significant handicaps in social, occupational, or other important areas of function.

E. Symptoms are not better explained by an intellectual developmental disorder or global developmental delay. Although intellectual disability and ASD frequently co-occur, comorbid diagnoses require social communication that is deficient compared to the expected general developmental level.

Neurogenetic comorbid conditions and intellectual disability have also been found to be associated with ASDs, although the most recent data indicate the percentages to be much less than previously thought, estimated at 10% and 50%, respectively. Clinicans must consider in the differential diagnosis any neurogenetic syndromes that may play a causative role in ASDs or otherwise may be associated, as well as other PDDs (Table 54–1).

Table 54–1 • NEURODEVELOPMENTAL CONDITIONS ASSOCIATED WITH AUTISM SPECTRUM DISORDERS		
Condition	Etiology	Characteristics
Rett syndrome	X-linked dominant disorder (fatal to male fetus)	Microcephaly, seizures, and hand-wringing stereotypies
Childhood disintegrative disorder	Unknown	Normal development until 2-4 y, then severe deterioration of motor and social functioning
Fragile X syndrome	Most common genetic cause of AD and intellectual disability in males	Intellectual disability, macrocephaly, large pinnae, large testicles, hypotonia, and hyperextensible joints
Tuberous sclerosis	Autosomal dominant, but most cases are new mutations	Hypopigmented macules, fibroangio-mata, kidney lesions, CNS hamartomas, seizures, intellectual disability, ADHD
Neurofibromatosis	Autosomal dominant, half of cases are new mutations	Café-au-lait spots, axillary freckling, neurofibromas, ocular Lisch nodules
Phenylketonuria	Inborn error of metabolism	Routinely tested for by newborn screening; intellectual disability/AD preventable with dietary modification
Fetal alcohol syndrome	Exposure to alcohol in utero	Characteristic facies; associated with AD and other developmental disorders
Angelman syndrome	Loss of maternally expressed ubiquitin-protein ligase gene	Global developmental disorder, hypotonia in early childhood, wide-based ataxic gait, seizures, and progressive spasticity
Childhood schizophrenia	Unknown	Thought disorder, delusions, and hallucinations

Treatment

The key to successful management of ASD is early diagnosis leading to early intervention. **Surveillance for ASD should occur at every preventive visit throughout childhood utilizing standard developmental screening tools.** The Ages and Stages Questionnaires are common standardized tools that assess developmental milestones from 2 months through 6 years of age. This includes eliciting a family history of ASD, parental and other caregiver concerns, developmental history, and making accurate observations of the child. **All children should also be screened with the Modified Checklist for Autism in Toddlers (M-CHAT) at the 18- and 24-month visits.** If concerns for an ASD are raised during well-child visits, a screening tool specifically designed for ASD should be used. Prior to 18 months of age, screening tools that target social and communication skills may be helpful for detecting early signs of ASD.

   Red flag symptoms indicating the need for immediate evaluation include

- No babbling or pointing by 12 months
- No single words by 16 months
- No two-word phrases by 24 months

- Loss of language or social skills, repetitive behaviors or speech, resistance to change, restricted interests, or unusual and intense reactions to sensation at any age

When a child demonstrates two or more risk factors or a positive screening result occurs, the clinician should take immediate action. The following steps should be accomplished simultaneously:

- Refer the child for a comprehensive ASD evaluation

- Refer the child to early intervention/early childhood education services

- Obtain an audiologic evaluation

Children with ASDs who begin treatment at a younger age have significantly better outcomes, making early identification and intervention critical. The goals of treatment are to improve language and social skills, decrease maladaptive behaviors, support parents and families, and foster independence.

CASE CORRELATION

- See Case 5 (Well-Child Care).

COMPREHENSION QUESTIONS

54.1 A mother brings her 5-year-old son to your office because his teacher is concerned that he has attention deficit hyperactivity disorder (ADHD). The teacher has noticed that the child frequently makes long-winded speeches about boats in class and is often rocking back and forth in his seat. On further history taking, the child's mother states that he is very independent, with few friends, and has always been interested in boats, preferring them over all other toys. You observe that his speech is monotone, restricted in volume and rate, and he never makes eye contact with you or his mother. Which of the following statements is most accurate regarding this child?

    A. An ASD-specific screening tool appropriate for the child's age is the next important step.

    B. The most important issue for today's visit is to screen the child for abuse and neglect.

    C. This child should be started on oral amphetamine salts, which will lead to improved behavior.

    D. This parent should be reassured, as this child's behavior and development is most likely a normal variant.

    E. It is probable that one of his vaccinations is responsible for this child's clinical findings.

54.2 Which of the following statements is a correct statement regarding development in children?

A. A previously healthy, normally developing 3-year-old child begins to lose bladder control and will no longer speak in sentences due to normal toddler developmental regression.

B. No use of single words by 12 months of age in a child is reason for immediate referral to speech therapy.

C. Children with ASDs will rarely grow up to be independent adults.

D. The parents of a 6-year-old son with autism are counseled that their second child is at increased risk for having an ASD.

54.3 Which of the following observations during a clinical examination is concerning for the presence of an ASD?

A. You walk into the examination room and find a 36-month-old child pretending to have tea with her imaginary friend.

B. A 12-month-old child walks over to the sink and points toward the faucet, but only utters "Uh," and does not say water.

C. A 2-year-old child is holding tightly to a tattered old blanket, without which his mother says he will not leave the house.

D. You tap an 18-month-old child on the shoulder and say, "Look!" and point to a toy in the room, but the child ignores you and continues to spin the wheels on his toy car.

ANSWERS

54.1 **A.** While at first glance the concerns of this child's teacher and mother may sound typical for ADHD, your clinical suspicion should be that the child has ASD (previously Asperger syndrome) based on a history of monotone, restricted speech limited to only one topic of interest, lack of eye contact, lack of peer relationships appropriate to developmental age, and the repetitive, nonfunctional, atypical behavior of rocking and twirling. Appropriate steps at this time include a complete history and physical examination accompanied by an Asperger-specific screening tool and immediate referral to a developmental pediatrician for a complete evaluation. You should reassure the child's mother that immunizations are not implicated in the cause of developmental disorders and administer any vaccines needed (answer E). You should not delay your diagnostic workup for a developmental disorder for any reason. Although immunizations are important, for this child's situation, evaluation of the developmental problems is of higher priority. Abuse and neglect (answer B) are always important to consider, but there are no red flags for abuse or neglect in this child. Answer C (start oral amphetamines) should not be done without a diagnosis. Answer D (reassurance) is not the correct response since this child's behavior is not within developmental expectations.

54.2 **D.** Family studies estimate a recurrence risk of as much as 5% to 6% when there is an older sibling with an ASD. Red flag symptoms indicating the need for an immediate evaluation for an ASD include loss of language or social skills at any age and no use of single words by 16 months of age (not 12 months, as in answer B). Although most children with an ASD will retain their diagnosis and exhibit residual signs of their disorder into adulthood, children with ASD who begin treatment at a younger age have significantly better outcomes, and one of the goals of treatment is to foster independence (answer C). Answer A (regression of bladder and speech) is not necessarily a normal developmental pattern and should be investigated.

54.3 **D.** This child demonstrates a deficit in joint attention, one of the most distinguishing characteristics of very young children with ASDs. It is the lack of pretend play skills, rather than their presence (answer A), that is concerning for an ASD. As demonstrated in answer B, at about 12 to 14 months of age, a typically developing child will begin to request a desired object that is out of reach by pointing, and, depending on the child's speech skills, the child may utter simple sounds or actual words. Similar to answer C, during their early development most children will form attachments to a stuffed animal, special pillow, or blanket. However, children with ASDs may prefer hard items such as ballpoint pens, keys, or flashlights.

CLINICAL PEARLS

▶ Screening tools for ASD and developmental delay are simple and easy to use in the office setting.

▶ Common features shared by all the ASD include severe deficits in social skills and limited, repetitive, and stereotyped behavior patterns.

▶ Red flag symptoms indicating the need for immediate evaluation for an ASD include no babbling or pointing by 12 months, no single words by 16 months, no two-word phrases by 24 months, and loss of language or social skills at any age.

▶ When a child demonstrates two or more risk factors or a positive screening result occurs, take immediate action.

REFERENCES

Ages and Stages Questionnaires. http://www.agesandstages.com. Accessed January 1, 2019.

Centers for Disease Control and Prevention. Diagnostic criteria for 299.00 autism spectrum disorder. http://www.cdc.gov/ncbddd/autism/hcp-dsm.html. Accessed January 1, 2019.

Centers for Disease Control and Prevention. Prevalence of autism spectrum disorder among children aged 8 years—Autism and Developmental Disabilities Monitoring Network, 11 sites, United States, 2014. *MMWR Morb Mortal Wkly Rep.* 2018;67(6);123. http://www.cdc.gov/mmwr/volumes/67/ss/ss6706a1.htm. Accessed January 1, 2019.

Harrington JW, Allen K. The clinician's guide to autism. *Pediatr Rev.* 2014;35(2):62-78.

Hurley AM, Tadrous M, Miller ES. Thimerosal-containing vaccines and autism: a review of recent epidemiological studies. *J Pediatr Pharmacol Ther.* 2010;15(3):173-181.

Johnson CP, Myers SM; American Academy of Pediatrics, Council on Children with Disabilities. Identification and evaluation of children with autism spectrum disorders. *Pediatrics.* 2007;120:1183-1215.

Johnson CP, Myers SM; American Academy of Pediatrics, Council on Children with Disabilities. Management of children with autism spectrum disorders. *Pediatrics.* 2007;120:1162-1182.

Modified Checklist for Autism in Toddlers (M-CHAT). http://www.m-chat.org/mchat.php. Accessed January 1, 2019.

Raviola GJ, Trieu ML, DeMaso DR, Walter HJ. Autism spectrum disorder. In: Kliegman RM, Stanton BF, St Geme JW, Schor NF, Behrman RE, eds. *Nelson Textbook of Pediatrics.* 19th ed. Philadelphia, PA: Saunders Elsevier; 2016:176-183.

Sanchack KE, Thomas CA. Autism spectrum disorder: primary care principles. *Am Fam Physician.* 2016;94(12):972-979.

Screening Tool for Autism in Toddlers and Young Children (STAT). http://vkc.mc.vanderbilt.edu/vkc/triad/stat/. Accessed January 1, 2019.

Smeeth L, Cook C, Fombonne E, et al. MMR vaccination and pervasive developmental disorders: a case-control study. *Lancet.* 2004;364:963-969.

A 46-year-old woman presents to your office complaining of a right-hand tremor that has been steadily worsening over the past 2 years. She works as a literary agent and states that this tremor is increasingly impairing her ability to work since it affects her dominant hand. She tells you in a slightly quivering voice, "I am often required to take my clients out to lunch, and I get embarrassed when I cannot eat and drink normally. Sometimes, I cannot even drink from a cup without shaking." She finds that a glass of wine with her meal sometimes helps minimize the tremor. On examination, her blood pressure is 125/85 mm Hg, her pulse is 84 beats/min, and her respiratory rate is 16 breaths/min. Neurologic examination reveals a mild head tremor but no resting tremor of the hands. However, when she holds a pen by its tip at arm's length, a coarse bilateral tremor becomes readily visible and is more pronounced on the right side. The rest of her examination is unremarkable.

▶ What is the most likely diagnosis?
▶ What further evaluation needs to be performed?
▶ What pharmacologic interventions may be beneficial?

ANSWERS TO CASE 55:
Movement Disorders

Summary: A 46-year-old woman presents with

- A classic essential tremor, manifesting during action and remitting when the limb is relaxed (unlike the tremor of Parkinson disease)
- Great concern about the tremor, as it is leading to a great deal of social embarrassment, often interfering with her work
- Symptom of tremor reduced with alcohol
- Neurologic examination revealing a mild head tremor but no resting tremor of the hands
- Unremarkable rest of examination

Most likely diagnosis: Essential tremor.

Further evaluation: Ensure that medications, thyroid disease, alcohol, or other neurologic diseases are not causing the tremor.

Beneficial pharmacologic interventions: Propranolol and primidone.

ANALYSIS

Objectives

1. Become familiar with the presenting signs and symptoms of the most common movement disorders. (EPA 1, 2)

2. Become familiar with the management of common movement disorders. (EPA 4)

3. Be able to gauge the severity of disease and understand potential side effects of therapies. (EPA 1, 2, 4)

Considerations

Essential tremor is the most common of all movement disorders, affecting 0.4% to 6% of the population. A complete history is crucial in making an appropriate diagnosis of essential tremor. It can present in early adulthood, but its prevalence significantly increases in persons over the age of 70. It often interferes with common tasks and activities of daily living. Close to one-half of all patients with an essential tremor have a family history of tremor, although this is not a strict criterion for diagnosis. Tremor is often attenuated with the use of alcohol. It is important to ask about the consumption of caffeine, cigarette smoking, and stimulant use (eg, pseudoephedrine) and to inquire about prescription medications (eg, fluoxetine, lithium, theophylline, valproic acid, haloperidol, metoclopramide) that are known to cause or enhance physiologic tremor.

When essential tremor is suspected, the patient should be observed while performing goal-directed tasks such as finger-to-nose testing or reaching for and drinking from a glass. Evaluating handwriting samples can help to identify the time of tremor onset and progression of disease. Tremor occurs with action (postural and kinetic), is usually bilateral, and is easily observed in the wrists and hands. However, it may also affect the head, voice, tongue, face, and lower limbs; half of patients report multiple affected body parts. In evaluating patients who present with tremor, thyroid and liver function tests are indicated. Additional testing includes serum ceruloplasmin and copper levels when patients are under age 40 years for evaluation of Wilson disease, a disorder of copper metabolism.

Pharmacotherapy constitutes the main approach to treatment of essential tremor. First-line therapies include the beta-blocker propranolol and the anticonvulsant primidone, which are equally efficacious in reducing tremor symptoms. The patient's report of symptoms and functional ability, rather than the severity of tremor detected on physical examination, should serve as guides for adjustment of therapy. It is also important to monitor patients for side effects of these medications. Propranolol is associated with fatigue, headaches, bradycardia, impotence, and depression. Primidone can cause an acute reaction consisting of nausea, vomiting, confusion, or ataxia in many patients. Therapies used for Parkinson disease, such as deep-brain stimulation and ablation of the ventral intermediate nucleus of the thalamus (Vim nucleus) and focused ultrasound may be considered for patients with intractable tremor.

APPROACH TO:
Movement Disorders

DEFINITIONS

CHOREA: Unpredictable, involuntary, irregular, brief movements that are jerky, writhing, or flowing.

HYPERKINESIAS: Movement disorders characterized by extra or exaggerated movements.

HYPOKINESIAS: Movement disorders characterized by overall slowness of movement (bradykinesia), lack of movement (akinesia), or difficulty in initiating movement.

CLINICAL APPROACH

Definition and Classifications

A movement disorder can be defined as any condition that disrupts normal voluntary movement of the body or that consists of one or more abnormal movements. They can be classified as hypokinesias or hyperkinesias (Table 55–1). Although less frequently encountered by family health providers than other chronic diseases, they are fairly common, especially in the aging population. Parkinson disease, for example, affects 1% of those over 60 and 4% of those over 80 years of age.

Movement disorders present a special challenge for many reasons. Signs and symptoms can often be subtle and may not be detected on routine physical examinations.

Table 55–1 • CLASSIFICATION OF MOVEMENT DISORDERS	
Hypokinetic Disorders	Hyperkinetic Disorders
Parkinson disease	Tremor (essential tremor, dystonic tremor,
Secondary or acquired parkinsonism (can be caused by neuroleptics, hydrocephalus, head trauma)	drug-induced tremor, physiologic tremor)
	Tic disorders (Tourette syndrome)
Progressive supranuclear palsy (PSP)	Chorea (Huntington disease)
	Myoclonus
Multiple system atrophy (Shy-Drager syndrome, olivopontocerebellar atrophy, striatonigral degeneration)	Dystonia
	Ataxia

The normal process of aging is associated with changes in movement that may be mistaken for a more serious problem. **Laboratory and radiologic testing are often of limited value in the diagnosis of movement disorders.**

Management of tremor is equally challenging. Movement disorders have a great impact on other medical conditions as well as on the psychological well-being of patients and their families. Educating both the patient and the family about the disease process and available treatment options can provide better understanding and management of the disorder. Although pharmacotherapy and surgeries are often administered by specialists, family health care providers play an integral role in helping patients to cope with the broad impact of their disease.

Parkinson Disease

Pathophysiology. Parkinson disease is the most common neurodegenerative disease and can cause significant disability and decreased quality of life. Symptoms appear as neurons and dopamine are lost from the substantia nigra (part of the basal ganglia) and intracytoplasmic inclusions (Lewy bodies) proliferate. Dopamine depletion in the substantia nigra ultimately leads to increased inhibition of the thalamus and decreased excitation of the motor cortex, which gives rise to parkinsonian symptoms such as bradykinesia. The **cardinal physical signs of the disease are distal resting tremor, micrographia, cogwheel rigidity, bradykinesia, postural instability, shuffling gait, and asymmetric onset.** Expressive language is typically not affected, but clarity and volume of speech may be compromised.

Treatment. Pharmacotherapy is the mainstay of treatment for Parkinson disease and has been shown to reduce both morbidity and mortality. The goals of treatment are to slow progression and symptomatic therapy. For symptomatic early disease, first-line treatments are levodopa for motor impairment, dopamine agonists such as pramipexole and ropinirole to lower risk of motor complications, and monoamine oxidase type B (MAO-B) inhibitors. Amantidine may be used early on in the disease course but has limited evidence in improving outcomes. Anticholinergics (eg, benztropine, trihexyphenidyl) can also be utilized in young patients with severe tremor, but their use is often limited by side effects.

Tremor is best treated with dopamine agonists, levodopa, and anticholinergics. For motor fluctuations and dyskinesia, dopamine agonists and/or MAO-B inhibitors (eg, selegiline, rasagiline), or catechol-O-methyl transferase (COMT) inhibitors (eg, entacapone, tolcapone) can be added. Deep-brain stimulation of the subthalamic nucleus has been shown to ameliorate symptoms in patients with advanced disease. Physical therapy and exercise may have modest benefits in slowing a patient's functional disability in Parkinson disease.

Complications. Common comorbid problems associated with Parkinson disease include depression, dementia, fatigue, excessive daytime sleepiness, and psychosis. Depression and dementia are common in patients with Parkinson disease. Psychosis is usually drug induced and can be managed initially by reducing the dose of antiparkinsonian medications. In patients with debilitating psychotic symptoms and hallucinations, antiparkinsonian drugs may be discontinued in the reverse order of their effectiveness. Anticholinergics should be stopped first, followed by amantadine, then COMT inhibitors and dopamine agonists. Discontinuing levodopa is typically not an option for most patients with Parkinson disease; however, dose reduction may be considered as a last resort to minimize symptoms. Consultation with a subspecialist for optimal medical management is often required. Since the functional impairment of Parkinson disease is progressive, discussion of advance directives is appropriate with all patients. Education and support are important ways patients can cope with their illness.

Tourette Syndrome

Pathophysiology. **Tourette syndrome (TS) is the most common tic disorder,** usually developing during childhood or early adolescence. Inheritance through an autosomal dominant pattern is thought to play a major role in its etiology. The diagnosis requires the presence of vocal tics such as grunting and multiple motor tics occurring several times a day for at least 1 year, onset generally between 2 and 15 years of age but no later than age 21, and having tics that cannot be explained by other medical conditions or medication side effects. Additionally, a family history of tics or similar symptoms also supports the diagnosis of TS. There are a number of different types of tics, ranging from simple noises to echolalia (repetition of words), coprolalia (excessive use of obscene words), and palilalia (repetition of phrases or words with increasing rapidity). Tics may be temporarily suppressed during mental concentration but generally worsen during periods of stress, excitement, boredom, or fatigue. The majority of affected children also suffer from coexisting attention deficit hyperactivity disorder (ADHD), obsessive-compulsive disorder (OCD), a learning disorder, conduct disorder/oppositional defiant disorder, or migraine headaches.

Patient Education. Education and counseling of patient and family are most important and may be the only treatment necessary. Explanation of tics, obsessions, and compulsions and appreciation that these are not voluntary are often very helpful to patients, family, teachers, and coworkers. Patients frequently will suppress tics most of the day and need to "release" tics upon return from school or work.

Pharmacotherapy. Pharmacotherapy should be considered if there is continued functional impairment despite education and behavioral therapy. Treatment of comorbid ADHD and OCD can reduce Tourette symptoms. Clonidine is considered the first-line treatment due to its long-term safety and its ability to improve symptoms of comorbid ADHD and OCD. Another alpha-receptor blocker, guanfacine, appears safe and effective for tics in patients with ADHD but can cause significant hypotension and must be dosed cautiously.

Neuroleptics such as risperidone, olanzapine, pimozide, and haloperidol are more effective for tics than clonidine but have a greater risk of long-term side effects. Botulinum toxin injection into the affected muscles may be effective for the treatment of refractory phonic tics. Deep-brain stimulation surgery is a final option available for refractory symptoms and requires subspecialty evaluation.

Huntington Disease

Pathophysiology. The most common cause of chorea among adults is Huntington disease. **Huntington disease is inherited in an autosomal dominant pattern** and affects men and women in equal numbers. It is caused by a trinucleotide (CAG) expansion in the huntingtin gene located on chromosome 4. Onset may be at any age, although symptoms first appear between 25 and 45 years of age, with progressive neuronal loss and dysfunction over the following 10 to 20 years.

Clinical Presentation. The two types of movement abnormalities pathognomonic for Huntington disease are **chorea** and **abnormal voluntary movements**. The presence of chorea is required at the time of diagnosis of Huntington disease. Initially, chorea involves mostly the face, trunk, and limbs. With time, the chorea becomes more widespread and affects the diaphragm, larynx, and pharynx. Abnormal voluntary movements include uncoordinated fine-motor movements, gait disturbances, abnormal eye movements, dysarthria, dysphagia, and rigidity. Difficulties with voluntary movements get worse with time. Weight loss and cachexia are common among Huntington disease patients and are caused by the hyperkinetic movements and altered cellular metabolism leading to increased energy expenditure. Cognitive problems include difficulties with memory, visuospatial abilities, and poor judgment. A global dementia may be present in patients with advanced disease. The most common psychiatric problem is depression, which affects up to one-half of patients. Patients with Huntington disease are at significantly higher risk for suicide.

Treatment. There is **currently no treatment available to slow the progression of Huntington disease.** Treatment should target the prevalent signs and symptoms and be adjusted according to disease severity. Physiotherapy for gait and balance issues, a high-calorie diet for increased metabolic requirement, and speech and swallowing therapy for managing dysphagia and aspiration are a few of the supportive measures available for Huntington disease patients. Tetrabenazine, a dopamine-depleting agent, can be helpful for chorea but has limited outcome data. Side effects of tetrabenazine include depression, sedation, akathisia, and parkinsonian symptoms. Chorea that is unresponsive to tetrabenazine can be treated with neuroleptics. Benzodiazepines and antidepressants may be indicated for insomnia, anxiety, and depression. The primary counseling responsibility of the family care provider is to understand the role of genetic testing and to offer it to affected and asymptomatic individuals in a responsible manner. Optimal care usually requires input from a multidisciplinary team that includes neurologists and therapists.

CASE CORRELATION

- See Case 25 (Major Depression and Other Mood Disorders).

COMPREHENSION QUESTIONS

55.1 An 18-year-old young man is noted to have motor tics and involuntary, obscene vocalizations. Which of the following medications is indicated in the treatment of this disorder?

A. Trihexyphenidyl

B. Phenytoin

C. Carbamazepine

D. Haloperidol

E. Levodopa

55.2 A 21-year-old previously healthy woman has been hospitalized for 3 weeks for psychiatric reasons. She developed auditory hallucinations and persecutory delusions over the course of 3 days. Since hospitalization, she was started on haloperidol 2 mg three times daily. Within a week of treatment, she developed stooped posture and a shuffling gait. Her head was slightly tremulous, and her movements became slowed. Her medication was changed to thioridazine, and trihexyphenidyl was added. Over the next 2 weeks, she became much more animated and reported no recurrence of her hallucinations. Which of the following is the most likely diagnosis responsible for the gait and posture condition?

A. Hyperparathyroidism

B. Adverse effect of neuroleptic

C. Encephalitis

D. Hypermagnesemia

E. Tourette syndrome

55.3 Which of the following represents the decrement in speech commonly exhibited by the patient with parkinsonism?

A. Progressively inaudible speech

B. Neologisms

C. Expressive aphasia

D. Receptive aphasia

E. Word salad

55.4 A 67-year-old woman with known Parkinson disease is brought to the clinic by her health care provider. She is confined to a wheelchair and completely dependent on others. You notice large, grossly abnormal movements in both arms and legs. The patient has to be strapped to the wheelchair to avoid falling out and cannot keep her shoes on due to the jerking movements. Bed rails have had to be installed on her bed to prevent her from falling out at night. She is not able to tell the correct month or the year. She has not had a change in her medication in 6 months. Which of the following medication adjustments would benefit her most?

A. Add haloperidol

B. Decrease levodopa/carbidopa

C. Increase levodopa/carbidopa

D. Add donepezil

E. Add entacapone

ANSWERS

55.1 **D.** The clinical scenario described is associated with TS. A variety of drugs may help suppress the tics that are characteristic of this syndrome. These include haloperidol, pimozide, trifluoperazine, and fluphenazine. Antiepileptics such as carbamazepine (answer C) and phenytoin (answer B) are not useful. Levodopa (answer E) is the drug of choice in treating advanced Parkinson disease. Trihexyphenidyl (answer A) and benztropine are useful in suppressing the parkinsonism that may develop with haloperidol administration but are not useful in the management of TS.

55.2 **B.** Butyrophenones, the most commonly prescribed of which is haloperidol, routinely produce some signs of parkinsonism if they are used at high doses for more than a few days. This psychotic young woman proved to be less sensitive to the parkinsonian side effects of thioridazine than she was to haloperidol. Adding the anticholinergic drug trihexyphenidyl may have also helped to reduce the patient's symptoms. Hyperparathyroidism (answer A) manifests as bony pain, fatigue, disorientation, confusion, abdominal pain, and kidney stones. The patient did not have any of these medical problems. Answer C (encephalitis) presents as confusion, photophobia, fever, and nuchal rigidity. Answer D (hypermagnesemia) presents as shallow respirations, somnolence, and muscle weakness. Answer E (TS) presents with normal cognitive function without hallucinations but with physical or vocal tics.

55.3 **A.** Language is not disturbed in Parkinson disease, as it is with aphasias (answer C, expressive aphasia; and answer D, receptive aphasia). The clarity and volume of speech is what suffers. Handwriting is similarly disturbed, as the patient has increasingly smaller and less legible penmanship as he or she continues to write. This is referred to as micrographia. Neologisms (answer B) are made up words or phrases. Word salad (answer E) is a confused mixture of random words or phrases that make no sense.

55.4 **B.** The patient is suffering from dyskinesias from too much levodopa/carbidopa. Stopping levodopa/carbidopa is usually not an option for most patients; however, a reduction of the medication would be most beneficial to her. Increasing the levodopa/carbidopa (answer C) would likely worsen her symptoms. Haloperidol (answer A) would be a good choice if the patient were suffering from hallucinations. Donepezil (answer D) is a medication used primarily for Alzheimer dementia and has no use in Lewy body dementia. Entacapone (answer E) is a medication used to enhance levodopa/carbidopa.

CLINICAL PEARLS

▶ Movement disorders have a profound impact on the quality of life of patients and their families. Providers should become adept at counseling patients about prognosis and the availability of support groups and community resources.

▶ The management of certain movement disorders, including Parkinson disease, is rapidly changing. It is important to find the latest information about emerging and alternative therapies and to seek the help of a specialist when required.

▶ Huntington disease presents as chorea (dance-like movements) and progressive cognitive decline when the patients are in their 20s or 30s.

▶ The pathophysiology of Huntington disease is too many trinucleotide repeats of CAG, affecting the huntingtin gene on chromosome 4.

▶ Tourette syndrome is the most common type of tic disorder in children.

REFERENCES

Crawford P, Zimmerman EE. Tremor: sorting through the differential diagnosis. *Am Fam Physician.* 2018;97(3):180-186.

Gazewood JD, Richards DR, Clebak K. Parkinson disease: an update. *Am Fam Physician.* 2013;87(4):267-273.

Haubenberger D, Hallett M. Essential tremor. *N Engl J Med.* 2018;378:1802-1810.

Kurlan R. Tourette's syndrome. *N Engl J Med.* 2010;363(24):2332-2338.

Novak MJ, Tabrizi SJ. Huntington's disease. *BMJ.* 2010;340:c3109.

Olanow C, Klein C, Obeso JA. Tremor, chorea, and other movement disorders. In: Jameson J, Fauci AS, Kasper DL, Hauser SL, Longo DL, Loscalzo J, eds. *Harrison's Principles of Internal Medicine.* 20th ed. New York, NY: McGraw Hill; 2018: Chap. 428. http://accessmedicine.mhmedical.com/content.aspx?bookid=2129&sectionid=192532409. Accessed December 14, 2018.

Olanow C, Klein C, Schapira AV. Parkinson's disease. In: Jameson J, Fauci AS, Kasper DL, Hauser SL, Longo DL, Loscalzo J, eds. *Harrison's Principles of Internal Medicine.* 20th ed. New York, NY: McGraw Hill; 2018: Chap. 427. http://accessmedicine.mhmedical.com/content.aspx?bookid=2129&sectionid=192532363. Accessed December 14, 2018.

A 28-year-old man presents to your office complaining of a 3-month history of rhinorrhea, itchy eyes, and exertional cough and wheezing. These symptoms have been progressively worsening over the past few months. His past medical history is significant for seasonal allergies to pollen and ragweed. His family history is significant only for hypertension in both parents. His siblings and children are in good health without allergies or respiratory illness. He does not smoke or use illicit drugs and only drinks alcohol rarely. He has worked as an animal laboratory technician for the last 6 months. On questioning, his symptoms were initially more severe toward the end of the work week but are now continuous. He has been taking over-the-counter antihistamines, which helped initially but no longer relieve his allergic symptoms. On review of systems, he has noted hives that are less prominent now that he has been taking the antihistamines on a regular basis. On examination, he is afebrile, his body mass index is 23 kg/m², blood pressure is 120/75 mm Hg, pulse is 72 beats/min, and respiratory rate is 18 breaths/min. His conjunctivae are injected, there is mild clear ocular discharge, and his nasal turbinates are boggy without visible polyps. His lung examination reveals a prolonged expiratory-to-inspiratory ratio and end-expiratory wheezing at the bilateral bases. His heart examination is unremarkable, and there is no peripheral edema.

▶ What is the most likely diagnosis?
▶ What further evaluation should be considered?
▶ What are the initial steps in therapy?

ANSWERS TO CASE 56:
Wheezing and Asthma

Summary: A 28-year-old man presents with

- Classic signs and symptoms of asthma
- A constellation of ocular, nasal, and pulmonary symptoms temporally related to work and environmental conditions, which is suspicious for occupational-related asthma and allergy
- Injected conjunctivae, mild clear ocular discharge, and boggy nasal turbinates without visible polyps
- Lung examination revealing a prolonged expiratory-to-inspiratory ratio and end-expiratory wheezing at the bilateral bases

Most likely diagnosis: Occupation-related allergic asthma, allergy mediated.

Further evaluation: Peak flow measurements pre– and post–beta-agonist treatment. Further workup should include a chest radiograph if concerned about alternative etiologies, pulmonary function testing with bronchodilator challenge, and consideration of allergen testing.

Initial steps in therapy: Initial treatment with a short-acting inhaled beta-agonist (SABA) such as albuterol. A short course of oral steroids should be considered if the patient continues to have wheezing, decreased pulse oximetry, and decreased predicted peak flow measurements after beta-agonist therapy. Antihistamines should be considered for allergic symptoms. This patient should be removed from his current duties of working with laboratory animals.

ANALYSIS

Objectives

1. Recognize the presenting signs and symptoms of the common causes of wheezing. (EPA 1, 2)
2. List the etiologies and pathogenesis of asthma. (EPA 2)
3. Describe the clinical evaluation, diagnosis, and staging of asthma. (EPA 1, 3)
4. Implement the treatment and management of asthma in children and adults. (EPA 4)

APPROACH TO:
Wheezing and Asthma

DEFINITIONS

ASTHMA: A chronic pulmonary disease characterized by inflammation and hyperreactivity of the airways.

EXERCISE-INDUCED ASTHMA: A form of asthma that is intermittent in nature, and associated with activity. Spirometry is normal in between exacerbations.

INTERMITTENT ASTHMA: Symptoms of asthma occurring less than two times a week, nocturnal awakening less than two times a month, the need for oral corticosteroid treatment less than two times in a year, and *no* limitations in normal activities.

PEAK EXPIRATORY FLOW (PEF): An easily reproduced age- and gender-controlled measure of pulmonary function that is used as an indication of current levels of pulmonary obstruction and can be used to monitor and manage asthma.

PERSISTENT ASTHMA: Signs and symptoms greater than those given previously in this section. There are three classifications of persistent asthma: mild, moderate, and severe.

REACTIVE AIRWAY DISEASE: Irritant-induced asthma usually associated with significant environmental exposures to chemical irritants and allergens.

CLINICAL APPROACH

Epidemiology

Asthma is one of the most common chronic diseases in the United States. It is accountable for a substantial number of emergency department evaluations and hospitalizations, many of which are preventable with appropriate management. It affects approximately 10% of adults and 15% of children, with an increasing prevalence in economically developed countries. Genetic and environmental factors play a significant role in the development of asthma. Work-related asthma is implicated in approximately 10% of asthma cases in young adults.

Pathophysiology

In asthma, pathologic changes to the airways reflect inflammatory and remodeling changes, including inflammatory cell infiltration, basement membrane thickening, shedding of epithelial cells, proliferation and engorgement of blood vessels, mucus plugging, smooth muscle hypertrophy, and fibrosis. A differential diagnosis for wheezing is included in Table 56–1.

Classification of the severity of asthma is imperative to direct appropriate acute and maintenance care and to minimize future exacerbations (Tables 56–2 and 56–3).

Table 56–1 • DIFFERENTIAL DIAGNOSIS FOR WHEEZING
Allergic rhinitis and sinusitis
Foreign body in trachea or bronchus
Vocal cord dysfunction
Vascular rings or laryngeal webs
Laryngotracheomalacia, tracheal stenosis, or bronchostenosis
Enlarged lymph nodes or tumor (benign or malignant)
Bronchiectasis of various causes, including cystic fibrosis
Viral bronchiolitis or obliterative bronchiolitis
Cystic fibrosis
Bronchopulmonary dysplasia
Pulmonary infiltrates with eosinophilia
Chronic obstructive pulmonary disease (chronic bronchitis or emphysema)
Pulmonary embolism
Heart failure
Cough secondary to drugs (angiotensin-converting enzyme [ACE] inhibitors)
Aspiration from swallowing mechanism dysfunction or gastroesophageal reflux
Recurrent cough not due to asthma

Data from Health Care Guideline: Diagnosis and Management of Asthma. *9th ed. 2010. Copyright © Institute for Clinical Systems Improvement.*

Clinical Presentation

History. **The characteristic history of asthma includes dyspnea, wheezing, productive or nonproductive cough, and chest tightness or discomfort.** Depending on etiology and patient characteristics, the symptoms can be perennial or seasonal, be episodic or continuous, and/or have a diurnal pattern. Suggestive symptoms include episodic wheezing and cough with nocturnal, seasonal, or exertional characteristics in the absence of an acute upper respiratory tract illness. Frequent episodes of "bronchitis" are seen in young children who are likely to have asthma. Positive family histories for asthma and patient history of atopy (allergies, eczema) when associated with symptoms are correlated with the diagnosis of asthma. It is important to realize that **asthma can occur in all age groups, can present with a varied spectrum of signs and symptoms,** and may be coupled with allergic symptoms.

Physical Examination. The examination may be normal in between symptoms and exacerbations. The variable presentation and often normal examination can account for delays in diagnosis. The eyes and nose should be examined for signs of allergies, including conjunctivitis and nasal polyps. The neck should be evaluated for accessory muscle use in respiratory distress or lymphadenopathy, which may signify an infectious etiology. The lung examination may reveal wheezing heard predominantly on end expiration or forced end expiration with prolongation of expiration compared to inspiration. The heart examination can reveal tachycardia and pulsus paradoxus during exacerbations. The skin should be examined for signs of atopy, eczema, or urticaria, which are all associated with an allergic process.

Acute Exacerbations. An acute asthma exacerbation presents with worsening of the classic symptoms and documented decrease from expected peak flow. Emergency treatment should be considered for

Table 56–2 • CLASSIFYING ASTHMA SEVERITY IN CHILDREN 5-11 YEARS					
		Classification of Asthma Severity (Children 5-11 y)			
			Persistent		
Components of Severity		Intermittent	Mild	Moderate	Severe
Impairment	Symptoms	≤ 2 d/wk	> 2 d/wk but not daily	Daily	Throughout the day
	Nighttime awakenings	≤2×/mo	3-4×/mo	> 1×/wk but not nightly	Often 7×/wk
	Short-acting beta-2 agonist use for symptom control (not prevention of EIB)	≤ 2 d/wk	> 2 d/wk but not daily	Daily	Several times per day
	Interference with normal activity	None	Minor limitation	Some limitation	Extremely limited
	Lung function	• Normal FEV_1 between exacerbations • FEV_1 > 80% predicted • FEV_1/FVC > 85%	• FEV_1 = > 80% predicted • FEV_1/FVC > 80%	• FEV_1 = 60% to 80% predicted • FEV_1/FVC = 75% to 80%	• FEV_1 < 60% predicted • FEV_1/FVC < 75%
Risk	Exacerbations requiring oral systemic corticosteroids	0-1/y	≥ 2 in 1 y		
		Consider severity and interval since last exacerbation; frequency and severity may fluctuate over time for patients in any severity category.			
		Relative annual risk of exacerbations may be related to FEV_1.			

Abbreviations: EIB, exercise-induced bronchoconstriction; FEV₁, forced expiratory volume in 1 second; FVC, forced vital capacity.
Source: Reproduced with permission, from National Asthma Education and Prevention Program Expert Panel Report 3. Guidelines for the Diagnosis and Management of Asthma. National Heart Lung and Blood Institute. NIH Publication number 08-5846. October 2007.

- Peak flow less than 50% predicted normal (based upon age, gender, and height) and hypoxia

- Failure to respond to a beta-2 agonist

- Severe wheezing or coughing

- Extreme anxiety due to breathlessness

- Gasping for air, sweaty, or cyanotic

- Rapid clinical deterioration over a few hours with worsening hypoxia

- Severe retractions and nasal flaring

- Posture with shoulders hunched forward

Signs and symptoms for patients who are particularly at risk for poor control of the disease and outcomes, including death, are listed in Table 56–4. Other risk

Table 56–3 • CLASSIFYING ASTHMA SEVERITY IN YOUTH AND ADULTS

Components of Severity		Classification of Asthma Severity (Youth > 12 y and adults)			
		Intermittent	Persistent		
			Mild	Moderate	Severe
Impairment Normal FEV₁/FVC: 8-19 y 85% 20-39 y 80% 40-59 y 75% 60-80 y 70%	Symptoms	≤ 2 d/wk	> 2 d/wk but not daily	Daily	Throughout the day
	Nighttime awakenings	≤ 2×/mo	3-4×/mo	> 1×/wk but not nightly	Often 7×/wk
	Short-acting beta₂-agonist use for symptom control (not prevention of EIB)	≤ 2 d/wk	> 2 d/wk but not >1×/d	Daily	Several times per day
	Interference with normal activity	None	Minor limitation	Some limitation	Extremely limited
	Lung function	• Normal FEV₁ between exacerbations • FEV₁ > 80% predicted • FEV₁/FVC normal	• FEV₁ ≥ 80% predicted • FEV₁/FVC normal	• FEV₁ > 60% but < 80% predicted • FEV₁/FVC reduced 5%	• FEV₁ < 60% predicted • FEV₁/FVC reduced > 5%
Risk	Exacerbations requiring oral systemic corticosteroids	0-1/y	≥ 2/y		
		Consider severity and interval since last exacerbation; frequency and severity may fluctuate over time for patients in any severity category. Relative annual risk of exacerbations may be related to FEV₁.			

FEV_1, FEV_1/FVC, $beta_2$

Abbreviations: EIB, exercise-induced bronchoconstriction; FEV_1, forced expiratory volume in 1 second; FVC, forced vital capacity.
Source: Reproduced with permission, from National Asthma Education and Prevention Program Expert Panel Report 3. Guidelines for the Diagnosis and Management of Asthma. *National Heart Lung and Blood Institute. NIH Publication number 08-5846. October 2007.*

Table 56–4 • SIGNS AND SYPTOMS OF POOR ASTHMA CONTROL

At Regular Ambulatory Visits	At Presentation With Symptoms
• Previous admission for intensive care or intubations • Three or more emergency department visits for asthma in the last year • Two or more canisters of short-acting beta-agonists in a month • Failure to use controllers (inhaled corticosteroids) despite symptoms • Current or recent cessation of oral corticosteroids • Multiple courses of oral corticosteroids in the past year for asthma exacerbations • Large fluctuations in peak flow	• A chest examination with minimal sounds on auscultation • Distress and difficulty speaking on examination • Tachycardia • Elevated carbon dioxide (CO_2) on arterial blood gas with hypoxia. Typically, arterial carbon dioxide is low during an asthmatic attack due to increased respiratory rate. Normalization of carbon dioxide may be a sign of a severe exacerbation indicating CO_2 retention and impending respiratory failure requiring intubation

factors include a low socioeconomic status in an urban environment, mental disorders, and substance abuse.

Diagnostic Studies. Accurate spirometry is recommended for every patient 5 years of age or older at the time of diagnosis. Additional studies, tailored to the specific patient and symptoms, include

- Bronchial provocation (eg, methacholine challenge) testing is the "gold standard" test for the diagnosis of asthma for patients with normal or near-normal spirometry

- Allergy testing (eg, skin testing, serum allergen [radioallergosorbent test, RAST] testing, immunoglobulin [Ig] E antibody testing)

- Chest radiography, to exclude alternative diagnosis

- Arterial blood gas measurement

- Computed tomographic (CT) scan of sinuses

- Evaluation for gastroesophageal reflux disease

- Complete blood count with eosinophils, total IgE, sputum culture

Treatment

Treatment for asthma always begins with education and counseling, environmental controls, and management of comorbid conditions. Proper use of inhalers is paramount for minimizing morbidity, including hospitalization. Reduction in exposure to causative or aggravating environmental exposures, including allergens, occupational exposures, smoking, and other irritants and allergens, is paramount in limiting the long-term remodeling and damage associated with this chronic disease. **The chief cause of poor control in asthma is due to lack of adherence to environmental controls and prescribed medications.** Education in asthma self-management involving self-monitoring by PEF or symptoms, along with regular monitoring and a written plan, improves outcomes for patients.

Pharmacologic measures to treat and manage asthma are instituted in a stepwise fashion based on the staging of asthma (Table 56–5). Subcutaneous immunotherapy is an option for any patient with persistent allergic asthma in stages 2 to 4.

Medications—Fast-Acting Agents

Short-Acting Beta-2 Agonists. **Short-acting beta-2 agonists** are the most effective therapy for prompt relief of asthmatic symptoms. Albuterol, levalbuterol, and pirbuterol are the SABAs used in the United States and are generally considered equally effective in onset and duration of action. They have an onset of action of 5 minutes or less, peak in 30 to 60 minutes, and last 4 to 6 hours. They should be used only as needed for relief of symptoms or before anticipated exposure to known asthmatic triggers (eg, animals, exercise). Dose-dependent side effects include tremor, anxiety, heart pounding, and tachycardia (but not hypertension).

Table 56–5 • TREATMENT FOR ASTHMA BASED ON SEVERITY

Classification	Days With Symptoms	Nights With Symptoms	PEF or FEV₁*	Treatment[a] (for Persons ≥ 12 y)
Severe persistent	Continual	Frequent	≤ 60%	Preferred: high-dose inhaled steroid and long-acting beta-agonist and consider omalizumab in patients with allergies
				If needed, high-dose inhaled steroid, long-acting beta-agonist, and oral steroid and consider omalizumab in patients with allergies
Moderate persistent	Daily	> 1×/wk but not nightly	> 60% to < 80%	Preferred: low-dose inhaled steroid and long-acting beta-agonist or medium-dose inhaled steroid
				Alternative: low-dose inhaled steroid and leukotriene modifier, theophylline, or zileuton
				Additional treatment if needed (particularly in patients with recurring severe exacerbations):
				Preferred: increase inhaled steroid within medium-dose range and long-acting beta-agonist
				Alternative: increase inhaled steroid within medium-dose range and add leukotriene modifier, theophylline, or zileuton
Mild persistent	> 2 d/wk but not daily	3-4/mo	≥ 80%	Preferred: low-dose inhaled steroid
				Alternative: cromolyn, nedocromil, leukotriene modifier, or theophylline
Intermittent	≤ 2/wk	≤ 2/mo	≥80%	No daily medication needed; short-acting beta-agonist as needed for symptoms
				Severe exacerbations may occur, separated by long periods of normal function and no symptoms; a course of systemic corticosteroids is recommended

*PEF is % of Personal Best; FEV₁ is % of Predicted.

[a]All patients: short-acting bronchodilator as needed for symptoms.

Data from National Asthma Education and Prevention Program Expert Panel Report 3. Guidelines for the Diagnosis and Management of Asthma. *National Heart Lung and Blood Institute. NIH Publication number 08-5846. October 2007.*

Metered-Dose Inhalers. **Metered-dose inhalers** (MDIs) are the delivery mechanism of choice for all SABAs, and the use of spacers is encouraged. **Nebulizer** treatments with SABAs are an alternative in those who cannot use an MDI, yet MDIs with spacers work as well as nebulizers when used correctly. MDI actuations can be taken in 10- to 15-second intervals, and nebulized treatment doses can be given continuously in severe cases. Increasing use or using them more than 2 days per week for symptom relief (not for prevention) generally indicates inadequate control of asthma or persistent asthma. If patients are not controlled with MDIs, the clinician should ensure that the medications are being used in the appropriate dosing intervals.

Anticholinergic Bronchodilators. **Anticholinergic bronchodilators,** such as ipratropium, combined with a SABA are more beneficial in treating severe asthmatic attacks or those induced by beta-blockers in the urgent care setting compared to treatment with a SABA alone.

Medications—Long-Acting Agents

The long-term daily use of control medications is indicated for persistent asthma to prevent symptoms and eventually hospitalizations. These medications are **inhaled corticosteroids** (ICSs), **leukotriene receptor antagonists** (LRAs), and **long-acting beta-2 agonists** (LABA).

Inhaled Corticosteroids. **When ICSs are used consistently, they improve asthma symptoms more effectively than any other medications in both children and adults.** Except with long-term, high-dose use, systemic side effects of ICSs may occur but are rare. Dysphonia, sore throat, and thrush can occur but are generally managed well with the use of a spacer, and rinsing out the spacer with water after use. **Oral corticosteroid** treatment is recommended for moderate-to-severe exacerbation dosed 1 to 2 mg/kg per day for 3 to 10 days in children or 40 to 60 mg per day in one or two divided doses for 5 to 10 days in adults. Tapering steroid doses for short courses is typically not necessary.

Leukotriene Receptor Antagonists. The two most widely available LRAs are montelukast and zafirlukast. In patients who are unable or unwilling to use ICSs, montelukast and zafirlukast are appropriate alternative therapies for mild persistent asthma, and they have the advantages of ease of use. They also play a role in controlling many symptoms of allergic rhinitis. Combining LRAs and ICSs is a viable option for moderate persistent asthma.

Long-Acting Beta-2 Agonists. The LABAs **salmeterol** and **formoterol** are beta-agonists with a duration of action of more than 12 hours. They have low rates of tremor and palpitations or tachycardia. However, the inhibition of exercise-induced asthma rapidly wanes with regular use. There appears to be an increase in severe exacerbations and deaths when LABAs are added to usual asthma therapy. It is recommended that **LABAs should never be used as monotherapy for long-term control of persistent asthma** and should only be used in combination therapy. Increasing the dose of an ICS should be considered before adding a LABA if the initial dosage of the ICS is not effective.

Omalizumab. Omalizumab is a monoclonal anti-IgE antibody that should be instituted only in collaboration or consultation with an asthma subspecialist for highest risk patients 12 years or older. It is used as additive therapy in patients with severe persistent asthma who have demonstrated immediate hypersensitivity to inhaled allergens. Additional antibodies that block interleukin (IL) 5 or its receptor have been developed; these antibodies reduce eosinophil counts and decrease exacerbations in patients with persistently elevated eosinophils despite being on maximal ICS therapy.

Acute Management of Asthma

In the acute care setting, immediate treatment with a SABA with monitoring of vitals and PEF is indicated. If within 20 minutes a patient has an **incomplete response** (PEF 40% to 69% predicted), then three more SABA treatments within 1 hour (via MDI or nebulizer) should be given. If there is a **poor response** (PEF < 40% or oxygen saturations < 90%), then the addition of oral or intravenous corticosteroids is indicated. If the patient continues to have an inadequate or poor response, then inpatient management with continuous oximetry and close monitoring should be considered.

Additional Measures

All asthmatics should be given a dose of the pneumococcal polysaccharide vaccine (PPSV 23) and should have a yearly influenza vaccination. They should also remain up to date with age-appropriate pertussis and pneumococcal conjugate vaccine (PCV 13) immunizations.

CASE CORRELATION

- See Case 2 (Dyspnea [Chronic Obstructive Pulmonary Disease]), Case 19 (Upper Respiratory and Ear Infections), and Case 24 (Pneumonia).

COMPREHENSION QUESTIONS

56.1 A 25-year-old woman who is training for a competitive marathon complains of "hitting a wall" and "getting short of breath quicker than [she] should." She complains of coughing at the end of her training runs and states that she may be expecting too much of herself. She does not smoke and has no significant family history or history of occupational or environmental exposures. Her physical findings, including lung examination, are unremarkable. Spirometry reveals normal values both pre- and postalbuterol treatment. What would be the most reasonable first step in the treatment of this patient?

A. Trial of albuterol MDI before exercise

B. Chest radiograph

C. Chest CT

D. Counseling for athletic burnout or stress

E. An echocardiogram to rule out pulmonary hypertension or cardiac disorder

56.2 A 34-year-old man with a 20-year past history of asthma presents to an acute care clinic with an asthmatic exacerbation. Treatment with nebulized albuterol and ipratropium does not offer significant improvement, and he is then admitted to the hospital. He is afebrile and has a respiratory rate of 24 breaths/min, pulse rate of 96 beats/min, and oxygen saturation of 93% on room air. On examination, he has diffuse bilateral inspiratory and expiratory wheezes, mild intercostal retractions, and a clear productive cough. Which one of the following is the best next step in the management of this patient?

A. Chest physical therapy

B. ICSs

C. Azithromycin orally

D. Theophylline orally

E. Oral corticosteroids

56.3 A 13-year-old boy has a nonproductive cough and mild shortness of breath on a daily basis. He is awakened by the cough at least 5 nights per month. Which one of the following would be the most appropriate treatment for this patient?

A. A LABA daily

B. A SABA daily

C. Oral prednisone daily

D. An oral leukotriene inhibitor as needed

E. ICS daily

ANSWERS

56.1 **A.** Exercise-induced asthma or bronchoconstriction is a common, underdiagnosed condition in athletes. Many of the athletes are unaware of the problem. It is defined as a 10% lowering of the forced expiratory volume in the first second of expiration (FEV_1) when challenged with exercise. It is much more common in high-ventilation sports and in cold, dry air. The incidence among cross-country skiers is as high as 50%. A physical examination and spirometry evaluation at rest will be normal unless there is underlying asthma. Methacholine challenge testing can be ordered, but if it is not available, a trial with an albuterol inhaler is reasonable. Pulmonary or cardiac dysfunction not found during the physical examination is much less likely; therefore, an echocardiogram (answer E), chest x-ray (answer B), and CT (answer C) would not be indicated until common etiologies have been ruled out. Psychologic causes (answer D) are also a less likely etiology.

56.2 **E.** Hospital management of acute exacerbations of asthma should include inhaled short-acting bronchodilators and systemic corticosteroids. The efficacy of oral versus intravenous corticosteroids has been shown to be equivalent. Antibiotics (answer C) are not needed in the treatment of asthma exacerbations unless there are signs of infection. Chest physical therapy (answer A) and theophylline (answer D) are not recommended for acute asthma exacerbations. ICSs (answer B) are not sufficient in this acute hospitalized episode; systemic corticosteroids are required.

56.3 **E.** This patient has moderate persistent asthma. The most effective treatment is daily ICSs. A leukotriene inhibitor (answer D) would be less effective and, when used as an asthma controller, should be used daily. Oral prednisone daily (answer C) is problematic due to the risk of adrenal insufficiency. LABAs and SABAs (answers A and B, respectively) are not recommended as daily therapy because they are considered rescue medications rather than asthma controllers.

CLINICAL PEARLS

▶ Use the rule of twos to differentiate between intermittent and persistent asthma. Intermittent asthma involves: two or less symptoms or SABA use a week, two or less nocturnal awakenings a month, or two or less need for oral steroids in a year.

▶ The chief causes of inadequate control are poor adherence to medication plan, to appropriate MDI utilization, and to environmental control.

▶ As with any chronic disease, continuous education and follow-up are essential for optimal management.

▶ Persistent asthma should have controller therapy. ICSs are the first-line controller.

▶ In adults with new-onset asthma, it is important to take a good occupational and allergy exposure history.

REFERENCES

Barnes PJ. Asthma. In: Jameson J, Fauci AS, Kasper DL, Hauser SL, Longo DL, Loscalzo J, eds. *Harrison's Principles of Internal Medicine.* 20th ed. New York, NY: McGraw Hill; 2015: Chap. 281. http://accessmedicine.mhmedical.com/content.aspx?bookid=2129&Sectionid=186950288. Accessed November 14, 2018.

Falk NP, Hughes SW, Rodgers BC. Medications for chronic asthma. *Am Fam Physician.* 2016; 94(6):454-462.

National Institute for Health and Care Excellence. Asthma: diagnosis, monitoring and chronic asthma management. https://www.nice.org.uk/guidance/NG80/evidence. Accessed March 3, 2019.

Pollart SM, Compton RM, Elward KS. Management of acute asthma exacerbations. *Am Fam Physician.* 2011;84(1):40-47.

Tarlo SM, Lemiere C. Occupational asthma. *N Engl J Med.* 2014;370(7):640-649.

Tarlo SM, Liss GM. Prevention of occupational asthma. *Curr Allergy Asthma Rep.* 2010;10(4):278-286.

Weiler JM, Anderson SD, Randolph C, et al. Pathogenesis, prevalence, diagnosis, and management of exercise-induced bronchoconstriction: a practice parameter. *Ann Allergy Asthma Immunol.* 2010;105(6 suppl):S1-S47.

A 55-year-old man presents to your office accompanied by his wife. She reports that while he has snored heavily for years, recently she believes that he stops breathing in his sleep several times every night. Over the last year, he reports increasing daytime somnolence and increasing dependence on caffeine, with some difficulty concentrating on his work tasks. He admits that he has almost fallen asleep while driving on several occasions. He sleeps 6 to 8 hours per night but does not feel rested in the morning. He smokes a pack of cigarettes daily and drinks a few beers on the weekends. On examination, he is an obese man with a short, wide neck. His body mass index (BMI) is 36 kg/m², blood pressure is 167/96 mm Hg, pulse is 88 beats/min, and respiratory rate is 16 breaths/min. On HEENT (head, ears, eyes, nose, and throat) examination, you can only see his hard palate when he opens his mouth and says "ahhh." His cardiac, pulmonary, abdominal, and extremity examinations are unremarkable.

► What condition is most likely to be responsible for his sleepiness?
► What should be the first step in his evaluation?
► What would be the most effective initial management?

ANSWERS TO CASE 57:

Obstructive Sleep Apnea

Summary: A 55-year-old man presents with

- Snoring and possible apnea
- Excessive daytime sleepiness, falling asleep while driving, and difficulty concentrating at work
- Examination showing an obese and hypertensive male with a short, wide neck
- Only his hard palate visible when he says "ahh" on HEENT examination
- Blood pressure of 167/96 mm Hg and other vital signs within normal limits
- Unremarkable cardiac, pulmonary, abdominal, and extremity examinations

Condition most likely responsible for his sleepiness: Obstructive sleep apnea (OSA).

First step in his evaluation: Comprehensive sleep evaluation including the Epworth Sleepiness Scale and a polysomnogram (PSG). If the PSG is positive, then continuous positive airway pressure (CPAP) titration is indicated.

Most effective initial management: CPAP for nighttime use and lifestyle modifications, including weight reduction, control of hypertension, and smoking cessation.

ANALYSIS

Objectives

1. Identify patients at risk for OSA, the common signs and symptoms of OSA, and indications for conducting a comprehensive sleep evaluation (EPA 1, 3)

2. Explain the pathophysiology and differential diagnosis of OSA. (EPA 2)

3. Describe the diagnosis and management of OSA and the importance of patient support and education. (EPA 4)

4. Identify comorbid conditions associated with OSA. (EPA 12)

Considerations

The patient in this case presents with a history and examination that suggest a diagnosis of OSA. The first step in his management is advising him not to drive, for the safety of himself and others, pending further evaluation and treatment. A comprehensive sleep evaluation includes a thorough sleep history, medical history, and physical examination. **The gold standard for diagnosis of OSA is determined by overnight PSG.** The initial treatment approach should include patient education, weight reduction, hypertension management, smoking cessation, and CPAP with close follow-up.

APPROACH TO:
Obstructive Sleep Apnea

DEFINITIONS

APNEA: Defined in adults as breathing pauses lasting at least 10 seconds accompanied by a 90% or more drop in airflow.

APNEA HYPOPNEA INDEX (AHI): Number of apnea and hypopnea episodes per hour of sleep.

HYPOPNEA: A 50% reduction in airflow lasting at least 10 seconds with a 3% drop in oxygen saturation, or a 30% reduction in airflow lasting at least 10 seconds with a 4% drop in oxygen saturation.

POLYSOMNOGRAPHY: A noninvasive procedure that monitors sleep stages and cycles as well as limb movements, breathing, and cardiac parameters (also called a sleep study).

RERA: Respiratory effort–related arousal. This is a breathing disorder characterized by upper airway reduction of air flow, and resolves with arousals. The patient's condition does not meet the criteria for apnea or hypopnea.

RESPIRATORY DISTURBANCE INDEX (RDI): Number of apnea, hypopnea, and RERA episodes per hour of sleep.

CLINICAL APPROACH

Pathophysiology

OSA is a chronic disease that affects 2% to 9% of adults and 2% to 5% of children. Its prevalence has increased dramatically in the last few decades in proportion with obesity. People with OSA experience repetitive collapse of the upper airway during sleep, leading to hypopnea, apnea, and RERA episodes. During normal sleep, decreased tone of oropharyngeal muscles and supine positioning increase susceptibility of the airway to collapse, leading to reduced or absent airflow despite continued respiratory effort. Anatomic and pathologic factors that increase the risk of OSA are listed in Table 57–1.

This phenomenon is demonstrated on PSG by lack of airflow despite abdominal and chest wall movement during an obstructive event. In contrast, central apnea is defined as reduction of breathing due to lack of respiratory effort, evidenced by absence of chest wall or abdominal wall movement on PSG. In OSA, airway obstruction (often preceded by snoring) results in hypoxia and hypercapnia. Untreated OSA is associated with significant morbidity, including excessive daytime sleepiness, cognitive impairment, increased risk of motor vehicle and work-related accidents, low mood, and impaired relationships. In addition, OSA is associated with

Table 57-1 • PATHOPHYSIOLOGIC FACTORS ASSOCIATED WITH OSA
• Anatomy that predisposes to narrow airway and obstructed airflow
• Micrognathia—abnormally small mandible
• Retrognathia—posteriorly displaced mandible
• Enlarged tonsils or adenoids
• Obesity, causing increased adipose tissue
• Nasal polyps
• Thyroid enlargement and acromegaly, both of which narrow the upper airway with increased tissue
• Decreased tone of upper airway, dilating muscles
• Arousal threshold: arousal from sleep is a protective mechanism to restore airway patency; patients with OSA are less able to restore airflow without arousal

increased mortality related to a variety of metabolic and cardiovascular conditions, including sudden cardiac death (Table 57–2).

The diagnosis of OSA is based on a comprehensive sleep evaluation, which includes a sleep-related history and physical examination. If OSA is suggested by the history and physical, a PSG with CPAP titration should be performed to confirm the diagnosis, determine severity, and guide treatment. A differential diagnosis for OSA is included in Table 57–3.

Clinical Presentation

History. A comprehensive sleep history includes asking the patient and their bed partner about snoring, daytime sleepiness not explained by other causes, witnessed apneas, choking or gasping during sleep, sleep amount, nocturia, decreased libido, morning headache, insomnia, frequent awakenings, impaired concentration and memory, alertness, and history of falling asleep at the wheel.

Several standardized scales are available to assess fatigue and sleepiness. The Epworth Sleepiness Scale is a useful tool to help determine the extent of sleepiness, although a low score does not rule out sleep apnea. Positive results on an OSA-specific questionnaire (ie, STOP-Bang Questionnaire) or physical examination merit further evaluation.

Table 57-2 • CONDITIONS ASSOCIATED WITH OSA
Obesity
Atrial fibrillation
Resistant hypertension
Acute coronary syndrome, including acute myocardial infarction (MI)
Heart failure
Type 2 diabetes
Stroke
Nocturnal dysrhythmias
Pulmonary hypertension
Sudden cardiac death

Table 57–3 • DIFFERENTIAL DIAGNOSIS FOR OSA
Snoring
Narcolepsy
Pulmonary disease
Periodic limb movements of sleep
Shift work sleep disorder
Obesity hypoventilation syndrome (obesity and hypoventilation in the absence of other conditions that could account for hypoventilation; evidenced by a $Pco_2 > 45$ mm Hg while awake; most people with this condition have concomitant OSA)

Physical Examination. The physical examination should include evaluation for features suggestive of the presence of OSA. They include BMI over 30 kg/m², hypertension, retrognathia (abnormal posterior positioning of the mandible), obesity, thick neck (likely correlated to a Mallampati class 3 or 4 score), macroglossia (large tongue), acromegaly, thyroid enlargement, tonsillar hypertrophy, enlarged uvula, enlarged nasal turbinates or polyps, and narrow or high-arched palate. The appearance of the oropharynx may be assessed using the Mallampati Classification (Figure 57–1).

Polysomnography. According to the American Academy of Sleep Medicine, in-lab PSG and home testing with portable monitors are both acceptable objective tests for OSA. PSG includes the following physiologic assessments: electroencephalogram, continuous telemetry, electrooculogram, chin electromyogram (EMG), airflow, and oxygen saturation. Additionally, anterior tibialis EMG can help assess for

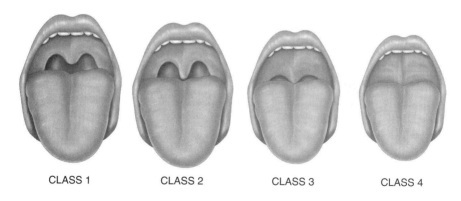

CLASS 1   CLASS 2   CLASS 3   CLASS 4

MALLAMPATI CLASSIFICATION
CLASS 1: Soft palate, fauces, uvula, pillars
CLASS 2: Soft palate, fauces, portion of uvula
CLASS 3: Soft palate, base of uvula
CLASS 4: Hard palate only

Figure 57–1. The Mallampati classification. (*Source:* Reproduced with permission, from Brunicardi FC, Anderson DK, Billiar TR, et al., eds. *Schwartz's Principles of Surgery,* 11e. 2019. Copyright © McGraw Hill LLC. All rights reserved.)

periodic limb movements, which can coexist with sleep-related breathing disorders. The diagnosis of OSA in adults is confirmed by the following:

- AHI or RDI ≥ 15, defined by at least 15 obstructive events (apneas, hypopneas, RERAs) per hour on PSG with or without symptoms

Or

- AHI or RDI ≥ 5, defined by five or more obstructive respiratory events per hour on PSG in a patient who has symptoms of
  - Daytime sleepiness
  - Unrefreshing sleep
  - Fatigue
  - Insomnia
  - Nighttime awakenings associated with gasping, choking, or breath holding, or witnessed loud snoring and/or breathing interruptions

Severe OSA is defined as having more than 30 RDI per hour; moderate OSA is defined as 15 to 30 RDI per hour, and mild OSA is defined as 5 to 14 RDI per hour.

Most patients will require a full night study for diagnosis, with a follow-up study to determine the level of positive airway pressure (PAP) required for appropriate treatment. In the unlikely event that a patient demonstrates AHI ≥ 20 during the first 2 hours of a diagnostic study, the technician may convert to a split-night study in which diagnosis and PAP titration can be accomplished in a single night.

Treatment

The medical, behavioral, and surgical therapies for OSA should involve a multidisciplinary approach. PAP is the treatment of choice for OSA of all severities, although alternative therapies may be indicated based on the patient's anatomy and severity of OSA.

Risk Reduction Strategies. All patients should be counseled on risk reduction strategies and supported with evidenced-based health behavior modification resources as needed. These include weight loss, smoking cessation, avoidance of alcohol and sedating medications, and driving precautions. Some individuals have elevated AHI or RDI in the supine position but not in other positions and may benefit from sleep-position measures to prevent sleeping in the supine position. After significant weight loss, the need for continued therapy or for CPAP adjustment should be evaluated.

Positive Airway Pressure. PAP acts as support to maintain patency of the upper airway and reduces the AHI. Different modes of PAP delivery include CPAP, bilevel (BiPAP), and automatic titrating (APAP). PAP can be applied using a full-face mask, oral mask, nasal mask, or nasal pillows. Proper fitting of these appliances is key to efficacy and patient experience. Heated humidification can assist in patient comfort. Adverse effects include nasal congestion or dryness, nosebleeds, claustrophobia, air swallowing, skin rash, or minor trauma from the mask.

Surgery. Surgical therapy, such as uvulopalatoplasty, may be considered in patients who are resistant to PAP and possess a reversible anatomical cause of obstruction. However, there is insufficient evidence to support any particular surgical treatment of OSA. In contrast, bariatric surgery has been shown to improve symptoms in obese patients with OSA. Tracheostomy is curative and can be considered in extremely advanced cases refractory to treatment. There is no pharmacologic therapy for OSA aside from treating underlying diseases, such as acromegaly or hypothyroidism, that are causative etiologies. All patients with OSA require individualized care and regular follow-up to assess symptoms, treatment response, and side effects, and to treat medical conditions associated with OSA.

CASE CORRELATION
- See Case 2 (Dyspnea [Chronic Obstructive Pulmonary Disease]) and Case 56 (Wheezing and Asthma).

COMPREHENSION QUESTIONS

57.1 A 47-year-old obese woman presents complaining of excessive daytime sleepiness, snoring, and frequent awakenings from sleep. She is having difficulty concentrating, and her sleepiness is affecting personal and professional relationships. She smokes a pack of cigarettes per day, averages two glasses of wine per night, and has hypertension and hyperlipidemia. You perform a comprehensive sleep history and physical examination. You suspect OSA. Which of the following physical examination findings is most suggestive of OSA?

A. Mallampati score of 2
B. Obesity
C. Acanthosis nigricans
D. Peripheral edema
E. Elevated blood pressure

57.2 You decide to perform an overnight PSG study to confirm the diagnosis for the patient in Question 57.1. The study is converted into a split-night study because her AHI was found to be over 40 (normal < 5) in the first 2 hours of the study. What is the most likely diagnosis?

A. Mild OSA
B. Moderate OSA
C. Severe OSA
D. Positional OSA
E. Central apnea

57.3 What is the next step in management of the patient in Questions 57.1 and 57.2?

    A. Dobutamine stress echocardiogram

    B. Treatment with PAP

    C. Referral for uvulopalatoplasty

    D. Pulmonary function testing

    E. Dental evaluation for oral appliance

57.4 A 54-year-old man comes to your clinic for a follow-up for OSA. He has been using PAP with a nasal mask for the last 3 years since he was diagnosed. He has recently purchased a CPAP machine and tells you he has been unable to use it because of facial discomfort and nasal congestion. You check the machine and all the parts are in good condition. What is the next most appropriate step in the management of this patient?

    A. Decrease the airway pressure

    B. Refer for surgery

    C. Refer for an oral appliance

    D. Change the mask

    E. Add heated humidification

ANSWERS

57.1 **B.** People who are obese are considered to be at high risk for OSA. A Mallampati score of 3 or more suggests increased risk for OSA (not Mallampati score of 2, as in answer A). Acanthosis nigricans (answer C) is suggestive of insulin resistance. Peripheral edema (answer D) has a broad differential diagnosis, and further evaluation is warranted. Elevated blood pressure (answer E), in contrast to resistant hypertension, is not a risk factor for OSA.

57.2 **C.** This patient has severe OSA based on an RDI over 30 episodes per hour. The other answer choices (answer A, mild OSA; answer B, moderate OSA; answer D, positional OSA; and answer E, central apnea) are not correct based on these findings.

57.3 **B.** PAP is the treatment of choice for OSA, and since this patient had an AHI over 40 per hour for 2 hours of the study, it should be converted into a split-night study, meaning PAP was applied and titrated in the same night. Surgery (answer C) and oral appliances (answer E) are alternative treatment options, but for this patient the initial treatment should be PAP. Pulmonary function testing (answer D) and cardiac stress testing (answer A) are not indicated.

57.4 **E.** Heated humidification is indicated to improve patient comfort while using PAP. If the patient remains uncomfortable despite this addition, other measures should be taken, such as a trial of a different type of mask (answer D), such as nasal pillows or pressure relief. If all modifications and patient comfort interventions fail, then an alternative treatment (such as surgery [answer B]) may be necessary.

CLINICAL PEARLS

▶ OSA is a chronic disease that, if left untreated, is associated with increased risk of cardiovascular disease and sudden death.

▶ A diagnosis of OSA should be considered in people with associated medical conditions or suggestive features on history (smoking) or physical examination (obesity).

▶ Polysomnography is required to confirm the diagnosis of OSA, determine the severity, and guide treatment.

REFERENCES

Greenstone M, Hack M. Obstructive sleep apnoea. *BMJ.* 2014;348:g3745.

Krishnan V, Dixon-Williams S, Thornton JD. Where there is smoke . . . there is sleep apnea: exploring the relationship between smoking and sleep apnea. *Chest.* 2014;146(6):1673-1680.

Myers KA, Mrkobrada M, Simel DL. Does this patient have obstructive sleep apnea? The Rational Clinical Examination systematic review. *JAMA.* 2013;310(7):731-741.

Qaseem A, Holty JC, Owens DK, et al. Management of obstructive sleep apnea in adults: a clinical practice guideline from the American College of Physicians. *Ann Intern Med.* 2013;159:471-483.

Ramar K, Olson EJ. Management of common sleep disorders. *Am Fam Physician.* 2013;88(4):231-238.

Semelka M, Wilson J, Floyd R. Diagnosis and treatment of obstructive sleep apnea in adults. *Am Fam Physician.* 2016;94(5):355-361.

US Preventive Services Task Force. Screening for obstructive sleep apnea in adults: recommendation statement. *Am Fam Physician.* 2017;96(2):122A-122C.

Wellman A, Redline S. Sleep apnea. In: Jameson J, Fauci AS, Kasper DL, Hauser SL, Longo DL, Loscalzo J, eds. *Harrison's Principles of Internal Medicine.* 20th ed., New York, NY: McGraw Hill; 2018: Chap. 291. http://accessmedicine.mhmedical.com/content.aspx?bookid=2129&Sectionid=189408390. Accessed May 26, 2019.

A 72-year-old woman presents complaining of moderate right-sided chest pain and difficulty breathing deeply after she accidentally stumbled and fell against a railing while walking the previous day. She has no significant medical history or hospitalizations and is taking no medications or supplements. Her parents died of "old age" in their 90s, and her siblings and children are in excellent health. She has never smoked, only drinks on rare occasion, has lactose intolerance, is a vegetarian, and exercises several times weekly by walking. She denies recent illness and has an unremarkable review of systems. On examination, her blood pressure is 108/75 mm Hg, pulse is 72 beats/min, respiratory rate is 15 breaths/min, pulse oximetry is 97%, and body mass index (BMI) is 19.5 kg/m^2. The general; head, ears, eyes, nose, and throat; neck; heart; abdominal; and extremity examinations are all unremarkable, although she appears rather frail. The chest examination reveals normal lung sounds bilaterally, but inspiration is limited secondary to pain. There is significant point tenderness and a moderate-size bruise in the right anterior and lower ribs where she sustained trauma. An electrocardiogram (ECG) reveals normal sinus rhythm without abnormality. Chest and rib radiographs reveal a nondisplaced fracture of the anterolateral right ninth and tenth ribs corresponding to the site of injury.

▶ What additional diagnoses should be considered?
▶ What is the most likely underlying cause?
▶ What would be your next steps in evaluation and treatment?

ANSWERS TO CASE 58:

Osteoporosis

Summary: A 72-year-old woman presents with

- Fractured ribs after a low-velocity trauma
- Significant point tenderness and a moderate-size bruise in the right anterior and lower ribs where trauma was sustained
- Frailty and a BMI below normal
- No signs of cardiopulmonary compromise and a normal ECG
- Clinically stable appearance
- Normal lung sounds bilaterally but limited inspiration secondary to pain

Additional diagnoses: Underlying causes of pathologic fracture.

Most likely underlying cause: Osteoporosis.

Next steps: Pain management; evaluation for pathologic fractures that include primary and secondary causes of osteoporosis, including chronic systemic diseases, endocrine disorders, metabolic disorders, malignancies, adverse drug effects, and nutritional deficiencies.

ANALYSIS

Objectives

1. Identify the primary and secondary causes of osteoporosis. (EPA 12)
2. Understand the recommendations for screening of osteoporosis in women and men. (EPA 12)
3. Describe a rational evaluation for osteoporosis. (EPA 3)
4. List the nonpharmacologic and pharmacologic options for prevention and management of osteoporosis. (EPA 4)

Considerations

This 72-year-old patient presents with a rib fracture from a low-impact trauma. Her age, weight, frailty, and dietary restrictions place her at an increased risk for developing osteoporosis. Caucasian and Asian ethnicity would also increase her risk of osteoporosis. After treating her pain and preventing complications, assessment and management of the various causes of osteoporosis would significantly reduce this patient's risk for future fractures and disability.

The evaluation of this patient should include a dual-energy x-ray absorptiometry (DEXA) scan. Considerations for laboratory testing to rule out secondary causes of osteoporosis include serum alkaline phosphatase, calcium, and 25-hydroxy vitamin D. Additional testing of thyroid, liver, and kidney function to rule out hyperthyroidism, chronic liver disease, and renal insufficiency, respectively, should be considered. A complete blood count (CBC) should be considered if anemia, blood cell malignancy, or malabsorption syndromes are considered.

> # APPROACH TO:
> ## Osteoporosis

DEFINITIONS

OSTEOMALACIA: A defect in bone mineralization that can lead to osteoporosis, usually due to calcium or vitamin D deficiency.

OSTEOPENIA: The World Health Organization (WHO) defines osteopenia as "a hip or spinal mineral density (T score) of 1.0 to 2.5 standard deviations below the mean for 'young normal' adult."

OSTEOPOROSIS: A low-density, mass, and structural deterioration of bone that leads to an increased risk of fracture. The WHO defines osteoporosis as "a hip or spinal mineral density (bone mineral density [BMD]) of 2.5 standard deviations or more below the T score (mean) for 'young normal' adult."

Z SCORE: The BMD compared with an average healthy individual of same gender and age. A Z score of −2.0 or less is generally used with clinical signs in premenopausal women and men less than 50 years of age.

CLINICAL APPROACH

Epidemiology

Based on an overall 10.3% prevalence of osteoporosis, it is estimated that 10.2 million adults over 50 years of age have osteoporosis, and overall low bone mass prevalence is estimated at 43.9%. **The US Preventive Services Task Force (USPSTF) recommends that all women aged ≥ 65 and those < 65 years with risk factors that are equal to or greater than the risk of a healthy 65-year-old Caucasian woman should be screened for osteoporosis (Grade B).** This 10-year risk is 9.3% based on the WHO's Fracture Risk Assessment Tool (FRAX) (https://www.shef.ac.uk/FRAX/). The USPSTF states that there is insufficient evidence to assess the balance of benefits and harms of screening for osteoporosis in men. The National Osteoporosis Foundation (NOF) recommends that all men aged 70 and older and those aged 50 to 69 with risk factors should undergo screening. The preferred screening modality for osteoporosis is via DEXA scan of the femoral neck and lumbar spine.

Pathophysiology

Diagnosis. A DEXA T score of −2.5 or lower of the femoral neck and lumbar spine is the standard radiographic diagnostic criteria for osteoporosis. A clinical diagnosis of osteoporosis can present with low-impact fractures (eg, a fall below standing height) or by spontaneous fractures due to bone fragility. Patients who present with these fractures should undergo thorough evaluation to rule out secondary causes of fracture.

Secondary Causes of Osteoporosis. In postmenopausal women, secondary causes of osteoporosis are presumed unusual, and in the absence of other symptoms, additional testing may not be indicated. Approximately 50% of pre- and perimenopausal women and men of any age with osteoporosis may have a secondary cause. Common secondary causes include hyperthyroidism, primary hyperparathyroidism, vitamin D deficiency, amenorrhea (eg, female athlete triad, anorexia), and chronic corticosteroid use. Tobacco use and alcohol use of greater than two drinks per day are also significant risks. Serologic testing, including a CBC, comprehensive panel with serum calcium, thyroid-stimulating hormone, and 25-hydroxy vitamin D levels, should be considered standard components of the workup for the patient with suspected or diagnosed osteoporosis. When appropriate, estradiol levels in women and testosterone levels in men can screen for hypogonadism, as there is a direct correlation between osteoporosis and menopause and testosterone deficiency/late-onset hypogonadism.

Treatment Recommendations

Prevention. The NOF recommends that all men and women 50 years of age or older should be counseled on risk of fractures from osteoporosis, be screened for possible secondary causes of osteoporosis, have adequate daily intake of calcium (1200 mg) and vitamin D (800-1000 IU), and perform regular weight-bearing exercise. Smoking cessation and alcohol reduction can further reduce risk. Additional Food and Drug Administration (FDA)–approved pharmacologic options for preventive treatments include hormone therapy, selective estrogen receptor blockers, and bisphosphonates.

Treatment Recommendations. Recommendation for treatment varies between organizations. The NOF recommends treatment for postmenopausal women and men aged 50 and older presenting with

- Hip or vertebral fracture
- T score of −2.5 or less (more negative) at femoral neck or spine after appropriate evaluation to exclude secondary causes
- BMD T score −1.0 to −2.5 at femoral neck or spine and ≥ 3% 10-year risk of hip fracture and ≥ 20% 10-year risk of major osteoporosis fracture based on the WHO FRAX algorithm.

Treatment should be considered in patients with elevated risks or BMD above and below these recommendations and based on patient preferences.

Nonpharmacologic Treatment. Nonpharmacologic treatments include fall prevention along with treatments to mitigate risks from impaired vision, balance, gait, cognitive impairment, and presyncope. Smoking cessation and avoidance of excessive alcohol consumption should be encouraged. Home safety evaluations for hazards and durable medical equipment (eg, grab bars, walkers) needs should be undertaken. Hip protectors and lumbar braces have not been shown to be effective in the prevention of falls in patients with osteoporosis.

Calcium and Vitamin D Supplements. A universal recommendation in post-menopausal women and patients with osteoporosis is calcium and vitamin D intake supplementation, although in recent years the latter has become controversial. It is recommended that patients with osteoporosis consume at least 1200 mg of calcium a day in divided doses (no more than 500 mg per dose). A dose of at least 800 to 1000 IU of vitamin D should be used in conjunction with the calcium. In proven vitamin D deficiency, loading doses of ergocalciferol (vitamin D_2) 50,000 IU weekly for 4 to 8 weeks is recommended, followed by maintenance dosing of 50,000 IU monthly or cholecalciferol (vitamin D_3) 1000 to 2000 IU daily. The treatment goal serum level of 25-hydroxy vitamin D is > 30 ng/mL. The Institute of Medicine recommends against routine screening of vitamin D levels in the general population.

FDA-Approved Pharmacologic Therapy

Bisphosphonates. Oral bisphosphonates are the first-line agent for treatment of osteoporosis. Alendronate, risedronate, and ibandronate inhibit osteoclastic activity and have antiresorptive properties. These medications have excellent evidence for reduction in fractures in the hip and spine. Depending upon the agent, they can be dosed daily, weekly, or monthly. Intravenous bisphosphonates can be given four times a year (ibandronate) or yearly (zoledronic acid). **Oral agents must be taken on an empty stomach with a full glass of water and the patient must stay in an upright or standing position for at least 30 minutes after dosing due to a risk of esophagitis.** The optimal length of treatment continues to be debatable, as there are concerns about atypical bone fractures in patients taking bisphosphonates for 5 years or greater. There are also rare reported cases of osteonecrosis in the jaw (mostly with intravenous bisphosphonates in cancer patients). Combining bisphosphonates with other agents has not been well studied, the cost may be prohibitive, and the potential for adverse drug effects is unknown.

Hormone Replacement Therapy and Selective Estrogen Receptor Modulators. Estrogen replacement is FDA approved for prevention of osteoporosis in women with significant menopausal vasomotor symptoms, yet this recommendation is fraught with controversy due to the increased risks of thrombosis and breast cancer. It should be used at the lowest effective dose and for the shortest possible time duration. Women taking estrogen who have not had a hysterectomy should also take progesterone to limit the risk of endometrial cancer. Raloxifene, a selective estrogen receptor modulator (SERM), is FDA approved for the prevention and treatment of osteoporosis, especially of the lumbar spine. Raloxifene has been shown to reduce the risk of breast cancer, yet it increases vasomotor symptoms and risk of deep venous thrombosis. This medication may be best reserved for postmenopausal women who do not tolerate bisphosphonates, who do not have vasomotor symptoms, and who have a high risk for development of breast cancer. Outcomes with testosterone replacement therapy for treatment of osteoporosis in men are conflicting and should only be considered when reviewing risks and benefits.

Calcitonin. Calcitonin is an antiresorptive medication that is administered as a nasal spray. It has evidence for prevention of vertebral compression fracture reduction as well as a modest analgesic effect. It is considered a second-line agent, as more effective medications are available.

Teriparatide. Teriparatide is a recombinant human parathyroid hormone that causes bone density growth through its effect on osteoblasts. It is administered as a daily subcutaneous injection for up to 2 years. Because of its osteoblastic activity, it is contraindicated in patients at risk for osteosarcoma, such as patients with Paget disease, a history of bone radiation, or unexplained elevated serum alkaline phosphatase levels (which can be fractionated via isoenzymes to discern origin of tissue). It is approved for patients with severe osteoporosis and in those who have not benefited from or cannot tolerate bisphosphonates.

Denosumab. Denosumab is approved for women with severe risk of osteoporotic fracture who are intolerant of bisphosphonates. It is a monoclonal antibody that prevents osteoclast differentiation and limits bone turnover. It has evidence in prevention of all forms of osteoporotic fractures and has similar efficacy to bisphosphonates. Denosumab is given as a subcutaneous injection once every 6 months and has a warning of increased risk of serious infection due to its immunosuppressive properties.

Monitoring of Treatment Success. Little evidence is available to indicate how often and what kind of follow-up testing is needed for monitoring effectiveness of treatment for osteoporosis. The **NOF recommends repeat BMD testing every 2 years.** Biochemical markers of bone turnover can be used early on to assess effectiveness of treatment but are of limited usefulness due to biological and laboratory variability. Reduced BMD after treatment usually indicates patient adherence issues but could indicate inadequate calcium and vitamin D intake, an undiagnosed secondary cause of osteoporosis, or treatment failure.

CASE CORRELATION

- See Case 12 (Musculoskeletal Injuries), Case18 (Geriatric Health Maintenance and End-Of-Life Issues), and Case 53 (Acute Low Back Pain).

COMPREHENSION QUESTIONS

58.1 According to USPSTF guidelines, which of the following patients should be routinely screened for osteoporosis via DEXA scan?

A. A 65-year-old African American man who takes hydrochlorothiazide for hypertension

B. A 53-year-old postmenopausal Caucasian woman who takes hormone replacement therapy for hot flashes

C. A 67-year-old Caucasian woman who takes 1500 mg of calcium and 800 IU of vitamin D daily

D. A 45-year-old Asian woman who broke her hip by falling off of a ladder while cleaning her gutters

E. A 55-year-old African American woman who used inhaled steroids for 10 years for the management of asthma but never took oral steroids

58.2 A 60-year-old woman presents for follow-up for a wrist fracture that she sustained when she tripped while walking her dog. Follow-up DEXA scanning revealed a T score of −2.9. She has been postmenopausal for 10 years and has not had a hysterectomy. Which of the following interventions is most appropriate for reducing her risk of subsequent osteoporosis-related fractures?

A. Daily exercise

B. Estrogen replacement therapy

C. Vitamin D and calcium supplementation with a follow-up DEXA in 2 years

D. Alendronate

E. Calcitonin

58.3 A 51-year-old newly menopausal, physically active woman of mixed Asian-European origin presents inquiring about bone density testing. Her BMI is 20.9 kg/m², and she has a history of lactose intolerance and a 15-year use of low-dose inhaled corticosteroids for allergy-induced asthma. She has no history of fracture, oral steroid use, heavy alcohol use, or smoking. Based on the USPSTF and NOF recommendations and FRAX calculations, which of the following statements is true for this patient?

A. Her risk as an Asian is greater than her risk as a Caucasian.

B. DEXA scanning is recommended.

C. Inhaled steroids significantly increase her risk of osteoporosis.

D. Calcium and vitamin D supplementation are recommended.

E. Low-dose bisphosphonate therapy is recommended.

ANSWERS

58.1 **C.** The USPSTF recommends routine osteoporosis screening for women 65 years of age or older without previous known fractures or secondary causes of osteoporosis. They also recommend routine screening for women < 65 years old whose 10-year fracture risk is greater than or equal to that of a 65-year-old white woman with no additional risk factors. A hip fracture that occurred with a significant traumatic injury (answer D) would not be an indication for bone density screening, but a hip fracture associated with a minor injury, such as falling from a standing position, would be. Inhaled steroids (answer E) are not considered a risk factor for osteoporosis. Men over the age of 70 (answer A) are usually offered screening, or earlier if risk factors. Women over the age of 65 (answer B) without risk factors are offered screening.

58.2 **D.** This patient meets the criteria for the diagnosis of osteoporosis. Bisphosphonates, such as alendronate, are the first-line treatment in this situation based on their effectiveness at reducing fracture risk. Supplementation with calcium and vitamin D (answer C) along with daily weight-bearing exercise (answer A) are appropriate but not likely, by themselves, to increase her bone density sufficiently to reduce her fracture risk. Estrogen therapy alone (answer B) is not recommended in women with an intact uterus, as there is an increased risk of endometrial cancer. Calcitonin (answer E) would be reserved for consideration in a patient who does not tolerate or has contraindications to the use of bisphosphonates.

58.3 **D.** Calcium of at least 1200 mg per day and vitamin D of at least 800 IU per day is a universal recommendation for menopausal women. The FRAX calculator shows that Caucasian and Asian women in the United States have a 10-year risk of 4.5% and 3.3%, respectively (answer A). DEXA scans for screening (answer B) are recommended by USPSTF when women aged 50 to 64 have a 10-year risk of 9.7% or greater. Low-dose inhaled steroids (answer C) are not associated with a significantly increased risk of osteoporosis. Bisphosphonates (answer E) are not indicated unless the DEXA scan shows a significantly decreased BMD.

CLINICAL PEARLS

▶ Calcium supplementation is considered a universal recommendation for prevention and treatment of osteoporosis in postmenopausal women.

▶ The outcomes data on benefit for vitamin D supplementation remain controversial, but the risk of harm is limited.

▶ The DEXA scan is considered the diagnostic test of choice for both screening and diagnosis of osteoporosis and osteopenia.

▶ There is no universal agreement on screening for osteoporosis in men, but if a male patient has significant risk factors, screening should be conducted since approximately 20% of patients with osteoporosis are men.

REFERENCES

Buckley L, Humphrey MB. Glucocorticoid-induced osteoporosis. *N Engl J Med.* 2018;379:2547-2556.

Gourlay ML, Fine JP, Preisser JS, et al. Bone-density testing interval and transition to osteoporosis in older women. *N Engl J Med.* 2012;366:225-233.

Jeremiah MP, Unwin BK, Greenwald MH, Casiano VE. Diagnosis and management of osteoporosis. *Am Fam Physician.* 2015;92(4):261-268.

Lindsay R, Cosman F. Osteoporosis. In: Jameson JL, Fauci A, Kasper D, Hauser S, Longo D, Loscalzo J, eds. *Harrison's Principles of Internal Medicine.* 20th ed. New York, NY: McGraw Hill; 2018: Chap. 404. https://accessmedicine.mhmedical.com/content.aspx?sectionid=192530678&bookid=2129&Resultclick=2. Accessed April 24, 2019.

National Osteoporosis Foundation. *Clinician's Guide to Prevention and Treatment of Osteoporosis.* Washington, DC: National Osteoporosis Foundation; 2010.

US Preventive Services Task Force. Osteoporosis to prevent fractures: screening. June 16, 2018. https://www.uspreventiveservicestaskforce.org/Page/Document/RecommendationStatementFinal/osteoporosis-screening1. Accessed April 24, 2019.

Wright NC, Looker AC, Saag KG, et al. The recent prevalence of osteoporosis and low bone mass in the United States based on bone mineral density at the femoral neck or lumbar spine. *J Bone Miner Res.* 2014;29(11):2520-2526.

A 36-year-old single man who works in an office arrives at your office to establish care. He has a 3-year history of low back pain and is requesting a refill of medications. He had to change health care providers due to a change of job and insurance. The pain started 3 years ago with a motor vehicle accident in which he broke ribs and developed disabling low back pain. The patient has been on naproxen and oxycodone regularly since then. He also takes cyclobenzaprine at night as needed for sleep and muscle relaxation. He brings old medical records, which include a report of magnetic resonance imaging (MRI) of the lumbar spine without noted pathology, a copy of a pain contract, and a problem list that shows a history of tobacco use disorder and a family history of alcohol use disorder. His previous physician had recommended a referral to chronic pain management due to worsening pain and increasing requests for oxycodone. On intake, the patient completed a screening, brief intervention, referral for treatment (SBIRT) evaluation, showing a nine-question Patient Health Questionnaire (PHQ9) score of 15 (indicating moderate-to-severe depression) and ASSIST (Alcohol, Smoking, Substance Involvement Screening Test) score of 32 for use of prescription opiates obtained from friends. He states he finds himself looking forward to taking the oxycodone and doubling his dose more often recently. He admits that he was given the option of leaving or being fired from his previous job due to sleepiness at work and poor performance. The Prescription Monitoring Program showed increasing urgent care visits with prescriptions for opiates in the past year. On reviewing the SBIRT screen results with the patient, he admits that he feels out of control and that he tried to cut back on his oxycodone recently but felt empty, isolated, and unable to sleep without the medication. He would like to stop using the medication but does not know how.

▶ How do you address the increasing desire for opioids?
▶ How can you address his depression?
▶ How can you address his chronic pain?

ANSWERS TO CASE 59:
Opioid Use Disorder and Chronic Pain Management

Summary: A 36-year-old man presents with

- Self-admitted escalating and uncontrolled use of opioid pain medication for chronic pain syndromes with social and economic consequences
- Moderate-to-severe depression and chronic pain
- An SBIRT screen showing a PHQ9 score of 15 (indicating moderate-to-severe depression) and ASSIST score of 32 for use of prescription opiates obtained from friends

Addressing the increasing desire for opioids: Express understanding and present the patient with options for medication-assisted therapy (MAT) for stabilization versus outpatient detoxification. Depending on circumstances, this can be done in a substance use disorder (SUD) clinic or in a primary care office with a Drug Enforcement Administration (DEA) waiver.

Addressing depression: Contract for safety (whether verbal or written) and treatment with antidepressant, counseling, support groups for SUD, and frequent follow-up.

Addressing chronic pain: As part of his treatment plan, include nonnarcotic pain management using nonsteroidal anti-inflammatory drugs (NSAIDs), acetaminophen, muscle relaxers, topical pain rubs, physical therapy, cognitive behavioral therapy, and consideration for alternative therapies, such as acupuncture.

ANALYSIS

Objectives

1. Describe ways health care providers can minimize the risk of causing, as well as manage, opioid use disorder (OUD). (EPA 12)

2. Describe an appropriate evaluation of a patient presenting with chronic pain. (EPA 1, 2)

3. List treatment modalities for chronic malignant and nonmalignant pain syndromes. (EPA 4)

Considerations

This case represents a common primary care scenario of the management of a patient with chronic pain due to trauma that has led to OUD. For patients with no history of addictions (including tobacco) or family histories of SUDs (see Case 41), the risk of development of OUD is low with short-term use of opioid pain management. However, approximately one-quarter of patients with chronic pain have a history of SUDs and are considered higher risk for development of OUD. This patient demonstrates the four Cs of addiction: (1) loss of **control** over use, (2) **craving** for the addictive substance, (3) **compulsive** use, and (4) **continued** use despite knowledge of consequences, including failure to fulfill obligations and loss of occupational activities.

The management of chronic, nonmalignant pain syndromes can be challenging. **The treatment of chronic, nonmalignant pain should be multidisciplinary** and should utilize the biopsychosocial model of care to maximize outcomes. The use of pain medications is one option, with other modalities, including exercise, physical rehabilitation, counseling, nonnarcotic medications, and complementary/alternative therapies, as other viable options. The overall goals of chronic pain management should be to maximize function while minimizing pain and treatment side effects.

APPROACH TO:
Opioid Use Disorder and Chronic Pain Management

DEFINITIONS

INFLAMMATORY PAIN: Pain due to the release of inflammatory agents, such as prostaglandins, in response to an illness, injury, or inflammation-causing condition (eg, rheumatoid arthritis).

MECHANICAL/COMPRESSIVE PAIN: Most commonly musculoskeletal pain aggravated by activity and improved by rest and limitation of physical activity.

MUSCLE PAIN: Local or regional pain involving soft tissue of the musculoskeletal system.

NEUROPATHIC PAIN: Pain caused by damage or dysfunction of a nerve or of the nervous system.

OPIOID USE DISORDER: Chronic, relapsing disease in which cognitive, behavioral, and physiologic symptoms indicate that opioids are continually used for ≥ 12 months despite problematic consequences.

PSYCHOPHYSIOLOGIC DISORDERS (PPDS): Chronic noncancer pain that does not have an easily identifiable physical source, often with a psychological overlay, and therefore is difficult to "fix" with simple interventions. These disorders include fibromyalgia, myofascial pain syndromes, chronic headache, irritable bowel syndrome, chronic dyspepsia, and chronic pelvic pain syndromes.

CLINICAL APPROACH

Pathophysiology

Acute pain is pain associated with an illness or injury that has a generally accepted time course and progression—the pain starts with the onset of the illness/injury, the pain may be constant or intermittent, and the pain improves as the illness/injury improves. Acute pain can often be managed with nonopioid medications, including

NSAIDS, acetaminophen, topical pain relievers, and thermotherapy (ice and heat). In contrast, **chronic pain is persistent pain that negatively impacts the person's quality of life and functioning.** The pain can be constant, intermittent, or recurrent and may be associated with an illness or injury but lasts longer than would be expected with the improvement of the condition.

Psychophysiologic Disorders. Dealing with the chronic pain of PPDs can be frustrating for the patient. Patients with chronic pain may have difficulties with personal and professional relationships due to their pain, may not be able to perform required or desired functions, and often feel inadequate pain relief. Health care providers can be a trusted single source of care for the patient, making sure appropriate testing is provided (no more, no less), partnering with the patient to have reasonable goals of restoring function as much as possible and having more good days than bad over a period of time. Numerous guidelines and recommendations for the management of chronic, nonmalignant pain are available. The overall goal of chronic pain management is to create a comprehensive plan utilizing the biopsychosocial model with a specific emphasis on managing pain, minimizing dependence, and improving function while limiting disability and side effects.

Clinical Presentation

Initially, an assessment should be made to identify the type and cause of the pain through a thorough history and physical examination. The history should focus on the location, duration, intensity, and type of pain (eg, neuropathic, musculoskeletal, etc). Time should be spent performing detailed psychological and social histories to evaluate for comorbid depression, other psychiatric conditions, or evidence of substance abuse. **Chronic pain is often seen in patients who have experienced physical and emotional trauma as children and young adults.** Clinicians should reflect on this fact with patients and offer additional resources if questioning reveals trauma. Since it is legal for medicinal uses in many states, inquiring about marijuana use is paramount, as use of this drug may limit a clinician's ability to prescribe opioid-based therapy.

It is important to understand how the chronic pain condition has interfered with the patient's personal life, relationships, occupation, and other functioning. A detailed physical examination should be performed and documented at every visit. Functional assessment utilizing a standardized tool should also be performed, as this can establish a baseline and provide an objective way to measure improvement or deterioration over time. When available, previous medical records should be obtained and reviewed to avoid duplication of testing. If the history and examination suggest the presence of a treatable condition, and if the test has not previously been performed, then focused diagnostic testing should be performed.

Treatment

Nonpharmacologic Management. The comprehensive management of chronic pain should involve both pharmacologic and nonpharmacologic treatments (see Table 59–1). The patient, family, and clinician should start by **establishing realistic**

Table 59–1 • TREATMENT APPROACHES FOR CHRONIC PAIN

First-Line Treatments	Second-/Third-Line Treatments	Comments and Resources
Chronic Low Back Pain (CLBP)		
Education on self-care, including staying active as tolerated, safe exercise, posture, ergonomics, limit sitting to 30 min at a time. Somatics and other mind/body treatments	**SNRI** such as duloxetine (modest benefit)	**Differentiate subtypes of CLBP to ensure proper treatment.** Avoid diagnosis and treatment of CLBP solely by imaging
If suffers from PPD, then individualized treatment program	**Tramadol** to treat flares if not responsive to first-line treatments	Sparse evidence of efficacy for most modalities overall; therefore, use most benign modalities first. Emphasize activity as tolerated, modalities such as yoga, tai chi; mindfulness-based stress reduction, other relaxation techniques
Psychotherapies, such as CBT and others	**Gabapentinoids** not shown effective for *nonspecific* CLBP. Improvements for radicular symptoms are small	
Nonopioid analgesics such as NSAIDs, curcumin	**Nonbenzodiazepine muscle relaxants** (eg, cyclobenzaprine) for flares. Avoid long-term use because of narrow therapeutic window and side effects	**Avoid benzodiazepines** in almost all cases of CLBP due to their strong addictive potential and side effects
Manual therapies: massage (short-term benefits) or manipulation (modest short-term benefits)	**Spine interventional modalities** in carefully selected patients (eg, epidural glucocorticoids in persistent radiculopathy); no evidence supporting epidural steroid injections in nonspecific CLBP or acute lumbosacral radiculopathy or spinal stenosis	**Avoid chronic opioids** in most cases of CLBP, as there is little evidence of efficacy and much potential harm
Acupuncture (moderate benefits < 3 mo)	**Surgery** if lumbar disk prolapse radiculopathy with severe or progressive neurologic deficits or other serious lesions	**Refer intractable severe CLBP** cases to a multidisciplinary pain center
Chronic Neck Pain		
Individualized treatment program if PPD	If symptoms persist, trials of trigger point injections, acupuncture, TENS	Conservative treatment is adequate in majority of cases
Posture, ergonomics, neck pillow; limit sitting to 30 minutes at a time; gentle exercise; qigong/tai chi	If severe facet joint symptoms, trial of cervical medial branch blocks or percutaneous radio-frequency neurotomy	Avoid prolonged use of cervical collars
PT; gentle neck mobilization; NSAIDs or botanical analgesics	Surgery if alarm or significant neurological symptoms	

(Continued)

Table 59–1 • TREATMENT APPROACHES FOR CHRONIC PAIN (continued)		
First-Line Treatments	**Second-/Third-Line Treatments**	**Comments and Resources**
Osteoarthritis		
Exercise: aerobic and strengthening (strong evidence of benefit) **Nonopioid analgesics:** start with topical NSAIDs, capsaicin, or oral botanicals such as curcumin **Acupuncture:** moderate benefits (conflicting evidence) **Walking and other aids** **Psychological support/therapy**	**Oral NSAIDs**, especially for flares **Supplements:** Glucosamine/chondroitin sulfate (not HCl form), ASU, SAMe (S-adenosyl-methionine; also may help mood) may be worth a 3-mo trial **Surgical options if severe:** Joint replacement effective No evidence of benefit for arthroscopic knee surgery	**Treat related regional myofascial dysfunction** with myofascial release or dry needling techniques **Limit steroid injections**, perhaps maximum of 4 injections per joint per lifetime (overuse associated with cartilage thinning) Intra-articular hyaluronic acid may have small benefit (controversial)
Shoulder Pain (eg, Impingement, Rotator Cuff, Frozen Shoulder)		
PT tailored to problem or home rehabilitation Individualized treatment program if PPD	**Steroid injections** if severe pain may be of short-term benefit and help patients succeed at PT **Surgery** may be indicated in rotator cuff severe tears or recalcitrant frozen shoulder	PT guided by diagnosis will help resolve majority of shoulder pain syndromes Consider addressing "pain body memories" with mind/body therapies such as somatics and psychotherapies
Myofascial Dysfunction		
Individualized treatment program if PPD Emphasize self-management programs, including self-help guides for deactivation of trigger points	Practitioner-dependent myofascial release techniques (eg, strain-counterstrain, muscle energy, dry needling, manipulation)	Research is sparse. Individualize modalities to needs of patient. Adequate sleep, exercise, posture, and mental health are key Treat underlying cause if possible
Fibromyalgia		
Individualized treatment program for PPD **Education:** stress reduction, improving mood and sleep hygiene, creative outlets, and adequate self-care. Empathic listening and affirmation through regular visits **CBT and other psychotherapies** **Graded exercise** (especially water based) **Mind/body:** yoga, tai chi, biofeedback, daily meditation **Optimize nutrition:** vitamin D; avoid excitotoxins like MSG, aspartame	**Medications** have only modest benefit, often used in combination (eg, SNRIs, amitriptyline, and/or pregabalin) **Acupuncture** may be helpful (limited evidence) Less researched options include low-dose naltrexone, memantine, cannabinoids, and anti-inflammatory botanicals such as turmeric, ginger (weak evidence) Treat comorbidities such as depression	**Foundational and multidisciplinary approaches** are key NSAIDs generally are not helpful in fibromyalgia Opioids should be avoided. Tramadol can be used for severe flares (avoid chronic use) For difficult cases, consultation with fibromyalgia expert/multidisciplinary team. Pain clinics that focus on interventions without a well-rounded psychological/mind/body approach are generally not very helpful

(Continued)

Table 59–1 • TREATMENT APPROACHES FOR CHRONIC PAIN (continued)		
First-Line Treatments	Second-/Third-Line Treatments	Comments and Resources
Headache (Tension, Chronic Daily Headache) or Migraine		
Individualized treatment program if PPD **Behavioral self-management,** including stress reduction, relaxation, biofeedback, posture, ergonomics **Focus on preventive measures and medication while minimizing acute medications** (can lead to chronic daily headache)	**Migraine preventive therapies:** **Natural agents:** butterbur, magnesium, riboflavin **Pharmaceuticals:** beta-blockers (eg, nadolol, propranolol), amitriptyline, topiramate, botulinum toxin type A injections **Acupuncture, myofascial release** (limited evidence)	**Search for and treat common comorbidities** (depression, anxiety, insomnia, IBS) Many patients with chronic headache are medication sensitive—**start low, titrate up slowly** **Avoid opioids and barbiturates** in most chronic headache syndromes
TMJ Syndrome		
Individualized treatment program if PPD **Stress reduction**, relaxation **Occlusal splint**, exercises if bruxism	**NSAIDs, muscle relaxants** for flares Consider surgery in severe, recalcitrant cases	Rule out serious dental causes
Chronic Neuropathic Pain		
First-line neuropathic pain medication: TCAs, gabapentin, pregabalin, SNRIs, topical lidocaine **For diabetes-related neuropathic pain:** prevention with anti-inflammatory low glycemic load diet and glycemic control **For postherpetic neuralgia:** TCAs, gabapentin, pregabalin, SNRIs; if local, lidocaine patches, capsaicin **For trigeminal neuralgia:** carbamazepine or oxcarbazepine	**Prevention/early treatment:** alpha lipoic acid (conflicting evidence), gamma linolenic acid (eg, evening primrose oil)	Combination of medications is often needed Low-dose opioids often added for severe neuropathic chronic pain

Abbreviations: ASU, avocado soybean unsaponifiables; CBT, cognitive behavioral therapy; IBS, irritable bowel syndrome; MSG, monosodium glutamate; PPD, psychophysiologic disorder; PT, physical therapy; SNRI, serotonin-norepinephrine reuptake inhibitor; TCA, tricyclic antidepressant; TENS, transcutaneous electrical nerve stimulation; TMJ, temporomandibular joint.

and achievable goals. The initial management should include nonpharmacologic therapies, including targeted exercise such as physical therapy or occupation-specific rehabilitation programs, psychologic interventions such as counseling or cognitive behavioral therapy, and complementary or alternative modalities such as spinal and musculoskeletal manipulations, acupuncture, and meditation. Patient acceptance and participation are mandatory for success in reducing chronic pain. Unfortunately, third-party payers may not cover some of these treatment options, and inability for patients to pay may limit access.

Pharmacologic Management. Initial pharmacologic management options should be based on the type, location, and severity of pain; the presence of comorbid conditions; and the need to minimize interactions with other medications that the patient may require. **Nonnarcotic analgesics, such as acetaminophen or NSAIDs, should be considered as first-line agents.** However, these may not be viable options in the presence of significant liver (acetaminophen) or renal (NSAID) disease. Topical agents can be tried to minimize gastrointestinal, hepatic, and renal effects. Neuropathic pain may be relieved or reduced by the use of anticonvulsants, and musculoskeletal pain may benefit from the judicious use of muscle relaxants. Antidepressant therapy (eg, selective serotonin reuptake inhibitors) is also a beneficial adjunct to other therapies to help improve mood, sleep, and overall function. Benzodiazepines should be avoided in patients receiving chronic opioid analgesics to minimize the risk of oversedation and respiratory depression.

Treating Patients With Terminal Illnesses. As treatment modalities for cancer improve, many people are living longer with cancer that would have been fatal in the past. Cancer can cause pain from direct invasion of organs or inflammation at the site of either the primary tumor or the metastases, with bony pain from metastatic disease being a common and especially painful complication. Some cancer treatments, such as surgery or radiation therapy, can be painful as well. Many persons experience significant pain in the final months of life. In addition to wanting to preserve as much quality of life as possible, most patients express a preference to die outside of institutional settings.

A key element to achieving these goals is adequate pain control. A stepwise approach to pain management with frequent pain assessment in the patient with terminal cancer can help patients and their families achieve the goal of dying at home with minimal pain. Pain should be assessed regularly in all patients with terminal illness, including those with cognitive impairment. Providers should begin with nonopioid analgesics and progress to more potent analgesics until pain is relieved. In some cases, interventional procedures, such as nerve blocks or epidural infusions, will be needed. Many patients with terminal illnesses require immediate opioid therapy or have contraindications to common nonopioid analgesics. In patients with constant pain that responds to opioids, scheduling opioids with adequate breakthrough doses provides optimal analgesia. When patients develop opioid tolerance, rotating to an alternative opioid may improve analgesia. Tricyclic antidepressants, serotonin-norepinephrine reuptake inhibitors, and anticonvulsants are first-line therapies for neuropathic pain associated with chemotherapy and malignancy.

Opioid Use Disorder

Opioid use disorder often starts with an injury or surgical procedure for which opioids were prescribed to manage the acute pain. In the recent past, clinicians and hospitals were encouraged to manage nonmalignant pain with opioid analgesics to address the "fifth" vital sign of pain. This led to overprescribing and an increase in the development of OUD in patient populations. Providers can minimize this risk by using nonopioid pain management options first and by limiting opioid use for acute pain to 3 to 5 days since dependence can develop in as few as 5 days of opioid pain management. If longer term opioid pain management is deemed appropriate, prescribers should use

- the Opioid Risk Tool to assess risk for opioid use disorder

- pain contracts

- pill counts

- urine toxicology testing

- prescription monitoring programs

- good communication with other providers who are involved in the patient's care

Screening Tools. Those on higher doses of opioids should be provided with naloxone and should avoid the use of benzodiazepines due to the high risk of overdose and respiratory arrest associated with the combination. Patients on long-term opioid therapy often develop constipation, so stool softeners are often coprescribed. The SBIRT screen has the ASSIST tool, which aids in assessing risk and determining whether brief interventions in the office or referral for stabilization through MAT at an SUD treatment center would be most beneficial. Table 59–2 describes MAT.

Methadone may be preferred for patients with recent use of opioids, relative lack of social structure and support, or failure to follow recommendations for

Table 59–2 • MEDICATION-ASSISTED THERAPY
Methadone
• Oral liquid, usually 60-120 mg/d
• Cannot be prescribed by physicians for opioid-use disorder; can be dispensed only through licensed opioid-treatment program
• Requires daily program attendance during early phases of treatment
• Is the standard in pregnancy but may cause neonatal abstinence syndrome in infants
Buprenorphine–naloxone
• Sublingual tablet or film, or buccal film formulation
• Typical dose is 4-24 mg/d
• May be available at providers' offices and at opioid-treatment programs
• Must be prescribed by a physician who has obtained a waiver and training from the Drug Enforcement Agency (DEA)
• Requires the patient to be opioid-free for 8-12 hours before administration of short-acting opioids and for more than 36 hours before administration of long-acting opioids
• Is contraindicated in pregnancy (however, buprenorphine by itself can be used in this situation)
Naltrexone
• Oral tablet (50-100 mg/day) or Injectable IM (380 mg/mo)
• Tablet is not a controlled substance; can be prescribed by a physician, nurse practitioner, or physician assistant
• Injection: DEA waiver needed.
• May be initiated only in patients who have been opioid-free for 7-10 days

formal treatment of an SUD, as the structure provided at an opioid treatment program may be beneficial. Buprenorphine/naloxone may be most appropriate for patients who are motivated to receive treatment, have a higher level of social functioning despite drug use, and have expressed interest in outpatient monthly visits. Naltrexone is an excellent option for patients with alcohol use disorder, as it can be effective for both. A patient should not be started on this unless the patient has negative drug screens and can reliably claim not to have used opioids in the last 7 days.

> ## CASE CORRELATION
> - See Case 41 (Substance Use Disorder).

COMPREHENSION QUESTIONS

59.1 A 45-year-old diabetic patient presents for a routine follow-up. His diabetes has been uncontrolled, although he is making good efforts to comply with his diet, exercise, and medication regimens. He has a long history of burning pain in his feet that has been uncontrolled by over-the-counter medications and is now worsening in severity such that he can no longer work. Your examination of his feet reveals no skin ulcerations, diminished but present and symmetrical pedal pulses, and reduced sensation on monofilament testing bilaterally. Along with aggressive management of his diabetes, which of the following interventions would be most appropriate at this time?

    A. An NSAID

    B. A long-acting opioid agonist

    C. A short-acting opioid agonist

    D. Gabapentin

    E. Acupuncture

59.2 A 59-year-old man has terminal pancreatic cancer with metastases to the spine and bony chest. He has severe cancer pain. Opioid therapies provide the greatest analgesic relief for most patients with a terminal illness. Concerns about which one of the following can limit the use of opioids in this setting?

    A. Dementia and delirium

    B. Respiratory depression

    C. Gastrointestinal upset

    D. Renal failure

    E. Hypotension

59.3 A 68-year-old man with prostate cancer metastatic to the bone is going to be started on long-acting morphine for his pain. He denies depressed mood or insomnia. Which of the following adjunctive therapies should be considered along with long-term use of opioid agonists?

A. Bisacodyl

B. Trazodone

C. Tramadol

D. Gabapentin

E. Nortriptyline

59.4 A 32-year-old married woman presents with a history of panic disorder and posttraumatic stress disorder resulting from sexual trauma. She began using opioids when a friend gave her oxycodone to help her to "relax." Currently, she uses opioids daily "just to function." Despite ongoing use, she has been able to continue working as a receptionist. She says that she has a support system, although few people are aware of her use. She has begun individual therapy and started taking citalopram after meeting with her psychiatrist. She attempted non–medication-assisted detox last year but had horrible withdrawal symptoms. She relapsed soon after detox was completed. She is interested in medication to help with her OUD. She cannot take much time off work, and she is currently on long-term birth control. Which option would be the best choice for this patient's medical condition?

A. Methadone

B. Buprenorphine/naloxone

C. Naltrexone

D. Continued use of oxycodone with slowly tapering dosage

E. Lorazepam

ANSWERS

59.1 **D.** Diabetic neuropathy is the most common type of peripheral neuropathic pain. In many patients, it can be extremely painful and debilitating. Aggressive management of the patient's diabetes is extremely important, but improvement in neuropathic symptoms from diabetic control may take months, and in some patients, the neuropathy does not improve in spite of ideal diabetic control. An anticonvulsant, such as gabapentin, is often effective at alleviating or minimizing neuropathic pain. Antidepressants, especially tricyclic antidepressants, and NSAIDs (answer A) may also be effective. Physical therapy and acupuncture (answer E) have no proven benefit in reducing symptoms of neuropathy. Opioid agonists (answers B and C) are not indicated as first-line agents.

59.2 **B.** Concerns about addiction and respiratory depression often limit the use of opioids or lead to inadequate dosing in patients with a terminal illness who are experiencing pain at the end of life. Sedation usually precedes respiratory depression. Dementia and delirium (answer A) usually are not concerns since patients can still indicate whether they are in pain. Answer C (gastrointestinal upset) can occur, but there are delivery systems other than oral (eg, transdermal) to avoid this. Answer D (renal failure) is not a concern in most cases since metabolism takes place primarily in the liver. Answer E (hypotension) is not common with opioids.

59.3 **A.** Constipation is a common side effect of narcotic medication use. Establishing a bowel regimen for a patient who will be on a chronic narcotic program is an important adjunctive treatment. None of the other options (answer B, trazadone; answer C, tramadol; answer D, gabapentin; and answer E, nortriptyline) is likely to be effective for chronic pain management due to metastatic disease to the bone.

59.4 **B.** Buprenorphine/naloxone would be most appropriate for this patient. She is motivated to receive treatment, has a high level of social functioning despite her drug use, is on birth control, and does not want to go through prolonged detox. Methadone (answer A) could be used but would require daily treatment at a specialized clinic, interfering with her job. Naltrexone (answer C) could also be used but would require 7 to 10 days off opioids with withdrawal symptoms. Benzodiazepines (answer E) should be avoided when a patient is also on opioids. Answer D (tapering opioids) has not been shown to be effective for the vast majority of individuals trying to abstain from opioids; medication-assisted programs have the highest success rates.

CLINICAL PEARLS

▶ The management of chronic pain is best performed by using a multidisciplinary approach that utilizes the biopsychosocial model of care. Medications are only one aspect of this model.

▶ Anticipate common side effects of your treatments, such as constipation associated with opioid agonists, and prophylactically provide your patient with the tools needed to address the problem.

▶ Prior to providing opioid pain management, screen for risk for developing addiction and check prescription monitoring programs.

▶ If using an opioid for acute pain management, limit prescriptions to 3 to 5 days to reduce the risk for developing tolerance and addiction.

REFERENCES

Department of Family Medicine at Oregon Health and Science University. SBIRT OREGON. https://www.sbirtoregon.org. Accessed May 8, 2019.

Groninger H, Vijayan J. Pharmacologic management of pain at the end of life. *Am Fam Physician.* 2014;90(1):26-32.

Remde A. Chronic pain. In: Usatine RP, Smith MA, Mayeaux EJ Jr, Chumley HS, eds. *The Color Atlas and Synopsis of Family Medicine.* 3rd ed. New York, NY: McGraw Hill; 2019: Appendix B. http://accessmedicine.mhmedical.com/content.aspx?bookid=2547&Sectionid=206790688. Accessed May 8, 2019.

Rodriguez CP, Vaidya A, Tishler LW, Suzuki J. An interactive clinical case: a painful subject. A Case from Brigham and Women's Hospital. *N Engl J Med.* 2015;373:e32. doi:10.1056/NEJMimc1505316.

Schug SA, Goddard C. Recent advances in the pharmacological management of acute and chronic pain. *Ann Palliate Med.* 2014;3(4):263-275.

World Health Organization. WHO's pain relief ladder. http://www.who.int/cancer/palliative/painladder/en/. Accessed May 8, 2019.

A 52-year-old healthy man presents to your office complaining of a 2-year history of bilateral leg swelling and intermittent heaviness that has become more bothersome over the past 3 months. He works in a factory and states that this heaviness is increasingly impairing his ability to finish a 10-hour shift. He tells you, "The swelling in my legs is worse in the evening, especially when I have been standing all day." By the end of the day, he has swelling up to his midcalves, and the top of his socks leave deep indentations in his skin. He complains of brown spots, dryness, and itching on his feet and ankles. He denies shortness of breath on exertion, fatigue, or sleep disturbance but states he has been using over-the-counter ibuprofen for several months for knee pain. On examination, his blood pressure is 130/85 mm Hg, pulse is 72 beats/min, respiratory rate is 16 breaths/min, and body mass index (BMI) is 23 kg/m^2. His heart, lung, and abdominal examinations are unremarkable. On examination of his extremities, he has symmetrical bilateral edema to his midcalves with pitting, prominent varicose veins, and brown-pigmented 2-mm size macules on his feet and ankles. His posterior tibialis and dorsalis pedis pulses are 2+ bilaterally, and his feet are warm.

▶ What is the most likely diagnosis?
▶ What diagnostic evaluation should be considered?
▶ What are the treatment options?

ANSWERS TO CASE 60:

Lower Extremity Edema

Summary: A 52-year-old man presents with

- Classic signs and symptoms of peripheral venous insufficiency causing edema
- Edema that is bilateral, chronic, dependent, and without significant constitutional, cardiac, or pulmonary symptoms
- Physical examination revealing varicosities and venous stasis dermatitis
- Edema often interfering with and aggravated by his work
- Posterior tibialis and dorsalis pedis pulses 2+ bilaterally with warm feet

Most likely diagnosis: Chronic venous insufficiency, aggravated by use of nonsteroidal anti-inflammatory drugs (NSAIDs).

Diagnostic evaluation: The diagnosis is made clinically, yet it is important to ensure an absence of comorbid conditions. If further information suggests possible underlying etiologies, the following can be obtained: polysomnogram and echocardiography if obstructive sleep apnea and pulmonary hypertension are considered, respectively; echocardiogram, chest radiograph (CXR), electrocardiogram (ECG), brain natriuretic peptide (BNP) if heart failure (HF) or other cardiac cause is considered; serum electrolytes, serum creatinine, and urinalysis if renal causes are considered; serum albumin if malnutrition or malabsorption states are considered; liver enzymes if hepatic dysfunction is considered; and thyroid-stimulating hormone (TSH) if thyroid disorders are considered. Ankle-brachial index (ABI) testing should be considered if symptoms suggest peripheral arterial disease (PAD).

Treatment options: Leg elevation, compression stockings, low-sodium diet, and avoidance of medications that may cause edema. Appropriate skin care should be performed with use of emollients for hydration to prevent skin breakdown and risk of cellulitis.

ANALYSIS

Objectives

1. Describe the presenting signs and symptoms of common causes of lower extremity swelling. (EPA 1)
2. Explain the clinical evaluation used to define and diagnose low- versus high-risk lower extremity swelling indicative of severe comorbid conditions. (EPA 1, 3)
3. Describe the management of common causes of lower extremity swelling. (EPA 4)

Considerations

In older people, chronic venous insufficiency is the most common cause of bilateral lower extremity swelling, and it increases in prevalence with age and obesity. Although venous insufficiency can often be diagnosed clinically without extensive testing, in older patients there is an increased risk of **pulmonary hypertension** (most commonly secondary to obstructive sleep apnea) and **HF** as the etiology of the lower extremity swelling. Many **medications are also associated with fluid retention** and should be considered in the differential diagnosis as a potential cause of or contributor to lower extremity swelling.

APPROACH TO:
Lower Extremity Edema

DEFINITIONS

DEEP VEIN THROMBOSIS (DVT): thrombus or blood clot that forms in the deep veins of the body, usually the lower extremity.

LIPEDEMA: A form of fat maldistribution with fat deposits under the skin that can appear to be leg swelling with sparing of the foot; it is not a true form of edema.

LYMPHEDEMA: An excess of protein-rich interstitial fluid within the skin and subcutaneous tissue.

MYXEDEMA: A dermal edema secondary to an increased deposition of connective tissue components (mucopolysaccharides) in the dermis seen in various forms of thyroid disease.

STASIS DERMATITIS: Inflammation of the skin of the lower legs that involves dry skin, itching, scaling, hyperpigmentation, and possible ulceration caused by chronic venous insufficiency. It is diagnosed clinically, and treatment is aimed at reducing chronic venous insufficiency to prevent progression and cellulitis.

WELLS CRITERIA FOR DVT: A clinically validated scoring system to assess pretest probability of having a DVT.

CLINICAL APPROACH

Pathophysiology

Edema is defined as a visible and palpable swelling due to an accumulation of interstitial fluid when there is disequilibrium between the hydrostatic pressure gradient and oncotic pressure gradient across the capillary and the interstitial space. When edema develops rapidly, diagnosis and management should occur promptly since edema can be a sign of systemic disease. The most common cause of leg edema in North American patients older than 50 years is venous insufficiency.

Venous insufficiency develops due to venous dilation of the dependent veins or damage to veins or their corresponding valves. The mostly likely cause of leg edema in women younger than 50 is idiopathic edema, which may be confused with obesity.

Clinical Presentation

History. The most important element of the history in evaluating the patient with lower extremity edema is the **duration of edema** (acute [≤ 72 hours] vs chronic). Acute swelling may suggest DVT, cellulitis, compartment syndrome after trauma, ruptured popliteal cyst, or adverse drug reactions. Chronic progression of edema suggests chronic venous insufficiency, HF, pulmonary hypertension, renal disease, hepatic disease, protein-losing enteropathy, and generalized malnutrition. Other elements to assess from the history include presence of pain, overnight improvement when sleeping or when elevated (indicating dependent edema, often seen in venous insufficiency), signs or symptoms of obstructive sleep apnea, and history of chronic medical conditions, including heart, liver, kidney, and thyroid disease.

The clinician should inquire about **past history of pelvic or abdominal malignancies** or radiation therapy, as these can lead to destruction of lymphatics. Certain **medications** (eg, calcium channel blockers) may cause salt and water retention, increasing capillary hydrostatic pressure, whereas loop diuretics cause reflex stimulation of the renin-angiotensin system due to volume depletion. Family history of clotting disorders, varicosities, and lymphedema are also important to document.

Physical Examination. The key elements of the physical examination in the patient with lower extremity edema include evaluating the edematous area and assessing for systemic signs of disease. Clinicians may grade edema on a scale of 1+ to 4+, which can be useful in tracking changes in edema over time. Pitting edema occurs when the etiology of edema leads to low protein in the interstitial fluid. Unilateral leg swelling is commonly seen with venous insufficiency, lymphedema, DVT, and complex regional pain syndrome. Bilateral leg swelling is commonly seen with bilateral venous insufficiency, adverse drug reactions, lipedema, and idiopathic or systemic causes. Generalized edema is seen in advanced systemic diseases, including HF, renal failure, and liver failure. Tenderness of the edematous area can be seen with DVTs, complex regional pain syndrome, and lipedema; lymphedema is usually painless. Warmth and erythema over the edematous area can be associated with DVTs and cellulitis.

Common skin changes in lower extremity edema include hemosiderin deposition (brown-pigmented spots), dry scaling dermatitis, and brawny induration in chronic venous insufficiency. **Lymphedema** can cause a warty texture with papillomatosis. Varicose veins are common in patients with chronic lymphedema and venous insufficiency.

In assessing systemic disease, findings such as jugular venous distention, hepatojugular reflux, and rales on pulmonary examination may suggest HF. BMI > 30 kg/m² and a thick neck circumference (> 17 inches [42 cm]) may suggest obstructive sleep apnea. Jaundice, ascites, and spider hemangioma may suggest

Table 60–1 • ADAPTED WELLS CRITERIA FOR DEEP VENOUS THROMBOSIS
Step 1: Give 1 Point for each of the following (THE VOICES): **T**enderness (localized along distribution of deep veins) **H**istory of DVT or PE previously **E**ntire leg swollen **V**eins (collateral superficial, varicose) **O**n bedrest (due to surgery) **I**mmobilization (paralysis) **C**ancer (active within 6 months) **E**dema (pitting one leg) **S**welling (entire leg)
Step 2: Subtract 2 points for: There is another diagnosis as likely or more likely that DVT
Step 3: Total score (add steps 1 and 2): If score ≥ 3 points, means high risk (75%); if score is 1-2 points, means moderate risk (17%), and if score < 1 point = low risk (3%)

hepatic disease, while exophthalmos, tremors, and weight loss may indicate thyroid disease.

Diagnostic Studies. **The majority of patients older than 50 years who present with leg swelling have venous insufficiency.** If the etiology is unclear, a complete blood count (CBC), comprehensive metabolic panel, and TSH can potentially rule out common systemic diseases associated with leg swelling.

If the clinical history and examination indicate a cardiac etiology, an ECG, echocardiogram, BNP, and CXR should be obtained. A normal BNP can rule out HF with a sensitivity of 95%. If renal disease is suspected, a creatinine level and urinalysis should be obtained. Proteinuria and serum albumin < 3 g/dL are diagnostic for nephrotic syndrome. If hepatic etiology is suspected, liver enzymes and albumin values should be obtained.

If a DVT is suspected (as in cases of acute, unilateral edema), one should establish pretest probability for a more strategic approach to diagnosis using clinical gestalt and studied tools such as the Wells criteria (Table 60–1). For patients with low-to-moderate pretest probability for a DVT, a D-dimer level should be obtained. Due to its high sensitivity and low specificity, **a normal D-dimer level essentially rules out a DVT, but a positive D-dimer is not diagnostic of DVT.** If the D-dimer is positive, then compression venous ultrasonography of the lower extremities with or without Doppler should be obtained. For patients with high pretest probability of DVT, D-dimer should not obtained, and you should proceed directly to ultrasonography. In patients with intermediate-to-high pretest probability of DVT, negative ultrasonography alone is insufficient to exclude the diagnosis of DVT. Further assessment is recommended, including repeating ultrasonography in 1 week if the D-dimer is elevated. If malignancy is suspected, then an abdominal and pelvic examination and computed tomographic scan should be considered. Tumors commonly associated with lower extremity edema include prostate cancer, ovarian cancer, and lymphoma.

Treatment

Venous Insufficiency. In patients with venous insufficiency, diuretics should be avoided unless comorbid conditions require treatment. Nonpharmacologic therapies include compression stockings and leg elevation. Often, compression levels of 30 to 40 mm Hg at the ankle are required to adequately control the swelling, especially if there is ulceration. Compression stockings are contraindicated in patients with PAD; ABI with arterial Doppler ultrasonography should be performed to assess for arterial insufficiency prior to application of stockings. Higher compression stockings can be difficult for some patients to put on, so patients should be instructed to put them on upon awakening before the leg swelling progresses. Advising the patient to roll the stockings off at the end of the day so that they can be rolled back on in the morning is also helpful. **Promoting good skin care is important for patients with chronic venous insufficiency** to prevent skin breakdown, which can cause dermatitis and cellulitis. If stasis dermatitis develops, daily emollients and short courses of topical steroid creams should be used.

Lymphedema. Patients with lymphedema should be educated regarding the chronic nature of the condition. Reasonable expectations for treatment must be set and understood, as this condition is often difficult to manage. **Treatments include exercise, elevation, compression stockings, intermittent pneumatic compression devices, manual lymph drainage massage, and surgical procedures.** Diuretics are typically not helpful for lymphedema. Patients with chronic lymphedema are at a great risk of development of cellulitis. Patients should use topical antibiotics after small breaks in the skin. For patients with recurrent cellulitis, prophylactic antibiotics should be considered.

Deep Vein Thrombosis. Acute DVT requires prompt treatment with anticoagulation. **Treatment options include low-molecular-weight heparin, warfarin, and direct Xa inhibitors to prevent clot progression.** The therapeutic goal for warfarin therapy should be a target international normalized ratio (INR) of 2.0 to 3.0. The duration of anticoagulation therapy varies based upon cause and recurrence rate of the DVT. In initial cases of uncomplicated DVT, 3 months of anticoagulation are warranted. In cases of recurrent DVT and/or concomitant pulmonary embolism, then long-term anticoagulation is the standard of care. If anticoagulation therapy is contraindicated, then inferior vena cava filter placement may be indicated to prevent life-threatening pulmonary embolism.

Idiopathic Edema. Lifestyle modifications necessary to manage idiopathic edema include intermittent recumbence or leg elevation, avoidance of heat, low-sodium diet, decreased fluid intake, and weight loss. Loop diuretics should be avoided due to a higher risk of electrolyte abnormalities (eg, hypokalemia) and renal insufficiency. Compression stockings are less successful with this condition.

CASE CORRELATION

- See Case 27 (Heart Failure).

COMPREHENSION QUESTIONS

60.1 A 60-year-old woman presents for follow-up of lymphedema that developed following a mastectomy and lymph node dissection for breast cancer. She finds the swelling to be very uncomfortable and limits the use of her right arm. Which of the following treatment options is recommended?

A. Intermittent pneumatic compression

B. Oral warfarin

C. Oral furosemide

D. Oral hydrochlorothiazide

60.2 Which patient would have the most benefit from a diagnostic testing evaluation for systemic disease as a cause of lower extremity swelling?

A. A 35-year-old woman has cyclic bilateral ankle swelling without significant pain. She is taking over-the-counter ibuprofen for her menstrual cramps. On examination, she has +1 pitting at the ankles.

B. A 42-year-old woman has a 3-year history of bilateral, pain-free, moderate swelling in her calves that is worse at the end of the day. She has a normal BMI, no daytime somnolence, and no constitutional symptoms. She is not taking any over-the-counter or prescription medications. On examination, she has mild varicosities and hemosiderin skin deposition on both legs with nontender +1 pitting edema.

C. A 58-year-old man has +2 bilateral lower extremity edema that has slowly been worsening over the last year. He has a history of hypertension and is taking hydrochlorothiazide, lisinopril, and amlodipine. On review of systems, he complains of daily fatigue, somnolence, and constipation. He has a BMI of 32 kg/m².

D. A 55-year-old man who works in a factory develops swelling in both legs by the end of his shift after he is on his feet all day. The swelling usually improves overnight.

60.3 A 65-year-old man with a history of prostate cancer and radiation therapy 3 years ago presents with chronic left leg swelling. He denies dyspnea, chest pain, orthopnea, or wheezing. He denies daytime somnolence or snoring. On examination, he has nonpitting edema to his left calf with wart-like hyperplasia and dermal thickening of the left foot. What is the most likely diagnosis?

A. Deep vein thrombosis

B. Secondary lymphedema

C. Myxedema

D. Venous stasis

E. Hypoalbuminemia secondary to prostate cancer

ANSWERS

60.1 **A.** In chronic lymphedema management, options include exercise, elevation, compression stockings, intermittent pneumatic compression devices, manual lymph drainage massage, and surgical procedures. Diuretics (answers C and D) are not typically used in chronic venous insufficiency alone; they can be used in patients who have comorbid medical conditions. Anticoagulation (answer B) is indicated for patients with a DVT.

60.2 **C.** Older patients with lower extremity edema and systemic signs such as fatigue, somnolence, and constipation require an evaluation for systemic disease as a cause for lower extremity swelling. A CBC, comprehensive metabolic panel, urinalysis, TSH, and serum albumin level would be reasonable in this patient. Sleep studies and an echocardiogram would also be useful due to the increased risk for pulmonary hypertension as a cause of edema in patients with large neck circumference and BMI > 30 kg/m². Medications associated with edema include NSAIDs (5% risk of edema), calcium channel blockers (50% risk of edema), and oral contraceptives. Answer A (35-year-old with cyclical bilateral ankle swelling) likely has symptoms due to menstrual hormones and not DVT. Answer D (55-year-old factory worker) likely has dependent edema of the lower extremities. Answer B (42-year-old woman with a long history of pain-free moderate swelling in calves worse at the end of the day, an otherwise uncomplicated history, and mild varicose veins) most likely has venous insufficiency and not systemic disease.

60.3 **B.** The most common cause of lymphedema is that secondary to malignancy (prostate, ovarian, lymphoma); surgery; and radiation therapy. Chronic bilateral lower extremity swelling is unlikely to represent a DVT (answer A). Myxedema (answer C) is associated with thyroid disorders. Hypoalbuminemia (answer E) is seen in advanced malignancies, nephrotic syndrome, protein-losing enteropathies, and liver disease.

CLINICAL PEARLS

▶ Venous insufficiency and idiopathic edema are the most common causes of lower extremity swelling in patients without systemic disease and often can be diagnosed with history alone.

▶ Pulmonary hypertension secondary to sleep apnea should be considered in older patients presenting with leg swelling who have a BMI > 30 kg/m², a neck circumference > 17 inches (42 cm), daytime somnolence, and a history of snoring.

▶ If there is an unclear etiology of the lower extremity swelling, look for signs of systemic illness, including HF, renal disease, hepatic dysfunction, and thyroid disease. Lipedema and lymphedema should also be ruled out.

▶ Options for anticoagulation in the treatment of DVT include low-molecular-weight-heparin, warfarin, and direct Xa inhibitors.

REFERENCES

Braunwald E, Loscalzo J. Edema. In: Jameson JL, Fauci A, Kasper D, Hauser S, Longo D, Loscalzo J, eds. *Harrison's Principles of Internal Medicine.* 20th ed. New York, NY: McGraw Hill; 2018: Chap. 37. https://accessmedicine.mhmedical.com/content.aspx?sectionid=192012582&bookid=2129&Res ultclick=2. Accessed May 3, 2019.

Buller HR, Prins MH, Lensin AW, et al.; EINSTEIN-PE Investigators. Oral rivaroxaban for the treatment of symptomatic pulmonary embolism. *N Engl J Med.* 2012;366(14):1287-1297.

Eberhardt RT, Raffetto JD. Chronic venous insufficiency. *Circulation.* 2014;130:333-346.

Raju S, Neglen P. Chronic venous insufficiency and varicose veins. *N Engl J Med.* 2009;360:2319-2327.

Rockson SG. Current concepts and future directions in the diagnosis and management of lymphatic vascular disease. *Vasc Med.* 2010;15(3):223-231.

Trayes KP, Studdiford JS, Pickle S, Tully AS. Edema: diagnosis and management. *Am Fam Physician.* 2013;88(2):102-110.

Review Questions

REVIEW QUESTIONS

R1. A 52-year-old obese man presents for follow-up of his hypertension. His blood pressure is well controlled on a daily dose of hydrochlorothiazide. You notice that he has thickened, velvety skin circumferentially around his neck. The result of a random glucose test performed an hour after he ate lunch was 130 mg/dL. Which of the following test results is diagnostic for diabetes mellitus?

A. This test is diagnostic (no further testing is needed)

B. A hemoglobin A_{1c} level of > 6%

C. A fasting plasma glucose of 120 mg/dL

D. A random plasma glucose of 220 mg/dL and symptomatic polyuria

E. A plasma glucose of 130 mg/dL drawn 1 hour after a 50-g glucose challenge

R2. For the patient in Question 1, appropriate testing confirms the diagnosis of type 2 diabetes mellitus. Along with diet and exercise modifications, which of the following is the most appropriate initial management?

A. Oral glyburide

B. Oral metformin

C. Oral pioglitazone

D. Mealtime injections of short-acting insulin

E. Single daily injection of long-acting insulin

R3. A 38-year-old African American man is evaluated for the new diagnosis of hypertension. His workup has revealed multiple elevated blood pressure readings in the range of 150/95 mm Hg over the past few months but no evidence of any other medical conditions. You plan to initiate an antihypertensive medication. Which of the following is the best initial choice for this patient?

A. Amlodipine

B. Lisinopril

C. Losartan

D. Carvedilol

E. Doxasozin

R4. A 45-year-old man presents for a routine physical examination. He has no known medical history and has not seen a doctor in several years. He is a nonsmoker. His blood pressure is 130/80 mm Hg. On a screening lipid panel, he is found to have a total cholesterol of 320 mg/dL, high-density lipoprotein (HDL) cholesterol of 50 mg/dL, triglycerides of 100 mg/dL, and low-density lipoprotein (LDL) cholesterol of 220 mg/dL. According to the American Heart Association/American College of Cardiology guidelines, in addition to therapeutic lifestyle changes, which of the following management options is most appropriate?

A. Repeat lipid panel in 3 months

B. Ezetimibe

C. Aspirin 81 mg daily and repeat lipid panel in 3 months

D. Statin

E. Gemfibrozil

R5. A 50-year-old woman with hypertension presents for a routine well-woman examination. Medical record review shows a negative Papanicolaou and human papilloma virus testing last year and a negative mammogram 6 months ago. She has no other chronic conditions besides hypertension, has not had any surgeries, has never smoked cigarettes, and is postmenopausal. For which of the following conditions would you routinely recommend screening at this encounter?

A. Cervical cancer

B. Ovarian cancer

C. Colon cancer

D. Osteoporosis

E. Lung cancer

R6. A 2-year-old girl is brought in by her mother for a routine well-child visit. Per her mother, the child has had no significant medical illnesses and is up to date on her vaccinations. The patient's mother is concerned because she thinks that the child looks "cross-eyed" when she is showing her pictures in a book or watching TV. On examination, the child has appropriate growth and development for a 2-year-old. Careful examination of her eyes reveals an asymmetric corneal light reflex. When you cover and then uncover her right eye, the light reflex on the left eye does not change. When you cover the left eye, the light reflex appears to move more central on the right cornea. When you uncover the left eye, the light reflex moves laterally on the right cornea and is central on the left. What is your recommendation to the child's mother?

A. The child should be referred to a pediatric ophthalmologist.

B. This finding is common in 2-year-olds and will normalize as the child gets older.

C. Hold picture books to the child's right side to try to improve her rightward gaze.

D. The child will most likely require surgery to correct this problem.

E. No intervention is needed at this time, but the child will likely need glasses when she starts school.

R7. A 24-year-old woman presents for prenatal care at 10 weeks' gestation of her first pregnancy. Which of the following recommendations is appropriate counseling?

A. She should avoid sexual activity, as it may precipitate early labor.

B. She should not undergo radiographs during her pregnancy because of the risk to the fetus from ionizing radiation.

C. She should delay any vaccinations until the postpartum period.

D. She may use any over-the-counter medicine, if needed, as they are safe during pregnancy.

E. She should be screened for gestational diabetes at 24 to 28 weeks' gestation.

R8. A 40-year-old woman presents with a palpable lump in her anterior neck that has slowly enlarged over the past year. She has no pain in the area and no trouble swallowing. She denies palpitations, weight change, or changes in her skin or hair. On examination, you palpate a nodule in the left lobe of the thyroid. An ultrasound reveals a 2.5-cm solid nodule in the thyroid, and blood tests reveal normal thyroid function. Which of the following is the next step in the evaluation of this finding?

A. Fine-needle biopsy of the nodule

B. Nuclear medicine thyroid uptake scan

C. Computed tomographic (CT) scan of the neck

D. Referral for thyroidectomy

E. Careful observation with repeat blood tests and ultrasound in 6 months to assess for change

R9. A 62-year-old woman presents with 1 week of low back pain. She denies any injury but states that the pain started the day after she planted her vegetable garden, which she has done for many years without problem. She has no history of back problems in the past. The pain is mostly in the left lower back and gets worse when she bends forward. She has no neurological symptoms, fever, or weight loss, and she otherwise feels well. Her general examination and vital signs are normal. She has left-sided paraspinal tenderness but no midline tenderness to palpation. She has limited forward flexion and rotation but normal extension of her back. A straight leg raise test is negative, lower extremity reflexes are symmetric, and lower extremity strength testing is normal. Which of the following interventions is appropriate at this time?

A. Radiograph of the lumbar spine

B. Referral for physical therapy

C. Recommendation for 3 to 5 days of bed rest

D. Narcotic pain medication at bedtime to help her sleep

E. Recommend normal daily activities as much as possible

R10. A 2-year-old child is brought in to your office as a new patient for the evaluation of a cough and fever. Your history and examination are consistent with a viral upper respiratory infection, and you counsel the parent appropriately. However, you note that during the encounter the child does not interact with you or his mother. He seems extremely focused on the toy motorcycle in his hands. On questioning, his mother states that he often sits by himself while holding the motorcycle and does not interact much with other children. He has not yet started talking, but she thinks that it is because he is "confused" because the family speaks both English and Spanish at home, so he does not know which words to use. Along with arranging for a hearing evaluation, you also recommend which of the following?

A. Comprehensive developmental screening

B. Reassurance that children from multilingual households develop speech at later ages, so this is likely normal

C. Assessment by child protective services for child abuse and neglect

D. Taking the toy motorcycle away to force him to interact with others around him

E. Speaking only English or Spanish at home to reduce his language confusion

R11. A 7-month-old baby boy presents for his first well-child examination. His mother states that she never brought him to the doctor because they did not have insurance and he was doing fine at home. She said that he had a vaccine in the hospital on the day after he was born but otherwise has had no vaccines. Which of the following vaccines would be contraindicated in this child?

A. Hepatitis B

B. Influenza

C. Pneumococcal conjugate

D. Rotavirus

E. Inactivated polio virus

R12. A 24-year-old nulliparous woman presents for a pregnancy test. She has not had a menstrual period in 4 months. She has a history of chronically irregular menstrual cycles since menarche. She usually will have a period every 3 months and sometimes will go 6 months in between periods. On examination, she is a comfortable-appearing obese female with a body mass index of 41 kg/m^2, and her blood pressure is 138/90 mm Hg. She has some visible dark hair growth on her chin. The remainder of her general examination is normal, and a urine pregnancy test is negative. Which of the following is required to make the diagnosis of polycystic ovary syndrome (PCOS) in this case?

A. A pelvic ultrasound showing 15 or more follicular cysts

B. Elevated serum estrogen level

C. Elevated serum androgen level

D. Menstrual bleeding induced after taking oral medroxyprogesterone for 10 days

E. No specific testing is needed for this diagnosis

R13. An 80-year-old man is brought in by his daughter out of concern for reduction in his hearing. He has worn hearing aids in both ears for several years, but she says that his hearing has become acutely worse in his right ear in the past 3 weeks. She had the battery in the hearing aid replaced, and it seems to be functioning normally. She is requesting a referral to an audiologist for repeat testing for her father. What is the most likely cause of this acute hearing reduction?

A. Presbycusis

B. Cerumen impaction

C. Battery or hearing aid failure

D. Stroke

E. Brain tumor impinging on the eighth cranial nerve

R14. A 36-year-old gravida 2, para 2 woman presents to discuss options for con-traception. She is generally healthy but smokes a pack of cigarettes per day and is not ready to quit. She is unsure if she wants to have more children but wants an effective contraception option with ease of administration. Which of the following would be her best option?

A. Combined oral contraceptive pills

B. Progesterone only "minipills"

C. Subdermal etonogestrel secreting implant

D. Tubal ligation

E. Natural family planning

R15. A 48-year-old woman with chronic migraine headaches presents for an acute visit with the "worst migraine" she has ever had. She describes her typical migraines as a one-sided, throbbing pain with nausea and photophobia that resolve after she takes sumatriptan. However, she states that this headache feels different. It came on suddenly, is "15 out of 10" in intensity, involves her whole head, and even her neck hurts. On examination, she is lying very still on the examination table with the lights off. She can flex and extend her neck with some increase in her pain. She has no papilledema but has moderate photophobia. Her neuro-logical examination is otherwise nonfocal. Which of the following is the most appropriate next step in the management of this patient's headache?

A. Give her another dose of sumatriptan, as she may not have reached ther-apeutic threshold.

B. Give her an injection of intramuscular ketorolac in the office to see if you can reduce the headache intensity.

C. Order a magnetic resonance imaging of her head and follow up in the clinic tomorrow.

D. Order an outpatient CT scan of the head and follow up in the clinic tomorrow.

E. Activate emergency medical services to arrange for ambulance transport to the emergency department.

ANSWERS

R1. **D. 220 mg/dL and symptomatic polyuria.** There are four diagnostic criteria for the diagnosis of diabetes, yet only one is required:

- Fasting plasma glucose of 126 mg/dL or greater

- Hemoglobin A_{1c} of 6.5% or greater

- Plasma glucose of 200 mg/dL or greater 2 hours after a 75-g glucose challenge

- Random plasma glucose of 200 or greater and typical symptoms of hyper-glycemia (polyuria, polyphagia, or polydipsia)

When possible, the result should be repeated to confirm the diagnosis. In this question, none of the other answer choices meets these criteria: answer A (the test is diagnostic and no further testing is needed); answer B (hemoglobin A_{1c} > 6%); answer C (fasting glucose of 120 mg/dL); and answer E (plasma glucose of 130 mg/dL drawn 1 hour after a 50-g glucose challenge). (For more information, see Case 51, Diabetes Mellitus)

R2. **B. Metform.** This patient has type 2 diabetes. A healthy lifestyle, including regular physical activity, and weight loss of 5% to 10% are very important. If not contraindicated, metformin should be the first-line treatment for type 2 diabetes mellitus in most cases. In January 2017, the American College of Physicians listed metformin as a first-line agent. It is associated with improvement in hemoglobin A_{1c} levels and lipid levels. Studies have shown an improvement in outcomes, including reduction in mortality risk, in those taking metformin. It also does not induce hypoglycemia and is generally well tolerated. The safety, efficacy, and outcomes data generally make it the initial treatment of choice. Most experts believe that insulin (answers D and E) and sulfonylurea agents (answer A) are secondary agents, and glitazones (answer C) are reserved as third-line agents. (For more information, see Case 51, Diabetes Mellitus)

R3. **A. Amlodipine.** African American patients have a higher prevalence of hypertension and cardiac disease. There is also a higher rate of low-renin physiology. That said, it is important not to make "all-inclusive" presumptions. Studies deal with trends and populations and not individuals. According to the Eighth Joint National Committee (JNC 8) recommendations for treatment of hypertension, thiazide diuretics, angiotensin-converting enzyme inhibitors (answer B), angiotensin receptor blockers (answer C), and calcium channel blockers (answer A) are the recommended initial medications for most patients with hypertension. The JNC 8 recommendations state that thiazide diuretics or calcium channel blockers are likely to be more effective than other medications in African Americans; therefore, amlodipine, a calcium channel blocker, would be the best choice out of the options provided. Carvedilol (answer D) is a nonselective beta-blocker and an alpha-1-blocker that acts on both the heart and the kidneys, decreasing renin secretion. Answer E (doxasozin) is not a first-line agent and is used mainly in patients with benign prostatic hyperplasia. (For more information, see Case 30, Hypertension)

R4. **D. Statin agent.** The American College of Cardiology/American Heart Association 2018 guidelines for the management of hyperlipidemia recommend the use of HMG CoA (beta-hydroxy-beta-methylglutaryl coenzyme A) reductase inhibitors ("statins") as the appropriate treatment for hyperlipidemia in the settings listed next. This patient has an LDL cholesterol exceeding 190 mg/dL (criteria 2) and therefore should be on a high-intensity statin agent, as this has been shown to reduce mortality. The other answer choices (nonstatin agents or watching) would not be appropriate. (For more information, see Case 35, Hyperlipidemia)

1. Anyone under the age of 75 with established atherosclerotic cardiovascular disease (ASCVD) should be on high-intensity statin therapy.

2. Anyone with LDL cholesterol greater than 190 mg/dL should be on a high-intensity statin.

3. Anyone between the age of 40 and 75 with a 10-year ASCVD risk of 7.5% or greater should be on a moderate- or high-intensity statin.

4. All diabetics age 40 to 75 with an LDL cholesterol of 70 mg/dL or greater should be on a moderate- or high-intensity statin.

R5. **C. Colon cancer.** The United States Preventive Services Task Force recommends colon cancer screening for all persons age 50 and above. This patient is up to date on her cervical cancer screening (answer A), so she does not need that at this visit. Osteoporosis screening (answer D) would routinely be recommended at the age of 65. Ovarian cancer screening (answer B) in asymptomatic women is not recommended, and lung cancer screening (answer E) is only recommended in those between the ages of 55 and 80 years who have a history of smoking cigarettes for 30 pack-years and currently smoke or who have quit within the past 15 years. (For more information, see Cases 1 and 11, Health maintenance)

R6. **A. Ophthalmology referral.** Examination of the eyes and vision screening is an important part of routine well-child care. Eye examinations should start in the newborn nursery. Children usually have a conjugate gaze by the time they are about 6 months old. This child is showing signs of strabismus, a misalignment of the eyes. Strabismus is the most common cause of amblyopia, an impairment of vision in one of the eyes. Children with suspected strabismus should be referred to a pediatric ophthalmologist as soon as the condition is suspected for evaluation and management. Thus, answers B (finding is benign and will normalize with age), C (holding picture books to the side), and E (no intervention) all are incorrect, since permanent visual loss may occur if strabismus is not treated. While surgery (answer D) is sometimes necessary to correct the problem, this is not common and would not be an initial appropriate recommendation. (For more information, see Case 5, Well-child care)

R7. **E. Diabetes screening at 24-28 weeks.** Counseling and anticipatory guidance are very important components of routine prenatal care. The American College of Obstetricians and Gynecologists, along with the United States Preventive Services Task Force, recommends the routine screening of pregnant women for gestational diabetes at 24 to 28 weeks' gestation, as the identification and management of gestational diabetes can improve outcomes. There is no evidence that sexual activity may precipitate early labor in normal pregnancy (answer A), although there are some conditions in which counseling to avoid sexual activity may be warranted. Radiographs during pregnancy (answer B) may be done when the benefit outweighs the risk.

Shielding of the pregnant abdomen would be recommended, when possible. While live virus vaccines should be delayed, other vaccines (answer C) are not contraindicated during pregnancy. Influenza vaccine and tetanus, diphtheria, and acellular pertussis (Tdap) vaccines are recommended routinely. Finally, pregnant women should be advised to discuss the use of all medications, including over-the-counter medications and supplements (answer D), with their clinician prior to use. (For more information, see Case 4, Prenatal care)

R8. **A. FNA biopsy.** A patient with normal or reduced thyroid function (eg, normal or high thyroid-stimulating hormone [TSH]) and a thyroid nodule 1 cm in size or larger should have the nodule biopsied to assess for malignancy. Approximately 5% to 6% of solitary thyroid nodules are malignant. The workup of a thyroid nodule should include an assessment of thyroid function by obtaining a TSH level and an ultrasound to assess the size of the nodule. Hyperfunctioning nodules (low TSH) are usually benign adenomas that are assessed with a radioactive iodine uptake study (answer B). Answer E (waiting for 6 months) would be unwise because if the thyroid nodule is malignant, then it may spread and continue to grow. CT imaging of the neck (answer C) can be performed if the biopsy returns as malignant but is not indicated at this time. Answer D (referral for thyroidectomy) is not indicated until the etiology of the mass is characterized; in other words, a benign thyroid nodule would not necessarily need to be removed. (For more information, see Case 15, Thyroid disorders)

R9. **E. Normal Activities.** This patient's presentation is a very typical case of acute low back pain that is likely due to lumbosacral strain. This patient has no "red flag" signs or symptoms that would warrant immediate imaging studies (answer A). Some of those red flags include bladder or bowel dysfunction, fever, trauma, unexplained weight loss, parenteral drug abuse, or cancer history. The treatment of this common condition includes the use of anti-inflammatory medications, heat, and early mobility. Bed rest (answer C) should be avoided, and narcotic pain medications (answer D) have shown no benefit in this setting. Physical therapy (answer B) may have some short-term benefits, but studies have not shown long-term benefit. (For more information, see Case 53, Acute low back pain)

R10. **A. Developmental screening.** While not diagnostic, this child's behaviors, lack of interaction with others, and speech delay are very concerning for autism spectrum disorder or other possible developmental conditions. While children in multilingual households may have some mild delays in speech at young ages (answer B), the lack of any words at the age of 2 is a significant red flag that should lead to further testing. This testing should include both an assessment of hearing and a comprehensive developmental assessment. Answer C (child protective services referral) is not indicated since there is no history of injury or neglect. Answer D (taking the toy away) would likely cause the child to become upset and unnecessarily combative and emotional.

Answer E (speaking only one language at home) is what experts believed was best 40 to 50 years ago, but today, we know that speaking multiple languages at home is positive for all parties involved, and it may be an asset for the child to be bilingual. (For more information, see Case 54, Autism Spectrum Disorders)

R11. **D. Rotavirus vaccine.** Review of current immunization guidelines and patient records is paramount. In this case, the rotavirus vaccine is contraindicated. Rotavirus vaccines should not be initiated after the age of 15 weeks. All other vaccines (answer A, hepatitis B; answer B, influenza; answer C, pneumococcal conjugate; and answer E, inactivated polio virus) can be given, and "catchup" schedules provided by the Centers for Disease Control should be followed. (For more information, see Case 5, Well-child care)

R12. **E. No specific test.** This patient has evidence of PCOS clinically and meets the Rotterdam criteria for the diagnosis without further testing. The Rotterdam criteria are as follows:

- Hyperandrogenism, evidenced by hirsutism or elevated serum androgen levels (eg, testosterone, androstenedione, or dehydroepiandrosterone [DHEA])

- Oligomenorrhea with cycle length greater than or equal to 35 days

- Multifollicular ovaries on pelvic ultrasound, defined as 12 or greater small follicles in an ovary (and not 15 follicular cysts, as in answer A)

Answer B (elevated estrogen level) is often found but not a strict diagnostic criterion. Answer C (elevated androgen level) is often found, but hyperandrogenism can be clinical. Answer D (vaginal bleeding with oral progestin) is often found with PCOS but is not a diagnostic criterion; sometimes the hyperandrogenism can inhibit vaginal bleeding.

Her evidence of hirsutism (evidence of hyperandrogenism) and her oligomenorrhea are enough to meet the diagnostic criteria. Management would include working with her to try to lose weight, considering the use of medroxyprogesterone or combined contraceptives to regularize her menses, and considering the use of metformin or a thiazolidinedione agent to reduce insulin resistance. (For more information, see Cases 33, Obesity and 50, Menstrual cycle irregularity)

R13. **B. Cerumen impaction.** This patient complains of acute hearing loss over 3 weeks. Acute hearing reduction is most likely caused by a cerumen impaction, an often-overlooked condition. Examination of the external auditory canal may show near-complete, or complete, blockage with wax. Removal of the wax will often return the patient to his baseline level of hearing. Presbycusis (answer A) is the most common cause of hearing reduction in the elderly population. It is a slowly progressive condition and is a diagnosis of exclusion. The patient's change of hearing over 3 weeks is not consistent with this etiology. Answer C (battery or hearing aid failure) is not likely since these were both recently checked. Answer D (stroke) is always a possibility, but it is usually associated with other findings, such as facial or extremity weakness or numbness. A brain tumor impinging on the eighth cranial nerve (answer E) would likely be an acoustic neuroma, which is also associated with tinnitus and dizziness/vertigo; it is much less common than cerumen occlusion. (For more information, see Case 18, Geriatric health maintenance and end-of-life issues)

R14. **C. Progestin implant.** Of the options provided, the subdermal etonogestrel implant (Nexplanon) would likely be this patient's best option. Both combined and progestin-only oral contraceptive pills (OCPs) (answers A and B) require regular compliance to be effective. The combined OCPs are also relatively contraindicated in a woman over the age of 35 who smokes cigarettes because of the increased risk of thrombosis and its complications, including myocardial infarction, stroke, and pulmonary embolism. A tubal ligation (answer D) would be appropriate only if she desired permanent contraception. Natural family planning (answer E) is less effective than other methods and requires significant effort on the part of the woman to be as effective as possible. (For more information, see Case 28, Family planning—Contraceptives)

R15. **E. Activate EMS.** This patient has the acute onset of "the worst headache of her life" that is significantly different from her chronic migraine headaches. She is reporting classic symptoms that are concerning for a subarachnoid hemorrhage (SAH). SAH is an emergency situation, and timely diagnosis and therapy can impact survival and neurological function. Thus, immediate transport to a hospital is mandatory. Imaging with follow-up in the clinic the next day would not be appropriate (answers C and D). While she does have a history of migraines, it is important not to assume that this headache is only a migraine and treat with sumatriptan (answer A) without further evaluation. Answer B (injection of intramuscular ketorolac) utilizes a nonsteroidal anti-inflammatory agent that is useful in tension and migraine headaches. It is of critical importance not to miss alarm symptoms of headaches that require urgent evaluation. (For more information, see Case 34, Migraine and other headache syndromes)

Page numbers followed by *f* or *t* indicate figures or tables, respectively.

G

GABS. *See* group A beta-hemolytic streptococcus
galactocele, 559
galactorrhea, 559, 563
galantamine (Razadyne), 356t
gamma-hydroxybutyrate. *See* GHB
GAPS guidelines, 326
GAS infection. *See* group A streptococcus
gastroesophageal reflux disease (GERD)
  clinical approach, 535–536
  complications of, 540–541
  definition of, 536
  description of, 225t
  management of, 540–541
  upper respiratory infections and, 212
gastrointestinal bleeding, lower. *See* lower gastrointestinal bleeding
gastrointestinal obstruction, 344–347
GBS. *See* group B streptococcus
gemfibrozil, 393t
gender, 3
gender diversity, 327
gender identity, 325
generalized anxiety disorder, 277
genetic counseling, 49
genital examination, 6
genital herpes, 514
gentamicin, 248t
GERD. *See* gastroesophageal reflux disease
geriatric anemia
  analysis, 104–105
  case study, 104
  clinical approach, 105–108
  clinical pearls, 110
  clinical presentation, 107
  comprehension questions, 108–109
  definitions, 105
  epidemiology, 105
  laboratory values for, 106t
  treatment, 107–108
Geriatric Depression Scale, 272
geriatric health maintenance
  activities of daily living, 201, 202t
  algorithm for, 202f
  analysis, 200
  cancer screening, 206
  case study, 200
  clinical approach, 201–206
  clinical pearls, 209

  cognitive screening, 204
  comprehension questions, 207–208
  definitions, 201
  depression, 205
  end-of-life issues, 206–207
  fall assessment, 204
  functional assessment, 201
  hearing screening, 203–204
  hypertension screening, 205
  immunizations, 206
  incontinence, 205
  instrumental activities of daily living, 201, 202t
  nutrition screening, 205
  osteoporosis screening, 206, 659–660
  presbycusis, 201, 203
  preventive services, 201
  screening tests, 201–206
  stroke prevention, 205
  vision screening, 201–203
gestational diabetes, 55–56, 582
GFR. *See* glomerular filtration rate
GHB (γ-hydroxybutyrate), 459t
GI bleeding. *See* lower gastrointestinal bleeding
Giardia, 113
Gilbert syndrome, 523
ginkgo biloba, 357
glaucoma, 203
glitazones, 586
glomerular filtration rate (GFR), 236
glomerular hematuria, 158
GLP-1 agonists, 586
gluconeogenesis, 583
glucose tolerance test (GTT), 56, 582
glucosuria, 580
glycoprotein IIb/IIIa inhibitors, 222
glycosylated hemoglobin (HbA$_{1c}$), 365, 580
gonorrhea, 513
gouty arthritis. *See also* joint pain
  classification, 40
  clinical presentation, 40
  definition, 39
GP inhibitors. *See* glycoprotein IIb/IIIa inhibitors
grapefruit, 597
Graves disease, 166–170
Grey-Turner sign, 6
gross hematuria, 157–159